LOGIC, SIGNS AND NATURE
IN THE RENAISSANCE
The Case of Learned Medicine

How and what were doctors in the Renaissance trained to think, and how did they interpret the evidence at their disposal for making diagnoses and prognoses? *Logic, Signs and Nature in the Renaissance* addresses these questions in the broad context of the world of learning: its institutions, its means of conveying and disseminating information, and the relationship between university faculties. The uptake by doctors from the university arts course, which was the foundation for medical studies, is examined in detail, as are the theoretical and empirical bases for medical knowledge, including its concepts of nature, health, disease and normality.

The book ends with a detailed investigation of semiotic, which was one of the five parts of the discipline of medicine, in the context of the various versions of semiology available to scholars at the time. From this survey, a new assessment is made of the relationship of Renaissance medicine to the new science of the seventeenth century.

IAN MACLEAN is Senior Research Fellow at All Souls College, Oxford, and Titular Professor of Renaissance Studies at the University of Oxford. His many publications include *The Renaissance Notion of Women* (1980), *The Political Responsibility of Intellectuals* (edited, with Alan Montefiore and Peter Winch; 1990), *Interpretation and Meaning in the Renaissance: The Case of Law* (1992) and *Montaigne Philosophe* (1996).

IDEAS IN CONTEXT

Edited by Quentin Skinner (*General Editor*), Lorraine Daston,
Dorothy Ross and James Tully

The books in this series will discuss the emergence of intellectual traditions
and of related new disciplines. The procedures, aims and vocabularies that
were generated will be set in the context of the alternatives available within the
contemporary frameworks of ideas and institutions. Through detailed studies of
the evolution of such traditions, and their modification by different audiences,
it is hoped that a new picture will form of the development of ideas in their
concrete contexts. By this means, artificial distinctions between the history of
philosophy, of the various sciences, of society and politics, and of literature may
be seen to dissolve.

The series is published with the support of the Exxon Foundation.

A list of books in the series will be found at the end of the volume.

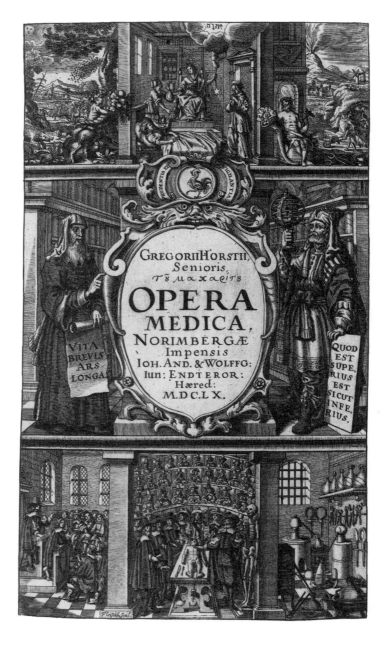

GREGORII HORSTII,
Senioris,
τȣ μακαϱιτȣ
OPERA
MEDICA,
NORIMBÉRGÆ
Impensis
IOH. AND. & WOLFFG:
Iun: ENDTEROR:
Hæred:
M.DC.LX.

VITA
BREVIS
ARS
LONGA.

QUOD
EST
SUPE,
RIUS
EST
SICUT
INFE,
RIUS.

F.leisch.scul.

LOGIC, SIGNS AND NATURE IN THE RENAISSANCE

The Case of Learned Medicine

IAN MACLEAN

All Souls College, Oxford

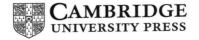

CAMBRIDGE
UNIVERSITY PRESS

PUBLISHED BY THE PRESS SYNDICATE OF THE UNIVERSITY OF CAMBRIDGE
The Pitt Building, Trumpington Street, Cambridge, United Kingdom

CAMBRIDGE UNIVERSITY PRESS
The Edinburgh Building, Cambridge CB2 2RU, UK
40 West 20th Street, New York, NY 10011-4211, USA
477 Williamstown Road, Port Melbourne, VIC 3207, Australia
Ruiz de Alarcón 13, 28014 Madrid, Spain
Dock House, The Waterfront, Cape Town 8001, South Africa

http://www.cambridge.org

First published 2002

Printed in the United Kingdom at the University Press, Cambridge

Typeface Baskerville Monotype 11/12.5 pt.   *System* LATEX 2ε   [TB]

A catalogue record for this book is available from the British Library.

Library of Congress Cataloguing in Publication data
Maclean, Ian, 1945–
Logic, signs and nature: learned medicine in the Renaissance/Ian Maclean.
p.   cm.   (Ideas in context: 62)
Includes bibliographical references and index.
ISBN 0 521 80648 8
1. Medicine – Europe – Philosophy – History– 16th century.
2. Medical education – Europe – History – 16th century.
3. Medicine – Europe – Philosophy – History – 17th century.
4. Medical education – Europe – History – 17th century.
5. Renaissance – Europe – History.   I. Title.   II. Series.
R484.M33   2001
610′.94′09031– dc21   2001025612

ISBN 0 521 80648 8 hardback

For my long-suffering family

Contents

Illustrations

Frontispiece: Titlepage of Gregor Horst's *Opera medica*,
Nuremberg, 1660

FIGURES

The frontispiece and fig. 4.3b are reproduced by kind permission of the
Provost and Scholars of the Queen's College, Oxford; figs. 4.1 and 4.4
are reproduced by kind permission of the Warden and Fellows of All
Souls College, Oxford; figs. 4.2, 5.1, 5.2, 5.3, 5.5 and 5.6 are reproduced
by permission of the Bodleian Library, University of Oxford; and fig. 5.4
is reproduced by kind permission of the Principal and Fellows of Jesus
College, Oxford.

Acknowledgements

It is a great pleasure here to acknowledge the numerous scholarly debts I have incurred in writing this book. The greatest of these I owe to those heroic scholars who undertook to read the whole typescript, and make extensive comments on it, offering references to an immense amount of additional material and countless suggestions for improvement, which are not all individually acknowledged in the notes. Nicholas Jardine and Brian Vickers read the first draft for the Cambridge University Press; Sachiko Kusukawa, Michael McVaugh and Nancy Siraisi did so at my request. I received valuable assistance from Andrew Wear (who generously let me have a copy of his thesis on a cognate subject); Vivian Nutton; from my colleagues in All Souls, especially Robin Briggs, Miles Burnyeat, Eleanor Robson, Peregrine Horden, Scott Mandelbrote and Charles Webster; from Constance Blackwell, Laurence Brockliss, Richard Cooper, Peter Corlett, Chiara Crisciani, Sylvia de Renzi, Eckhard Kessler, Gillian Lewis, Bob Lowrie, Christoph Lüthy, Ewen Maclean, Jan Papy, Margaret Pelling, Martin Porter, David Sackett, and Ron Truman. To the audiences at the Wellcome Unit of the History of Medicine, University of Oxford, the Department of the History and Philosophy of Science, Cambridge, and the participants in the Summer School on the History of Learned Medicine in the Renaissance, who patiently listened to drafts of what follows and submitted me to shrewd but kindly questioning, I am deeply grateful. I owe a special debt to the infinitely patient and resourceful Librarians of the Bodleian Library, the Herzog-August-Bibliothek, Wolfenbüttel, and the two Oxford college libraries where much of this research was done: Queen's and All Souls. The time-honoured formula (that the virtues of the text are theirs, and the remaining errors mine) of course applies. To the same two colleges I am also grateful for indispensable material and financial assistance. I owe special thanks to my copy-editor,

Virginia Catmur, through whose vigilance this *opusculum* has been (to use the formula so frequently abused on Renaissance title pages) 'ab innumerabilibus mendis purgatum'. It goes without saying that I owe an immeasurable debt to my family for their encouragement and moral support, and for having patiently endured the painful and protracted gestation of this volume.

Notes on the text and its modes of reference

I have followed the Harvard conventions for bibliographical reference except where I have not myself seen an original text, and have felt constrained to cite its full title. In chapter 2, which discusses formats and books as such, I have sometimes included bibliographical details in the footnotes where they are germane to the argument. I have cited Greek as it occurs in quotations; elsewhere I have transcribed it according to the usual conventions for distinguishing long and short vowels.

I have left a number of Latin words in their original form as they are terms of art: 'scientia', 'circumstantiae', 'experientia', 'practica', 'theoria', 'quaestio/quaestiones', 'differentia/differentiae', 'spiritus', 'locus'. I have used both 'semiotic' and 'semiology' to designate this area of medicine; the former is the more common in humanist texts, but the latter has become subsequently dominant. For the form of names (whether vernacular or latinised), I have consulted (but not always adopted) the form given in the published Wellcome Library catalogue; I have where appropriate adopted the modern distinction between 'i' and 'j', 'u' and 'v', and have omitted accents on Latin words where these do not contribute to the sense. There is a great inconsistency in usage in the transcription of surnames (even between the published Wellcome catalogue, and its www version); this I have perpetuated, as my major concern has been to ensure that the reader can locate copies of the texts to which I refer in library catalogues, especially in difficult cases such as Dubois/Sylvius, du Chesne/Quercetanus, Giachini/Jacchinus/Iacchinus and da Monte/Montanus. In cases where it is relevant, I give the dates of the most important authors when these are first mentioned in the text; but it would be wrong to suggest that one could create out of these a simple chronology of influential writers. Not all texts were made available to the wider public at the time of their composition. Some were first published a long time after the death of their authors, but were well known to the academic community before their death; the treatises of Pomponazzi on incantations and fate are good examples of this. Other authors taught generations of students who disseminated their views before they appeared in printed form; a few were 'discovered' after their demise by other scholars or entrepreneurial publishers. The story of the reception of medical ideas is therefore very complex, except in some very striking cases such as those of Vesalius and Fracastoro; this fact (together with the other reasons given above) led me to adopt an ideal-typical rather than chronological approach to Renaissance semiology, although I do offer broad accounts of the development of theories in this area over the period under investigation here.

I have cross-referenced to numbered sections rather than pages throughout. All the longer quotations in Latin in the text (but not in the notes) have been translated, in a freer style than that used in the rendering of the Greek Galen by the assembled scholars whose versions go to make up the standard Giunti edition (1541–2; 9th edition 1625). In some but not all cases, these translations were adopted in the Kühn edition of Galen, 22 vols., Leipzig, 1821–33; I have where possible made reference to this edition also (K, followed by volume number and page); but not all the references and quotations found in Renaissance texts can be easily located there. I refer also to the *Patrologiae cursus completus, series latina*, ed. J. P. Migne, 222 vols., Paris, 1844–1904, via the abbreviation PL.

Introduction

This book is conceived as the companion volume to *Interpretation and meaning in the Renaissance: the case of law* (1992); it is concerned with the extraction of sense from words and signs in medicine, and the rules used to regulate such extraction. In the case of medicine, the emphasis is less on the recovery of intention from words than on the practice of drawing deductive inferences from complex evidence. Like the study of law, this book does not start from great names and great innovations, although these may be seen to have a greater role to play, given the degree of innovative thinking in medical faculties. Some of the figures who broke new ground were celebrated (or reviled) in their own day, such as Girolamo Fracastoro, Jean Fernel, Paracelsus, and Andreas Vesalius; some were commemorated in the following century (Girolamo Cardano, Santorre Santori (Sanctorius Sanctorius), Jan van Heurne (Heurnius), Daniel Sennert); some have had to wait until more recent times to enjoy recognition (Giambattista da Monte (Montanus), Giovanni Argenterio, Leonhart Fuchs); some may still not be adequately recognised (Girolamo Capo di Vacca (Capivaccius) and Guillaume Rondelet being two of these). Rather than be drawn into establishing a revised medical pantheon, however, I have chosen here to concentrate on writers whose modes of thought and expression were widely known in the medical community. Through a selection of their published writings I hope to be able give an ideal-typical account of the range of what was thinkable and knowable to the members of that community who had enjoyed much the same education and training.

It would have been much easier to have taken a microhistorical approach, and chosen one or a number of thinkers who could have been subjected to Geertzian thick description.[1] But it still seems to me that the ideal-typical approach I adopted before has its place, provided that there

---

[1] Geertz 1973.

is a broad justification for the parameters within which it is set. In this case, the choice of learned medicine in the age of medical humanism (or hellenism) and its aftermath (from 1530 to about 1630) can be, and has been, argued for on several grounds.[2] It is a century of linguistic stability (that is, Latin remained the dominant form of communication); of consolidation; of textual continuity; of conciliation (initially of the medieval tradition with the new Greek medicine, as in the work of Giambattista da Monte; latterly of the marriage of Paracelsianism with Aristotle and Galen, as in that of Daniel Sennert). The closing date of 1630 marks the sharp decline in *peregrinatio medica* because of the Thirty Years War, and the consequent decline of academic exchange, which was weakened further by the disruption to the Frankfurt Book Fair.

This study is intended to reveal the ways in which the medical profession were predisposed to view human beings and the natural world by the way they were trained to think in universities, and through the doctrine with which they were inculcated. The questions which have driven this enquiry are the following: through what instruments did learned physicians think? What were their operative concepts, and how coherent were they? What did they disagree about, and in what terms? How did medical discourse relate to, and distinguish itself from, other learned discourses (theology, law, natural philosophy, philosophy itself)? I have set it out in a way similar to the book on law; it begins with a brief history of learned medicine in the Renaissance (chapter 1), followed by accounts of the modes of transmission of medical knowledge (chapter 2), and the interaction of medicine with other related disciplines (chapter 3). I then offer an extensive examination of the arts course and its complex relationship to medical logic and method (chapters 4 and 5); an account of the theory and practice of the interpretation of medical texts (chapter 6) and of the philosophical content of medical thought (chapter 7); all of which is designed to serve as an introduction to the last chapter of the book, which is a critical examination of the doctrine of signs and evidence. In the postscript I shall return briefly to the issues I have mentioned in this introduction, and offer some suggestions about the relationship of the medical discourse studied in this book both to its medieval forebear and to the emergence of experimental philosophy after 1630. Because this work sets out to survey some rather technical areas of Renaissance thought, a brief account of these is given in footnotes as background to the discussion in the text.

[2] Siraisi 1997: 3–4.

There has in recent years been much distinguished writing about late medieval and early modern medicine and science. Scholars such as Nancy Siraisi, Andrew Wear, Vivian Nutton, Iain Lonie, Andrew Cunningham, Roger French, Charles Schmitt, Nicholas Jardine, Charles Webster, Jerome J. Bylebyl, Ole Peter Grell, Luis García Ballester, Don Bates and many others whose works are listed in the bibliography have transformed the received history of medicine and scientific practices in this period in a number of ways, and have drawn attention to a new range of problems and questions; and the field has benefited also from the work on the theory and methodology of such history done by Ludwik Fleck, Thomas S. Kuhn and others. Whole new areas of research have also been explored, among them what might broadly be called the social history of medicine, seen through the experience of patients (especially women), the activities of non-learned practitioners, the organisation of medical institutions, the collection and display of scientific objects, the production, diffusion and consumption of medical and scientific knowledge, the interaction of learned and popular medicine, and the influence of patrons, towns and courts.[3] These investigations have been related to grander narratives, charting the 'Entzauberung' or 'disenchantment' of the world, the collapse of monolithic theories (notably Aristotelian physics), the rise of scepticism and rationalism, the switch of (Kuhnian) paradigm from a qualitative to a mathematised and probabilistic approach to nature, or (Foucauldian) episteme from a grid of correspondences to a theory of representation.[4] All this is testimony of what Paul Veyne has called the 'extension of the historical agenda'.[5]

It would not be appropriate to review here all of this work: but some of its liveliest areas of debate are relevant to the present investigation and may be noted here. A great deal of attention has been paid to the relationship of Renaissance natural philosophy to the new scientific outlook of the seventeenth century. On the one hand, there is the claim (known from the work of Sarton and Crombie) that humanism impeded the progress of experimental science, which was further advanced in the fourteenth century than in the sixteenth; against this, there are those who propound the view that the source of scientific progress is to be found in the low sciences (alchemy and occultism) of the Renaissance period, and

---

3 Webster 1979b; Eamon 1994; Palmer 1983; Findlen 1994; Daston and Park 1998; Ashworth 1990b; Blair 1997; Bono 1995; Céard 1996; Barona 1994.
4 Weber 1991: 151, 351–3; Henry 1997; Kuhn 1970; Foucault 1966.
5 Veyne 1978: 141–56.

that the magus is the prototype of the modern experimental scientist.[6]
This latter party also has its critics, among them Brian Vickers, who has
argued strongly that the occult (alias hermetic, or alchemical) sciences
of the Renaissance relate to a quite different mind-set from the scientific
mentality that emerged in the seventeenth century.[7] A different account
of Renaissance natural philosophy and medicine asserts that Galenism,
which, according to García Ballester, had 'attractive complexity' for the
fourteenth-century mind, was 'threadbare' and 'academic' by 1600; that
a growing number of its adherents were manifesting serious unease about
its claims; and that the Aristotelianism with which it was associated had
declined with it into a text-based sterility, suffering from over-complexity
and lack of explanatory power.[8]

Owsei Temkin attributes this alleged decline to a number of factors:
the challenge of Paracelsus and his followers to the moral, political and
scientific validity of learned medicine; the humanist attempt to liber-
ate Galen from his systematisation by the Arabs; the rise of practical
medicine outside the universities; the breakthrough in anatomical studies, and the practice of autopsy.[9] Such a view is consistent with the representation of Aristotelianism in the polemic of the new scientists of the
seventeenth century as the most sterile of all intellectual areas, impris-
oned inside peripatetic metaphysics and logic. It is consistent also with
the periodisation of Renaissance Galenic studies in particular, and medical hellenism in general, suggested by Vivian Nutton: after a first, heroic,
period of textual discovery, edition and commentary (say 1500–50), there
followed a period of consolidation and critique, during which the metaphysical and methodological underpinnings are explicit and operative
(say 1550–1600); the eventual failure to reconcile all the authorities, to
incorporate the new empirical findings into the doctrine, and maintain
the coherence of the medical art marked its decline, which occurred
between 1600 and 1630.[10] This model of a doctrine's life cycle (familiar,
in the history of ideas, through the work of Lovejoy)[11] is not professed
by all historians; in their account of wonders and the order of nature,
Lorraine Daston and Katharine Park prefer a cyclical pattern, in which

---

[6] Sarton 1953; Crombie 1994; Cochrane 1976; Yates 1967: 255; Meinel 1992: 40; Vickers 1984b:
   1–55; Bennett 1998.
[7] Vickers 1979; 1984b.
[8] García Ballester 1993b: 38; Siraisi 1987a: 349; Galilei 1998.
[9] Temkin 1973: 136. Zanier 1983:1–4, 39–43 says that Galenism's extreme eclecticism is the cause
   of its decline.
[10] Nutton 1993a; Siraisi 1987a: 349–55.
[11] Lovejoy 1936.

is manifested a return to favour of discredited doctrines or elements of them.[12]

There are those also who oppose the thesis of a decline in medical and natural-philosophical doctrines towards 1630, and are willing to attribute some impulsion towards scientific advance to developments in Renaissance Aristotelianism. According to J. H. Randall, Paduan Aristotelianism marks a step forward on the path to the secular and naturalistic scientific outlook of the seventeenth century;[13] this view has been strongly challenged, and a different, less progressivist, reassessment of Aristotelian natural philosophy has been proposed by Charles Schmitt, who lays more emphasis on the conceptual (as opposed to experimental) developments in both theory and practice.[14] Ian Hacking propounds a more negative view: according to him, not only is there no concept of evidence in the Renaissance in the sense of 'that by which one thing can indicate contingently the state of something else', but also this lack is aggravated by a commitment to privileging the final cause as the true explanans of any event (as opposed to the efficient and material causes, espoused by the new science of the seventeenth century).[15] This contention may be linked both to that which asserts that all testimony is based on the credibility of the witness, not the intrinsic value of the facts he adduces; and to that which sees 'facts' as we understand them emerging for the first time in the late seventeenth century.[16] Steven Shapin's *Social history of truth* develops the former view of testimony with respect to the association of credibility and social status in seventeenth-century witnesses to scientific events.[17] Others have proposed a similar view about the reception of philosophical ideas in the Renaissance, especially as mediated by the practice of commonplace books; this is said to have the effect of dissociating 'facts' from their original context, and thus of fragmenting knowledge into individual pieces (loci) which are then available to be reconfigured and given new functions in an argument.[18] According to one historian of philosophy, this fragmentation predisposes Renaissance thinkers to a nominalist outlook.[19]

[12] Daston and Park 1998: 9–12.
[13] Randall 1961; Randall 1976: 271–82.
[14] Schmitt 1983b; Wear 1981: 238 offers yet another view, suggesting that Leoniceno's characterisation of art as a utilitarian practice can be seen as 'a primitive move towards a free-standing science'.
[15] Hacking 1975: 37.
[16] Shapiro 1999.
[17] Shapin 1994.
[18] Moss 1996; Goyet 1996.
[19] Kessler forthcoming.

Another contention concerns the status of particulars and singular cases. Paula Findlen has argued that the exceptional case or oddity takes on a new role in Renaissance thinking: not that of a deviation from the general rule but as an object in its own right. Lorraine Daston and Katharine Park have also supported this view in their work on the emergence of a group of 'praeternatural historians' (figures such as Marsilio Ficino, Cornelius Agrippa, Girolamo Cardano, Scipion Dupleix and Giambattista della Porta) in the early modern period. These are said to espouse a new kind of enquiry into the occult forces and aberrant manifestations of nature, characterised by the abandonment of the medieval concentration on the normal and the regular.[20] The switch from an interest in the general to an interest in particular instances parallels the switch traced in the various writings of Peter Dear from the scholastic reliance on 'experience' (that is, generalised statements about how things usually occur based on sensory evidence available to all) to the practice of 'experiment'.[21] Both praeternatural historians and experimenters are associated with the rise of technology, because art is a form of praeternatural activity by which man imposes his own order on nature.[22] Their articulate spokesman is Francis Bacon, who instructs the readers of his *Advancement of learning* to engage in the study of 'nature erring' and 'nature wrought' as well as 'nature in [her ordinary] course', and to begin their reclassification of natural objects by an inductive process, which privileges the individual case.[23] Bacon it is also who explicitly poses the question of the expansion of the field of knowledge. Whereas in the Middle Ages, according to Edward Grant, the limited range of 'quaestiones' which were permitted in disputations restricted the possibility of enquiry (a claim made also by Paula Findlen about natural philosophy in the Renaissance),[24] Bacon is able to assert that having discovered new lands, new seas and new stars, it would be disgraceful for men of his age to allow the world of the mind ('globus intellectualis') to remain circumscribed by the same boundaries as before.[25] Knowledge also manifestly

---

[20] Findlen 1994; Daston and Park 1998; Grafton and Siraisi 1999.

[21] Dear 1987; 1990; 1995.

[22] Newman 1997.

[23] Bacon himself acknowledged however that some effort, albeit wrongly focussed, had gone into the recording of praeternatural events: Bacon 2000: 63.

[24] Grant 1978; Findlen 1994: 4.

[25] Bacon 1878: 277 (*Novum organum*, i.84): 'Neque pro nihilo aestimandum, quod per longinquas navigationes et peregrinationes (quae seculis nostris increbuerunt) plurima in Natura patuerint, et reperta sint, quae novam philosophiae lucem immittere possint. Quin et turpe hominibus foret, si globi materialis tractus, terrarum videlicet, marium, astrorum, nostris temporibus immensum aperti et illustrati sint: globi autem intellectualis fines, inter veterum inventa et angustias cohibeantur.'

increases in the sphere of medicine in the course of the sixteenth century; not only knowledge of new diseases and new materia medica, but also new discoveries in anatomy. This poses a problem which was already explicit to the minds of fifteenth-century thinkers, and which is posed anew by learned doctors in the Renaissance: is the mind the measure of all things, or can man aspire to knowledge of the universe beyond this constraint and the limitations and uncertainty of information obtained through the senses?[26] These questions add immediacy to the philosophical discussions about classification and the relative value to be placed on empirical information and existing theory; the presence of elaborate accounts of logic in medical treatises at the end of the sixteenth century is as much due to them as to a devotion to theory for its own sake.

In attempting to give historical accounts of medicine in the early modern period, one encounters also more general questions of theory and method. A much debated area concerns the alternative hypotheses of realism and social construction.[27] This is a dichotomy whose shortcomings have been widely discussed, and which Ian Hacking has called to be replaced by 'richer tools with which to think'.[28] When Jon Arrizabalaga, John Henderson, and R. K. French's *The great pox: the French disease in Renaissance Europe* was reviewed in the *Sunday Times*, its reviewer, betraying a trust in modern scientific categories which is not shared by all its modern practitioners, called for the reader's 'objective interest in the condition and its agent' to be satisfied, which the authors of this study in the cultural reception of a complex phenomenon had declined to do.[29] A more extreme constructivist position would involve the claim that it would be inappropriate to talk of plague before the date of the discovery of the plague bacillus;[30] this affirmation of the impossibility of achieving an objective account of past phenomena (such as witches)[31] rests on the broader assumption that there is no such thing as a meta-discourse or an extra-linguistic space in which to adjudicate between the 'objective facts' of the past and the past's own account of such facts.[32] Even a cure can be seen as a construction of the profession or the community in

[26] Blair 1997: 4; Bacon 1878: 210–11 (*Novum organum*, i.41).
[27] This debate has become involved in the so-called 'science wars': for a judicious account of these, see Jardine and Frasca-Spada (1997).
[28] Hacking 1999: 1; Wear 1995a: 151 sees a more complex split in the historiography of medicine: both between internal and external, and epistemic and sociological.
[29] *Sunday Times*, 19 January 1997, Book Section, 6.
[30] Cunningham 1992.
[31] Clark 1997: 6–7; cf. Jones 1940: 178: 'if the law says sorcery exists, then it exists'.
[32] This is an assumption already voiced in the Renaissance by Juan Luis Vives in respect of the mind's ability to know itself: Vives 1555: 2.516.

which it occurs.[33] Such a view does not imply necessarily a thorough-going relativism,[34] only the proposition that knowledge and meaning are negotiated by the communities in which they arise, by a process which Don Bates has called 'coherencing'.[35] Such negotiation also has connections with the claims made by Quentin Skinner and others on the one hand that rhetorical, dialectical and topical argumentative procedures affect the whole mental universe of the Renaissance[36] and, on the other, the more radical claim that there can be no such thing as objective or pure description; every statement is theory-laden, or impregnated with interpretative procedures and premisses.[37]

Three claims are made about the conditions intrinsic to thought which are relevant to here. The first, by T. S. Kuhn, is too well known to be rehearsed at length. It involves the contention that paradigms of science are incommensurable; that they are discontinuous; that they contain their own validation processes; that they are espoused by a scientific community; and that while the paradigm is in force, there is such a thing as 'normal science', which can be represented not only by the brightest minds of any generation, but also by scientists of the middle rank. Paradigms can of course co-exist; and it is implicit in Kuhn, and explicit in some of his followers, that there are two in the period of the Renaissance; one espoused in university circles intent on preserving received Aristotelian doctrine, another in new research fields such as chymistry, magnetism and the low sciences, which did not suffer that constraint.[38] A different distinction of paradigm is that which, according to Brian Vickers, separates the mentality of seventeenth-century adherents of the new science from Renaissance occult philosophers who eschew abstraction, jealously guard the secrecy of privileged knowledge for adepts, do not encourage others to repeat the experiments through which they establish their lore, are the victims of the anthropomorphic, socio-religious or occult categories by which they structure their knowledge, and look upon their activities as religious rather than secular in nature. Vickers sees the occult philosophy as failing to distinguish between words and things, between metaphor and literal meaning, and between the use of analogy which dominates the thought it is meant to enlighten by reifying

---

[33] Siraisi 1997: 35.
[34] Daston 1997: 6.
[35] Bates 1998.
[36] Kristeller 1988; Skinner 1996: 19–110; Mack 1990; Schmidt-Biggemann 1983.
[37] Gadamer 1962; a claim refuted by Engel 1990.
[38] Kuhn 1970; Eamon 1994: 6–7; see also Fleck 1979: 39 (on *Denkstil* as 'the given stock of knowledge and level of culture'); Iliffe 1998: 349.

it on the one hand, and on the other the scientific use of analogy as a heuristic tool.[39]

A second claim, not necessarily that of Kuhn himself, but certainly to be associated with the name of Gaston Bachelard, concerns the thinkability of propositions and theories. According to Bachelard, there is an 'epistemological obstacle' which prevents thinkers in a certain mindset from surpassing the limits of their thought; thus, for example, there could be no probabilistic thought before the elaboration of an appropriate notation and a community to operate it and make it their own mental property.[40] Lorraine Daston's statement in *Classical probability in the Enlightenment* that until the nineteenth century 'causeless events were unthinkable' is another example of this.[41] Karl Popper energetically opposed this view; while conceding that we are always within the prison-house of our mind-set, he argued that we are at any time able to transcend it by recognising its limits.[42] This argument has been developed by Graham Priest, among others.[43] My own investigation is in agreement with these claims for limited self-critique, which have implications also for historical semantics and the conditions under which it can be claimed that a proposition is indeed 'thought'. There is a risk in adopting Popper's position, which is that everything may become translatable into the past; by taking elements of past thought out of context, one can detect prior versions of nearly all modern thinking, not least (as we shall see) Popper's own falsification theory. The strictures of the Annales school against such anachronistic thinking and the demonstration by Stuart Clark in his excellent article on popular beliefs in France of the dangers of departing from the terms and categories by which actors in past events describe their participation in them are to be borne in mind here as salutary warnings.[44]

A third set of claims is associated with the name of Alexandre Koyré, and concerns the influence of metaphysical presuppositions on scientific thought, the role of mistaken theories in the progress of science, and the greater importance to be attributed to the emergence of problems than to the achievement of concrete results.[45] I believe that there is a risk that if the history of science is treated with this degree of abstraction from

[39] Vickers 1984b: 41–2, 95; also Clulee 1984: 57–9.
[40] Bachelard 1933; Fleck 1979.
[41] Daston 1988: 10.
[42] Popper 1970.
[43] Priest 1995; Pickering 1995.
[44] Clark 1983.
[45] Koyré 1958.

its context, it will under-represent the means by which thought comes to be propagated through institutions and through the various media of publicity available to thinkers. I have argued elsewhere that ideas are sustained and spread through human institutions such as universities; and that the speed with which they change (and whether they change at all) is dependent on the means available to teach them to others, to publicise and circulate them, and the willingness of sponsors to pay for such diffusion. In doing so such sponsors may be serving a variety of interests beyond the purely intellectual (if there is such a thing as a purely intellectual interest); and they may be engaging in a process which they do not fully control (indeed, which no one may fully control, for it is not possible accurately to predict the uptake by others of texts which are widely circulated). The ideas thus diffused may not be perfectly or completely comprehended, or may be taken up in contexts quite different from that in which they were first conceived.[46] Koyré himself acknowledged many of these points, although in practice he did not always employ them in his historical works.[47]

These are some of the issues which this study sets out to investigate; in discussing them, I should declare a commitment of my own, namely that Galenic medicine was not in the moribund state in which it is said to be by Temkin and O'Malley and by later seventeenth-century polemicists (which is not to say, of course, that it was not subjected to critique).[48] It seems to me to be animated by vigorous polemics, and to be informed by novel attempts to adapt its conceptual structures to emergent knowledge. Not least among the signs of this vigour is the doctrine of symptoms, signs, illness and cause of which this study shall speak. I shall argue that the part of medicine known as semiotic or semiology (about which some notoriously false claims have been made)[49] grows in importance towards the end of the sixteenth century, as does practical medicine in relation to the theoretical part. Both reflect the complex relations between the empirical and rational parts of

---

[46] Maclean 1998a, 1998c.

[47] Redondi 1987.

[48] Temkin 1973: 134ff.; O'Malley 1970: 101: 'it was in the latter sixteenth century that the medical students were exposed to the first stirrings of doubt and the first suggestions of overthrow of a complacent classical medicine, and its replacement, although in the distant future, by one more scientifically based'. Cf. also Wightman 1962: 263 (on Galenists as 'academic pedants' and slaves to authority' as opposed to forward-looking [al]chemists).

[49] Lehoux 1976: 483: 'il faut attendre 1650 pour rencontrer, chez Jean Henry, l'un des premiers traités de sémiologie'; cf. Dewhurst 1966: 59: 'Sydenham's revival of the Hippocratic method of studying the natural history of diseases by making a series of accurate and detailed observations set the clinical pattern for future progress.'

the discipline, and both testify to the persistence of modes of thought which are specific to medicine, separating its internal practices of argument, and the ways in which its adherents express disagreement and consensus with each other, from those of neighbouring discourses such as natural philosophy and from the rival higher faculties of theology and law.

Currently received opinion espouses an account of Renaissance Galenism which sees it rising, flourishing and declining in the course of the sixteenth century. I accept of course that there was a powerful renaissance of Galenic studies in the first few decades of the sixteenth century, as well as a growing critique of Galenism in those which followed, but there are two reasons why I do not see this in terms of a decline. The first is that such a view restricts the discourse of medicine to what at any one time can be conceptualised in terms of the discourse as a whole: whereas it seems to me that new ideas beyond the limits of the discourse, or in localised segments of the discourse, can be expressed, even if they cannot carry conviction with the entire medical community. The second reason for rejecting the thesis of decline, it seems to me, resides in the exclusion from the discourse of what might be called its operative knowledge, arising both from its practical application (therapy, surgery, anatomy), and its *bricolage* with mental procedures which can only be made to do the work required of them by transgressing against the very rules which govern them;[50] what I shall call protoprobabilistic thought and quantification are two examples of this. Through these acts of *bricolage* such questions as which of two diagnoses is *more likely* to be right, a question which is apparently excluded by the precepts of the medical art, can be asked and answered. I shall also take it as a methodological principle that the importance of a doctrine is not to be measured by the frequency of its allegation or the degree of elaboration of its discussion: in his *Pathologia*, Jean Fernel refers in only half a chapter to the 'morbus totius substantiae'; its subsequent importance is not however to be measured by the number of words he consecrated to the topic, but rather by the uptake it enjoyed in what Fleck would call the 'Denkkollektiv'.[51]

---

[50] The term is taken from Lévi-Strauss 1962: 23–6, on which see Derrida 1967: 417–19. This is not the same (progressivist) claim as that made by Findlen 1994: 10: 'while something we might approximately designate as the precursor to modern science was in the process of formation, it was arrested by, in fact derived from, a most "unscientific" world of philosophizing that did not privilege "science" because it had not yet identified it as a better, truer form of knowledge'.

[51] Siraisi forthcoming; Fleck 1979: 37, defining thought collective as 'a community of persons mutually exchanging ideas or maintaining intellectual interaction'. Kuhn 1970: x–xi offers two critiques of this idea: it functions like an individual mind; and 'what the thought collective supplies

As is implicit in the above, I shall proceed as though medicine is an embodied discipline, relying not only on its doctrines to define itself, but also its institutions, its curricula, and the means it uses to propagate and stabilise itself: its means of transmission of knowledge and its genres. In the words of the title of a recent work edited by Christopher Lawrence and Steven Shapin, it is a 'science incarnate';[52] to study it by excluding its social and institutional context would be to ignore its accommodations with the practical issues with which it deals. Even if one could just about do this using only the corpus of pedagogical texts of theory and practice I have examined below, it would be an egregious mistake to assume that their influence was felt only in university circles; they are addressed to, and taken up by, practitioners as well. This relationship between practice and the discourse of medicine marks a discontinuity with the modern discipline which I did not detect in comparing the discourse of Renaissance law with that of the present day: whereas a twentieth-century jurist shares many concerns about language, intention, and evidence that were expressed by his sixteenth-century predecessors, I doubt whether a modern doctor wedded to the cause of Evidence-based Medicine would recognise a prior version of himself in a late Renaissance Galenist.[53] In this sense, 'to think like a doctor' means something very different now from what it meant in 1800, let alone 1600, even if some constants, such as the Hippocratic oath, the patient–doctor relationship, the process of diagnosis and prognosis, can be said to be found at all three times. On the other hand, there does seem to be a greater degree of continuity from the ancient world to the late Renaissance; the universe of discourse which constitutes medicine in about 1620 includes, and indeed treats as contemporaries, Hippocrates, Sextus Empiricus, Galen, Arnau de Vilanova, Pietro d'Abano, Andreas Vesalius and Girolamo Fracastoro. It will be the task of this study to trace both the discourse which binds such texts together and the conceptual innovations which divide them.

As in the case of law, I have here to confess that I do not have a specialist grounding in the subject in hand. When I had finished the first

its members is somehow like Kantian categories, prerequisite to any thought at all. The authority of a thought collective is thus more nearly logical than social, yet it exists for the individual only by virtue of his induction into a group.' But Kuhn approves of Fleck's insistence (38–51) that scientific epistemology has to historicise both scientific thinking and scientific facts, and that such epistemology is not just a matter of a knowing subject and an object to be known, but also of the existing fund of knowledge which 'must be a third partner'.

[52] Lawrence and Shapin 1998. The metaphor of embodiment is prominent in cultural materialism and the study of the 'intersection of speculative and cultural formations across a wide range of contexts': Taub 1997: 80.

[53] Sackett, Richardson, Rosenberg and Haynes 1997.

draft of the book, I was pleased to note that the content of chapters 7 and 8, and to some degree also the ordering of material, was very close to that adopted by Franciscus Valleriola in his *Loci medicinae communes* of 1562, which I had only recently read: from which similarity I am emboldened to think that my study may not be a wholesale and anachronistic rewriting of Renaissance medical thought. The temptation to look at the semiology, diagnosis and hermeneutics of this period in the light of modern problematics and theories is very great, and has not been everywhere resisted; I hope however that I have not unwittingly impregnated texts of the sixteenth century with a suspect modern hue, and that the exotic nature of their embodied modes of thought and expression has not been wholly obscured. A thorough knowledge of the relevant ancient sources allowed the writers studied here to quote allusively from them, and to be confident that these allusions would be recognised by their contemporaries; I have no doubt failed to do this on many occasions, and have thereby attributed to a Renaissance thinker a concept or proposition which he had extracted without acknowledgement from an ancient source. I hope that those who detect such failures to recognise allusions will look indulgently on them; they can to some degree be excused, in that the concept or proposition in question has been actively incorporated into the thought of its user, and is not present as mere allegation or ornament: as Montaigne says, 'la verité et la raison sont communes à un chacun, et ne sont non plus à qui les a dites premierement, qu'à qui les dict apres'.[54]

---

[54] Montaigne 1965: 152 (i.26).

CHAPTER I

Learned medicine 1500–1630

Strange new illnesses produce strange new doctors.

(Severinus)[1]

I.I INTRODUCTION

It would be possible to record the history of learned university medicine in this period in a few sentences: its place in the whole field of medical activities, its adoption of medical humanism, its revision of curricula and teaching practices and development of clinical precepting, its involvement with outside institutions such as courts, guilds, colleges of physicians and hospitals, its extension into the fields of anatomy, botany and zoology, its relationship with neighbouring disciplines such as natural philosophy, law, and theology, its confessionalisation, its growing unease with, but continuing adherence to, the inherited Galenic and Aristotelian doctrines, its interaction with Paracelsianism, natural magic, astrology, alchemy, as well as surgeons and empirics. Not all of these topics are pertinent to this study. The excellent and comprehensive book *Medieval and early Renaissance medicine* by Nancy Siraisi happily dispenses me from attempting to offer a balanced view; I intend here to look at those issues only which provide a helpful context for later chapters. I shall thus discuss in turn the relation of learned medicine with the other parts of what we would now consider the medical world; the state of the discipline as this was inherited from the fifteenth century; the revival of Greek medicine, and the wider impact of humanism, seen both in the rejection of Arabic medicine and the exposure of errors in ancient texts and the development of nosology, anatomy, botany and zoology; the period of critique and innovation in theory in the middle years of the century; the changes in curricula and teaching practices; the varying uptake of these

[1] Severinus 1571: 3: 'paradoxi morbi paradoxos medicos peperere'.

14

innovations in Europe, and the relative importance of different teaching institutions; the networks and influences at work in the profession, both inside and outside universities; and finally the state of the discipline at the end of the period which I am considering. This approach will concentrate on those doctors whose doctrines were made widely available through publication; it does not set out to trace the evolution of medical thought in this period uniquely through the productions of the great innovating minds of the time – Andreas Vesalius (1514–64), Girolamo Fracastoro (1483–1553), Girolamo Cardano (1501–76), Jean Fernel (1497–1558), Giovanni Argenterio (1513–72) – and so may seem not to accord to them their due place in a history of intellectual achievement.

1.2 UNIVERSITIES IN THE BROADER MEDICAL CONTEXT

1.2.1 Guilds, surgeons, colleges

University medicine was not hermetically sealed off in a pedagogical ghetto; its professors took on other roles, interacted with local medical communities such as colleges of physicians, town and court physicians and surgeons, and were influenced by some of their attitudes and practices. It would seem that a group to which such professors were implacably opposed through the need to protect the interests of their profession are the empirics, by which I mean to designate all those who acted without licence: Jewish doctors, quacks, 'Landfahrer', cunning men and women, alchemistic or occult healers, charlatans. Such opposition is expressed in the statutes of both universities and colleges of physicians, as well as in pamphlets.[2] But even this hostility, which after 1560 comes to be associated also with Paracelsian medicine, is not uniform; Jakob Horst (1537–1600) addresses one of his early writings to 'Hausartzte, vernünfftige Weiber, gute Warterinnen und Apotheken',[3] and several historians have shown how difficult and fitful the regulation of this sector was.[4] Relations with court and town doctors were much easier, as they were nearly all university trained, and often widely respected

---

[2] This list is reminiscent of that produced in about 1312 by Henri de Mondeville: 'illiterati, sicut barberii, sortilegi, locatores, insidiatores, falsarii, alchemistae, meretrices, metatrices, obstetrices, vetulae, Judaei, conversi, Saraceni': Mondeville 1892: 65. See also Pagel 1935: 218 (quoting Freitag, *Noctes atticae*, 1616); Emericus 1552: R4r–v; Pelling 1995; Efron 1998; Sylvius 1539: a3v; Eamon 1994; Siraisi 1997: 25–6. See also below ch. 3, note 134.
[3] Horst 1574.
[4] Pelling 1995; Siraisi 1990c.

for their publications;[5] many moved in and out of university positions.[6] Universities often enjoyed close relations with colleges of physicians and other universities, although these could also be made fraught for reasons of non-recognition of each other's qualifications and competition for students.[7] The habit of thinking protectively leaves its mark on the training and image of the rational doctor, as I shall hope to show.

1.2.2 The state of the discipline before humanism

This rivalry involves also medicine in its guise as craft or 'ars factiva' and its protection of trade secrets. More than apothecaries, surgeons here come into question: they had acquired a high reputation in France and Italy in the late fourteenth century, and had counted among their number some of the foremost medical figures of their day, such as Guy de Chauliac and Jacques Despars.[8] In the early years of medical humanism, manuscripts of their works were sought by leading learned doctors, including Niccolò Leoniceno (1428–1524), Guillaume Cop (1460–1532) and Thomas Linacre (1460–1524);[9] and their stock gradually rose throughout the sixteenth century, partly on the coat-tails of anatomy, but also through the respect enjoyed by such figures as Ambroise Paré (1510–90), Wilhelm Fabry de Hilden (Fabricius Hildanus) (1560–1634), and Jacques Daléchamps (1513–88) because of their effectiveness as practitioners and their empirical approach. Although the majority of surgical works continued to be written in the vernacular rather than Latin, they were often translated into Latin for the international community, and efforts were made in the vernacular to provide surgeons with the rational basis which was seen to be enjoyed by their physician colleagues.[10] These developments are not uniform through Europe, but

---

[5] See Cardano 1583: a5r, who mentions Guillaume Cop, Jean Ruel, Thomas Linacre, Niccolò Leoniceno, Antonio Musa Brasavola by name. Franciscus Valleriola and Andreas Libavius are examples of doctors employed by municipalities who have a distinguished publishing record.

[6] Andreas Vesalius, Girolamo Cardano, Berengario da Carpi, and Giovanni Argenterio are some examples.

[7] Non-recognition was mostly at issue where Faculties of Medicine acted also as a licensing body for practitioners in a given area, as was the case in France and certain Italian cities. See also Herberger 1981: 278–80.

[8] Siraisi 1990c; García Ballester 1993b: 40; Jacquart 1998.

[9] Nutton 1985a: 78.

[10] *Ibid.*; Jean Canappe's *Opuscules* of 1552 are often quoted as the earliest instance of this: but Maittaire 1722: 421–37 has evidence of earlier medical publications in French in the 1540s. See also Eusèbe 1566; Schmitt 1977; Bylebyl 1979: 367.

they represent the trend;[11] although in 1601, Joannes Baptista Silvaticus (1550–1621) can still cast doubt on the status of surgeons as more than mechanicals, it would be safe to say that their stock had risen considerably by this time.[12] This development is one mark of the growing prestige of practical medicine over the period in question which has, I believe, a determinable effect on the rational claims of the discipline at a whole.

If one looks at the early publication of medical books (up to 1500), one can obtain an impression of the state of the discipline. It is marked on the one hand by the production of textbooks – the *Articella*, Pietro d'Abano's *Conciliator*, Avicenna's *Canon* – which set the agenda of questions governing the curricula, and have an enduring effect on these throughout the century, as Nancy Siraisi has shown;[13] and on the other by the appearance of the best practical manuals of the fifteenth century, of which Michaele Savonarola's is a good example. This is a work covering general pathology, therapy, dietetics, materia medica, prognosis and nosology (the longest section); it was produced for practising doctors as well as for teaching purposes; its contents and even to some degree the disposition of its material can in large part be found in the practica being taught and published in Italy in the early seventeenth century.[14] In similar fashion, the *Conciliator* is used as late as 1610 as the basic tool for covering the syllabus of theoretical as well as practical medicine.[15] There are even works of anatomy and mirabilia (by Mondino de' Luzzi (1270–1326), Berengario da Carpi (d. 1550), Antonio Benivieni (1443–1502)) which are published in this very early period, although it would be wrong to claim that they are typical products of their day. The group of texts concerning quantification of compound medicines and computation of qualities and humours reflects the uptake in late fifteenth-century Italian universities of the work of fourteenth-century Oxford mathematicians, and reveals an area of expertise which, as Crombie and others have claimed, became obscured by the medical humanism (see below 5.2);[16] and the issue of astrological medicine was also a live one, which finds

---

[11] Nutton 1990a: 238. In England, the first president of the newly founded Guild of Barber-Surgeons, John Chamber, was a doctor trained in Padua: Woolfson 1998: 80.

[12] Silvaticus 1601: 434 (xciv): 'an manufaciendae operationes ad medicum spectant, necne'.

[13] Siraisi 1987a; Avicenna was finally supplanted by Galenism in the 1550s; *ibid.*, 102. For an account of the contents of the *Articella*, see Arrizabalaga 1998.

[14] O'Neill 1975 argues that Savonarola is atypical, but not in respect of the contents of his writing, which is largely drawn from Avicenna. See Mikkeli 1999: 22; Siraisi 1990c; Wear 1973: 196.

[15] See Horst 1621 (for the University of Giessen); also the contents of Cardano 1565, Vallesius 1606, and even Ferdinandus 1611. See also Siraisi 1997: 46ff.

[16] See Iliffe 1998: 357; Clulee 1971; and McVaugh 1969 for the earlier manifestation of this interest.

echoes in other disciplines at the time (see below 3.6).[17] Some of these features will re-emerge in different contexts with different valencies in the later part of the sixteenth century.

1.3 HUMANISM

Humanism itself had a great effect on medical studies from the middle of the fifteenth century onwards. Its first and abiding contribution is seen somewhat peripherally in the elegant Latin of prefaces and to some degree translations, together with the use of antique poets for the purposes both of quotation and doctrine; it is also reflected in the enhanced awareness of history, including the history of medicine as a discipline and the biographical studies of prominent doctors of the near and distant past.[18] It contributes to the development of natural science as a whole; the revival of Platonic and neoplatonist studies in the fifteenth century had implications for the influence of the superlunary on the sublunary, the renewed interest in animistic accounts of natural philosophy, the greater respect shown for both the liberal and mechanical arts and for man's potential to rise above the constraints of the material world.[19] The rediscovery of mathematical and astronomical texts enriched the disciplinary environment of medicine. More narrowly, humanistic techniques were used to purify medical texts from accretions and restore them to their historical purity, to expand the classical sources for humoral therapy, and to make available both Galen and Hippocrates in far larger measure.[20]

---

[17] On this see Siraisi 1990c: 67–8; and for a characteristic text Hasfurtus 1533. See Copenhaver 1988: 283.

[18] On this see Momigliano 1985: 1–24; Barona 1994: 121–51; Siraisi 1999; Siraisi 2000 (who also mentions the place of the biography of doctors in Renaissance histories of Italian cities, and the broader role of history in medical studies, including anatomy and psychology); on the tendentiousness of this history see Siraisi 1987b: 122, who points out that the humanist Coluccio Salutati omitted the schools of Salerno and Montpellier from his history of medicine. See also Cardano 1663: 1.149, cited by Maclean 1999a: 28 (on the connection between history and medicine as textual disciplines).

[19] I shall use 'animistic' to refer to a dualistic (Platonic) account of the soul as separate from the body, and 'vitalistic' as a hylomorphic account, after Bono 1995: 85–108. The contemporary terms 'spiritus', 'facultas', 'vis', 'virtus' give rise to discussions of these two possibilities: see for example Valleriola 1562: 118–64.

[20] Joutsivuo 1999: 14–15; Mikkeli 1999: 23–4; on the influence of humanist Latin, see Nutton 1985a and Nutton 1995. Evidence of a historical sense is to be found in the title of Struthius: 1602, which cites how long ago Galen wrote; somewhat ironically, as for Galen the ancients ('antiqui' in the Latin) were those who wrote a hundred years before him whereas for Renaissance writers, 'neoterici' could have been writing as early as 1300: see Silvaticus 1601: 433–4 and Galen, *In aphorismos*, vi, K 18a.6–7. Arrizabalaga 1998: 23 argues that there are two distinct groups of hellenists at this time: neoplatonists and Aristotelians. It has also been suggested that the

Bylebyl claims that 'the emergence of a triumphant and uncompromising Galenism in the first half of the sixteenth century was probably a necessary precondition for the marked, if somewhat diffuse, Aristotelian revival [in medicine] that gathered force in some medical circles towards the end of the century';[21] this may be somewhat misleading in respect of Aristotelianism itself, which was transformed in the middle years of the century by the same mechanism – the emergence of Latin translations of hellenist commentators – as Galenism had been some fifty years earlier. The claims also that the new Greek discoveries and their mediation into Latin transformed medical science have also to be attenuated by the strong continuity that exists between the fifteenth and the sixteenth centuries, and by the excellence of some pre-humanist translations.[22]

1.3.1 Greek

A central issue which throws light on this problem is that of hellenism. The high value placed upon Greek studies, especially in the medical field, is well known: Nutton quotes Jason Pratensis saying in 1527 'the whole of the profession of medicine is an imposture if it does not have Greek';[23] and it is not difficult to show that those doctors who were fluent in Greek such as Jacques Dubois (Sylvius) (1478–1555) of Paris presuppose it in their readers.[24] It has been claimed that the publication of Greek authors such as Galen (whose edition in 1525 contained one hundred and six texts in all, of which forty-six had not previously been published),[25] Hippocrates, Paul of Aegina, and Aetius brought considerable enrichment to medicine: not only in the sphere of medicinal herbs and specific diseases and that of anatomical structures, but also in that of gynaecology, on which Hippocrates (but not Galen) had written a separate treatise that inspired the first collection of texts specifically

---

philological return *ad fontes* was a factor in the rise of the unmediated study of the human body through dissection.

[21] Bylebyl 1985a: 245.

[22] Durling 1961: 238–9 (on Niccolò da Reggio); according to Bylebyl 1991: 170, the hellenist Sylvius is scarcely better than his medieval predecessor Gatinaria.

[23] Nutton 1987: 38: 'sine graeco impostura est omnis istaec professio [medicinae]'. A similar sentiment is put by the doctor Rabelais into the mouth of Grandgousier in *Pantagruel*, viii: 'Grecque, sans laquelle c'est honte que une personne se die sçavant': Rabelais 1973: 246.

[24] Sylvius 1539; there is also strong support for Greek studies from Englishmen at this time: see Woolfson 1998: 79, 90.

[25] According to Durling 1961: 236 and Mikkeli 1999: 25, the most influential among the newly edited texts were *De atomicis administrationibus*, *De placitis Hippocratis et Platonis* and *Ad Thrasybulum*. I would add to this list *De crisibus* and the *De causis procatarcticis*. See also Joutsivouo 1999: 26; Nutton 1987: 37–42; Mani 1956: 45–6.

dedicated to the diseases of women.[26] But Nutton points out that these editions made little impact when they first appeared in the 1520s; that translations were swiftly put in train; and that as early as the late 1530s, the necessity of knowing Greek at all was being questioned. The Basle printer Andreas Cratander recognised that few physicians had any real command of Greek, but also saw this accomplishment as superfluous, since by that time most of the Greek texts had been translated and published in Latin.[27] It is not difficult to show that the impact of most Galenic texts unknown in the fifteenth century waited on their appearance in Latin, just as the influence of the hellenistic commentators of Aristotle can be dated from a similar act of publication.[28] (An exception to this would be the *De anatomicis administrationibus* in Paris.)[29] Later in the century, Joseph Justus Scaliger (1540–1609) unmasked the poor philology even of those doctors who had produced editions; and by the beginning of the next century, Greek words were being seen as little more than Ciceronian ornaments or terms of art: a humanist knowledge of the language was no longer being required by university teachers.[30]

1.3.2 Polemic against medieval doctors and Arabs

As well as bringing with it the positive acquisitions of philology and linguistic skills, humanism marked also a polemical phase in medical studies, found in destructive criticism of Arabic and medieval medicine, of that of the ancient world itself, and of new writings on the subject. Both Arabs and scholastics were described as 'barbari';[31] the former were impugned for their style, their tendentious transmission of Galenic doctrine, and their teaching methods, which sacrificed demonstration to system.[32] Some universities, such as Florence, Tübingen and Paris, were explicit in their preference for Galen, claiming that 'there is no

---

[26] Bylebyl 1979: 340f.; Mikkeli 1999: 134.

[27] Hieronymus 1995: 96.

[28] Schmitt 1987; Nutton 1997a: 158ff.; Bylebyl 1991: 175.

[29] Siraisi 1990c: 165; O'Malley 1964.

[30] Nutton 1993b: 19 (recording Joseph Justus Scaliger's supersession of the Parisian commentaries on the Hippocratic text *On wounds in the head*); Nutton 1995: 189: 'one might argue that it was in discussion of Latin terminology, far more than any other aspect of medical theory or practice, that the influence of hellenism was felt most deeply'; Laurembergius 1621: 5.

[31] Fuchs 1530: 6r; Struthius 1602: α3; Temkin 1973: 126–7 (quoting Servetus); Kusukawa 1995b: xxxii.

[32] Siraisi 1987a: 74; they were even accused of having recourse to redundant and unreal qualities ('supervacaneas quasdam et fictitias qualitates'): Vallesius 1606: 7.

one who would not prefer to teach medicine from Galen than from Avicenna'.[33] Scholastic doctors such as Giacomo da Forlì, Ugo Benzi, Gentile da Foligno are accorded the same treatment, and the translations of Galen by medieval masters were harshly, indeed sometimes unfairly, judged.[34] But it would be wrong to stress this rejection too much. Andrea Alpago after all bothered to produce a superior edition of Avicenna which appeared in the 1520s; Leonhart Fuchs (1501–66) admits that the Arabs are 'not to be condemned and rejected wholesale'; Cardano later praised them for their empirical knowledge, which was defended also by Santorre Santori (Sanctorius) (1561–1636), and Duncan Liddel (1561–1613) appreciated their computational skills.[35] Averroes enjoyed a revival in the middle years of the century, as Charles Schmitt has shown.[36] Their works were still lectured on in major centres, just as were the major pedagogical instruments of the Middle Ages, such as the *Conciliator*.[37]

1.3.3 Polemic against ancients

At the same time, errors were being discovered not only in ancient doctors but also contemporaries. Leoniceno probably set the trend of 'error' literature, with his attack on Pliny in the 1490s; Symphorien Champier (1472–1539), Erasmus, Giovanni Manardo (1461–1536), Fuchs and Cardano soon followed in his wake.[38] The middle years of the century saw the emergence of a number of powerful critics of Galen: Argenterio, known as 'Galeni censor', who attacked not only his style, but his self-contradiction, his sloppiness as a thinker, his claims to infallibility, and the weakness of his premisses and arguments; Pereira, whose remarkably bold anti-Galenic book was hardly

---

[33] Fuchs 1537b: titlepage: 'nemo [est] qui non potius ex Galeno quam Avicenna medicinam discere velit'; Fuchs 1530; Siraisi 1997: 28; also *Novae academiae Florentinae opuscula* 1534; Brockliss and Jones 1997: 85ff. The development away from the Arabs can be seen in changes of statutes in Tübingen (Roth 1877: 300–19 (Statutes of 1497 and 1538)) and Wittenberg (Friedensburg 1926: 45–51, 173–84, 537–54 (ending with anti-Ramism)).

[34] Siraisi 1997: 48; Nutton 1993b: 19.

[35] Fuchs 1530: 5r: 'non in universum damnandos atque rejiciendos'; Siraisi 1997: 48 on 'subtle Averroes, judicious Avicenna, grave Rhasis', on whom da Monte had lectured in the 1540s; Liddel 1628: 584; Siraisi 1990b: 225 (quoting Sanctorius).

[36] Schmitt 1979.

[37] Both Cardano and Argenterio quote medieval commentaries on Galen: Siraisi 1997: 60; Argenterio 1610: 167. See also Horst 1621, and his use of the Conciliator.

[38] Towaide 2000; Durling 1961: 237–8; Manardo 1536; Fuchs 1530; Maclean 1994: 313.

referred to after its publication; Cardano again, this time as a Bologna professor.[39]

1.3.4 Polemic against contemporaries

These critics also attacked each other; Argenterio attacking Fernel and Fuchs, others attacking and defending him, traditionalists at the end of the century turning on most of these figures.[40] These polemics, some more courteous than others, are indications of the vigour of medical argument; they are evidence of the existence of a form of pre-scientific debate where the falsification of the claims of others is seen as a path to truth. The *Methodi vitandorum errorum* (1630) by Sanctorius sets up a system which not only recognises that all previous doctors have made mistakes, but is designed to provide fail-safe processes.[41] It is hardly surprising that Hippocrates, with his terse aphoristic style and his consideration of individual cases rather than grand conceptual schemes, gains in reputation as the century progresses. According to Laurence Brockliss and Colin Jones, he was seen as one of the twin pillars of medical science in Paris by the middle years of the century; Thomas Rütten has shown how important his oath in its various versions was to the profession at this time; and Vivian Nutton has indicated how his texts escape the trend towards antiquarian and philological treatment which others suffer at the end of the period.[42]

1.4 NEW DEVELOPMENTS

I come now to the innovative aspects of medicine, some of which, but not all, flow from its humanistic phase: nosology, anatomy, botany, zoology, the input from alchemy, medicine and natural magic, quantification and instrumentation. In respect of nosology (the doctrine of diseases), it is pertinent to mention the general challenge to the Galenic account of disease

---

39 Siraisi 1990a; Gallus 1590 describes Argenterio as 'Galeni censor'; Pereira 1558; Barona 1993 argues that sixteenth-century Spanish medicine was characterised by a desire to be independent of Galenism. Siraisi 1997: 58, 62. For Galen's self-professed infallibility, see *De locis affectis*, iii.4, K 8.145–6.
40 Siraisi 1990a: 178; Argenterio 1578: 1.271; Riccoboni 1598: 71ff.; Verderius 1600; Herberger 1981: 288. Occasionally these writers had the grace to admit that they had themselves erred: Siraisi 1997: 35.
41 Wear 1973; Sanctorius 1630.
42 Brockliss and Jones 1997: 94ff.; Nutton 1993b; Rütten 1996. Cardano 1663: 1.107 declares that he intended to write commentaries on all the Hippocratic texts, in part to replace those of Galen which he saw as defective: see below 6.4. A version of the oath was known in the Middle Ages, being present in the *Articella*.

posed by epidemics of one kind or another, and a particular challenge faced by the medicine of the 1490s; namely the emergence of 'the great pox'. Medical doctors had always realised that they would not necessarily encounter in their own practice every possible presentation of an illness, and would have to rely on descriptions in the literature; but the outbreak of pox caused even the notion that medical knowledge was potentially finite to be challenged, and gave added weight to the explanation of disease as a form of divine punishment.[43] It also raised the metaphysical questions of the existence of an infinite class, and the nature of specific form (see below 4.4).[44] That the new illness gave rise to unorthodox medical thinking was noted by at least one Renaissance doctor.[45]

1.4.1 The expanding field of knowledge

In a more literal way, it struck a chord with the new discovery of America, and the consequent expansion in the numbers of known plant and animal species. The medieval view that Hippocrates closed the era of discovery (the 'ordo inventionis'), which was succeeded by one of explanation (the 'ordo doctrinae' of Galen) could now be challenged, even if it was bound up not only with the limitations on what is to be known but also what could be apprehended by the human mind.[46] The view of knowledge as accumulative within a closed disciplinary framework now was replaced with one which described 'veritas' as the 'filia temporis' and was prepared to seek for truth in different disciplinary areas (such as alchemy and occult medicine), revealing a new attitude to the products of 'art' in the sense of experiment.[47] It is not clear whether these discoveries were thought to be exclusively empirical in nature, or whether and when the view also arose that a new epistemology could be used heuristically to advance

---

[43] Arrizabalaga, Henderson and French 1997; Schleiner 1995: 170ff. Other Renaissance manifestations of new disease (the English Sweating Sickness, whooping cough) are referred to by Rondelet 1586: 642–3; see also Flood forthcoming.

[44] Vallesius 1606: 256: 'species perpetuae, carentes principio et fine'; Nutton 1983: 15n.

[45] Severinus 1571: 3: 'paradoxi morbi paradoxos medicos peperere'.

[46] Crisciani 1990: 120–5; Joutsivuo 1999: 46–7; Ingegno 1988: 242 (on Pomponazzi).

[47] Crisciani 1990; Brockliss 1993: 70 (quoting Fernel); Kühlmann 1992: 105 (quoting Croll); Debus 1991: 53–7 (quoting Du Chesne); Zwinger 1606: 13 ('Paracelsus Chymiae limites transcendit'); Argenterio 1606–7: 1.5ff.; Siraisi 1990a: 178 (on the question whether it is a new method, or logic which has brought about new knowledge); Roger 1960: 11–12 (quoting Fernel); Maclean 1999a: 24–8 and Siraisi 1997: 58 (on Cardano); Emericus 1552: Q3v: 'plurima namque inveniuntur hodie, quae apud maiores nostros non fuere inventa' (with reference to Vesalius); Polydore Vergil, *De inventoribus rerum*, on which see Margolin 1994, Céard 1994 and Siraisi 1999: 346. The idea of the present surpassing the past is also a topos among artists at this time: see Cellini 1956: 12 (Vasari), 31.

knowledge.[48] New illnesses and new cures may indeed have made the 'ars longa' of medicine an expanding discipline; but this effect was overborne by the theory of idiosyncrasy which makes it a subject of infinite study (see below, 4.4).[49] By the time Francis Bacon wrote about this, it is clear that he was speaking to a generation that had become used to the idea of the advancement of learning;[50] one could look back to the middle years of the century and find a number of clairvoyant medical thinkers (da Monte, Fernel, Cardano, Fracastoro, Argenterio, Pereira), but not perhaps in such numbers or achieving such widespread acceptance in the medical community that it would be possible to argue for an earlier *prise de conscience* of this idea.[51] The practical consequence of the notion of the expansion of knowledge can be seen in syllabuses and commentaries over the course of the century, which accumulate materials and propositions without, however, on the whole eliminating any; the experience of the widening horizons of experience and scholarship seems to have been that of aggregation in universities.[52]

1.4.2 Nosology

It is pertinent to mention the major revisions in nosology; the most important name in this context is that of Fracastoro whose notion of contagion and its fortunes have been examined in two seminal articles by Nutton. This is the one context in which Lucretian atomism finds strong echoes, although it would be unwise to exaggerate the radical nature of Fracastoro's physics as opposed to his explanation of disease. This theory had repercussions later in the century for fever theory.[53] There were also important developments of theory in France: Jean Fernel in Paris with his

---

[48] Wear 1995a: 151–5, 171 (on fixity of nature's rules and her constancy, which is discussed below 7.2–3).
[49] Valleriola 1554: 289.
[50] Bacon 2000: 113.
[51] This may be because the Platonic theory of forms set a sort of plausible limit on recoverable knowledge by deriving this from innate ideas: see *Meno*, 70, and Maclean 1996: 59–62 for Montaigne's discussion of this; Maclean 1999a: 26–8 (for Cardano on the infinite); on Bruno's radical switch to an infinite number of forms, see Koyré 1958: 39–55. Siraisi 1997: 158–9 shows that Fernel was looked upon as a 'neotericus' in Padua in 1587, and a sound author in 1600, which suggests that the *prise de conscience* occurs there about 1600; see also Bruyère 1984: 153 on Fernel seen as a heretic, and Siraisi 1997: 54, 68 on Cardano described by his Pavia colleague Camuzio as a heresiarch in 1563. Gallus 1590 passes a milder judgement on Argenterio. Lonie 1981: 36 points out that Joubert's *Paradoxa* of 1566 sets out divergent doctrines without suggesting the existence of an orthodoxy.
[52] Siraisi 1987a: 221ff.; Siraisi 1997: 13–14.
[53] Nutton 1983: 30–3; Nutton 1990c; Lonie 1981.

revisionary view of substantial form and his brief discussion of 'morbus totius substantiae', which had implications for occult causes deduced from sensory data, and Laurent Joubert (1529–83) in Montpellier, who espoused a quasi-ontological account of 'affectio' (see below 7.5.5).[54]

1.4.3 Anatomy, zoology, botany

Anatomy, zoology and botany are other areas of innovation: anatomy perhaps the most celebrated of all, because of the career of Vesalius. He had his predecessors (Berengario da Carpi, Alessandro Benedetti (1452–1512) and Gabriele Zerbi (1445–1505)) from an era before the publication of Galen's *De anatomicis administrationibus*.[55] Galen was already known to have argued for the need for anatomical knowledge (in *De locis affectis*, i.1, K 8.15–18); the appearance of his treatise dedicated to the subject occasioned a revival of anatomical studies in Paris, before passing with its most famous exponent to Padua. As well as being bitterly opposed by Vesalius's erstwhile tutor, Jacques Dubois (Sylvius), it attracted some valuable early support from Argenterio and Cardano, and the subject itself was dignified by Fernel by its prominent place in his *Physiologia* and by his use of anatomy in diagnosis. The hiring by the patrons of the University of Pisa of Gabriele Falloppio or Falloppia (1523–62), Realdo Colombo (*c.* 1515–59) and other prominent anatomists in the 1540s and 1550s is another sign of its growing prestige.[56] For all this, anatomical textbooks and broadsheets do not adopt a Vesalian form of presentation, probably because they were used only as a means of locating, not of accurately depicting, organs.[57] It is now widely accepted that the nature of the subject changed towards the end of the century, and became Aristotelian in character; and that this development was in turn changed by the growing emphasis placed on autopsy.[58] The Aristotelian phase of this development can be associated with the growing interest in the Stagirite's zoological works, with their looser concept of taxonomy and heuristic procedures of investigation by analogy (see below 4.4); the

---

[54] Fernel's theory was not entirely new: see Copenhaver 1988: 284n. (giving Galenic loci); Blum 1992: 60–1; Brockliss and Jones 1997: 128–38; Siraisi 1990a: 170; Siraisi 1997: 41, 168; Richardson 1985: 175ff.; Bylebyl 1991: 166 (on Joubert).

[55] Mikkeli 1999: 149–60; Conrad, Neve, Nutton, Porter and Wear 1995: 267–8; Park 1995.

[56] Bylebyl 1979: 357; Nutton 1993d; Cunningham 1997; French 1994: 38; Siraisi 1997: 68, 94–9, 110, 142.

[57] Siraisi (forthcoming) (quoting Fernel's 'anatomy is to medicine as geography is to history'); Carlino 1994a, 1995, 1999b.

[58] Cunningham 1985, 1997; not all autopsy involved dissection in public: see Platter 1961: 88ff., 110.

investigation of fish and animals by figures such as Guillaume Rondelet (1507–66) and Conrad Gessner (1516–65) come here to mind. At a similar period, herbals and other works investigating the plant kingdom were produced, bringing considerable revision to the Dioscoridean legacy; in their wake followed botanical gardens in Tübingen, Padua and Pisa. From an early date, students were trained in simples; a consequence of this was, according to Paula Findlen, a greater appreciation of the particulars of nature.[59] The motive force behind many of these developments was however not so much natural history as medicine, through its practical concern with materia medica.

1.4.4 Alchemy and natural magic

Two other importations into medical studies from the late medieval period need to be mentioned: alchemy and natural magic. The first has the longer tradition; like medicine, it was an operative art dependent for its explanations on natural philosophy. The two arts were linked by analogies (such as that between sulphur and semen) based on function; analogies were made from medicine to alchemy and vice versa. Alchemy may have helped to raise the status of the doctor by attributing serious powers to experiment; and it may also have been one of the paths through which atomistic thought reached medical theoreticians.[60] Natural magic grew out of Renaissance neoplatonism; the image of the doctor as magus bringing about cures is found in Ficino, and reinforces the view that art is the handmaid of nature, not its pale imitator. It manipulates phenomena which are known only by their effects (such as magnetism and sympathy);[61] it brings together thereby the practical and the mysterious. Its combination of sublime speculative theorising with deduction and hypothesis is not easy to comprehend from a modern perspective; the apparent sterility of its theories of correspondence of plants, zodiacal signs, planets and illnesses, of signatures, and more generally of the macrocosm and the microcosm has to be seen in the context of its ability to offer satisfying explanations of the spiritual dimension of life, which, it is argued, must have a divine origin, and of the occult powers at work in

---

[59] Reeds 1991; Findlen 1994; Joutsivuo 1999: 29; Grafton and Siraisi 1999. In spite of Tübingen's precedence in time, it seems that the most influential model for a university botanical garden was Padua; Luyendijk-Elshout 1991: 344, 353. See also Schmitt 1972, 1974.

[60] Crisciani 1996a: 13 (her term is 'instrumental analogy'); Newman 1996.

[61] Copenhaver 1988: 264 (quoting Agrippa); see also Rice 1976; Goldammer 1991: 19–58.

nature (see below 8.8.6).[62] Signatures are also linked to the natural signs of the world (seen in hands, faces, foreheads) and are the subject matter of the conjectural arts of chiromancy, physiognomy and metoposcopy which were much discussed in the sixteenth century (see below 8.8).

1.4.5 Paracelsus and Paracelsianism

Mention of alchemy and natural magic evokes the name of Paracelsus (1493?–1541); but he represents more than just these. He was at once a radical empiric who argues that doctors should not engage in prognosis and can only effect cures through reliance on their own experience of nature, a mechanical and an alchemist who supplanted Galen with these skills and sketched both an ontological account of disease and the first treatise on occupational illness, and an astrologer and a popular theologian rejecting sterile rationalism, whose perception of the doctor's role and of nature itself was in large part derived from the Bible: a fact recognised in his own time, if forgotten by some of his later emulators. He writes in the vernacular, and his style is more homiletic than expository; there are few examples of sustained argument, and even the three principles (sulphur, salt and mercury) can only be extracted with some difficulty from his works.[63] His impact dates from his translation into Latin and publication by Adam von Bodenstein (1528–77), Gerhard Dorn and others in the 1560s and 1570s; this was accompanied by explanation, lexica (which Paracelsus, as a proponent of the 'claritas verborum', would have not seen as necessary) and assimilation into the very discourses – Galenism and Aristotelianism – which he had rejected by Petrus Severinus (1542–1602), Dorn, Joseph du Chesne (Quercetanus) (1544?–1609), Johannes Albertus and their like, some of whom associate him with Hippocrates.[64] This wave of publication is

---

[62] Arber 1986: 247–63; Copenhaver 1988: 274–5 (on Ficino); *ibid.*, 264; Bianchi 1987; Kühlmann 1992: 114–17 (on Agrippa's views on signatures and spiritual elements); see also Fernel 1610a: 70 (on divine origin of occult properties); du Chesne 1609; Blum 1992: 59; Henry 1997: 48–55. On the mixture of personal and impersonal elements in magical thought, see Pittion 1987: 124 (quoting Mauss).

[63] Webster 1995: 407; Webster 1998: 68; Gallus 1590; Siraisi 1997: 15. Copenhaver and Schmitt 1992: 306–7 (on the three principles).

[64] Severinus 1571: 30ff. (a new definition of medicine, followed by the use of words such as 'facultates', 'symptomata', 'semina' with new meanings and by an adapted employment of the opposition act/potency); Albertus 1615: C7ff. (on consistency of Paracelsianism with 'rationes scientificae' and 'experientia'; Crusius 1615: 188, on Paracelsus being known indirectly through commentators, and on the clarity of his text ('quando enim Paracelsi mens non satis percipitur id non fit

accompanied predictably enough by some more forthright denunciations of his claims to medical knowledge. It seems that the only universities which actually adopted his teachings did so through pressure from outside their medical faculties; Paracelsianism was stronger in courts than in academe.[65] The most sustained consideration of the competing claims of his and Galenic medicine is to be found at the very end of our period in the writings of Daniel Sennert (1572–1637); it coincides with his rejection further south in Europe.[66]

1.4.6 Quantification, mathematics, instrumentation and astrology

A last aspect of innovation to be mentioned is the rise of mathematics, instrumentation and the ongoing debates about the influence of the superlunary world on health. As has been said, there are several attempts at a mathematical approach to quantification in the late fifteenth century: these are taken further after 1560 both in respect to dosology and humoral theory (see below 5.2). Their expression seems closer to the debates about practical medicine (e.g. the debate about the best site for bloodletting) than to theoretical issues.[67] The issue of astrology is debated mainly in respect of its relation to the Platonic doctrine of the continuity of the superlunary and sublunary worlds: this doctrine, which is supported by apparently forward-looking doctors such as Cardano and Fernel on the authority of the Galenic tract *De diebus decretoriis*, attracts an

---

ob vocabulorum obscuritatem sed legentis inhabilitatem'). Also Guinther von Andernach 1571; Dorn 1584; Aubéry 1585: 53–4 (who tries to use Fernel as a bridge between Galen and Paracelsus); Aubéry 1585: 16ff. (for an attempt at the conciliation of Paracelsianism and Galenism through a parallel of the principles salt, sulphur and mercury with indications 'ex morbo ipso, ex corporis temperamento, and ex ambiente aere'); Zwinger 1606; Du Chesne 1609; Zanier 1983: 100 (quoting Sennert): 'Petrum Severinum qui dogmata hinc inde disiecta in artis formam redigere conatus est, potius quam ipsum Paracelsum sequuntur. Hinc hodie nova quasi secta nata est, quae severiana dici potest'; Debus 1991; Conrad, Neve, Nutton, Porter and Wear 1995: 319; Flood and Kelly 1995: 104.

[65] Zwinger 1606; Erfurt, Copenhagen and Marburg were the three universities which for varying amounts of time permitted the teaching of Paracelsian doctrine: see Grell 1993; Zanier 1983: 110. On Paris, see Debus 1991 and Brockliss and Jones 1997: 119–28. Pumfrey 1998: 51 points out that 'frequently Protestant courts concerned about inter-confessional tensions, often patronized Paracelsian studies as part of the late sixteenth- and early seventeenth-century trend of promoting reformed, unifying, spiritual philosophies. When they failed . . . the trend was abandoned.'

[66] Sennert 1650: 3.699–862; Bartolettus 1619. See also Palmer 1985 and Zanier 1985, on the uptake of certain remedies as opposed to theories in parts of Italy.

[67] Bylebyl 1991: 157 (on the debate about phlebotomy). Wear 1973: 166 argues against the truly quantitative character of these discussions.

increasing number of opponents as the century progresses.[68] The issues of mathematics and astrology are linked not only because 'mathematici' can designate adherents of either science, but also because of the computational aspect of the Ptolemaic corpus, which Cardano claims is in itself a separate and coherent mode of dialectic.[69] Instrumentation is a feature of the very end of our period, and is most properly associated with the name of Sanctorius, who not only developed a primitive thermometer and pulsilogium, but also a weighing device to measure insensible respiration.[70]

1.5 MEDICINE IN THE UNIVERSITIES

1.5.1 The content of courses

I come now to the history of teaching of medicine over the sixteenth century. A strong claim is generally made for the continuity of the subject, seen in its curricula, textbooks, pedagogical methods, and, often, subjects of debate.[71] While it is possible to identify a 'long list' of Hippocratic and Galenic texts which were taught in a certain order from the Alexandrian period onwards, in fact the dominant texts were the first parts of Avicenna's *Canon*, Galen's *Ars parva* and Hippocrates's *Aphorisms* and *Prognosis*.[72] As Siraisi has shown, the importance of the first cannot be underestimated: the Galenic anthology of the middle of the century was calqued on the order of *Canon*, i.1.[73] The twofold division of theoria and practica which was popular at the beginning of the century gave way to the five- (or sometimes three-) fold division into physiology, pathology, therapy, hygiene (in this case, the doctrine of the conservation of health), and semiotic or semiology (in Heidelberg the last two were subsumed into the first three): this was popularised by da Monte in the 1541–2 Latin edition of Galen, where it is set out in the *Introductio seu*

---

[68] Siraisi 1990a: 165; Siraisi 1997: 119, 158–9; Grafton and Siraisi forthcoming; Wear 1981: 243–50; Nutton 1990b: 207 (on Fracastoro's opposition to this tract); also Liddel 1624: 600: 'nonnulli ad praedictiones astrologicas confugiunt, et indicia temporis mortis, ex remotioribus causis, astris nimirum sumunt, quae medicae considerationis non sunt'. See also 3.6.2, and 8.6.3.

[69] Cardano 1663: 11.307.

[70] Sanctorius 1642 (first edition 1614).

[71] Siraisi 1987a: 16.

[72] Nutton 1993c; Bylebyl 1979: 339; Durling 1961.

[73] Siraisi 1987a: 167.

medicus, and is the foundation of the 'ausserordentlich stabiles Gebilde' in Germany and elsewhere at the end of the century. [74]

Of course, variations and developments can be detected as well. Universities differed very greatly in the size of their medical intake; Padua and Bologna being the largest Italian faculties, with the greatest power to attract foreign students.[75] They usually paid most to the holders of the senior theoretical chairs, the next highest sums to ordinarii of practica, and the least to anatomy and botany, in spite of the fact that by the end of the century, at least, it is the teaching in practica, anatomy and botany which constitutes the greatest attraction for foreign students.[76] Pisa seems to have spent most on hiring famous teachers from other institutions; Padua, which of all universities had the strongest teachers in logic and in natural philosophy, also led the movement to 'render medicine independent of philosophy and thus make it an autonomous discipline', in the words of Mugnai Carrara; it is also unique in denying its senior chairs to locally born candidates.[77] Salamanca insisted on four rather than three years of study; Montpellier is unusual in having no arts faculty to serve its propedeutic needs. This may account for the long tradition there of practical medicine which does not lay great stress on the logical basis of medical precepts, whereas in Italy the prominent role of logic in the arts faculties may have predisposed professors in the medical faculty to seek more actively for an accommodation of their discipline with Aristotle's Organon.[78] Italy as a whole did not have theological faculties (although teaching in metaphysics and theology was available), allowing one scholar to refer to '[its] free air unsullied by clericalism and authoritarianism', whereas in Germany, the natural philosophy of Philip Melanchthon (1497–1560) with its specifically Christian impregnation was adopted in several prominent universities.[79]

---

[74] Siraisi 1987a: 98ff., 221ff.; Herberger 1981: 246, 301–2 (on Helmstedt); Eckart 1992: 139 (here quoted); Nutton 1981: 173 (on the Galenic canon). A related issue is the revision of the natural philosophy course, on which see Schmitt 1985: 1–5.

[75] Nauck 1954.

[76] Bylebyl 1979: 365.

[77] Mugnai Carrara 1999: 253 (where Manardo's role is stressed in this movement); Lines forthcoming demonstrates that this claim needs severe qualification.

[78] McVaugh 1990; Siraisi 1990b. I am grateful to R. G. Lewis for this point, which will no doubt be treated at greater length in her forthcoming study of Montpellier.

[79] Schmitt 1969: 127 (on the 'free air' of Padua); Ottosson 1984: 14; Siraisi 1997: 100; Luyendijk-Elshout 1991; Castro 1614: 197 (on Salamanca); Bylebyl 1979: 338; Schmitt 1972, 1974; Koch 1998; Kusukawa 1995a. Some theology was taught at Padua: see Schmitt 1978, Jardine 1997: 189. Nancy Siraisi has kindly pointed out to me that the University of Bologna seems to be marked by a quite strong presence of censorship, and that the 'freedom from clericalism' may not apply everywhere, nor at all times, in Northern Italy.

In terms of course content, a similar range of variations may be noted: after 1538, Arabic medicine was relegated to second place at Tübingen; Pisa, where Avicenna was not taught at all, was dedicated to reconciling Aristotle and Plato, and this policy spills over into natural philosophy and medicine; Bologna saw Cardano lecturing on some unconventional Hippocratic texts in the 1560s; Celsus seems to be taught nowhere else than Louvain;[80] Padua, which did not teach the otherwise popular Hippocratic *Prognosis*, is famous for its precepting;[81] Basle evinces a bias towards practical medicine, even in its disputations on theoria; some universities (Freiburg, Ingolstadt) banned the use of modern textbooks, 'compendia, epitomae, brevarii, synopses, institutiones'.[82] But this variation is not great enough to threaten the community of disciplinary discourse, or make *peregrinatio medica* an incoherent exercise.

Most studies of learned medicine in this period rightly stress the primordial role of Northern Italy, and especially Padua: it was the first place to introduce clinical precepting, and is often seen as the cradle of the new anatomy and botany as well.[83] It is also widely assumed that Basle played a leading role. These assumptions need qualification. The importance of Florence/Pisa and Paris in the attack on Arabic medicine in the 1530s, and the earlier development of anatomy at Paris and botany at Tübingen reveal that Padua was jealous of its reputation and sensitive to challenges from elsewhere, causing it promptly to adopt the innovations of other universities, in which it was aided by the policy of reserving the most senior medical professorships to those born outside the Veneto. Basle on the other hand was a tiny faculty with very few students until the last quarter of the century, when it benefited from the peregrinations of Calvinists and Philippists from Germany; its fame rests on its publishing industry and Paracelsus's brief and stormy passage through town and university in 1527–8. In the field of medicine most relevant to this study (semiology), Padua in fact reflects one of the most conservative approaches: da Monte based his lectures on this subject on Avicenna's *Canon*, i.2, and this model

---

80 But 'flosculi medicinales ex Celso' appear in the *Articella*: Arrizabalaga 1998: 28.
81 O'Malley 1970: 95 points out that clinical teaching must have begun before Giambattista da Monte, although its introduction is usually attributed to him; it was widely copied by the end of the century; it is part of Lange's ideal university, on which see Nutton 1985a: 95–6 See also Ongaro 1994 and Linden 1999: 23 (on Zerbi and precepting).
82 O'Malley 1970: 101; Mikkeli 1999: 38; Joutsivuo 1999: 22; Siraisi 1997; Siraisi 1990a: 163–6; Schmitt 1972, 1974, 1976b; Bylebyl 1979: 339; Bylebyl 1991: 186; Husner 1942 (on Basle theses).
83 Woolfson 1998; Italian medicine had its detractors also: e.g. Thriverus in Laurembergius 1621: *4v (his remarks are directed also against Spain). The awareness of Italian doctors of their high status is reflected in the celebration of doctors in histories of cities and of famous doctors; see below 3.7.

persists throughout the century in the newly established lectureship first
filled by Antonio Negri in 1551, and in the writings of Girolamo Capo di
Vacca (Capivaccius) (1523–89) and Emilio Campolongo or Campilongo
(1550–1604).[84] Elsewhere, new distributions of the subject were made
directly from the republished Galenic texts first by a certain Stephanus
Dutemplaeus or Dutemple in Lyon, then, a few years later, separately by
Jacques Dubois (Sylvius) in Paris and Leonhart Fuchs in Tübingen (see
below 8.1). A picture of the teaching in this area at Basle, which is more
closely allied to practica than elsewhere, can be gained from Johannes
Nicolaus Stupanus's (1541–1621) systematic coverage of the subject by
disputations between 1607 and 1612.[85] An important revisionary figure
is Argenterio, who offers a more systematic redistribution of Galen in
his lectures in Pisa which were published in the 1550s, and who attracted disciples.[86] The attention paid to this part of medicine is clearly
connected to the reassessment of the relationship between practica and
theoria to the benefit of the former.[87]

1.5.2 Networks and disciples

In mentioning disciples, I have raised the question of networks and proso-
pographical links; these have a very important role to play in medical studies, linking the court, the town and the university in various
countries. There are local circuits, such as that at Naples recorded in
Joannes Donatus Santorus's correspondence at the end of the century,
the earlier, smaller, English network at evidence in David Edwardes's
book on signs, the later range of epistolary contacts evinced by
Sigismund Schnitzer in the *Cista medica* of 1626, the group of Parisian and
Montpellier Paracelsians investigated by Allen Debus. Johannes Crato
von Krafftheim's (1519–85) circle and its continuation through Lorenz
Scholze (1552–99), and Johannes Jessenius's (1566–1621) contacts seem

---

[84] Siraisi 1987a: 27–79, 346–8; Facciolatus 1757: 2, 383ff. At the same time, in anatomy and especially
natural philosophy and zoology, Padua has a less Galenist hue: Wear 1981 and Cunningham 1997.

[85] These disputations cover in turn the status and principles of the discipline, the principles of
physiology, pathology (on causes, symptoms and diseases), general semiology (the five sources of
diagnostic signs) and particular semiology (from the head to the genitalia), which is usually seen
as a part of practica: Stupanus 1614. Galen's own recommendations for the study of semiology are
set out in his *Ars parva*, and include *inter alia De locis affectis*, the four treatises on the pulse, and *De
causis procatarcticis*, as well as the texts on diseases, symptoms and pulse which were dichotomised
by Fuchs and Sylvius. Galen also recommends Hippocrates's *Aphorisms*: Bylebyl 1991: 185.

[86] For new translations of Galen, see Durling 1961; Baudrier 1895–1921; Fuchs 1537a; Sylvius 1539;
Siraisi 1990a: 169–70 (a full comparison of Argenterio's chapters and Galen's texts); Le Thielleux
1581; and Jessenius's preface in Campilongo 1601:)(1. Later an attempt at distributing the
Paracelsian doctrine of signs was made by Fabricius 1626.

[87] See Alessandrini in Siraisi 1990a: 179 for an early manifestation of this reassessment.

to be more international, perhaps because these scholars felt themselves more isolated at the Eastern end of Europe.[88] There seems also to be some extension of the influence of Spain by such contacts: Bologna and Salamanca are said to be in close contact; there is a stream of Spanish professors in Toulouse who are taken up into French medical circles; and Franciscus Emericus even records that it was a 'hispanus quidam' who brought the news of Vesalian anatomy to Vienna.[89] *Peregrinatio medica* also linked various centres: Tübingen and Leiden with Padua, Altdorf and Basle; the most energetic travellers include Montpellier, Pisa, Paris, Vienna and Bologna in their wanderings, often staying with the most prestigious professors in each place.[90] It cannot however be contested that Italian universities, and especially Padua, were the most important of all academic centres to be visited, as the Italians themselves were proud to stress.[91] The implications of this for pedagogy are considerable: it is in no small part due to this influence that university medicine achieved its quasi-homogeneous state in the early years of the seventeenth century.

1.6 THE STATE OF MEDICINE IN 1630

One way to gauge this state is to look at the judgements of doctors of the time about the leaders of their profession: this can be inclusive of the past (thus Albertus praises the 'solida brevitas' of Hippocrates, the 'subtilitas' of Aristotle, the 'labor immensus' of Galen, the 'dexteritas' of Vesalius,

---

[88] Scholze 1598b; Nutton 1990b: 224; Campilongo 1601:)(5v; Capivaccius 1606: A2r (both Jessenius); Schmitt 1977.

[89] Santorus 1597; Edwardes 1532; Hornung 1626; Debus 1991; Schleiner 1995: 61; Pittion 1987: 121–2; Emericus 1552: Q3v. Crusius 1615:)(4v recommends a mixed set of Galenists and Paracelsians, from Basle and various parts of Germany; see also Kühlmann 1992: 110.

[90] For the influence of Italians, see Pittion 1987: 122ff. Struthius 1602: α2v (on the connection between Capivaccius and Bauhin); Luydendijk-Elshout 1991: 347–50 (Mercuriale, Colombo, Fernel, Falloppia, and Gessner); *ibid.*, 340–4 (Forest, Pauw, Heurnius and Vorstius in Padua); Zwinger 1606:)( )( )(1ff. (on the connections of Libavius); Joutsivuo 1999: 161. A model case of peregrination (motivated by the desire to see for himself) is afforded by Gryllus 1566, who seems to have gone to all famous centres except those in Switzerland; see also Platter 1961 and Grell 1993: 90 (on Caspar Bartholin). Three typical examples (of whom only one is famous) are Leonhard Rauhoff (1535–96), who visited Tübingen, Wittenberg, Montpellier and Padua; Oswald Gäbelchofer (1539–1616), who went to Tübingen, Padua and Bologna; and Caspar Bauhin, who went to Basle, Padua, Bologna, Montpellier, Paris and Tübingen before taking up a chair where he began; see Fichtner 1972–3. The practice of *peregrinatio medica* was so common by the end of the seventeenth century that the Danish doctor Thomas Bartholin devoted a book to it, in which he claimed that any doctor in a position of authority simply had to have had training abroad ('nostro saeculo tanta peregrinationis utilitas ad Medicum redundare videtur, ut Medici autoritatem tueri nemo possit, qui extra patriam vestigia non protulit': Bartholin 1674: 9).

[91] Siraisi 1997: 137; Riccoboni 1598. There is local pride in other centres: e.g. Milan, with which Silvaticus associates the names of Pietro d'Abano, Cardano, Lacuna and Vallesius (not all were natives): 1601: A2r.

the 'iudicium singulare' of Cardano, the 'labores' of Rondelet);[92] or it can merely mention the most recent, as does Bartolettus of Bologna in his predominantly Italian list; or it can be more international in character, as is Petrus Laurembergius's (1585–1639) selection, intended for Leiden students; he includes Liddel, Caspar Bauhin (1560–1624), André du Laurens (1558–1609), Franciscus Valleriola (1504–80), Jean Riolan the Elder (1538–1605) and Fuchs.[93] These lists very often reflect the availability and currency of broad teaching manuals, although it would be unwise to assume that these replaced completely earlier forms of textbook and commentary.[94] The names cited above all accept the new botany and the new anatomy, and with it an increasingly empirical and descriptive approach; most have adapted or rejected scholastic methods of teaching and pay more attention to the particularity of cases; most have absorbed the input of medical humanism, and most give greater weight than was hitherto the case to practical studies in environments such as the anatomy theatre which enhanced the dignity of such studies.[95] There is a distinction to be made between those who follow Aristotle and those who follow Galen, but this is, according to Temkin, a crude antithesis by 1600.[96] The most advanced form of synthesis, indeed the last of its kind to be written, is that of Daniel Sennert, who in the late 1610s attempts to reconcile a version of Paracelsianism with Galenic medicine. His essays on natural principles, occult qualities, atoms and procreation are however sharply attacked by Freitag as early as 1650.[97] More orthodox Galenic medicine goes on being taught at Padua into the eighteenth century, but the advent of mechanical philosophy, the advances in iatrochemistry and a range of empirical advances all take their toll on the credibility of the subject. I do not believe however that this is already the case in 1630: there still seems to me then to be a coherent body of doctrine, with appropriate metaphysical and epistemological

---

[92] Albertus 1615: B7v; he also mentions Georg Agricola and Gessner.

[93] Bartolettus 1619; Laurembergius 1621. Crusius 1615 classifies his near-contemporaries as 'clarissimi' (Platter, Bauhin and Hartmann), 'mediocres' (Brendel, Horst and Sennert) and 'obscuri'. The common bias towards one's own teachers is here very clear. See also Gallus 1590, Schenck 1609b; Horst 1574: 6r–7v, and such indicators as the Bodley catalogue. A specialist list of anatomists is given by Sennert: see Wear 1973: 289.

[94] Siraisi 1987a: 116.

[95] Siraisi 1990a: 162; Siraisi 1997: 15 (where four important advances in medical science are identified); but on the anatomical theatre as not necessarily progressive, see Ferrari 1976 and Rupp 1990.

[96] Temkin 1973: 150; Wear 1981 argues much the same case (that both Aristotelians and Galenists are traditionalists); but see Cunningham 1985, 1997.

[97] Eckart 1992: 141–3.

underpinning, which had evolved over the course of the preceding
100 years away from theory and towards practice, and still offered coherence and explanatory force to justify its existence.[98] Whether it possessed
the 'attractive complexity' which had endeared it to the thirteenth and
fourteenth centuries according to García Ballester is debatable; but it
does not in my mind deserve the harsh epithets of 'sterile' and 'threadbare' which have recently been attributed to it.[99]

---

[98] For a survey undertaken in 1628 by Caspar Bartholin in his *De studio medico*, see Grell 1993: 94–5.
[99] García Ballester 1993b: 39; Siraisi 1987a: 349; O'Malley 1970: 101.

CHAPTER 2

The transmission of medical knowledge

2.I INTRODUCTION

This book deals with the field of medical learning in the period 1500 to 1630 in Europe; it is pertinent therefore to ask whether its principal modes of transmission affect in any way the evolution of that field over this period. I shall offer here an ideal-typical description of these modes of transmission, which is intended to serve as a heuristic device by which to recognise the most important features of the field, even if it will not be able to account completely for each individual event. It is informed by the following questions: into what broad periods does medical publication fall in the late Renaissance? What relation is there between the publication of books, the diffusion of learning, and the various networks of the republic of letters of the time? How international, or local, was the market for learned medical books? How was the market sustained, what drove it, and under what controls did it operate? Was the medical book market seen to be an entity, and if so, how was it related to other parts of the learned book market? Who paid to produce medical books, saw to it that they were distributed, and what interests were they serving? How quickly did fashions, with respect to both content and presentation, change in the world of medical books? Did the operation of the market over time bring about a unification of medical knowledge? How did scholars get access to the books they cite in their manuals and monographs, and how did they classify them? Accordingly, I shall first attempt to break down the period into meaningful sections; then look in turn at transmission of medical knowledge in general, the authorship of medical and related books (2.2), the role of the book fairs and of active publishers and other agents (2.3), format and genre, illustrations and diagrams (2.4), and the organisation of the field of medical knowledge in real and ideal libraries (2.5). I shall attempt in a conclusion to suggest in what ways the transmission or mediation of medical knowledge affects its content.[1]

2.1.1 Periodisation

I cautiously propose the following tripartite division of the period under discussion, which is consonant with that sketched out in chapter 1; first, the period before 1525, in which year the Aldine Galen in Greek was published. In this period, as Osler's bibliography of medical incunabula to 1480 shows, many of the features of later medical publication already appear: these include standard medical authors and textbooks (Avicenna, the *Articella*,[2] Pietro d'Abano's *Conciliator*, lexica, including Latin–German lexica); some works of practical medicine by medieval authors; some popular works on regimen and plague. The vast majority of this material was published in Italy; it is predominantly produced in folio, perhaps reflecting the size of the manuscripts which it gradually came to replace; much of it came from one source, the presses of Ottaviano Scoto and later his heirs.[3] It seems however that various humanist attempts to publish the standard Greek texts of medicine (including Callierges and Vlastos's Galen edition of 1500) failed, and that even the publication in 1478 of Celsus, whose *De medicina* is one of the most elegant and lucid pieces of writing on this topic, seems not to have had a very great pedagogical impact.[4] There are several indications of unsatisfactory book distribution outside Italy at the end of this period.[5]

The second period would run from 1525 to 1565, during which Galen, Hippocrates and other classical texts were published in Greek and translated into Latin; the main genres of the medical book market

---

[1] Maclean 2000a is an earlier version of this chapter.

[2] See Arrizabalaga 1998, in which he lists the contents of the *Articella*, shows the relationship to the different editors and markets (Montpellier and Pavia), and accounts for the text's decline through the rise of medical hellenism, anatomical studies, the reformist programmes in medical schools and the competition of other medical compilations and manuals.

[3] Osler 1923; Arrizabalaga 1998: 4n. The collection of tracts in Jesus College, Oxford, Library shelfmark R 9.9 Gal bears witness to the close involvement of Ottaviano Scoto of Venice in early medical and scientific publication. On Osler's evidence, about twice as many folio books were produced as 4to up to 1480; and very few 8vos at all. On book production and financing at this time see Mardersteig 1967.

[4] Celsus's work appeared in florilegium form in part in the *Articella*, and was published fairly frequently, but does not seem to have been influential in pedagogical contexts.

[5] Nutton: 1993c cites the complaint of Leonhart Schmaus of Salzburg in 1519 that he could only get access to books if his friends from Vienna or Augsburg sent them to him. See also Nutton 1987: 27–8; Nutton 1993b: 20–3; and Andrea Alciati's letter to Bonifatius Amerbach of 1543 reproduced in Flood and Shaw 1997: 190–1.

emerged and became stable; new trends in publication, including studies of new diseases, divination, astrology and alchemy, had been absorbed into the subject area; and methods of diffusion and protection of books were regularised.[6] The final period would run from 1565 to 1625, and would mark the heyday of the Frankfurt Book Fair.[7] This rough division accommodates quite well the emergence of Paracelsianism around 1565, through the efforts of Adam von Bodenstein and others, who saw to the publication in a decade of some eighty books of Paracelsus's writings, thirty of them in Latin;[8] the conclusion of the Council of Trent (1563), and the development from 1561 onwards of the Catholic Indices of forbidden books;[9] the dominance of a number of entrepreneurial humanist printer-publishers specialising in medical literature: Guillaume Rouillé of Lyon, Heinrich Petri and his heirs of Basle, Pietro Perna and Konrad Waldkirch, also of Basle; the Giunti in Lyon and Venice, and Paolo and Roberto Meietti in Venice and Padua; André Wechel, his heirs in Frankfurt and Hanau, and the presses which are associated with his name although independent of him (Johann Wechel and Zacharias Palthen); even perhaps Jacques Chouet of Geneva, who specialised in reprinting.[10] By 1565 also, the most important scholarly apparatus of medicine – Latin translations of Galen and Hippocrates, post-Dioscoridean herbals, Brasavola's index to Galen and other similar intellectual tools – were generally available. So also were better editions of the prominent Arab authors and systematisers; these continue to be read, in spite of widespread criticism of them.[11] 1625 saw not only the apogee (in terms of the number of titles advertised) of the book fair, but publication of the ninth and last Giunti edition of Galen's complete works in Latin which had first appeared in 1541–2. Between 1590 and 1625, as a sign of the consolidation of the subject, at least three specialist bibliographies of medical writing were published, which owed much to the pioneering work on general bibliography undertaken by Conrad

---

[6] Siraisi 1997: 15; for a general account of the trade at this time, see Kapp 1886.
[7] This periodisation fits well with that offered by Durling 1961, 242.
[8] See Sudhoff 1894.
[9] See Putnam 1906–7. The dates he records of the introduction of Indices are as follows: Bavaria 1561, Rome 1566, Antwerp 1569, Parma 1580, Lisbon 1581, Madrid 1583, Toledo 1584, Naples 1588; the published Roman Index first appeared in 1590.
[10] These names emerge from an analysis of the holdings of a major library such as the Herzog-August Bibliothek Wolfenbüttel. See also Evans 1975 (on the Wechel presses); Hieronymus 1995; Hieronymus 1997 (for the medical publications of Heinrich Petri); Pettas 1997 (on the Giunti).
[11] Siraisi 1987a: 361–6, and Schmitt 1979.

Gessner and his successors.[12] The end of the period is marked by the collapse of the Frankfurt market, due in large part to the effects of the Thirty Years War, which impinged directly on Frankfurt in 1631. There were however other significant factors, both intrinsic to and extrinsic to the book trade. I have argued elsewhere that even if the war had not come to Frankfurt in that year, the market, which after 1631 declined by more than half in numbers of declared books in the learned disciplines, would have collapsed anyway, because of market saturation and legal, institutional and economic factors intrinsic to its operation.[13] This decline coincides with certain other occurrences in Europe which reduce the free exchange of books and people, such as the North Italian plague outbreak and the economic crisis in France.[14]

2.1.2 Language

There are three language categories in which nearly all medical books were written: Greek; Latin; and the various vernaculars. In respect to the first, the appearance of Galen, Hippocrates, Aetius and Paul of Aegina in the 1520s had the same effect as the Aldine of Aristotle of 1495, in respect of stimulating new translations and commentaries;[15] it even caused new plain texts to be produced, such as that which François Rabelais produced in 1532 of several shorter works by Galen and Hippocrates.[16] But the points made above about the nature of medical hellenism (1.3.1) have also to be borne in mind; as with Aristotle, the full impact of new texts and new ancient commentaries is felt only after their translation into Latin (which in the case of Galen is apparently the subject of a competitive race).[17]

In respect of Latin, it remains universally true that a writer in the vernacular, such as Paracelsus, had to be translated into this language to achieve an international readership, no matter what the author in question might have thought of such a procedure; this even happens

---

[12] Gallus 1590; Spachius 1591; Schenck 1609b. Under the rubric 'medicinae scriptores', Draut 1625a: 941 also names the continuator of Conrad Gessner's *Bibliotheca universalis* of 1545, Michael Neander, 'in bibl. sua universali, quam Grammaticae Graece suae praefationis loco praefixit, medicinae scriptores extantes et latitantes: Impressi, et M.S, Veteres luculenter recenset', Basle, 1565.

[13] Maclean 1991.

[14] Biraben 1975–6; Chaunu and Gascon 1977: 329–35; Le Roy Ladurie and Morineau 1977: 727–818.

[15] Nutton 1987, 1993b, 1997a, 1990b: 207 (on Aetius); Durling 1961.

[16] Durling 1961.

[17] Between the Italian and N European translators: see Nutton 1987.

late in the century, in the case of surgical works by Ambroise Paré and others.[18] Vernacular medical writing offers a somewhat different picture. Vivian Nutton has suggested that this is more likely to treat of drugs, surgery, practical remedies and astrology, but my own sampling indicates that there is a very great difference between vernaculars in this respect, and that Germany, France, Italy, England and Spain have very different readerships in the vernacular at this time. A cursory glance at the vernacular entries in Draut's *Bibliotheca classica* of 1625 shows that regimen books on plague and syphilis are common to all vernaculars;[19] but also that there are clear differences between the vernacular output of the first three countries. The French entry is by far the largest for the period 1565 to 1625, and reflects not only the aspirations of surgeons to acquire the arts course training of university doctors through vernacular guides to dialectics,[20] but also the receptive market for occult writing, astrology and the conjectural arts (best exemplified through the work of Antoine Mizauld (1520–78)), as well as books on midwifery and female ailments and the continuing French tradition of vernacular guides to surgery, including popular guides to phlebotomy. Connected with these publications is a specifically protestant project, that of making available the higher disciplines and new philosophy to those unable to read Latin: evidence of this is to be found in the works of Philippe Canaye (1551–1610) and Claude Aubéry (d. 1596) and, in the sphere of medicine, in Abraham de la Framboisière's (1559–1634) *Les Loix de la medecine* (1608), a book that he had already published in Latin thirteen years before under the title *Canones medicinales*. These acts of publication are also connected, as Richard Durling and Natalie Zemon Davis have shown, with the issue of trade or guild secrets and control: vernacular publishing acted as a means of regulation of surgeons and lay healers.[21] Although they were mainly printed in 8vo, one or two works were produced in folio,

---

[18] Ambroise Paré was attacked by the Medical Faculty of Paris for publishing in French: see Keynes 1968: xix; on Bernard Palissy's rejection of Latin in favour of the vernacular, see Daston and Park 1998: 217–21, who also make the point that as texts are produced at this time in both Latin and the vernacular, it is not a question of passive reception of Latin works into the vernacular.

[19] Gallus 1590 lists them separately.

[20] E.g. Eusèbe 1566; see also Brockliss and Jones 1997: 99–104, who claim that publication of surgical and other medical treatises in the vernacular from the mid-sixteenth century onwards is aimed both at surgeons and apothecaries and at the general public. But see the following footnote for evidence of earlier French-language publication.

[21] Draut 1625b: 64–74; Mizauld 1572: FI–4 advertised his own books in both Latin and French, including those forthcoming; Maittaire 1722: 421–37 (Chrétien Wechel's catalogue of 1544, with French-language books on phlebotomy and surgery); Durling 1961: 240–1; Davis 1975: 222–5, 258–67.

including the translation of André du Laurens's book of anatomy in 1621. The German vernacular medical book at this time also dealt with children's illnesses, pharmacopoeia and herbals: its authors even cited unlettered pharmacists as sources. In this respect, it is worth remembering that fourteenth-century vernacular sources in this field had been seen as being more advanced than their Latin counterparts which had borrowed freely from them.[22] German herbals are among the most lavish productions of their age, and are clearly produced more with the court than the university in mind.[23] Works of an innovative kind on therapy and astrology mark the English vernacular tradition in the sixteenth century; and Josep Lluís Barona has noted that in Spain (at least until the measures taken in 1558–9 to control the dissemination of ideas) vernacular medical writing seems to be more anti-authoritarian in nature than it is in Italy at the same period.[24]

2.2 MODES OF DIFFUSION

Medical knowledge was disseminated in a number of ways, and falls into various classes. First, there is knowledge not widely diffused, and not published (this is the category of local beliefs and practices, transmitted orally or by manuscript; this category, although much praised by Paracelsus, is not relevant to this investigation); second, there is knowledge initially unpublished but widely diffused, and often made more widely known through correspondence in the world of letters and students returning from foreign universities; third, there is knowledge published in book form but not widely diffused (e.g. books produced for local consumption in given universities, or markets such as Spain, England, and certain small German printing centres); fourth, there is the knowledge published and more widely diffused, through such offices as the Frankfurt Book Fair, which is the main focus of this study. The last alone affords the chance of sketching an ideal type of transmission.

[22] Keil 2000.

[23] Arber 1986; Reeds 1991; a survey of the entries under the various languages in Draut 1625a which contains, with other materials, most of the books declared at the Frankfurt Book Fair between 1564 and 1624 suggests that there is a very great difference in the nature of medical publication in the various vernaculars. It remains universally true, however, that a writer in the vernacular, such as Paracelsus or Ambroise Paré, had to be translated into Latin to achieve an international readership. On the national traditions, see Schmidt 1996: 116–50; Slack 1979; Stone 1953; Barona 1993.

[24] Barona 1993: 10–12. Blair 1999: 182 suggests that in the course of the sixteenth century, the gap between Latin and vernacular publication narrowed in respect of the relative degree of learning.

2.2.1 Peregrinatio

The second category of transmission mentioned above – travelling students – is a very significant factor in medical learning, especially in Germany. The list of German students at Padua, Bologna, and Ferrara between 1550 and 1630 is impressively long; Basle and Montpellier can also claim to have an international student body who take away with them just as positive an impression of their teachers. A cursory glance at the matriculation and disputation lists of Paris, Heidelberg, Wittenberg, Vienna, Helmstedt, Oxford and Cambridge shows a character which is more markedly local. Whatever the reasons for the popularity of some centres rather than others, it seems to me indubitable that their impact on the European medical world is very great.[25] *Peregrinatio medica* is mainly associated with Basle, Tübingen and Leiden, whose students travel to Padua, and Altdorf whose students travel to Basle and Montpellier; it is rare to find French students in Italy after 1500 however. The most energetic travellers include Pisa, Paris, Vienna and Bologna in their wanderings, often staying with the most prestigious professors in each place (see above 1.5.2).

2.2.2 Correspondence and dedications

The correspondence of doctors, especially in the same period, also reveals the range and liveliness of academic exchange. It seems that letters could be said to fall into two broad classes; those written with an expectation of later publication, and those which are written (at least initially) for the eyes of one recipient only. The first category is an established genre by 1550; fifteenth-century Italian humanists had used the letter form with classical models in mind to settle informally philosophical and philological questions, and their Northern counterparts were happy to continue this tradition, and to adapt it for the specific purposes of medicine (such as consilia, or specific questions of natural philosophy). Giovanni Manardo's early example in this was followed by Johann Lange (1485–1565), Johannes Schenck von Grafenberg (1530–98), Lorenz Scholze, Johannes Crato von Krafftheim and a host of others.[26] It is my impression that as a professional body these doctors are much more cosmopolitan than

---

[25] See Bertolaso 1959–60; Bertolis 1956–7; Bonuzzi 1975–6; Bosatra 1955–6; Brigi and Andrich 1892; Bylebyl 1979; Fichtner 1972–3; Dulieu 1979; Husner 1942; Martellozzo and Veronese 1969, 1971; Matsen 1968; Pesenti 1984; Piaia 1973; Premuda 1961–2, 1963, 1987–8; Ceseracciu 1978.

[26] See Nutton 1990b: 223 (on Crato, Fracastoro and Mercuriale).

their faculty rivals the lawyers, and more up to date with developments in medicine and natural philosophy throughout Europe; but this generalisation applies less well to Spain and England than to France, Switzerland, Germany, Italy and the Low Countries.

It is possible to detect networks inside the world of learning, not only in respect of places such as Padua, but also of people such as Andreas Libavius (*c.* 1546–1616) and Johannes Crato von Krafftheim; some of them are informed by ideologies linking the court, the town and the university in various countries. One such is the irenic and encyclopaedic version of Calvinism whose activities have been revealed by Robert Evans, Menna Prestwich and others.[27] There are both local, and more cosmopolitan circuits, some of which have been alluded to above (1.5.2). One of the clearest impressions left by humanism on medical books is the paratextual material: dedications, liminary poems, additional prefatory material. The Latin (or in some case Greek, or even Hebrew) is more carefully, often pretentiously, written, and a great deal of effort expended in the poems on the rhetoric of imitation.[28] These pieces of writing also reveal the connections of the author of the volume: his patrons, teachers, colleagues, friends, and pupils. Monographs and larger-scale works are often dedicated to grand patrons, who may or may not have had a part in financing the volume; the liminary poems may celebrate the family of the doctor in question; letters may act much as blurbs today, being solicited from a well-known professor to give dignity to the publication.[29] This practice is of course shared with other faculties such as law: as in that case, the two major classes of dedicatee seem to be patrons and colleagues. It is very common to find in prefaces generous acknowledgement made to erstwhile tutors: Paduan and Basle professors seem to be among the most often praised in this way.

2.2.3 Local publication

Local dissemination of knowledge through the medium of print occurs in various forms. It can reflect cultural isolation, which seems to be the case in England with very rare exceptions, and is certainly the case

---

[27] On which see Prestwich 1985; Evans 1975.

[28] The same humanist influence is sometimes revealed also by the form of the text itself: whether dialogue or verse. For examples see Fernel 1610a, Fracastoro 1574, Guinther von Andernach 1571, Suterus 1584; see also Nutton 1983: 8.

[29] Kleinfeld 1598 was advertised in the Book Fair Catalogues and includes a (solicited) testimonial letter by Jan van Heurne.

with Spanish doctors residing in Spain after the 1559 ordinances.[30] It also occurs in places such as Erfurt which specialised in discreet and inexpensive reproduction of learned books previously offered for sale at the international book fairs.[31] It may involve no more than the printing of almanachs, prognostications, calendars, and recipe books of various kinds; but it is also directly connected with the institution of the university, through the production of pedagogical materials such as the anatomical broadsheet[32] or the thesis, disputation or dissertation. These last were printed in some but not all centres (Paris produced them as broadsheets). By the end of the sixteenth century, however, they appeared in many German and Dutch universities in the form of a single gathering in octavo or in quarto. Many were written by the professor as 'praeses' of the disputation; they were defended there by a 'respondens' or supplicant for a higher degree.[33] They are very informative about the issues debated in the various institutions; some are even thought worthy to be republished in collections of dissertations, which then have a wider dissemination through advertisement at the book fairs.[34] Universities were also outlets for lucrative 'libri scholastici' or plaintexts, some of which were produced locally, some imported from centres such as Lyon, Basle and Frankfurt. These textbooks hardly ever figured in book fair catalogues.[35] They were brought out for the most part in small formats (8vo, 12mo and 16mo), and represented the staples of the medical book market. Galen's *Ars parva* or *Ars medica* and his *Methodus medendi* were printed, for example, at least thirty-one times between 1500 and 1550, forty-five times in the next fifty years, and twenty-nine times between 1600 and 1630.[36] Hippocrates's *Aphorisms* enjoyed at least fourteen editions between 1500 and 1550,

---

[30] Lynch 1964–9: 1.237–41; Slack 1979.

[31] Evidence for this in the first half of the sixteenth century is in Hase 1968.

[32] Carlino 1994a, 1995, 1999a; Cardano 1663: 1.118 (on his 'chirographia foliata'); Dale 1962: nos. 286–98 (the anatomical sheets from Paris (1539), Verona (*c.* 1550), Wittenberg (1573), and London (1540)); Nutton 1990c; Maittaire 1722: 35 (the *Tabulae de venis et arteriis* in Wechel's catalogue).

[33] Evans 1981; Duncan Liddel of Helmstedt produced two more or less identical disputations entitled *De praesagiis* for different respondents in 1598 and 1604, and used the same text in his own manual: Liddel 1628: 558ff. He did the same for the disputation *De signis* defended in 1598 (1628: 511ff.).

[34] *Decas* (1618–31). These were published by a printer (Johannes Jacobus Genathius) for both medicine and law; it is noteworthy that he was a bookseller, that there are three times as many theses in law than in medicine, and that of the medical theses about seven-eighths discuss practical rather than theoretical topics. See also Husner 1942.

[35] On evidence of multiple purchasing of copies and long use see Leedham-Green 1986 and Kusukawa forthcoming b.

[36] I have taken these figures from Lipenius 1679: 36–40, 51–4. Similar lists of editions can be found in the *Paris, Bibliothèque nationale, catalogue des sciences médicales*, Paris, 1857, s.vv.

thirty-three between 1550 and 1600, and twenty-four in the first thirty years of the seventeenth century. Certain editions survive to this day in large numbers, indicating that they were course books: an example of a less prominent text would be Joannes Guinther von Andernach's (1487–1575) edition in Paris of Galen's *De sectis* of 1528.[37] These textbooks vary in their forms of presentation, from plaintexts to rhymed mnemonic versions (there are at least eight different versions of the *Aphorisms* in this form between 1575 and 1634).[38] It would be wrong to suggest, however, that university students only purchased books linked directly to syllabuses: when Joseph Struthius's book on the pulse, the *Ars sphygmica*, was published in Padua in 1540, it was reported that 800 copies were sold in a single day.[39]

2.2.4 *Barriers to diffusion: confessionalisation*

It is worth considering whether there are any barriers in the free flow of this sort of information around Europe. There seems to be none in respect of specifically medical material until the Reformation, although I believe it to be true that very few Italian authors are cited in Paris, indicating perhaps a sense of insecure superiority. After the introduction of Catholic censorship in the years following the Council of Trent, a number of prominent figures (Paracelsus and Libavius among them) find their way on to the various Indices; but other doctors continue to be cited in spite of what could have been taken to be their religious affiliation. Among these are Rondelet, Fuchs, Paré, Bauhin, Liddel and Fernel. Fortunio Liceti (1577–1657) cited material from north of the Alps from news sheets rather than originals.[40] On the other hand, it is not uncommon to find the professional disagreement of a Catholic doctor

---

37 Nutton 1985a: 79.
38 The relevant shelfmarks in the catalogue of the Bibliothèque Nationale, Paris, are Td⁶ 64–74. See also Siraisi 1987a: 50; Carruthers 1997: 80; and Sanctorius 1630: 791–2 (xii.5) (the verse for circumstantiae).
39 Christian Gottleib Jöcher, *Allgemeines Gelehrtenlexikon*, Leipzig, 1750–1, iv.892, quoted in Durling 1961: 237. Laurent Joubert, *Opera latina*, Lyon, 1599: 2.154–5 records that 1,600 copies were printed in 1573 of a pirate Paris edition of Guillaume Rondelet's book on therapeutic method; the first volume of his own *Erreurs populaires* appeared in four different towns (Paris, Lyon, Bordeaux and Avignon) in a print run of 6,400 in all: see Barthélemy Cabrol's introduction to Joubert, *La Seconde Partie des erreurs populaires*, Paris, 1579: † 3r. The price rose sharply from 10–12 sous to 4 francs in a very short time. I am grateful to Dr R. G. Lewis for this information. Cf. the claim made by Mattioli, below note 44.
40 Liceti 1612; see also Fabritius Bartolettus 1619, from Bologna, who refers to the author of the *Opus paramirum* (i.e. Paracelsus) allusively as 'hermeticus' throughout his book. In general on this issue, see Göpfert, Vodosek, Weyrauch and Wittmann 1985. On Paracelsus, see Bogner 1994.

reinforced by mention of the heresy of the writer in question: the Jesuit Laurentius Forerus, in rejecting Goclenius's ideas about sympathy and antipathy, feels obliged to add of him that he had worn up to then the mask of a Calvinist heretic and a philosopher, but now was wearing that of an idolater and cabbalist; Simone Simoni is tarred with a similar brush.[41] Protestant doctors do not have the same inhibitions about citing their Catholic counterparts: indeed those who were once their pupils go as far as to edit them, and cause them to be printed locally. In this respect it is correct to claim that the Reformation in Northern Europe hardly affected medical study;[42] but in another, that of the teaching of medicine in the arts course, and the inflection given to medical study by the Lutheran and Philippist view of the human body as a potent argument in favour of God's design and providence, it would not be true to make this claim (see below 3.6).

2.3 BOOK FAIRS, AUTHORS AND PUBLISHERS

2.3.1 International publication

I move now to the fourth and largest category of transmitted knowledge, the field of freely circulated medical publication itself. The core of this field of knowledge may be taken to be editions of classical medical texts, monographs, scholarly works, and pedagogy, all in Latin. Although both town physicians and court doctors produced learned works, the majority of new publications came from the pens of university teachers.[43] It is very difficult to assess the print runs of these publications; there are indications that best-sellers such as Pier Andrea Mattioli's (1500–77) edition of Dioscorides sold in very large numbers (Mattioli himself claims that the first ten editions amounted to 30,000 copies);[44] other authors who give very full accounts of their publishing careers, such as Cardano,

---

[41] Forerus 1624: 276: 'iste Goclenius hactenus Philosophi haeretici, hic etiam Idololatriae personam suscepit. Antea Calvinista, nunc factus est caballista'; on Simoni see Madonia 1988. But Ulisse Aldrovandi 1599: 4v commends Bauhin and Rondelet to his readers. On the Inquisition and authors, see Palmer 1993; García Ballester 1993a: 151–91 (on Spain and its preoccupation with *conversos* and Jews).

[42] Grell and Cunningham 1993: 5.

[43] Unusual examples of town physicians who published are Franciscus Valleriola of Arles, who is a prolific producer of learned material as well as casebooks, and Jakob Horst in the early part of his career, who seems consciously to have published medical works to be read (in German) by the very categories of unlearned doctors and healing women which his later university colleagues were so grimly devoted to suppressing.

[44] Findlen 1999: 374.

are however silent on this matter, and may well not have known what the print runs of their books were.[45] The books came in a range of genres and forms: commentaries; monographs; pedagogical materials relating to the whole field of theoretical and practical medicine; lecture series, produced either with or without the consent of the lecturer, sometimes during his lifetime, sometimes after his death. Paduan professors were given an especially high profile through this form of publication, both at home and abroad;[46] one example is provided by Hercules Saxonia (Ercole Sassone) (1551–1607), whose *Tractatus triplex, de fe[b]rium putridarum signis et symptomatibus, de pulsibus et de urinis* was edited by Peter Uffenbach, the town physician of Frankfurt, and produced in 8vo at the expense of Johann Theobald Schönwetter in 1600. Three years later Uffenbach brought out at the expense of the publisher Zacharias Palthen the *Pantheum medicinae selectum* of Sassonia in folio, inspired, as he says, by four other Germans (Johannes Hartmann Beyer, Johannes Baumann with Johannes Munster, and Peter de Spina), who had edited the lecture notes of Hieronymus Capivaccius, Alessandro Massaria (1510–98) and Girolamo Mercuriale (1530–1606) respectively.[47]

2.3.2 The book fair

It is pertinent to mention here the institutions and commercial and practical aspects of publication, which contribute to the mediation of medical ideas.[48] A potent institution which drove the market for all learned books was the book fair. My comments on this institution will necessarily be germanocentric, because the survival of consolidated catalogues of the Frankfurt and Leipzig Book Fairs makes it easy to produce crude statistics and to get some feel for the universe of discourse it reveals; but I

---

[45] Maclean 1994.

[46] One might mention Johannes Jessenius a Jessen's edition of Emilio Campilongo, and the edition of Giambattista da Monte's works by Martinus Weinrichius (unusually complete, according to Bylebyl 1991: 174), and of Hieronymus Capivaccius (by Henricus Osthausius) in 1593. Alessandro Massaria, Girolamo Mercuriale undergo the same fate, sometimes more than once, with varying degrees of fidelity in the transcription.

[47] A further folio volume by Sassone (the *De pulsibus*) was edited by Uffenbach in 1604, following its appearance in Padua in 1603, 4to. Part of these works, all based on lecture notes, then appeared in folio, also from the Palthen presses, in 1610 with the title *Prognoseon practicarum*, edited this time by an ex-student from Cremona, Leander Vialatus, with an introduction by Johannes Jessenius a Jessen (University of Wittenberg). In 1620, the Venice publisher Francesco Bolzetta reprinted this volume in Vicenza, in folio.

[48] In a letter addressed to their authors dated 20 January 2000, the Presses Universitaires de France identified five métiers of the modern trade as 'éditeur, diffuseur, distributeur, libraire, imprimeur'. The functions of 'diffuseur' and 'distributeur' were less well distinguished in the Renaissance; both were connected with the operation of the book fairs.

hope to be able to throw some light, if only by analogy, on the operation of the French and Italian book markets. There is good evidence
that Italy operated both an internal market which satisfied local needs
and an export trade;[49] where there are editions of the same book of
the same date printed in Italy and Germany, it is often the case that
French libraries now hold the Italian copy, suggesting that the Italian
book trade with Paris and Lyon was more successful than the German
(a surprising finding, as the cost of paper, and hence of book production,
was much higher in Italy than in Germany).[50] The first consolidated
Frankfurt Book Fair catalogues appeared in 1564;[51] what I shall say will
be based on catalogues up to 1631, the year in which the Thirty Years
War impinged very directly on Frankfurt, after which the advertised
number of titles in Latin went into a marked decline. During this period,
the numbers of participating foreign publishers grew; by 1600, Venice
(mainly through the 'Societas' or consortium arrangements for export)
and Rome were well represented, as well as Switzerland, France and the
Low Countries. There were problem years for French publishers (from
1572 until about 1577), but the flight of Calvinist refugees after the St
Bartholomew's Eve Massacre to Frankfurt strengthened if anything the
representation of books from France.[52] The manner in which the fair operated meant that books were distributed in more that one way: not only
by direct purchase, but also by *Tauschhandel* (the swapping of the same
number of printed sheets between publishers), by the activities of the
bookshops, and by the presence of agents and colporteurs who bought
books speculatively to offer to known clients who were themselves unable
to visit the fair. By the 1590s, the twice-yearly pulse of the fair seems to
determine the course of public debates on contentious academic and
other issues: examples are afforded by the Erfurt debate over chemical

---

[49] Gehl 1997; *Catalogus* 1637.

[50] Pettas 1997. For evidence of market zoning, see Maclean 1990, 1994. On the cost of paper, see
Hirsch 1967: 71, Kapp 1886: 312. There is some evidence of poor standards of production in
Venice: see Maclean 1994: 314; the Lyon publisher's remarks in Capivaccius 1596; the parallel
editions of Alpini's *De praesagienda vita et morte* produced in 1601 in Venice and Frankfurt. On the
other hand, Giovanni Argenterio preferred to be published in Florence than Lyon or Basle, in
spite of tempting solicitations from publishers: Siraisi 1990a: 177. Gessner advised Crato von
Krafftheim in 1561 to have his book on distillations published in Lyon rather than Basle on the
grounds that 'Lugdunensis enim typographus facile praeter tuum privilegium, alterum a Rege
suo acciperet et ita libentius imprimeret': Gessner 1577: 8r. Sachiko Kusukawa kindly drew my
attention to this quotation.

[51] Fabian 1972–8; Schwetschke 1850–77 (whose analytical survey begins in 1565); Grosse 1600;
Clessius 1602.

[52] This is especially true of vernacular books: see Draut 1625b: 1–212 (by far the longest entry for
any vernacular other than German).

medicine involving Georg am Wald and Libavius, and the debate about the infamous case of the Silesian boy with the Golden Tooth.[53] A slower rate of polemic marks earlier decades of the century, but I do not think that it can safely be inferred from this that the rate of transmission of information was slower.[54]

2.3.3 Medicine and other disciplines

The rubric 'libri medici' (sometimes 'libri medici et chymici') appeared after theology and law, and before philosophical books, under which rubric books on natural philosophy were listed. Latin books were listed before those in vernaculars, which were usually relegated to the end of the catalogue.[55] Medical books invite comparison with law, and with natural philosophy: one being the professional rival, the other being the closest subject area. I shall not here give a detailed comparison of publication figures with natural philosophy, because they constitute a much smaller field of publication, with considerable fluctuations; many of the authors of this field are themselves doctors or become such (Cornelius Gemma (1534–74), Caspar Peucer (1525–1602), and Scipione Chiaramonte (1565–1652) among them), or have close contacts with medicine, such as Giambattista della Porta (1535?–1615). Trends are more easily gauged through the comparison with law. Throughout the period 1565–1631, the number of declared law books is more than twice that of medicine:[56] these being books that were (with very rare exceptions) only advertised once, and were in the main protected by privilege, and therefore in a certain sense 'new' publications.[57] The average annual

---

53 Details of the Erfurt debate are given in Gillespie 1970–80: 3.309–10. See also Müller-Jahnke 1994. The relevant publications in the case of the Golden Tooth are given in Maclean 2000a: 99. Sometimes controversial works (i.e. books involved in specific debates) are reissued if they fail to sell over a period of years: an example of this is Henning Rennemann's refutation (the *Responsio apologetica*) of Philippus Scherbius's *Dissertatio pro philosophia peripatetica, adversus Ramistas* of 1590, which first appeared in 1595, was reissued in 1599 and again in 1603.

54 Cf. the comments of Nutton 1990b: 215ff.

55 Publishers' lists were differently arranged: see Widmann 1984. Theology seems to have been recognised as the most lucrative market sector: see Gessner 1577: 139v (Gessner to Melchior Guilandino Borusso): 'typographus noster Froschouerus recusat amplius in re medica quicquam procudere, maius enim lucrum ex theologicis capit: quorum subinde aliquid Latine aut Germanice cudit'.

56 Paradoxically, however, in Draut's subject catalogue, law and medicine take up the same amount of space. The size of the law faculty in many universities was far larger than the faculty of medicine (which was sometimes subsumed into the faculty of arts).

57 For books to be advertised in the book fairs, they had to fall into one of the following categories: 'ganz neu'; 'sonstens verbessert'; 'auffs neu wieder auffgelegt'. The first category was often associated with legal protection of the book in question, on which see Eisenhardt 1970. On risk of piracy see Siraisi 1997: 55, and Gessner 1577: 8r, quoted in note 50.

Table 2.1

Decade	Medical books	Law books
1570–9	20	60
1580–9	33	68
1590–9	36	88
1600–9	52	123
1610–19	46	130
1620–9	50	86

number of medical and law books in Latin declared by decade is shown in table 2.1, which shows a sharp increase in production, not all of which was, of course, innovative publication; it is not clear that there was a concomitant increase in the numbers of students and practitioners over this period. The publisher or printer and the format were recorded with the titles that were declared. For the period 1596–1601 in Leipzig, on a sample size of 230, the percentages of medical books in the various formats are the following: folio, 23 per cent; 4to, 29 per cent; 8vo, 43 per cent; 12mo, 4.5 per cent; 16mo, 0.5 per cent. The small number of books declared in small formats gives support to my claim that 'libri scholastici', which were mostly produced in these sizes, were in general not advertised.

2.3.4 Active publishers and centres of publication

I should now like to move on to the role of printer-publishers in medical publication. For a book to be published, it required money in advance for the paper, payment of the printing workshop, advertisement in the right quarter, an envisaged readership; in this respect, Iain Lonie's reference to 'new genres prompted by the invention of printing [by which] an individual point of view might be addressed to the indeterminate audience created by printing' is misleading, for there is very little evidence that publishers or sponsors at this time were scholarly philanthropists willing to publish anything which might benefit mankind.[58] Titlepages often target the hoped-for purchasers and specify the intended readership: university teachers; practitioners; both medical doctors and natural philosophers; all of these and those of a curious disposition. Rodericus a

---

[58] Lonie 1981: 20; publishers are happy to make this claim however: see the Egenolff, Fuchs and Cornarius affair referred to in Kusukawa 1997.

Castro's (1546–1627) *Medicus-politicus* of 1614, a work broadly of medical ethics, suggests that it may be read with profit by all the following: doctors, patients, the friends and relations of patients, moral and political philosophers, and those who just like a good read. But this is as close as medical books come to advertising the economic interests which they serve.[59]

Even if publishers or sponsors at this time were not disinterested philanthropists, it cannot be doubted that many of them were scholarly; they often had to exercise a careful oversight over complex copy, as many authors lived too far away to supervise the production of their books.[60] This is of particular importance in the production of medical books, which contain clear evidence of the impact of hellenism, as I have already suggested. It is not difficult to illustrate how far the activities of publishers are important to the development of the scholarly world: the Wechels' policy of importing into the German-speaking world French (and later English, Italian and Central European) medical writers, including such figures as Jean Fernel (André Wechel's father-in-law), Girolamo Mercuriale, Tomas Jordán, Jean de Gorris, Nicolas Le Pois and Thomas Moufet, clearly made a difference to the field of medical knowledge, as did Valentin Voegelin's sponsorship of Jakob Horst, Peter Kopf's sponsorship of Andreas Libavius, Christophe Plantin's various acts of patronage of medical publication, Andreas Osiander's signing up of Girolamo Cardano for Johannes Petreius, and Cardano's later support from Guillaume Rouillé (Gulielmus Rouillius) and Heinrich Petri.[61] The locations of these publishers are worthy of note: Lyon, Basle, Venice/Padua, Paris, Frankfurt, Antwerp, Leipzig, Geneva. All are places which gave access to major book markets, and which had traditions of scholarship.

---

59 See also Temkin 1973: 150, who quotes the titlepage of Argenterio's *In artem medicinalem Galeni commentarii* (1578) proclaiming that they are 'non solum medicis et professoribus utiles et necessarii sed etiam philosophis et universis qui rerum scientiae delectantur summopere iucundi'. Publishers often specified the intended purchaser(s) on the titlepage. Examples are afforded by Campilongo 1601 and Castro 1614.

60 Cardano and others, for example, complain that they are unable to monitor the production of their works, and have to rely on the probity and thoroughness of the printer. The entrepreneurial Frankfurt publisher Sigismund Feyerabend, who published quite a number of medical books, could not read Latin, but he was exceptional: see Maclean 1994: 322; Pallmann 1881.

61 See Evans 1975; Maclean 1994, 1999a: 23–4; Rondelet 1586: ↑ 3r (Rouillé's advertisement of future medical publications by Hollerius and Pacotius). Dodoens 1583 and Wittesteyn 1588 are examples of Plantin's sponsorship of medical writing; on whom see *Fondscatalogus* 1988–9 and Voet 1969–72. A reference to commissioning is in Joannes Sinapius's letter to Simon Grynaeus dated 1534 (Flood and Shaw 1997: 173–4). Cf. Argenterio, who was approached by Basle and Lyon publishers but preferred to be published in Florence: Siraisi 1990a: 177; also the illicit publication of da Monte (Nutton 1990b: 207) and the immediate republication of Mercuriale in Basle after his Venice edition of 1577.

I would not myself wish to argue from this that the commercial sense of these publishers abandoned them when they adopted these authors. Indeed there is surviving testimony to show that they refused to publish works of very limited appeal or second editions of unsuccessful works, even by authors from whom they had greatly profited.[62] Further testimony to the hard-headedness of publishers is the phenomenon of the self-payer, the author who can find no sponsor at all, and has to finance the whole operation himself.[63] Printer-publishers also made decisions about which books merited reprinting (these being mainly, but not always, produced outside the zones of their licensed protection or after the lapse of a privilege). This was a speculative activity which reveals particularly clearly the symbiosis of commercial and intellectual interests in the medical book market; its results have sometimes been taken as a straightforward index of wide influence and popularity. Thus the intellectual impact of Manardo's letters has been gauged by the spread of editions, from Ferrara (in 1529), to Venice, Lyon (thanks to the initiative of Rabelais), Paris, Strasbourg, Basle and finally Hanau: a fine folio edition in 1611, a companion piece for the letters of Lorenz Scholze (1610) and Orazio Augenio (1597, first printed in Venice in 1592), and those of Johann Lange, first published in 8vo at Basle in 1554, then by the Wechel presses in 8vo in 1585, and in folio in 1605. Guinther von Andernach's *Institutiones anatomicae* begin life in Paris in 1536, and travelled via Basle, Venice and Padua to Wittenberg in 1585. Similar erratic trajectories can be traced for many successful textbooks and consilia; but they may reflect as much the protectionism of major international publishers who were willing to go to great lengths to preserve their monopoly of certain authors as the local needs of teaching institutions or academic enthusiasms. There is ample evidence of the successful protection of monopolies, such as that of Waldkirch and Perna in respect of Paracelsus (at least up to the 1590s, when Johann Wechel begins to publish Paracelsus at Frankfurt) and Petri in respect of Cardano; from this it is possible to infer that publication in Basle or in Frankfurt alone is an index not of narrow but of very wide international exposure.[64] In some cases, books appeared from the same publisher with different bibliographical

---

[62] Two examples of such refusal to publish are Wechel's of Camerarius's correspondence in Greek (Maclean 1988: 153) and Petri's of the second edition of Cardano's *De utilitate ex adversis capienda* (Maclean 1994: 321).

[63] One example of a self-payer is Ingolstetterus; see also Manlius, who does it to attract a patron who might give him preferment: Maclean forthcoming b.

[64] See Maclean 1990, 1994. The trajectories traced above are to be found in Nutton 1993c. Other examples of *Nachdruck* are deducible from Draut 1625a: 976–8.

addresses (e.g., Frankfurt and Cologne); this seems to have been a tactic employed to secure a sale in Southern Europe by naming a Northern town of known Catholicity in the imprint.[65]

2.3.5 Live authors, dead authors, editors: printing and reprinting

As Jon Arrizabalaga has shown, the percentage of live as opposed to dead authors being published rose from 0% in 1470–9 to 40% in 1490–9.[66] Thereafter they formed a significant part of the titles appearing in a given year. Whether authors were *re*printed seems however not to be determined by their topical currency as much as by decisions which were directly commercial in nature. Some later republication in other printing centres seems to be straightforwardly driven by speculation: thus Duncan Liddel's *Opera* were reprinted at Lyon in 1624, and thereafter at Hamburg in 1628, in response, I suspect, to his recommendation as a textbook in Leiden by Petrus Laurembergius.[67] The publishers of books which first appeared in printing centres which did not gain access to the book fairs often explicitly state that they have speculated on a gap in the market.[68] I am not suggesting that it was printer-publishers alone who determined what was reprinted, or that they were solely driven by the economics of the book trade, or that their support was a sufficient condition for success (although it seems to be a necessary one); but their influence is very considerable. It is able to be gauged *ex negativo* by noting that some excellent and highly innovative books have little or no European exposure (Pereira's *Novae veraeque medicinae, experimentis et evidentibus rationibus comprobatae, prima pars*, published in Medina del Campo in 1558, springs here to mind).

To what degree was the market sensitive to novelty? This is a difficult question to answer. The term 'neotericus' or '[auctor] recentior' is applied to more or less any post-1300 writer; and many medieval authors of secrets, of practical medical works and even of teaching materials were republished as 'neoterici' or 'recentiores' during the sixteenth century.

---

[65] Rhodes 1987; Maclean forthcoming a.

[66] Arrizabalaga 1998.

[67] Laurembergius 1621: 7.

[68] E.g. Lemosius 1598, which was first printed in Salamanca in 1585. The Italian publisher says in his note to the reader that he is reissuing this because it was inaccessible to Italian students (i.e. those studying at Padua) and presumably filled a gap; he advertised the book at the Frankfurt Book Fair, but it is the *Salamanca* edition which is found in Paris libraries and which presumably reached there via Medina del Campo and Lyon. Also Columba 1601, which first appeared in Messina in 1596.

To give a few examples: Alphonsus Betrutius's *Therapeutica* was reprinted in Mainz in 1534; three years later Marcus Gatinaria's complete works appeared in Basle;[69] Arnau de Vilanova's works were published in 1504, several times in the next three decades, and much later, in 1585, edited by Nicolaus Taurellus; Pietro d'Abano's *Conciliator* had at least sixteen reprintings in the century, and appeared in a digest form for students of Giessen University as late as 1621; the *Regimen sanitatis salernitanum* enjoys a similar fate.[70] Yet when the Venetian publisher Francesco Bolzetta published Franciscus Vicomercatus's (d. 1570) *De principiis rerum naturalium* in 1596, he felt constrained to apologise in a preface for producing a work that was written forty years ago, in the 1550s, as though the subject had moved on in the meanwhile.

Even though new authors did not always find it easy to accede to the world of print, once they were established, their writings appeared very quickly, suggesting that innovative writing was eagerly taken up by the profession.[71] The sense of novelty certainly seems to me to be very marked in some areas: not only in the demand for accounts of prodigious cases, but also in the area of iatrochemistry after 1570. By 1625, the foremost representatives of Paracelsian medicine were cited by one hostile commentator as Henning Scheunemann, Johannes Tanckius (1557–1609) and Oswald Croll (*c.* 1580–1609), all of whom wrote after 1600: the luminaries of the late sixteenth century, Gerhard Dorn, Joseph du Chesne (Quercetanus), and Petrus Severinus, seem to have slipped from view.[72] This state of affairs coexists however with commemorative posthumous publication: Felix Platter's (1536–1614) *Quaestiones medicae paradoxae et endoxae*, for example, were published after his death in 1625, some forty years after they had been written.

It is interesting to compare this situation with that which pertains about thirty years later in the 1650s, by which time the plethora of Renaissance publications on medicine, although no doubt still available on the second-hand market, had been reduced to a few reprinted titles, seen to be worthy of standing as the monuments of their age. One scholar actively involved in this triage was Charles Spon of Lyon, who between 1650 and 1665 selected Heurnius, Schenck, Cardano, Caspar Hofmann and Daniel

---

[69] Other editions in Venice, in 1516 and in Frankfurt, in 1604; see also Wear 1995b: 254.

[70] On the reprintings of Pietro d'Abano see Arrizabalaga 1998: 276.

[71] For the example of Cardano's publishing career, see Maclean 1994, 1999a; for the somewhat different case of Fracastoro, see Nutton 1990b.

[72] Wolf 1620: BIr. Nancy Siraisi has pointed out to me that Severinus was cited later in the century as a main representative of modern Paracelsianism by Hermann Conring in his *De hermetica Aegyptiorum vetere et Paracelsicorum nova medicina* of 1648 (2.1.179).

Sennert for folio editions which were produced by the entrepreneurial protestant firm of Huguetan and Ravaud.[73] Elsewhere, André du Laurens, Jacques Dubois (Sylvius) and Jacques Houillier (Hollerius) (d. 1562) had enjoyed similar celebration;[74] but I do not believe that the Paduans, Bolognans or Ferrarese fare so well. Even though, if we are to believe Georgi's *Bücherlexikon* which contains eighteenth-century prices, the value of these books seems to remain high long into the age of Enlightenment, there is little, if any, indication that these acts of republication had the effect of keeping their authors in the forefront of academic debate.[75] The break in international communications which was caused by the Thirty Years War marks also the end of a phase in intellectual activity as well.

2.4 FORMAT AND GENRE

2.4.1 Genres

I come now to the question of the genres of medical writing, which can be distributed according to various criteria. The distribution made by Pascal Le Coq (Gallus) in his bibliography of 1590 is based on subject; it begins with editions of and commentaries on classical texts; this is followed by surgery, anatomy, botany and pharmacy, after which come books of practica and consilia. Two more specialised classes – books on the regimen to be followed in times of plague, and books on venereal disease – close the sequence. I have chosen here to attempt a distribution by readership rather than subject, as this is more likely to show the effect of genre and format on the contents of the books in question. The student market is, as has been noted, partly local and partly international; some of the manuals produced for it respond not only to its needs, but also to that of practitioners, if evidence derived from the ownership of books is to be believed (below, 2.5.2). I am referring here to general manuals[76] and to treatises of practical medicine (pathology, therapeutics, pharmacopoeia), some of which had been given as lectures and still bear the

---

73 On Spon's activity, Pic 1911: 206ff.

74 Du Laurens's *Opera omnia anatomica et medica* appeared in 2 vols. in folio in Paris in 1627–8; Jacques Houiller's *Opera omnia practica* were reprinted in Geneva in 1623, 1635 and 1664. Jacques Dubois (Sylvius) enjoyed folio republication in Cologne in 1630: see Lonie 1985: 156.

75 Georgi 1742–58.

76 See Arrizabalaga 1998: 28 on the *Articella*, produced for students at Montpellier and Pavia as well as practitioners, and on the use of a smaller format (8vo) to secure this market; *ibid.*, 37–8, contains interesting speculations on the reasons for the demise of this textbook.

marks (Capivaccius, which is a mixture of theoria and practica; or da Monte's lectures on Rhazes); some of which have been reorganised by 'morbi', 'signa' and 'causae' (to which recommendations for treatment are occasionally added). These last follow the sequence of medical consultation, moving from observation to deduction: the works of writers of practica at the end of the sixteenth century such as Saxonia remain very close to the late medieval model of which Savonarola's *Practica* is an example.[77] The many books written on new diseases such as syphilis are also directed at this readership.

A paradox about textbooks and compendia is that their producers often claim that they are not suitable as a means of learning medicine (Fuchs), and universities often reject them as pedagogical tools (see 1.5.1); yet they not only continue to produce them, but even pen guides to writing and choosing textbooks, of which some striking examples are those by Janus Cornarius, Heurnius, Schenck and Bartholin.[78] The production of lecture series and of commentaries on both Greek and Arab set texts seems to be aimed at all levels of the university market; some are narrow in scope, some discursive if not actually digressive, having taken many years to evolve and acquire many accretions.[79] Two modes of writing are to be found here: that which is scarcely modified from its medieval roots, organised by quaestiones (into this category falls the much reviled but still used *Conciliator*);[80] and that which has humanist pretensions, or even humanist-inspired disposition in epitome, dialogue or commonplace form.[81] One should also mention here the compendia, lexica, and other academic instruments which are published throughout

---

[77] Saxonia 1603; Bylebyl 1991: 174 points out that Fernel's pathology covers only causes and signs until its 1679 edition. On Rhazes as a model for treatises on pathology see Wear 1995b: 258. See also Heyll 1534.

[78] Durling 1990: 181f.

[79] Oddi 1564 is an example of a very discursive commentary on the *Aphorisms*. See also Siraisi 1990a: 166. The first printed edition of a commentary (on Hippocrates's *Aphorisms*) is said to date from 1473; it was published by Ottaviano Scoto: Pesenti 2000.

[80] Bylebyl 1985a: 245. According to Fernel's biographer Guillaume Plancy (quoted by Bylebyl 1985a: 225), Fernel was opposed to quaestiones. On Argenterio's opposition to them, see Siraisi 1991: 169. Siraisi 1997: 51–2 refers to Cardano's preference for exposition; but Vallesius 1606 uses them, and Crusius 1615 adapts them to the scholia form. Lonie 1981: 19 points out that new quaestiones arise on the issue of fever from discrepancies between the various texts of Galen. Silvaticus 1601 lists as previous writers on controversiae Pietro d'Abano, Rorarius, Cardano, Lacuna (perhaps because of his Milan connections) and Vallesius. On the relationship of quaestiones to problemata see Blair 1997: 16, 35.

[81] Lacuna 1551; Valleriola 1562. Loci are rejected as an approach by Cardano, who prefers to present discrepancies in miscellany form: Cardano 1565, Siraisi 1997: 45, 55. See also Rorarius 1573 (treating discrepancies in a range of authors, including Celsus, Avicenna, Aetius, Paul of Aegina, Galen, and Hippocrates).

the century;[82] collective volumes on topics such as syphilis, childhood diseases, and gynaecology;[83] consilia, which are listed as a genre by Le Coq (Gallus), which, in so far as they do not inform the reader of the result of the advice offered, are distinct from texts recording rare medical events or celebrated cures performed by a given doctor.[84]

Of broader appeal is the class of books which fall between medicine and natural philosophy, such as those on certain Aristotelian texts such as the *Physiognomica*, the *De anima* and the *Libri naturales*, which are sometimes reduced to handbooks on natural principles;[85] there are also books on alchemy and natural magic, and on astrology and divination;[86] and best-sellers constituted by the secrets and remedies literature of the Middle Ages[87] and its sixteenth-century counterpart: works such as the *Regimen sanitatis salernitanum*, spruced up and made more agreeable to read by Johannes Curio and Jacobus Crellius;[88] Michael Puff von Schrich's book on herbal distillations, which was printed thirty-eight times in the course of the century; and Levinus Lemnius's (1505–68) *De occultis naturae miraculis*, which enjoyed multiple publication and translation in the second half of the period under consideration. I am myself inclined to include with this category of book the many volumes of mirabilia or remarkable cases (which are related to the genre of consilia), beginning with that of Antonio Benivieni (first published in 1507) and stretching to Schenck's immense compendium of *Observationes* published between

---

[82] These have a long history: Joannes de Sancto Amando, *Revocativum memorie* of the late thirteenth century lists 4,400 Galenic and Aristotelian statements organised in 528 alphabetically ordered topics: McVaugh in Arnau de Vilanova 2000: 132. Renaissance examples include the index to Andrea Alpaga's edition of Avicenna which appeared in 1526; Brunfels 1534; Brasavola 1556; Foesius 1588; Gorris 1601 (first edition 1564).

[83] On Luigi Linguini's collection of texts on syphilis, see Nutton 1990b: 225. There are collected essays also on children's illnesses (Sebastianus Austrius's *De puerorum morbis, et symptomatibus tum dignoscendis, tum curandis liber*, Lyon, 1549; Marius Zuccarus, *Tractatus de morbis puerorum*, Naples, 1604) and on women's ailments: *Gynaicea*, ed. Hans Kaspar Wolf, Basle, 1566, 1577; ed. Wolf and others, Basle, 1586–7; ed. Israel Spachius, Strasbourg, 1597. It is of note that this last was advertised under 'libri philosophici' in the Frankfurt Book Fair catalogue of Spring 1586.

[84] Agrimi and Crisciani 1994. Benivieni 1529 is an example of the recording of rare events (Daston and Park 1998: 145; Temkin 1973: 173 also thinks him innovative because he records reports of his own autopsies); Cardano 1663: 1.82–95 engages in the celebration of personal skills, on which see Siraisi 1997: 153–8; 196–213.

[85] On works connected with the *De anima*, see Schüling 1967. Some examples of handbooks on the *Libri naturales* are those by Biesius (1573) and Vicomercatus (1596). See also Herberger 1981: 233 (on the placita of Galen) and Webster 1990.

[86] E.g. Peucer 1593, Gemma 1575.

[87] See Eamon 1994; some rational doctors help propagate them (Jakob Horst translated Lemnius's *Occulta naturae miracula* into German); others attack them, as does Sylvius 1539a: a3v.

[88] See Gambacorta and Giordano 1983.

1584 and 1609.[89] An equally popular genre in both Latin and the vernacular is constituted by books of advice about the plague, of which literally hundreds were written. They are often quite local in character, and differ thus from monographs on specific diseases: this seems to have been recognised at the time, as Le Coq (Gallus) devotes a separate section to them (as he does to venereal disease) in his *Bibliotheca medica* of 1590.

2.4.2 Formats

Related to genre is the question of format, which I should like now to review in greater detail. In terms of a percentage of book production as a whole, there are many more law books than medical books published in folio throughout the period, reflecting perhaps the fact that lawyers practised amid their books, which were a sort of externalisation of their knowledge and of the competence and of the dignity of their calling; whereas doctors very often practised their profession, whether academically or therapeutically, away from their books, and did not need to be surrounded by them to impress their audiences or patients. At most they might have liked to have with them a manual of practica in pocket-book format, to consult discreetly during their clinical visit. There is still a considerable percentage of medical books produced in folio; they are made up of a mixture of standard editions of, and commentaries on, classic texts, the collected works of celebrated Renaissance doctors, books on anatomy, herbals, and the diagrammatic presentation of medical knowledge. While it is clear that the larger format is necessary to accommodate works of considerable length, this does not account for all volumes produced in folio: celebratory or commemorative publications such as *opera omnia, consilia*,[90] *epistolae* could as well have been produced in a smaller format; certain prestigious publishers used the larger format in series, no doubt to generate profit;[91] likewise Peter Kopf, the Frankfurt bookseller who funded the publications of Andreas Libavius, began (in 1595) by publishing him in 8vo, but moved to folio when he becomes well known (after 1600). Some genres also appeared in folio for apparently traditional reasons: Conciliators, for example, and the Renaissance

---

[89] See Maclean 1991, 1991b; Nutton 1993c. Daston and Park 1998: 116 (on the pseudo-Aristotelian *De mirabilibus auscultationibus* and the pseudo-Albertus *De mirabilibus mundi*), *ibid.*, 172 (on Nicolas Oresme's *De causis mirabilium*).

[90] See Crisciani 1996b: 7n and Siraisi 1997: 20, 203, 320 (on development of consilia from the thirteenth century); Bylebyl 1991: 169 (quoting Solenander).

[91] Heinrich Petri and his heirs at Basle published commentaries on Hippocrates and astrology in this format; André Wechel and his heirs at Frankfurt used it for consilia and collections of letters.

volumes of controversiae and contradicentia which are related to them, mainly followed the folio format of their ancestor, the *Conciliator* of Pietro d'Abano,[92] as did scholarly apparatus connected with an edition in folio (e.g. Brasavola's index to the Giunti Galen of 1550).[93] Publication in folio is also a matter of the physical expression of the excellence of the contents: Janus Cornarius reminded his reader in the preface to his translation of Galen of 1537 of Froben's old motto that a man who buys a good book at a high price gets a bargain, whereas someone who buys a bad book cheaply makes a loss.[94] Other folio printings are determined by the nature of the contents, such as books on anatomy, surgery and botany with splendid illustrations, of which Vesalius's *Fabrica* is the paradigm example.[95] It is pertinent to ask here who bought these fine editions. Elizabeth Eisenstein seems to think that they were accessible to students; but their cost was such that it is even doubtful whether any but the most prosperous professors of medicine or court doctor could afford them. Vesalius's illustrations can be shown to have had very little impact on anatomical illustration in cheaper formats or in broadsheet form, and indeed (for a variety of reasons) little impact on anatomical teaching. It seems that such lavish publication was aimed at the court and the institutional library more than any other market sector.[96] This would not be true, however, of plainer folio productions, which are to be found in abundance in the inventories of private libraries. A cursory glance at the distributions of various formats in the libraries of prominent and less prominent academic doctors confirms the percentages which my sampling of the Leipzig catalogues given above produced.[97] The dominant format for academic monographs in the case of France, Switzerland and Germany is 8vo, and in Italy and Holland is 4to.[98]

---

92 E.g. Vallesius, *Controversiae* (various editions from 1556 to 1606) and Joannes Baptista Silvaticus, *Controversiae medicae* (1601). There are other Conciliators: e.g. of Aristotle and Galen, and of Aristotle and Averroes: see Cranz 1976.

93 Lexica tend to match the size of the parent edition: the Giunti Galen is in folio; but Dorn's lexicon for Paracelsus (on which see Hieronymus 1995: 104f.) is in 8vo.

94 *Opus medicum practicum*, Basle, 1537, quoted by Hieronymus 1995: 100.

95 Other examples are Vidus Vidius's *Chirurgia* of 1544; Charles Estienne's *De dissectione* of 1542; and Leonhart Fuchs's *De historia stirpium commentarii insignes* of 1542, on which see Kusukawa 1997.

96 See Eisenstein 1979: 566–74; Nutton 1993c; and Cunningham 1997.

97 E.g. Kolb 1976: 45–56 (Peucer's library), and the inventory in the will of Francesco Martinez Polo (Valladolid, Archivo Histórico Provincial, Protocolos 1629). The Herzog-August-Bibliothek Wolfenbüttel contains the library of Wolfgangus Waldungus, which was acquired in the early decades of the seventeenth century, and which manifests the same features.

98 For different views, see Hieronymus 1995: 96 (8vo as standard) and Nutton 1993c ('the change in format from vast folio to smaller tract in the course of the sixteenth century is also partially wrong: the percentage of formats is relatively stable').

2.4.3 Illustrations and diagrams

There are two ways in which illustrations appear in medical writing. One is more or less representational; the other as a pedagogical tool for the visual display of knowledge. In the first category fall anatomical broadsheets and textbooks, as well as herbals and works of zoology; these have been investigated by Sachiko Kusukawa and others.[99] Andrea Carlino has argued that anatomical broadsheets were aimed at a public wider than that of medical students; this is to a degree true in Wittenberg, where they were recommended to students on the arts course, but I am less sure whether they can be said to target the general reader.[100] Anatomical textbooks, of which the most celebrated is Vesalius's lavish *Humani corporis fabrica*, fulfil multiple functions, as anatomical atlases, dictionaries of anatomical terms, dissection manuals, and detailed narrative descriptions of the human body, as Nancy Siraisi has pointed out.[101] The issue of the correctness of representation, which gives rise to some acrimonious exchanges in the 1540s both about the drawings and their plagiarised use, is one which principally concerns what the French call the 'imaginaire' of the period, and the book-historical question about the ways in which the illustrations of books were read. I do not wish here to offer a simple peremptory answer to a difficult topic, but I suspect that the fact that the illustrations in anatomy textbooks did not seem to have been influenced by the greater realism found in Vesalius's works and other such lavish productions may well be because they were principally produced to provide relative location of internal organs, not correct representation of them, which by the end of the century was being provided by dissections in anatomical theatres.[102]

The second category of illustration – the 'formula', 'paradigma', 'dispositio', 'anacephaleosis', 'tabella' – whose function is to provide visual aids to logical or taxonomic problems, is more germane to this study. Diagrammatic representations of knowledge are common in the medieval period: they are found in both logical manuals (squares of

---

[99] Kusukawa 1998; Carlino 1994, 1995, 1999. One might also mention here the collections of portraits of medical men (e.g. Joannes Sambucus, *Veterum aliquot ac recentium medicorum philosophorumque icones*, Antwerp, 1574; Erhard Cellius, *Imagines professorum tubinensium*, Tübingen, 1596), but I take the purpose of these to be either humanist, institutional or municipal pride: they are sometimes attacked as a sign of vainglory (as in the case of Fuchs: see Kusukawa forthcoming a). The issue of representation is very complex; sixteenth-century doctors can evince inconsistency in their attitude to it: for the case of Sylvius, see Kusukawa 1998: 135.
[100] Carlino 1995.
[101] Siraisi 1994b: 63.
[102] Nutton 1993c; Cunningham 1997.

contraries and Porphyry's trees) and in mathematics.[103] It is interesting to note in respect of the second that doctors were involved in the republication in the late fifteenth century of works by some of the 'Oxford calculators' (Burley, Swineshead, Bradwardine), which contained geometrical figures as well as tables of proportion, and representations of problems of velocity. Benedictus Victorius's (Vettori) (1481–1561) complex illustration of the latitude of health in his *Opus theorice latitudinum medicine* (1516), which sets out to show the consequences for medical doctrine of the 'lax' solution to the problem of the specific form of diseases (see below 5.2, 7.4.3), reveals how diagrams were adapted for medical purposes.[104] The presence of these diagrams reveals also the close affiliation of the mathematics of latitude of qualities, of proportion, and of quantity to medical thinking, and may even indicate an act of borrowing from one discipline to another.

As has already been pointed out by other historians, tree diagrams and dichotomies are found in works of natural philosophy such as Gregor Reisch's *Margarita philosophica* which date from the early years of the sixteenth century:[105] they appear in Parisian humanist textbooks in the late 1520s,[106] and became common in medical writing from the 1530s onwards, following the translation of Galen's semiological works in 1528 at Paris.[107] K. J. Höltgen's article of 1965 pointed to the tabular presentation of Galen's *De differentiis morborum* by Leonhart Fuchs published at Basle in January 1536/7 as the earliest large-scale case of such publication; but Fuchs himself acknowledges that a certain Stephanus Dutemplaeus preceded him, with his *Tabulae sex in sex Galeni libros de morbis et symptomatis*, which Baudrier records as being published by Sebastian Gryphius at Lyon in 1530.[108] This publication also stimulated Johannes

---

[103] Murdoch 1984.
[104] Kretzmann, Kenny and Pinborg 1982: 540–63; Ottosson 1984: 176–7; Schmitt 1983a: 56; Evans 1980; Höltgen 1965; Koch 1998; Joutsivuo 1999: 37, 241–2; Maclean 2001. There are numerous examples in the later part of our period, e.g. in the works of Taurellus 1581; du Laurens 1596; Campilongo 1601; Bartolettus 1619.
[105] Bylebyl 1990: 31.
[106] E.g. in Simon de Colines's *Grammatographia*, where the publisher comments on the use of diagrams for pedagogical purposes: see Kusukawa 1998: 133–4: 'et generales formae magnis chartis compinguntur, ut in abditioribus studii locis parietibus adfigi possint, quo semper domi, discentes habeant prae oculis quousque formae illae mente sint conceptae tenaciterque haereant, compinguntur et in libro cum formis tabulisque specialibus, ut foris etiam existentibus non desit proficiendi occasio'.
[107] The semiological works of Galen published in Latin by Simon de Colines in 1528 were the *De differentiis symptomatum* and the *De differentiis morborum*.
[108] The acknowledgement of Dutemplaeus is in the note to the reader on the first page of Fuchs's work: 'quum superioribus diebus post Galeni de Temperamentis atque simplicium medicamentorum facultatibus libros, eum quoque, qui de Morborum differentiis ab eodem

Agricola (Ammonius) (*c.* 1490–1570) to plan to produce at Augsburg a similar 'tabella' for a different work of Galen in 1534, and probably inspired Christophorus Heyll's limited use of visual dichotomies in his edition of the medieval medical writer Alphonsus Betrutius at Mainz in the same year.[109] One of the most elaborate early examples of such 'tabellae' is Sylvius's *Methodus sex librorum Galeni in differentiis et causis morborum et symptomatum in tabellas sex ordine suo coniecta*, published at Paris in 1539 by the Wechel publishing house, whom Ramus himself was later to employ.[110] This not only has a vast array of Galenic loci organised in bracketed dichotomies, but also has exhaustive combinatories (see below, 5.2), all employed to help the less able to grasp the subject under discussion.[111] Sylvius chooses not only to order miscellaneous dicta on signs scattered throughout the Galenic corpus in the endoxical mode, but to deal also with more restricted and even scientific (i.e. causally demonstrative) material in this work, which is only matched in its scale to my knowledge by Theodor Zwinger's (1533–88) *In artem medicinalem Galeni tabulae et commentarii*, printed in Basle in 1561.[112] Diagrams can also be used as a bridge between disciplines, as Johann Grün points out in introducing the 'skiagraphia' which he places in his adaptation of Melanchthon's syncretist *Liber de anima*.[113] Another motive for producing them is said to be clarity and brevity: Sylvius goes as far as to say that they are particularly helpful to the less intelligent reader.[114]

These and other examples had a marked effect on medical publishing which cannot, I think, be ascribed to the influence of Ramus, but to

---

inscribitur, ac reliquos quinque nunc sequentes publice enarrandos suscepissem: casu, neque tamen sine magno uestro (si quid iudico) commodo, in eas quas anno abhinc sexto Stephanus Dutemplaeus edidit tabellas indici, in quibus ferme totum, quod Galenus in sex libris de Morborum symptomatum atque differentiis et causis diffuse scripsit, mira breuitate complexus est'. See also Baudrier 1895–1921: 8.57; Maittaire 1722: 574.

[109] On Agricola Ammonius, see Dilg 1991: 194. See also Heyll 1534: 88–9, where the diagram is introduced by the words: 'quod ne obscurum sit methodicae artis studiosis (nam amethodos, et non diligentissimos prohibeo plane a librorum meorum lectione) placuit subiicere quae quibus locis inueniatur ad hunc modum'.

[110] On Wechel, see Maittaire 1722: 12ff. The differences between Fuchs's and Sylvius's dichotomies of the same works by Galen show how difficult the art of endoxical division was: cf. the comment by their Pisan colleague Argenterio 1610: 1463, written about a decade later: 'quantum enim difficile sit bene diuidere docet Aristoteles *initio operis de partibus animalium* tantoque profecto difficilior nobis est diuidendi ratio, quod nemo hactenus ex antiquis scriptoribus eam satis explicare sit conatus'.

[111] Akakia 1549: 59, 83 (the illustration is included 'ut [doctrinam] clarius intelligamus').

[112] See also Huggelius 1560.

[113] Quoted below in 3.4 from Kusukawa 1998: 133; Nutton 1993c.

[114] Sylvius 1539a: a 5r: 'ea [i.e. these materials] in tabellas coniecimus, ut iam possit etiam mediocriter doctis, cum opus erit, in usum uenire'.

developments internal to medical publication. By the 1570s, all major European medical publishing centres apart from those in Spain and Italy (which for some reason seem to eschew nearly all use of the tree diagram)[115] were making free use of the dichotomous table for a variety of purposes: both for anacephaleoses, and for divisions of material according to both scientific and endoxical principles.[116] Authors and publishers stressed the pedagogical usefulness of this mode of presentation, and there is even evidence that it was used in lectures.[117] A late and very ambitious use of the diagram in medical writing was that made by Ernestus Fridericus Fabricius in 1626, who sets out to reduce all of Galenic and Paracelsian medicine to comparative tables.[118] But just as in the case of law, discursive divisions are just as much used as visual representations,[119] and even one of the few medical texts to declare itself to be written in a Ramist mode (David Crusius's (1589–1640) *Theatrum morborum hermetico-hippocraticum, seu methodica morborum et curationis eorundem dispositio* of 1615, announced in 1612 as *Idea morborum hermetico-hippocratica methodo Ramea adornata*) contains in fact only one synoptic table, and a great deal of material presented in commentary or quaestio form.

2.5 BIBLIOGRAPHIES AND LIBRARIES

2.5.1 *The book market*

I come next to the issue of accessibility: how did a doctor find out about books on any given subject, and how did he get access to them? Before the production of book fair catalogues by the major Frankfurt and Leipzig booksellers, correspondence with colleagues and references in printed books were the principal ways of learning about recent productions;

---

[115] There are a few exceptions to this rule in Italy (Jacopo Zabarella's often reprinted *Tabulae logicae* of 1580 and Fabio Paolino's *Tabulae isagogicae* to Joannitius in the 1608 edition of Avicenna's *Canon* are two); it is surprising that a culture which began the century with copious use of mathematical diagrams should avoid the bracketed dichotomous table as though tainted by the pedagogical theories of Ramus. Note also the Wittenberg statutory prohibition of the use of Ramist modes of teaching: Friedensburg 1926: 537–54; but see note 117, below.

[116] See Maclean 2001.

[117] A surviving copy of a medical disputation delivered in Wittenberg in 1601 under the presidency of Jacobus Cocus contains manuscript notes which include not only the transcription of the dichotomies found in André du Laurens's *De crisibus* of 1596 but also a presentation by tree diagram of the disputation subject (*De signorum discretione*) by the praeses himself; the copy is to be found in the Universitäts-und Landesbibliothek, Halle.

[118] Fabricius 1626.

[119] Two examples of doctors eschewing the use of diagrams while using diairesis are Thriverus 1592 and Varanda 1620.

when a doctor found out about a book, he then sought to borrow it from a local source, or get some patron to buy it for him.[120] There were also some collections of books available for consultation in universities by the end of the century: the German nation in Padua had its own library, as is well known, and among the early acquisitions of the Bodleian Library in Oxford is a comprehensive collection of medical books.[121]

By 1612, furthermore, there had appeared a significant number of bibliographical guides either arranged by subject or specific to medicine.[122] These tend to be thorough and unselective, in the same way the fair catalogues are; indeed some of them are no more than organised compendia of catalogues available at fairs (including publishers' and booksellers' catalogues). The fair catalogues themselves were used by those wishing to build up collections: the professor at Heidelberg was in fact instructed by the revised university statutes of 1558 to attend the fair and make desirable purchases, and a similar practice was instituted at the Bodleian in its early years.[123] This ensured diffusion and accessibility in Northern Europe; the same does not seem to hold for Italy, and in the sale catalogues of book agents who obtain their second-hand material there in the early seventeenth century, it is extremely rare to find books from north of the Alps.[124] There seems to me to be more citation of recent Catholic authors by protestants than vice versa, although even authors of forbidden books (such as Paracelsus) are discussed (usually allusively and critically) by Italian doctors, as I suggested above (2.3). The editions of Italian and Spanish writers referred to by Northern protestants are often those produced outside Italy, and reflect the speculative publishing of works from abroad, which is a feature also of Italian publication.[125] It has often been said that Spain remains somewhat isolated from European intellectual debate after the measures of 1558–9 designed to control the importation of ideas, but the inventories of private medical libraries in Valladolid which I have seen suggests that more penetration of foreign books occurred than is generally thought.[126]

---

[120] Hornung 1626: 387 [ccv] (letter of Petrus Hofman to Sigismund Schnitzer about the books he has been recommended, dated 13 November 1602: 'istos in hoc genere authores, quos significas, non habeo, videbo tamen an ex clementissimi Nostri Principis Bibliotheca habere aut petere possim').

[121] Rossetti 1969; James 1605: 181–217.

[122] See above, note 12.

[123] Stübler 1926: 33–42; Pollard and Ehrmann 1965: 77, 66 (quoting W. D. Macray and Thomas Hearne).

[124] See for example *Catalogus* 1637.

[125] See for example Rhodes 1987.

[126] See Lynch 1964–9: 1.236–41; Rojo Vega 1997.

2.5.2 Book ownership

I come finally to the issue of the field of medical knowledge seen as a whole, and to the question of ownership and use of medical books. By the end of the period I am discussing, there seems to be a strong family resemblance between the real and ideal libraries which are recorded over a wide area of Europe. By ideal library, I mean a recommended reading list for students and practitioners: Rodericus a Castro of Hamburg produces one of these (which happens to exclude Paduan authors) in his *Medicus-politicus* of 1614; Petrus Laurembergius produces another for students at Leiden at 1621.[127] The bibliographies of Le Coq (Gallus) and Schenck are non-selective; there are also specialist bibliographies on dosage, sympathy and antipathy, mirabilia, and occult diseases.[128] Of real libraries, the collections of Caspar Peucer (1525–1602), Simone Simoni (1532–1602), Wolfgangus Waldungus, Gregor Horst (1578–1636), Sir William Paddy (1554–1634), Thomas Lorkin (1528?–91), and Caspar Bauhin all of about the same period give an indication of the assiduity with which new publications across the whole field of medical learning, including popular and vernacular works, were acquired,[129] and the possession of similar libraries is deducible from the writings of figures in universities such as Fortunio Liceti (1577–1657), the omnivorous reader and refuter of the opinions of others, town physicians like Andreas Libavius at Rothenburg an der Tauber, and court doctors such as Joseph du Chesne. Their libraries cover the whole range of medical writing; much of this would have been familiar to doctors living in 1500, although parts of the sections on anatomy, botany, chemistry and zoology might have been unfamiliar to them. In some cases, the collections which survive testify to the assiduity with which the books were read: this is the case with Waldungus's books, nearly all of which bear the marks of careful reading in the form of marginalia and summaries. It is of interest to note that the smaller formats, which are as much annotated as any others, are not always recorded in inventories and donors' books, suggesting that librarians of the time paid more attention to grand tomes than did the practically minded doctors who possessed both these and less impressive volumes.[130] It is interesting to note also that in some of the recorded

---

[127] Castro 1614: 84–91; Laurembergius 1621.
[128] Hasler 1578: 14–15 (dosage); Nutton 1985a: 89–90 (surgery); Eckart 1992: 150 (Sennert); Horst 1621 and Müncerus 1616 (occult disease); on a wider range of issues, Gallus 1590; Schenck 1609b; Dodoens 1581: a6–7 (on mirabilia literature).
[129] Kolb 1976 (Peucer); Madonia 1988 (Simoni); Nutton 1987: 14; Sayle 1921 (Lorkin); Gunther 1921; Fuggles 1975 (Paddy).
[130] Jones 2000.

libraries of practising doctors around 1600 (Bauhin, Horst, Waldungus, Paddy), there are still incunabula cited;[131] this is an index of the similarity of the field of medical learning over one and a half centuries. Another index is to be found in the 1625 student textbook version of Pietro d'Abano's *Conciliator*: new issues (such as the 'morbus totius substantiae' and the debates in anatomy and etiology) have been interpolated, but the general framework is the same.

2.6 CONCLUSIONS

I should now like briefly to return to the questions which I asked at the beginning of this chapter, and offer some tentative answers. I should wish to argue that the learned medical book was international rather than local in character by 1600, even if there seems to be little direct presence of books produced in the north of Europe in Italian libraries at this time; that its operation was considerably aided by the institutionalisation of the Frankfurt Book Fair in the 1560s, and given a new character by the dissemination of chemical medicine in the decade which followed, so much so that the heading of the book fairs was changed for a time to 'libri medici et chymici'; that it was sustained largely by speculative publication financed more by publishers or patrons than by the authors themselves; that it was omnivorous, consuming ancient and medieval medicine with the same appetite as new theories and new syntheses, and local productions as much as foreign ones; that over time instruments were elaborated to allow access to the whole field of production; and that it was reinforced by a very active network of correspondence, and given an international character by travelling students and academics. The features I should like here to stress are the role of the printer-publisher, whose mediation of learned books ties medical intellectual activity both to commercial interests and to patronage networks which are often ideological in character; and the coherence of the period 1470–1625 in broad outline, constituting a universe of discourse which allows by the end of the period an author to cite a classical authority, a medieval, and a modern in the same lemma.[132] Humanist medicine seems to me to have brought about aggregation, and some modification, but not a transformation of the field of medical knowledge. Knowledge was accumulated,

[131] Horst's library is printed in the introduction to his *Opera omnia* of 1641.; Bauhin's appears in Bauhin 1614: 12–36. Walding's library is now in the Herzog-August-Bibliothek, Wolfenbüttel; on William Paddy's library see Fuggles 1975.

[132] One example would be a marginalium from Crusius 1615: 3 citing Galen, Arnau de Vilanova and Giambattista da Monte on the same point.

and given an eclectic character by its preservation in libraries in which were juxtaposed ancient, medieval, humanist and more recent texts on the same subject.

A prominent printer-publisher (the Giunti) claimed early in the history of printing that it had the power to 'reconcile factions' by promoting works of collocation and conciliation; this claim has been repeated by Elizabeth Eisenstein, and associated by her with the newly discovered ease of conferring two printed editions with each other.[133] This is not how I see the situation: in respect to Eisenstein's point, I think she has underestimated the prodigious amount of textual information carried in the heads of medieval and early modern scholars who were perfectly capable of conferring these texts with each other without the invention of the 'fixity' of type; and in respect of Giunti's claim, it seems to me that the effect of printing was to generate an interpretation boom, further fuelled by ideological involvements such as crypto-Calvinism and Philippism (and its enemies), which is evinced in the steadily growing numbers of published books in the second half of the century.[134] But, if these were not the effects of printing, what were they, and how did its mediation of medical knowledge affect that knowledge? I should like tentatively to suggest the following: that the practice of printing medical books did not point up, but rather blurred, the distinction between classical and modern texts, even if contemporaries were able to cite the views of 'neoterici' as heterodox in respect of their ancient forebears; that there is evidence that doctors were voracious and attentive readers, in comparison to other professional groups; that diversity of opinion was fostered by the accessibility of a wide range of texts, at least in Northern Europe; and that a small group of rich and international publishers had much to do with the dissemination of medical knowledge beyond national frontiers, and may even have shared an ideological commitment to its increased accessibility, which was in harmony with the secular approach to medical and philosophical learning espoused by those Italian universities in which many of their authors had spent some time.

---

[133] Eisenstein 1979: 573–4; Tommaso Giunti, in his edition of the *Opera omnia* of Aristotle and Averroes of 1550–2, I.2–3, quoted by Cranz 1976: 125.

[134] Maclean 1991.

CHAPTER 3

The discipline of medicine

Of all arts, medicine is the most difficult.
(Camerarius)[1]

3.1 INTRODUCTION

In this chapter I set out to examine the university discipline of medicine
and its relationship with other disciplines, before looking at the professional status of the doctor. This will involve describing the composition
of the medical course, the status of medicine as a science and as an art,
the sects of medicine in relation to the intended product of the medical
course, the rational doctor, and the disciplinary interactions with natural
philosophy, law and theology.

3.1.1 Theory and practice

In medieval universities, the division between theoria and practica is
found universally; theoria involving a general understanding of the arts
course and the physiological principles specific to medicine; practica
constituting a body of information of proven medical usefulness. There
is an implied hierarchy here, in that all knowledge of causes is seen as
superior to the application of such knowledge; paradoxically however,
the practicus contains the theoricus, and not vice versa, as this Salernitan
syllogism indicates:

> Every master of practica is a master of theoria, but this proposition
> is not convertible
> The Salernitan master is a master of practica
> _____
> Therefore the Salernitan master is a master of theoria.[2]

---

[1] Camerarius 1626–30: 20 [i.32]: 'medicinam omnium artium esse difficillimum'.
[2] Herberger 1981: 162: 'omnis practicus est theoricus, sed non convertitur; sed magister Salernus
est practicus; ergo magister Salernus est theoricus'; see also Siraisi 1987a: 10 (on Avicenna,

Galen reinforces this implied hierarchy by describing practica (which is concerned with therapeutics) as inferior to the more theoretical parts of medicine such as physiology, pathology and semiotic;[3] but there is a marked trend from the fifteenth century onwards of revaluation of practica. Michaele Savonarola and later Giambattista da Monte argue that both practica and theoria are deployed to the same end, but are characterised by different habits of mind; they and others give precedence to Galen's *Methodus medendi* over theoretical texts, including the relevant sections of Avicenna's *Canon* and the *Ars parva*.[4] The movement to enhance the dignity of operative or mechanical knowledge is not confined to medical studies, being found in such disparate authors as Bernard Palissy and Petrus Ramus.[5] It is reflected, as has been noted (1.5.1), in universities; it may be connected to the growth in the numbers of published consilia; it can be detected at the end of our period in Gregor Horst's revisions to the relevant questions in the *Conciliator*.[6]

3.1.2 Other divisions

The twofold division of practica-theoria coexists with others which divide the field into either five divisions following the Alexandrian model: physiology, pathology, semiology, hygiene and therapy; or six, by the addition of etiology.[7] Therapy is seen to be the province of practica; it is characterised by the precept 'contraria contrariis curantur'; and it is usually calqued on Rhazes's ordering of illnesses 'a capite ad plantam pedis'.[8] Hygiene is separate from the others because of the difference in

Canon, i.1–2); Ottosson 1984: 72 (on Avicenna, *Canon*, i.1.1.1). The syllogism makes of practice the genus of which theoria is a species; but theoria precedes its genus in dignity and in pedagogical priority.

3 Bylebyl 1991: 159; Campilongo 1601: 1–4; Cesalpino 1593: 171ff.

4 Bylebyl 1991: 163, 169, 183 (citing Savonarola and da Monte); the same argument was used to promote clinical precepting by Capivaccius (*ibid.*, 163). On unity of medicine as a discipline see Galen, *Ad Thrasybulum*, K 5.848–9. See also Manardo cited by Mugnai Carrara 1999: 263 (opposing the distinction between theoria and practica).

5 Ramus attacks the distinction theoria and praxis (which he equates to that between analysis and synthesis) in the writings of Simplicius: see Bruyère 1984: 77. On Palissy see Henry 1997: 28 and Blair 1997: 53.

6 Horst 1621: 4 (a discussion of two senses of the distinction theoria and practica); see also Mikkeli 1992: 178.

7 Mikkeli 1999: 32ff.; for etiology, see Pseudo-Galen, *Introductio seu medicus* and Joutsivuo 1999: 101; this is divided in the Middle Ages between a general and a special study of causes, according to Ottosson 1984: 247ff. Sometimes etiology is substituted for pathology; *ibid.*, 70. For examples of the citing of five parts of medicine, see Capivaccius 1606: 1017; Horst 1609: 15; Sennert 1650: 1.261; Fuchs 1531: 8r (it is he who is responsible for promoting the division). See also Siraisi 1987a: 101.

8 Bylebyl 1991: 167.

the mode of intervention of the doctor, who in seeking to conserve health
follows the precept 'similia similibus conservantur';[9] hygiene, together
with physiology and pathology, are sometimes ordered by reference to
the 'res non naturales', 'res naturales' and 'res praeter naturam' (see
below 7.4) respectively.[10] Other classifications separate physiology, etiology and semiology (as theoria) from hygiene and therapy (as practica).[11]
Yet others point out that there can be no perfect division, as any of the
above versions excludes such issues as treating convalescents and the
old, the use of aliments, and prophylaxis.[12] For most doctors, semiology,
although clearly theoretical, is also involved both in the study of effects
and in reasoning from effect to cause (below 4.3.6), and is thereby to
be assigned to practica; it sits therefore on a sort of frontier, making it
particularly pertinent to the study of the range of interpretative methods
used in medicine, as will be seen (below chapters 6–8).

3.2 ART AND SCIENCE

Related to the division between theoria and practica is the question
whether medicine is an art or a science. It encapsulates the following
issues: the dignity of the discipline; its social usefulness; its epistemology
and its characteristic methods; its relationship to other disciplines; and
its relationship to truth. Hippocrates was credited with founding the rational 'art' of medicine, and Plato followed him (according to Hollerius)
in attributing to the 'practice' the three criteria of experience, prudence
and reason;[13] but it is Aristotle from whom the authoritative distinction of art and science in respect of disciplines derives. This is set out
in *Nicomachean ethics*, vi.4 (1140 a 1–24),[14] a passage which is cited by

---

[9] Liddel 1628: 11ff.
[10] Bartolettus 1619: 213. According to Mikkeli 1999: 35, Janus Cornarius claims that etiology
consists in both semiology and therapy, as both are linked to 'res praeter naturam'.
[11] Angelo Poliziano, cited by Mikkeli 1999: 34–5.
[12] Argenterio 1610: 85, cited by Mikkeli 1999: 36; Joutsivuo 1999: 100–5.
[13] See pseudo-Galen, *Introductio seu medicus*, cited by Siraisi 1990c: 223; Hollerius 1582: 3v; he seems
to be referring to *Laws*, 857 c–e. Myles Burnyeat has pointed out to me that the association
of 'empeiria', 'phronēsis' and 'logos' occurs in *Republic*, ix.8, 582 a, but without mention of
medicine.
[14] 'Let it be assumed that there are five qualities through which the mind achieves truth in affirmation or denial, namely art or technical skill, scientific knowledge, prudence, wisdom and
intelligence. Conception and opinion are capable of error . . . An object of scientific knowledge
exists of necessity. It is therefore eternal . . . All art deals with bringing something into existence . . . [It] is a rational quality, concerned with making, that reasons truly . . . Prudence
(practical wisdom) is not science, because matters of conduct admit of variation, and not art,
because doing and making are generically different . . . Wisdom must be a combination of
intelligence and scientific knowledge . . .'

Renaissance doctors,[15] together with the locus from *Metaphysics*, ii.1 (993 b 20f.) on the distinction between theoretical knowledge which relates to truth and being and practical knowledge which relates to action and coming-to-be. The same book contains a definition of art as both productive craft and knowledge of universals (i.1, 981 a 13f.) which attributes universality and teachability to the latter but not the former, and establishes a tripartite division of scientia into speculative, practical and productive modes (vi.1–2, 1025 b 20, 1026 b 6).[16] In a lay medical and non-philosophical context, Celsus produces a version of this combination of theory and practice by referring to the dual need in doctors for a method based on reason, drawing on information apprised directly by the senses.[17] This distinction is also that frequently cited between universals and scientific truth on the one hand and particulars and utilitarian knowledge on the other, which, according to ancient authority, is the source of all the arts and sciences.[18] Whether medicine is more the latter than the former had been debated from the time of Galen onwards;[19] in pseudo-Galen's *Definitiones medicae*, there is a division of the arts into theoretical, practical, productive and possessive, with medicine being placed in the third of these classes.[20] Galen also seems to have thought that it was only a science in a very broad sense of that word.[21] In the medieval period, Aquinas follows Boethius in seeing it primarily as art;

---

[15] Capivaccius 1606: 1009–10 follows the passage quoted in the previous note, and distinguishes between 'habitus principiorum' ('intellectus'), 'scientia' ('habitus conclusionis'), 'sapientia' ('habitus utriusque'), 'prudentia' ('habitus activus') and 'ars' ('habitus effectivus'). This last formulation is also used by Horst 1609: 11, citing *Nicomachean ethics*, vi.4, 1140 a 21–2 ('habitus animi effectivus cum vera ratione'). Cf. the use of 'lex sapientiae' by Ramus in his commentary on the conditions 'kata pantos', 'kath'auto' and 'katholou prōton' (*Posterior analytics*, i.4, 73 a 28ff.) in Ramus 1569: 31. See also Bruyère 1984: 267–75.

[16] Cited repeatedly by Argenterio 1606–7: 1.24–31, not only against Galen but also against Arabic commentators and neoterici such as da Monte. Argenterio downgrades even the trivium to 'peritiae' rather than arts.

[17] *De medicina*, Proemium, 74: 'rationalem quidem puto medicinam esse debere, instrui vero ab evidentibus causis, obscuris omnibus non ab cogitatione artificis sed ab ipsa arte reiectis'; cf. Liddel 1628: 605: 'definitur methodus curativa perfecta ratio et ordo inveniendi per intentiones et indicationes certa cuique morbo remedia, gratia sanitatis amissae restituendae'. Celsus also describes medicine as an 'ars coniecturalis': *De medicina*, Proemium, 48.

[18] Da Monte 1587: 13, cited by Wear 1973: 221; on the implicit distinction here between descriptive and prescriptive, see Herberger 1981: 223.

[19] Cardano 1565: 82v points out that Galen upbraids Hippocrates for saying that medicine was no more than a conjectural art; he records the latter as claiming in the *Liber de prisca medicina* that 'medicina non semper nec exacte verum continet', and gives three Galenic loci attacking this proposition (*In aphorismos*, i, K 17b.346–56; *In prognostica*, iii, K 18b.306–13; *Liber de venae sectione*, K 2.147ff.)

[20] Ottosson 1984: 69.

[21] Galen, *Ars parva*, i, K 1.307; Horst 1609: 11.

Avicenna sees it as both science and art in more or less equal measure; Averroes considers it to be no more than the highest form of art.[22] In the Renaissance edition of Arnau de Vilanova's exposition of the first aphorism of Hippocrates, there is an excursus (lifted from Avicenna's *Metaphysica*) which relates medicine to the speculative sciences (metaphysics, physics, mathematics), from which it draws its principles.[23]

3.2.1 Quaestiones

Per-Gunnar Ottosson, Nancy Siraisi and Heikki Mikkeli have given excellent accounts of this debate as it develops in the course of the Middle Ages and Renaissance, involving both doctors and natural philosophers; throughout this period it is determined by a set of quaestiones: does medicine take its principles from natural philosophy? How does the distinction between science and art relate to that between theory and practice? Does it contain certain knowledge, and can it aspire to apodictic demonstration? How does it relate to the mechanical arts? Is it a unified field of knowledge? What role do particulars play in it?[24] A number of new issues emerge in the Renaissance: one of these which is discussed by several mid-century doctors is the status of anatomy either as scientia (as a branch of natural philosophy) or as an empirical practice.[25] Another is the relationship between arts and sciences and doctrine or method, as Gilbert and others, who have examined the disagreements between the Italian scholars Niccolò Leoniceno, Giambattista da Monte and Giovanni Manardo, have shown.[26] Hieremias Thriverus of Louvain also comments on this latter issue: he bases his claim that medicine is a science on its use of both resolutive and compositive reasoning (see below 4.3.5), and compares the discipline to a building whose roof is 'sanitas', whose walls are 'remediorum discrimen' and whose foundations are 'corporum, morborum, signorum, causarum differentiae'.[27]

---

[22] McVaugh in Arnau de Vilanova 2000: 139–54; Aquinas, *In Boethium de trinitate*, 5.1 ad 5. On related issues see Mikkeli 1992: 167–79 (resolutive and compositive methods); Herberger 1981: 177 (on arts and infinites); Ferdinandus 1611: 14–15 (on the limits of art expressed in terms of Ockham's razor).

[23] Arnau de Vilanova 1585: 1680–90. I am indebted to Michael McVaugh (and through him, Alfonso Maierù) for the information recorded here about the interpolation.

[24] Ottosson 1984: 68–74; Siraisi 1981: 118–37, 314–17; Siraisi 1990c: 219–30 (referring to *Conciliator*, iii.7); Mikkeli 1992: 135–47 (tracing the views of Vernia, Achillini, Leoniceno, Manardo, Paterno, Zimara and Zabarella).

[25] Siraisi 1994b: 65, 67 (quoting Gessner); Cardano 1565: 110r (i.5.4).

[26] Gilbert 1960; Mikkeli 1992; Jardine 1997; for Manardo's views, see Mugnai Carrara 1999: 261–2.

[27] Thriverus 1592: 3.

This description gives the semiological part of medicine a fundamental role; it can be associated with the ancient descriptions of medicine, whether art or science, as conjectural; an art or science moreover which has to be satisfied with incomplete or even competing explanations of phenomena.[28] This does not mean, according to some, that the precepts of medicine are uncertain; only its practice, as Valleriola explains:

> medicine is not called conjectural through the precepts which are taught in it, as these possess perpetual and necessary truth, but through its practice and its work of healing, which, being uncertain and having an uncertain outcome, reduce the art to one of conjecture.[29]

For others, the conjectural part of medicine resides in the treatment of wounds and external lesions of the body, and the science in the contemplation of its complexion and diseases; a distinction which separates surgeons from physicians.[30] Argenterio's discussion of the topic is perhaps the most subtle of the century. He, like Thriverus, concentrates his attention on the semiological aspect of medicine; he describes this as a conjectural art, like mechanics, which deals with particulars (insofar as individuals, not classes of individuals, are cured by the art), with effects rather than causes, and with coming-into-being rather than being itself, which is the object of the highest science; yet medicine can aspire through its identification of causes to the status of a science by possessing some elements of apodictic demonstration.[31] These views are consistent with

[28] *Ars parva*, K 1.353; Wolf 1620: E4r (citing the formulation 'technikon stochasmon'); Taub 1997: 86–7. Cf. Aristotle, *De generatione animalium*, iv.3, 769 b 3–4: 'it is not easy by stating a single mode of cause to explain the causes of everything'; and Ptolemy's conjectural art (*Tetrabiblos*, i.2.9), which is unable to provide the full answer, and so can sometimes lead to error. Ptolemy explicitly compares astrologers, who, as well as using their knowledge of the stars, take into account nationality, country, upbringing and other accidental qualities, with doctors, who speak of both the sickness itself and the idiosyncrasy of the patient.

[29] Valleriola 1577: 558: 'non enim a praeceptis quae in ea [medicinali arte] traduntur, coniecturalis est dicta ut quae perpetua sint et necessariae veritatis, sed ab actione et medentium opera. Haec enim incerta et incertum eventum habentia coniectricem artem reddunt.' See also Cardano 1565: 82–3 (i.3.20: 'medicina an ars coniecturalis?'), where he records the Hippocratic claim that 'medicina non semper nec exacte verum continet', and creates the following division of arts: 'certa per se' (such as arithmetic), 'certa per se, coniecturalis exercitatione' (medicine and agriculture) and 'coniecturalis per se et in exercitatione' (divination). See also Joutsivuo 1999: 49n, citing Averroes, *Colliget*, i, on medicine as an 'ars operativa ex principiis veris'); Albanesius 1649: 7: 'ars' as 'habitus intellectus conceptus ex variis memoriis eorundem eventuum in operationibus directus ad simile operandum'.

[30] Josse Clichtove, *De artium scientiarum divisione introductio*, Paris, 1520, pp. 10–11, cited by Mikkeli 1998: 119.

[31] Argenterio 1606–7: 24–31; Siraisi 1990a: 174–5. Ferdinandus 1611: 5–7 attacks these views of Argenterio. On other revisions of the Conciliator's answers to his quaestiones on medicine as an art or science see Matthaeus 1603: 1ff. and Horst 1621: 1–9.

the art of medicine being seen as principally sign-based: 'The whole art has to begin from signs', as Vega put it; although this concern for signs has not a theoretical but a practical end ('curatio').[32]

Another conjectural feature of medicine is its having to deal with infinites and with chance events, as Cardano points out, following Hippocrates:

Among the best of us it is a form of knowledge which is extended not only to individual nations but even individual men, and individual operations, and fortuitous cases . . . and the knowledge of these infinites is in the realm of incorporeal things, into which fall fate, the causes of natural things, and the times, modes and occurrences of singular events, about which there is neither conjecture nor yet certain knowledge.[33]

Elsewhere, Cardano adopts a more novel stance by relating medicine to mathematics rather than natural philosophy. Basing himself on an untraditional set of Galenic loci, he argues that an art can also have the status of a science, that anatomy is such a science, and (against Argenterio) that medicine is an 'ars faciens'.[34] This emphasis is picked up by Sennert at the end of our period, who describes medicine as more 'factiva' through its completion or supplementation of the work of nature, than 'practica', borrowing this distinction from Aristotle. Medicine is for him an operative art; but it is also prescriptive and pedagogical, requiring its own dialectical rules. Its source is not only in 'sensus' and 'mens' but also 'memoria', which is the treasure house of individual instances of diagnosis, prognosis and cure.[35]

3.2.2 Factive art

Mikkeli claims that in the influential work of Jacopo Zabarella of the end of the century the divide between art and science is greater than it was

---

[32] Vega 1571: 159.

[33] Cardano 1663: 8.211–12: 'scientia est apud meliores nobis quae extenditur ad singulas gentes non solum sed etiam homines singulos, et singulas operationes, et casus fortuitos . . . et horum infinitorum ea scientia est apud incorporea, ex qua fatum et causae naturalium et singulorum et tempora et modi et eventus, de quibus nec conjectura est nedum scientia'.

[34] Siraisi 1987a: 51; his novel Galenic loci include a reference to *De elementis*, i, K 1.413ff. Where Argenterio denies that medicine is a 'habitus', Cardano claims that it is; for him 'ars experimentum praesupponit', and implies the passage from the understanding of singulars through the senses to the collection of singulars in the memory mentioned in *Metaphysics*, i.1, 980 b 28–981 a 1; he even speaks of 'artis vel prudentiae habitus', collapsing the distinction which Aristotle carefully makes in the *Nicomachean ethics* (see above note 14). The insistence on factive art is also related to the predominance of sense: see Cardano 1565: 20ff.; Siraisi 1997: 248 (quoting Cardano 1663: 6.360).

[35] Sennert 1650: 1.259–60. On art as the remedy of forgetfulness see Herberger 1981: 182; Wear 1973: 278 (quoting Mondino); Bylebyl 1991: 174 (quoting da Monte); Crisciani 1990.

at its beginning;[36] this claim is consistent with the far greater attention paid to the nature of medicine as an art around 1600. Liddel divides the principles of medical art into three classes: the 'principium inventionis' (which is 'experientia'); the 'principium constitutionis' (which is 'ratio et experientia') and the 'principium interpretationis et demonstrationis singulorum' (which is 'naturalis speculatio'). He follows Zabarella in subordinating medicine to natural philosophy: the natural philosopher has a pure gaze, where the doctor has an instrumental gaze, which makes his art factive ('poiētikē'). This stresses the practical and social dimension ('utilitas') of medicine, and shows that at one level at least the debate about the status of medicine is not a vain squabble over words, but has substantial effects in the real world, which can be associated with the rising value attributed to therapeutics, to clinical precepting, and to the design of hospitals at this time.[37]

3.2.3 Art and nature

The 'ars praestantissima' of medicine is associated with productivity in another way, being not only the minister of nature but also its 'corrector'.[38] This claim seems to contradict the doctrine that the doctor is bound by the laws of nature.[39] It is derived (inaccurately as it happens) from *Epidemics*, vi.5.[40] What is at issue here is the role given to art in respect of 'natura naturans' and 'natura naturata': of God and of nature. Aristotle states in *Physics*, ii.8 (199 a 19–21) that art both imitates nature and completes nature: this was taken to justify not only the practice of alchemy, but also that of the art of medicine, which 'brings about some things which are not possible for nature to bring about' (see below, 7.2.8).[41] The claim was also used to attack the Galenic medical art in so far as this art admits to its inefficacy through acknowledging

---

[36] Mikkeli 1992; Maclean forthcoming a (on the influence of Zabarella in Northern Europe); see also Pittion 1987: 123 on Mersenne's view of medicine in respect of the art/science divide.

[37] Liddel 1628: 3 (who does not acknowledge as sources either Galen, *De crisibus*, iii.8, K 9.735–40 or Cardano 1565: 22v (i.2.3)); García Ballester 1995: 145–7; Siraisi 1990c: 137; Joutsivuo 1999: 159–63.

[38] Liddel 1628: 3; Siraisi 1997: 228–9. This is an anti-Platonic view: see *Laws*, 888 e, cited by Montaigne 1965: 206c (i.31); see also Galen, *Ad Thrasybulum*, K 5.835, 853, 861–2 (giving the two senses of art as 'producer of an object' and 'restorer of an object'); Lucullus in Cicero, *Academica*, xi.7.21, refuted by Giulio Castellani, cited by Schmitt 1967: 25.

[39] Mikkeli 1992: 113–14, citing Zabarella 1597: 1162–3.

[40] Reference is also made to Galen, *Ars parva*, K 1.385; *De crisibus*, 3.viii, K 9.735–40. According to Montfort 2000, the true version should read 'naturae [i.e. individual natures] sunt medici morborum'. See also Cardano 1565: 83 (i.3.21); Ferdinandus 1611: 6.

[41] Newman 1997, 1998; Liddel 1628: 3: '[medicina] nonnulla efficit quae naturae possibilia non sunt'; Wear 1995a: 173 (quoting Edmundson).

the incurable nature of some illnesses.[42] Related to the same claim is the
view that arts are accumulative, and that they are a site of the extension
of human knowledge (see above 1.4).[43]

3.3 MEDICAL SECTS

3.3.1 Old sects and new tendencies

As well as being classified as theory and practice, art and science, rational
medicine is seen in contradistinction to a number of classically defined
sects (methodists and empirics), and, by the end of the century, a number of modern ones (Hippocratics, Paracelsians, and followers of figures
such as Fernel and Argenterio). The three ancient sects are described in
Galen's *De sectis*, which was issued as a plaintext, presumably for use at
the University of Paris in the 1520s, in his *De empirica subfiguratione*, and in
the pseudo-Galenic *Introductio seu medicus*.[44] Although Brasavola suggests
that in the time of Hippocrates, the rational sect relied on reason alone,
and the dogmatic sect on both reason and experience, he is unusual in
this: most of our writers identify the dogmatic with the rational sect, and
both with Galenism; its members are the products of university medical
faculties.[45] Methodists, the second sect, are said not to believe in long
training, experience or complexity of theory: theirs is based on a few
simple (rational) rules derived from three physical states: constricted, relaxed, and a mixture of the two; they do not practise prognosis.[46] They
are supported (perhaps in a less than fully serious way) by Agrippa in his
declamation against learned medicine, and after the end of the century
by Prospero Alpini (1553–1617), although his own account of methodism seems very close to one of practical medicine, and it is worthy of note
that he had previously written a work about prognosis (the *De praesagienda
vita et morte aegrotantium*).[47] Argenterio was accused of methodism by an

---

[42] Temkin 1973: 169.

[43] Agricola 1967: 209: 'artes omneis paulatim et per incrementa repertas esse'; Vega 1571: 893
(on Hippocrates, *Aphorisms*, vii.54); Siraisi 1997: 104.

[44] Siraisi 1990c: 3–5; 1990b: 224. The *De sectis* was issued by Guinther von Andernach in 1528,
together with the *Introductio seu medicus*, which also contains an account of ancient sects. These
are also lucidly described by Celsus, *De medicina*, Proemium, 6f., but his account does not seem
often to be quoted.

[45] Brasavola 1541: 10–11; Liddel 1628: 11.

[46] *Ibid.*; Victorius 1551: 9.

[47] Alpini 1611; 1601. On Agrippa, see Siraisi 1990b. A possible source for methodism is in
Hippocrates, *Nature of man*, ix.

opponent of his theories.[48] The third sect, the empirics, do not take account of hidden causes; they consider only the syndrome of signs evident to the senses. In many ways they seem to act as do practical (Galenic) doctors: but these, as we have seen from the Salernitan syllogism, do have recourse to theory and to hidden causes.[49] The upsurge in practical medicine in the fifteenth century has, however, much to do with the practice of accumulating sensory information about particulars.[50] It seems that the long survival of these labels in medical discourse can in part be ascribed to the need to define heterodox positions, much as heresies function in theology; indeed they are sometimes called heresies.[51]

Around the middle of the century new tendencies begin to appear. As one would expect, the humanist movement in medicine produced a palingenetic desire to identify Hippocrates as the true 'fons et origo' of medicine, from which since there had been a progressive decline. This led not only to the a growth of interest in certain books, notably the *Epidemics*, but also a renewed attention being paid to prognosis, to surgery, to case histories, and to aphoristic expression of medical doctrine (which found support in the humanist vogue for collections of 'loci communes').[52] Cardano was a key figure in this promotion of Hippocrates, but he was far from being alone.[53] Argenterio and Fernel can also claim in a certain way to represent new departures, although both can still be understood inside the discourse of Galen, as can Fracastoro, Vesalius and even the Melanchthonian doctors who associate the anthropology of Luther with rational medicine.[54] The upsurge of interest in scepticism is also linked to medicine, notably through Galen's *De optimo genere docendi*, which Erasmus translated into Latin in 1529, and through the publication of the Latin Sextus Empiricus in 1562 and 1569; but I do not follow Jean-Paul Pittion

[48] Siraisi 1990a: 174–5. He was also accused of being an academic and a Pyrrhonist.
[49] Liddel 1628: 11; Campilongo 1601: 14v; Hankinson 1995: 79.
[50] Daston and Park 1998: 138–42; it has been suggested by Eckart 1992: 157 that Sennert is the heir of this upsurge.
[51] Siraisi 1990a, 1990b, 1997: 27 (recording Andrea Camuzio's description of Cardano as a 'heresiarch'); Herberger 1981: 265–6 (quoting Colerus on medical heresy).
[52] Moss 1996; Goyet 1996; an early medical example is Otto Brunfels, *Theses seu communes loci totius artis medicae*, Strasbourg, 1532.
[53] See Daston and Park 1998: 146 (on Donati and Paré); Smith 1979; Lonie 1985; Nutton 1985a: 89; 1989; Crisciani 1990; Siraisi 1987a: 299–300; Siraisi 1997: 11, 45, 68, 138. Champier 1516a: A3r offers a list of epithets for Hippocrates ('gloriosus, divinus, sapiens, dialecticus medicus, rationalis medicus, clinicus medicus, inventor clinicae medicinae, dieticus medicus') but little else. Hippocrates is not to be equated with medical primitivists such as Leonardo Fioravanti: see Eamon 1993.
[54] Brockliss 1993: 71; Siraisi 1990a: 178–80 (on Alessandrini's claim that Fernel, Mattioli and Gessner all produced knowledge in the old matrix); Herberger 1981: 224; Kusukawa 1995a.

in identifying a strain of sceptical medicine in the early years of the
seventeenth century. The epistemological issues he sets out seem to me
to lead neither to medical empiricism nor to something yet more radical
which rejected the value of all sensory evidence and saw all arguments
as leading to a Pyrrhonist suspension of judgement; the battles being
fought in medical faculties were far more realist (or rather referentialist)
in character.[55]

Paracelsian and chemical or spagyrical medicine (they are sometimes,
but not always linked) is not however easily reducible to existing matrices
of thought, although some opponents try to claim that it is.[56] Paracelsus
recorded, it will be remembered, that others had referred to him as
the Luther of medicine,[57] but although he represented the same anti-
authoritarian stance and insisted in a similar way on the importance of
inner revelation or 'lumen naturae' (below 5.3.5), he diverged by not
being himself a new interpreter of purified texts. As Charles Webster
has shown, his central motivation is religious, and his union of spiritual
and physical medicine closely linked to his own faith and theology.[58]
It is more appropriate to associate the doctrine of hermetic medicine,
of the three principles (salt, sulphur and mercury), of powers, spirits,
correspondences and signatures with the first and second generations
of his popularisers, including Adam von Bodenstein, Gerhard Dorn,
Petrus Severinus, Joseph du Chesne and Oswald Croll.[59] Daniel Sennert,
who as the last great conciliator attempted to reconcile Galenism with
chemical medicine, had to purge it of many of the occult forces to which
it refers, but kept some of its most subversive features, including its
protoatomism.[60] These debates are more than theoretical; one social
consequence was that it had to be determined whether doctors declaring themselves to be Paracelsian should be supported and protected by
(or indeed prosecuted under) the imperial criminal code, the Carolina.[61]

---

[55] Pittion 1987: 106 (citing loci from Galen's *De facultatibus naturalibus* and *De simplicium medicinalium facultatibus*); Galen 1989.

[56] Bartolettus 1619: 259–63; Liddel 1628: 5–9 (who reduces Paracelsianism to empiricism); Horst 1609: 18–19 ('eadem secta, quatenus cum Empiricis convenit, intempestiva experientia peccet, prout autem cum Methodicis affinitatem habet, insufficienti ratiocinationis discursu utatur'). Some supporters (including Severinus 1571: 17–23) also express Paracelsianism in terms of empirical medicine.

[57] Paracelsus 1996: 8.43.

[58] Webster 1995.

[59] Pumfrey 1998; see also Eckart 1992: 146; Kühlmann 1992 (on Croll).

[60] Sennert 1650: 3.697ff.

[61] Sattler 1609.

3.3.2 The rational or dogmatic doctor

As I have already suggested, the discipline of medicine is accumulative: although it recognised deviancies, it did not always reject everything about them. The rational doctor, that is, the ideal product of the educational system of Renaissance universities, is characterised by his training in all parts of logic, astronomy, arithmetic, natural philosophy, pharmacopoeia and ethics, his reliance on 'experientia' both in the form of sensory particulars and in that of past experience and bookish knowledge, his inferential ability which extended where necessary beyond the construal of signs evident to the senses to the determination of hidden causes, his openness to hear indications (of the nature and quantity of remedies) by a sort of rational intuition, his knowledge of materia medica and its applications, and his prognostic powers.[62] He was, in other words, 'a man of judgement who gained understanding from careful observation of patients which then led to a reasoned choice of remedies'.[63] This ideal figure survives long into the seventeenth century, if not beyond, and does not seem to fit easily into Findlen's division of the natural philosophers in the seventeenth century into two tendencies: the old (sacred, occult, professional) and the new (secular, scientific, amateur).[64] In this sense, the guild interests of doctors, their close study of signs, and their rationalised empiricism mark not so much a transition as perennial features of their thinking.[65] Their combination of 'ratio' and 'experientia' which is everywhere proclaimed makes them in retrospect obvious candidates to be forerunners of the new science of the seventeenth century.

[62] Vallesius 1606: 279 (iv, preface), 353–4 (viii, preface: on more experienced doctors being better than young doctors, *caeteris paribus*); Barnes 1991; Cardano 1583: a6r; Siraisi 1997: 228–9; Bylebyl 1991: 174–89 (on da Monte); Castro 1614: 199ff.; Liddel 1628: 9ff., 605–7: 'medici rationales seu dogmatici cum ratione experientiam coniungunt, et causarum tam latentium quam evidentium, item signorum partium affectarum et caeterarum rerum naturalium et non naturalium cognitionem perquirunt'; cf. Celsus, *De medicina*, Proemium, 13, who defines rational medicine as 'abditarum et morbos continentium causarum notitiam, deinde evidentium post haec etiam naturalium actionum, novissime partium interiorum'; Wear 1995a: 165–6, citing John Cotta's view that books and reading are good although not as good as reason and judgement, which give 'daily new increase and light before untried and unexperienced truths'; Gryllus 1566: β4v (on a doctor being a 'technitēs aisthētikos'); Cardano 1565: 24–6 (i.2.4: 'experimentum an sit artis principium'); Bylebyl 1991: 167 (quoting Manardo); Wear 1995a: 163 (quoting Eleazar Dunk); Camerarius 1626–30: 30–9 (i.42–9).
[63] Siraisi 1990b: 225 (paraphrasing Mariano Santo).
[64] Findlen 1994: 10.
[65] See Siraisi 1987a: 111 (on Avicenna's account of the three functions of the doctor: understanding, healing, explaining).

3.4 MEDICINE AND OTHER DISCOURSES:
NATURAL PHILOSOPHY

3.4.1 Natural philosophy

I come now to the relationship of medicine to the disciplines most closely related to it: natural philosophy, law and theology. All of these have their own terms of art and their own discourse: it is part of the task of this book to define that of medicine. But they also have means of intercommunication, not just through the shared propedeutic of the arts course (chapters 4 and 5), but also through a certain grasp of the other discourses, and a recognition of their contiguity. This is indicated in this passage from Grün about his 'skiagraphia' or use of diagrams in his adaptation of Melanchthon's syncretist *Liber de anima*:

> Indeed these diagrams are neither anatomical nor medical, but philosophical, because they contain the first rudiments about the doctrine of the soul and its powers and actions insofar as it is usual and appropriate for philosophers to speak of these, and demonstrate that this part of philosophy is conterminous with theology, the medical art and ethics.[66]

This contiguity (which, as we shall see, poses particular ideological difficulties between medicine and theology: 3.6) is accompanied by a recognition that the discourses are specific to disciplines, and that the principles and procedures of one have to be translated into the notation of another. One example of this would be Clavius's attempt to translate geometry into syllogistic form for the purposes of regrading mathematics in the Aristotelian hierarchy of sciences;[67] another would be Gribaldus's offering of equivalences for terms of art ('regulae' in law becomes 'summae' for theology, 'theses' for logic and 'aphorismi' for physicians).[68]

It is recognised at this time that the higher disciplines have stronger affiliations with different elements of the arts course: theology relates most

---

[66] *Liber de anima in diagrammata methodica digestus*, Wittenberg, 1580, a5r, cited by Kusukawa 1998: 133n: 'haec vero diagrammata neque anatomica sunt neque medica, sed philosophica, quia prima doctrinae de Anima, eiusque viribus et actionibus rudimenta, quantum Philosophus de his dicere solet ac potest, continent, hujusque Philosophiae partis *pragmateian* cum Theologia Arte Medica et Ethica *sunoron* demonstrant'.

[67] Dear 1987: 136–7.

[68] Gribaldus, *De methodo ac ratione studendi*, 1541, 393r, quoted by Herberger 1981: 235. On division of disciplines and terminology see also da Monte 1587: 124–5, quoted in Maclean 1998b: 185; Rebuffi 1586: 3: 'Ne misceam sacra profanis, cum quaelibet scientia suos habeat terminos, theologis et medicis relinquam, et mea sorte contentus, iurisconsultorum verba interpretabor'; Glossa ad C 4.19.23 ('non ut physiologi sed iureconsulti disputamus'): Herculanus 1584: 4.19 (124); Pluta 1991.

closely to metaphysics, the law to moral philosophy, medicine to natural philosophy.[69] This is evident from the number of prominent doctors who interest themselves in matters of natural philosophy, the discipline derived from the various *libri naturales* of Aristotle (notably the *Physics*): one need only mention physicians who were zoologists and botanists such as Guillaume Rondelet, Ulisse Aldrovandi (1524?–1607), Conrad Gessner, Leonhart Fuchs, Pier Andrea Mattioli, and mathematicians and mechanists such as Cardano; and the natural philosophers who speak about medical matters, of whom Jacopo Zabarella (1533–89) is the most obvious case. The relationship in institutional terms is not always harmonious: university chairs of natural philosophy were less well remunerated than those of medicine throughout the period.[70] Galen had written a tract to establish that 'the best doctor is a philosopher' ('optimus medicus philosophus');[71] this suggests a sort of equality, whereas the other often-quoted tag, which states that 'where the natural philosopher leaves off, the physician takes over' ('ubi desinit philosophus, incipit medicus'), suggests (on one reading at least) that medicine may in some sense be subordinated to natural philosophy. It was often claimed that medicine took its 'praecognita', or dogmatic foundations (the elements, the humours, etc.), from natural philosophy, which enjoyed at the time the status of a science (insofar as it was based on the knowledge of causes).[72] This made natural philosophy's interest in things in themselves (its pursuit of 'veritas') superior to medicine's instrumental concerns (its pursuit of 'utilitas'), even if both disciplines were characterised by resolutive method (see below 4.3.6).[73] But it was also possible to argue that medicine was more advanced than natural philosophy in that its interest in the organs of the body and the rational calculus of diseases, causes, symptoms, cures, and prophylaxis is more evolved than natural philosophy; even

---

[69] Camerarius 1626–30: 28, citing Theodor Zwinger, *Theatrum Humanae vitae*, Basle, 1586–7, 1229 (v.2); Mikkeli 1992: 170–1 (quoting Zabarella). Unusually, Arnau de Vilanova 1585: 1694 had said that the study of ethics is not necessary for doctors.

[70] García Ballester 1993b: 41n; Daston and Park 1998: 224; Findlen 1996; Schmitt 1985: 4; Lines forthcoming; on the relative poverty of philosophy see the quotation of Keckermann in note 94.

[71] On these tags, see Schmitt 1985; Kristeller 1961: 45; Wallace 1988: 205; Truman 1994: 49; Sylvius 1539b: 6; Laurembergius 1621: 7; Mikkeli 1992: 180 (quoting Zabarella on 'physiologia' being properly part of natural philosophy).

[72] The Aristotelian locus is *De sensu et sensato*, 436 a 17–b 1. See also Ottosson 1984: 73 (quoting Avicenna); Mikkeli 1992: 132–3 (citing the Conciliator); Wear 1995a: 168 (citing Securis); Capivaccius 1603: 1017; Sennert 1650: 1.260; Blair 1997: 44 (citing Bodin).

[73] Edwards 1976: 294 (on Leoniceno); Joutsivuo 1999: 75 (quoting Agricola Ammonius: see also below 7.2); Jensen 2000: 204–6 (discussing Cesalpino's attack on medicine in respect of botany).

its empirical knowledge of singulars could be turned to its advantage.[74] Through its involvement with quantities and sensibles, it also was linked to 'scientiae mediae' such as optics, astrology, mathematics and mechanics, not all of which were prosecuted within the institution of the university.[75] What is at issue here, as Heikki Mikkeli has recently shown, is both the relative dignity of the disciplines, and the theory of disciplinary subalternation.[76]

3.4.2 Praecognita and procedures

Medicine's borrowings from natural philosophy take the form both of principles and of argumentation. In the case of the former, the many books on *principia naturalia* provide the relevant materials for comprehensive textbooks (see below 7.2).[77] A problem arises here, which Zabarella recognises: for if 'physiologia' belongs properly to natural philosophy and not to medicine, then the status of theoria is compromised. University teachers of medicine were understandably less keen than natural philosophers on abandoning an element of their course which enabled them to lay claim to the status of a science.[78] A further area in which principles are borrowed lies in the area of natural magic (astrology, sympathy and antipathy, transformation and spiritus).[79] The second sort of borrowing – ratiocination – is evident both in the subtlety and complexity of argument (seen best in the practice of distinctiones: see below 4.4.3),[80] and in the recourse to quaestiones. The Renaissance inherited these from various medieval sources, notably from Aquinas, Pietro d'Abano and the Plusquam commentator, Pietro Torrigiano. They may be publicly reviled, but they are very widely used to structure discussions of topics.[81] Their range was certainly extended in the course of the sixteenth century: not only to

---

[74] See Ottosson 1984: 73.

[75] Gabbey 1993: 134n.; Perfetti 1999a: 456 (quoting Pomponazzi on mathematics and medicine as 'scientiae mediae de sensibili').

[76] Mikkeli forthcoming. Capivaccius's *Opusculum de doctrinarum differentiis, sive de methodis, logicis, philosophicis, theologicis, iureconsultis atque medicis pernecessarium*, which addresses these issues, was published as a separate pamphlet in 1562 and 1594: see Capivaccius 1603: 1004–51.

[77] Sennert 1650: 1.1–14; Porzio 1598; Biesius 1573; Siraisi 1987a: 236–9 (on particles).

[78] Schmitt 1985: 5 records however Francesco Patrizi (a natural philosopher) as claiming that medicine does not need natural philosophy.

[79] See Porta 1588; Rice 1976 (on Lefèvre d'Etaples).

[80] See for examples of extreme nicety Horst 1621: 6: 'formale morbi non consistit in privatione, sed in positiva disconvenientia constitutioni sanae contraria'; Lonie 1981: 22, citing Sennert's distinctio between 'calidum innatum' and 'caliditas'.

[81] Bylebyl 1985a: 244–5: 'during the century figures such as Pietro d'Abano and Torrigiano may have suffered considerable abuse at the hands of medical humanism, but they continue to have

encompass some of the material in Aristotle's *Problemata*,[82] but also to formulate quaestiones which drew on newly discovered or re-evaluated texts. These often were theologically contentious, and concerned issues such as atoms and minima naturalia, the soul and its connection with matter, thinking processes, and sexuality.[83] These additions to the corpus of quaestiones still preserve the traditional form, even if they go beyond the traditional content. More radical thinkers claim that natural philosophy had let medicine down; speaking of the definitions of natural, praeternatural and contra-natural, Argenterio complains that these are obscure and uncertain, because the definitions and the principles are not set down, laying the blame for this on Aristotle's expositors.[84]

3.4.3 Aristotle and Galen

An area where this becomes particularly visible lies in the competing medical and physical claims of Aristotle and Galen, which is what inspired the work of the Conciliator in the first place. Pietro d'Abano was not altogether even-handed in his conciliation, preferring Aristotle's views on generation, and clearly dissenting from Galen's on decretorial days;[85] Jerome Bylebyl argues that the work of his Italian successors in the sixteenth century is marked by an initial phase during which Galenism was triumphant, followed by a diffuse Aristotelian revival.[86] This accords well with Andrew Cunningham's proposal that the anatomical project at Padua in the second half of the century was inspired by Aristotelian

a pronounced influence on the agenda and methods of medical controversy'; cf. Grant 1978; Severinus 1571: 7–8 attacks quaestiones as tired and boring. For their use in the discussion of fever, see Lonie 1981: 19; for their use in the genre of controversiae, see Vallesius 1606; for their use in natural philosophy see Porzio 1598 and Biesius 1573. On the adoption of quaestiones from theology, see Horst 1612, cited with parallels from Aquinas by Maclean 1998b: 183.

[82] On these see Blair 1999.

[83] See in general Horst 1621 (who uses the phrase 'sed nota' to mark new material, and has appendices for new quaestiones); on atomism, see Siraisi 1987a: 239–47; on thinking processes, there are new Galenic loci drawn from *De naturalibus facultatibus*, ii–iv, K 2.1–214: on which see Richardson 1985: 178; see also Fracastoro 1574: 1.124 (on 'subnotio'); on sexuality, Cadden 1986 (for medieval views); Maclean 1998b: 184 (citing da Monte 1587: 492–4 on the quaestio 'Venus an omnibus necessaria et quibus legibus usurpanda?', and Parisian theses defended between 1546 and 1620 from *Quaestionum series*, 1752: 'an Venus morbos gignat et expellat?' 'An Venus sit salubris?' 'An Venus virginibus, hystericis, pallidis, biliosis, ictericis, calculosis?'). As well as the passage in Galen's *Ars parva*, K 1.371–2, there are loci in *De locis affectis*, *De tuenda sanitate*, and Hippocrates, *Illnesses of women*; see also Blair 1997: 45f. (on Bodin's claims about new quaestiones).

[84] Argenterio 1610: 228: '[haec sunt] obscura et incerta, quia definitiones et principia eorum non sunt posita': also Patrizi cited by Schmitt 1985: 275n.

[85] Ottosson 1984: 232; Siraisi 1990c: 135–6.

[86] Bylebyl 1985a: 245; also Siraisi 1997: 63 (on the competing authority of Galen and Aristotle).

zoology.[87] It has also been argued that Galen and Aristotle are both seen as the bulwark of traditionalists;[88] I believe that this last view is best seen in the context of prevailing attitudes to all written authorities (see below 5.3). There is at least one other candidate for pre-eminence in authority among the ancients, namely Pliny, but his claims were never successfully pressed.[89] Most natural philosophers in the Italian schools are recognisably Aristotelian in their outlook, and impress their preference on the medical faculties of their universities.[90] This version of Aristotelianism did not exclude the use of empirical data where necessary, as Charles Schmitt has shown: and the naturalism and empiricism of the medical faculties probably owe some of these qualities to their natural-philosophical colleagues.[91]

3.5 MEDICINE AND OTHER DISCOURSES: LAW

I turn now to the uneasy relationship between law and medicine, which as higher faculties competed for the second place behind theology. The dignity of disciplines, and the question of precedence, were not seen as unimportant issues in the medieval and Renaissance period; they even have their place in academic politics today. In Italian universities, law was a faculty separate from the arts faculty, which included medicine: in Padua at least, it was much larger than the arts faculty, and attracted many more external students.[92] The dignity of the faculties was seen both in terms of ceremonial precedence and in respect of their relationship to Aristotelian conceptual categories of preeminence. These are linked to the epistemological status of the two disciplines (as either art, or science, or both), and to a range of positive and negative arguments which are rehearsed by most of those who write on this matter. The epistemological

---

[87] Cunningham 1997; but cf. Bylebyl 1979: 364 (who claims that Padua is solidly Galenist on the issue of anatomy).

[88] Wear 1981.

[89] Schmitt and Skinner 1988: 787 (on Pliny); Schmitt 1976b (on Plato). Walker 1958 has argued for a Platonic form of medicine seen in the work of Ficino and Fernel, but this has not got the elaborate structure and comprehensiveness of Galen and Aristotle.

[90] Schmitt 1985; Siraisi 1987a: 222f. (mentioning Zimara, Achillini, Nifo, Pomponazzi, Zabarella, Cremonini and Liceti).

[91] Schmitt 1969 on the use of experiment by Zabarella, who was 'an empirical Aristotelian in the sense that experience is almost always utilized to corroborate and verify the philosophical and scientific problems of Aristotle'; also Schmitt 1976a (on Girolamo Borro, and the Aristotelian loci supporting experiment in *De caelo*, iii, *Nicomachean ethics*, vi.8, and *De generatione et corruptione*, i).

[92] See Martellozzo and Veronese 1969.

status of the two disciplines can best be seen in their differing uptake from the arts course, which will be examined in detail below (chapters 4 and 5). It may be summarily said here that while both law and medicine are committed to accommodating the logic of the arts course to the practical aims which they serve, they approach the problem of subsuming the individual case under species and genera and of explaining that case in very different ways.

3.5.1 Polemic

It is appropriate here briefly to review the arguments deployed for and against the two faculties; these are somewhat modified in the fifteenth century by the attacks of Florentine humanists on the medical profession, but there is a great degree of continuity also.[93] In favour of law, it is argued that unlike doctors, who only treat the body and the individual human being, jurists deal with the whole body politic ('civitas'), and that they concern themselves with public as well as private good. Both faculties provide the means of enriching their adherents, as the popular couplet has it:

> dat Galenus opes et sanctio Justiniana
> ex aliis paleas, ex istis collige grana[94]

Doctors, however, are noted for their avarice, and for prolonging disease for their own gain or to benefit their reputation; it is alleged that even more than lawyers, they torture people with their remedies, and even can kill them with impunity. Furthermore they have a loathsome preoccupation with the excreta of the body. Doctors naturally respond to these arguments. Doctors are both philosophers and practitioners, whereas, as the saying goes, 'purus legista, purus asinus'; their art is God-given, and their operative powers quasi-divine; they have a privileged model in the figure of Christ the healer;[95] their action in the world is of a higher order, because in contrast to the lawyers, who argue from authority and who deal in accidents, circumstances, and particulars, doctors deal in

---

[93] Garin 1947; Bergdolt 1992.

[94] 'Galen brings riches and Justinian honour; from other disciplines you gather chaff, from these two grain'; cited by Temkin 1973: 131; Herberger 1981: 161–2. Sachiko Kusukawa pointed out to me that Keckermann 1608: 77 adapts this couplet in speaking of philosophers: 'nimirum [philosophiae] contemptu et praeposteris vulgi iudiciis, ex quo etiam orti sunt vulgati illi versiculi: dat Galenus opes, dat Justinianus honores, at nos Philosophi turba misella sumus'.

[95] Siraisi 1999: 360; Cardano 1568: 2.

ratiocination, in substance and in universals. Where the law is stipulative and prescriptive, medicine has an objective outcome, and is bound by the order of nature which it must not oppose.[96] In these exchanges, what is at stake is more than rhetorical advantage; social and institutional precedence had real effects in terms of recruitment, remuneration and privileges.

3.5.2 Medicine's legal rights and duties

The issue of the privileges peculiar to the medical profession and that of the legal functions of doctors are two areas where the two faculties interact more positively. Doctors enjoy certain immunities and privileges under the law, which are set out in books concerning medical ethics and the legal responsibilities of doctors at this time; they also are subject to certain forms of prosecution.[97] They have furthermore areas of expertise and special knowledge which the courts are able to call upon: the most important of these involve the determination (sometimes together with midwives or surgeons) of the material signs of virginity, rape, infanticide, and impotence; the assessment of evidence of simulation of illness, of poisoning, wounding and drowning; questions about legitimacy of children deduced from length of pregnancy, issues concerning plague, contagion, witchcraft and alleged miraculous abstinence; finally, in the case of Catholic countries, passing judgement on supernatural physiological

---

[96] Mikkeli 1992: 141 (quoting Manardo); Obicius 1605; Herberger 1981: 163, 195–7, 204–5, 211ff., 240ff. (quoting Christophorus Ehemius), 264, 267 (quoting Conradus Lagus as conceding that 'cum omnes casus non possunt legibus sigillatim comprehendi, necesse est ius ad Topicae artis subsidium confugere'), 284 (quoting the locus from Pliny, *Natural history*, xxix.1: 'experimenta faciunt [medici] per mortes hominum'); Pictorius 1558: 4; Castro 1614: 42–53 (borrowing much from André Tiraqueau's attack on doctors, but claiming against him that whereas lawyers depend on other writings and argue from grammar, doctors are bound by 'res suas'; that it is no detraction from the dignity of the profession to deal with bodies, and that medicine is not a mechanical but a liberal art: 'ac libere ag[it], cum ratio dictat, non tamen ex lege sed quae rationibus leges suas accommodat non rationes legibus'). On doctors and fatal errors see Juan Luis Vives, *De tradendis disciplinis*, Antwerp, 1531, iv.6 cited by Siraisi 1990b: 229: 'Nam si quem per ignorantiam aut pervicaciam inflexibilem occiderit, quomodo deinceps id damni sarciet? . . . Si quid ab uno theologo erratum sit, ab alio corrigitur; si a jureconsulto, succurritur aequitate judicis, restitutione in integrum . . . quod vero a medico, quis corriget? Homini extincto quis adferet remedium?' See also Camerarius 1626–30: 60 (i.40), quoting Robertus Feuinus, *De abusu medicinae coercendo*, Paris, 1574: 'Solis medicastis hominem impune occidere licet.' On earlier humanist attacks on medicine see Park 1985: 220–36.

[97] Hagecius ab Hagek 1596: 34–44 (citing C 10.52.6); Sattler 1609; García Ballester 1993b: 50. Castro 1614: 200 (on prosecuting bad doctors on the basis of D 1.18.3); on the duties of testimony, see Giovanni Battista Codronchi, *Methodus testificandi*, Frankfurt, 1597, cited by Schleiner 1995: 99; on medical mistakes punishable by law see de Renzi forthcoming (citing Zacchia 1630: vi).

states connected with the process of canonisation.[98] The fullest account of all this is to be found in Paolo Zacchia's compendium entitled *Quaestiones medico-legales*, which first appeared in 1621, and which grew considerably from edition to edition until 1630. The topics he covers determine partly also the nature of medical ethics in the Renaissance, which is most comprehensively covered by Castro's *Medicus-politicus* of 1614. Zacchia writes different introductions for his legal and medical readers, indicating their different expectations and discourses; Wolfgang Sattler's *Theses de iure et privilegiis medicorum* of 1609 was also included in the collected Basle theses of both law and medicine, but the emphasis here is more clearly legal. At issue here is the Constitutio Carolina Criminalis of 1532 and its provisions (35, 134, 149) concerning the medical profession, as well as the relevant parts of the Corpus Juris Civilis; Sattler covers the question of law, medical evidence and women, the interdict on quacks and empirics (which gives rise to the question mentioned above whether Paracelsians are to be penalised under this clause), judicial astrology, wrong treatment and negligence, and the duty to testify in certain cases.[99]

3.6 MEDICINE AND OTHER DISCOURSES: THEOLOGY

At least one of these issues – judicial astrology – concerns theology also, to which I shall now turn. The relationship between Christian theology and medicine had always been an uneasy one: on the one hand, doctors were dignified by the association of Christ with healing; on the other, according to Faith Wallis, 'Christian religious healing, based on relics, prayers and miracles, was radically set over against natural and scientific medicine, grounded in reason and experience.'[100] Belief in the supernatural (including diabolic) causation of disease persisted throughout our period.[101] There were some restrictions on the practice of medicine (or rather surgery) which were codified by a decree of the fourth Lateran Council in 1215.[102] Some of these were perpetuated into the Counter-Reformation: for example, no Jesuit schools taught medicine. Humanist

---

[98] Castro 1614: 251–63; Zacchia 1630 *passim*; Crawford 1994; Siraisi 1999; de Renzi forthcoming cites the Rota Romana as claiming that medical evidence is weak: 'oculus matronarum saepe fallitur . . . et iudicium medicorum similiter est fallax, ut experientia demonstrat'.

[99] Sattler 1609 has a comprehensive set of references to ancient and recent legal texts on these. On the recommendation that empirics who cause the death of their patients be themselves put to death see Ayrer 1592.

[100] Wallis 1995: 117. Nutton 1985b: 49–50 argues that 'from its inception Christianity offered itself as a direct competitor to secular healing'; cf. Amundsen 1996: 8ff., who espouses the opposite view.

[101] Gentilcore 1995; Clark 1997.

[102] Siraisi 1990c: 26.

educational programmes, on the other hand, such as Erasmus's *Ratio seu methodus ad veram theologiam* (1518), were adopted in places like Louvain where medical education also flourished. This contrasted with the rigorous separation of theology and philosophy which was a feature of contemporary Italian universities, making possible a certain freedom of debate. The doctrine of 'duplex veritas', which is associated with the Paris condemnations of natural-philosophical theses by Bishop Tempier in 1277, did not (as is sometimes supposed) prevent the discussion of such delicate issues as the mortality and materiality of the soul, the eternity of the world, the necessity of natural laws, the unicity of the intellect, and atomism: what is prescribed is the conclusion which has to be reached.[103]

3.6.1 Pomponazzi and Catholic Europe

The Pomponazzi affair of the 1510s, the requirement of the Lateran Council of 1513 that the immortality of the human soul be proved philosophically, and the papal bulls of 1516 and 1564 highlighted the conflict between the Church and the universities on these points.[104] The medical faculty in Padua seems to have remained staunchly Pomponazzian and to have insisted on the separation of the disciplines of theology and medicine: an enduring Italian attitude, it seems, if one looks at the work of da Monte, Argenterio, Bernardino Paterno (d. 1592), Francesco Buonamici (d. 1604), and Giulio Pace (1550–1635).[105] This separation allows for the discussion of the Galenic theory of complexion, of which a possible corollary is the materiality of the soul, and a naturalistic approach to sexual activity, deemed to be one of the 'passiones animi' not encumbered by any theological interdicts.[106] Similar views are also cautiously expressed in Paris.[107] Elsewhere, however, the incursion of the

---

[103] Wippel 1977; Niewöhner and Pluta 1999. One example of citation of these quaestiones is found in Agricola 1967: 208 (ii.6): 'est ne mundus aeternus an non? Est ne sol maior tota terra an non? Ecquid est immortalis anima?'

[104] Copenhaver and Schmitt 1992: 107–12; cf. Temkin 1973: 170 (citing Sir Thomas Browne's mention of 'an Italian doctor who could not perfectly believe in the immortality of the soul because Galen seemed to make a doubt thereof').

[105] Siraisi 1987a: 248ff.; Siraisi 1990a; Helbing 1989: 347 (on Buonamici); Schmitt 1987: 223; French 1994: 63 (on Pace). There seems to be an attempt by the Jesuit Pereira to save the situation by dividing metaphysics into two disciplines: Lohr 1988: 606–11; Blair 1997: 43. See also Papy 1999: 334 (on Thomas Fienus) and Maclean 1998b.

[106] Siraisi 1987a: 289ff.; below 7.4 (on sexual activity).

[107] Riolan 1610: 134–5, cited by Brockliss 1993: 81: 'faverem peripateticis, nisi religioni christianae Platonicoarum doctrina ex parte magis consentiret: malim errare cum ecclesia, quam cum philosophis bene sentire'.

ecclesiastical authority into medicine is more clearly to be felt: Alonso's *Medicorum incipientium medicina, seu medicinae Christianae speculum* of 1598 deals *inter alia* with the problem of prescribing remedies containing meat on fast days, and recognises the Church's right to draw the line between monstrous and non-monstrous births; and Codronchi's *De Christiana ac tuta medendi ratione* of 1591 shows a similar sensitivity to dogmatic issues.[108]

3.6.2 Protestant reactions

For those who do not see themselves as bound by the authority of Rome, the situation is somewhat different. As Sachiko Kusukawa has shown, the Lutheran doctrine of the relationship between soul and body caused Philip Melanchthon to introduce an element of medical teaching into arts course; at the same time, the argument of God's beneficence and the argument of providential design which can be made on the basis of medical evidence is deployed by Caspar Peucer and others as a bulwark against atomism and Pyrrhonism.[109] Later in the century, those who remain faithful to Philippism use these arguments to oppose the doctrine 'de naturalibus naturaliter' espoused by some Paduan doctors. Notable among these is Nicolaus Taurellus, a self-styled 'medicinae doctor et Christianae Philosophiae studiosus', who in 1581 announces in his preface to his *Medicae praedictionis methodus* that

The God of philosophy and of theology is the same God. Nor do we owe our faith to Christ and our mind to Aristotle, so that we believe as Christians and do philosophy as pagans. Christ claims all of me for himself, nor is anything to be attributed to Aristotle except what Christ himself has conceded [to him].[110]

---

[108] Alonso 1598: 510ff. (monsters born with two heads need to be nurtured, but not those with a cat's head or a dog's head, according to theologians); Schleiner 1995: 104ff., 182 (on Codronchi).

[109] Kusukawa 1995a; 1998: 129; Eckart 1998; Grell 1993 (on Bartholin); Nutton 1993b (on anatomy at Wittenberg being taught to reveal God's workings and promote Christian morality); Melanchthon 1999: 169–74. The same argument is found in the writings of some Catholics: e.g. Franz Titelmans (according to Pantin forthcoming) and Parisanus 1635: b5v. See also French 1994: 41.

[110] Taurellus 1581): (4r: 'idem enim Philosophiae Deus et Theologiae . . . Me sibi totum Christus vendicat: nec Aristoteli quicquam attribuetur, nisi quod Christus ipse concesserit, nec si quid obtulerit Aristoteles, id protinus excipiam, nisi quod Christo fuerit acceptissimum.' Chrisoph Lüthy has kindly communicated to me this extract from a letter of Taurellus to Theodor Zwinger dated 21 July 1581 (Universitätsbibliothek Basel MS Frey-Gryn II.26.5, 470): 'haec scholarcharum voluntas est, ut Philippi doctrinam in philosophia et Theologia sequamur: in hac educatus ego sum, quo fit ut res haec mihi merito sit gratissima'.

Similar statements about the unicity of truth may be found in Jean Bodin, Lambert Daneau, John Case and at least one Catholic (Vallesius);[111] but not all those sympathetic to Philippism and Calvinism follow this line. An example of a Northern doctor who highlights in an Italian way the frontier between theology and medicine is Duncan Liddel: and a similar approach may be sensed in the texts of Laurent Joubert and Guillaume Rondelet of Montpellier. On the other hand, the followers of Paracelsus, faithful to his theology, condemn both Galen and Aristotle as pagan, and insist on the unitary nature of the field of medicine and theology.[112]

3.6.3 God in nature

The issue of truth is linked by some thinkers to that of natural necessity and chance in nature (see below 7.3.2); those who espouse the one truth thesis are often led to assert God's direct intervention into nature, with the attendant doctrines of divinely ordained miracles and monsters. Jean Hucher gives coherent expression to this occasionalism in his *De prognosi medica* of 1602:

> The most high and great God, the lord of all of nature, freely administers, impels, hastens, delays, hinders or altogether prohibits the forces, actions and effects of nature . . . therefore Aristotle's disputations about chance and fortune as two unknown efficient causes are rightly refuted by pious men, for God is alone the author of all spontaneous events and their contingency.[113]

Such a view is often linked to the effective operation of various kinds of spirits and demons in this world: a view opposed both by the Counter-Reformation and by Lutheran authorities, who sought for different reasons to curb the animistic fervour of country-dwellers.[114] It is also linked to the issue of astrology, and the effect of the stars on the sublunary world.

---

[111] Blair 1997: 87, 94, 117, 143–4; Thorndike 1923–58: 6.339–62; French 1994: 54 (citing Charles Schmitt); Blair 2000 (on Vallesius).

[112] Temkin 1973: 167 (citing Edward Burney); Kühlmann 1992: 111–12 (on Croll and his contacts).

[113] Hucher 1602: **6v: 'Deus optimus maximus totius naturae dominus, vires actiones et effectus eiusdem libere administrat, impellit, urget, tardat, interpellat aut omnino prohibet . . . Merito igitur Aristotelis de casu et fortuna tanquam effectricibus duabus causis ignotis, disputationes a piis viris exploduntur; cum omnium spontaneorum casuum solus Deus sit author, eorumque contingentiae.' Cf. the Catholic Valerius 1573: 11: 'nihil temere aut fortuitu fieri in rerum naturae'. God has a 'potentia ordinata' (freedom to act); some Renaissance thinkers deduce from this that nature must be good in itself, and that as a consequence all disease is supernatural in origin: see Blair 1997: 123 (on Bodin); Siraisi 1997: 160 (on Fernel).

[114] See Clark 1997.

3.6.4 Astrology and divination

The issues which arise in the immense bibliography of this topic in the Renaissance are those of determinism, of occult cause, of the union of the sublunary and superlunary worlds or their separation, and the question of foretelling the future. It is of course theologically important to retain a space in the sublunary world for the freedom of the will;[115] it is equally important to ensure that divine providence is given a completely free hand; as Silvaticus says, 'it is not God and our reason together which are the authors of foretelling the future, but God alone'; and judicial astrology and all forms of vulgar divination are condemned on many sides, not least by papal bulls of 1586 and 1631.[116] Yet astrology is also a respected study of regularities in the heavens, and was recognised as having its own 'necessitas'.[117] It is even defended in Wittenberg as a path to the understanding of God's governance of the physical world.[118] Even if this is reduced to something less than necessity, doctors such as Valleriola and others argue that we must know as much as possible about the stars as about any other potential cause having effects on the human body.[119] A Paris edict ordained that every physician and surgeon must have a copy of the current almanach to use in their practice (of phlebotomy); and astrology was taught at Bologna, Paris and Montpellier as an aid to prognosis.[120] Many of its supporters were willing to condemn judicial astrology, but all defend the usefulness of the *De diebus decretoriis*, which is the only canonical Galenic text which takes astrology seriously; this is attacked by the growing number of opponents of astrology towards the end of the century as either flippant or only 'probable'.[121]

---

[115] Some (including Michael Scot) claim that astral determination acts only on the body: Canziani 1988: 214.

[116] Silvaticus 1601: 7: 'vaticinii autor non sit Deus simul et ratio nostra; sed Deus solus'; Siraisi 1997: 154–5 (citing Andrea Cattianus); Meinel 1992: 28. See also Dear 1987: 164; Walker 1958: 205–6; Daston and Park 1998: 126–9 (on the medieval background); Copenhaver 1988: 270–1, 287. Also Fulco 1560; Siraisi 1987a: 288–9.

[117] Gregory 1988 (on astrology as *scientia*); Blum 1992: 53–4.

[118] Kusukawa 1993: 38–9 (quoting Melanchthon).

[119] Valleriola 1577: 368–78; Rice 1976: 24 (on Ficino); Ferrier 1592: 107.

[120] Castellanus 1555: 11r–12v; Kusukawa 1993: 33ff.; Thorndike 1923–58: 4.141f.; Westman 1993: 2.

[121] Wear 1981: 245–50; Castro 1614: 57–64; Martinengius 1584: 25–9; Siraisi 1997: 114 (citing Cardano); Platter 1625: 72 (against prediction from eclipses); Horst 1621: 88 (iii.8: 'an sydera ad morborum generationem faciunt?'). An early refutation of the usefulness of astrology for medicine is by Polich von Mellerstadt (*c.* 1450–1513): see Kusukawa 1993: 55–6. Another Galenic text on astrology is alleged by Taisnierus 1583: 1–11 (*De ingenio sanitatis*, viii.20): but this text (a version of the *De methodo medendi*) was superseded in the Renaissance by the one of Greek rather than Arabic origin which did not contain the relevant passage.

3.6.5 The limits of knowledge

The issue of astrology and divination (linked by some to medical prognosis) raises the fundamental issue which concerns both medicine and theology, namely the limits to be placed on man's search for knowledge. Christian anti-intellectualism, which can be found from the Early Church onwards in theological writings, is much in evidence in the Renaissance on both sides of the religious divide; it is expressed through scholastic nominalism; it joins forces with the renascent scepticism of the middle years of the century; it is encouraged by certain inherent features of humanism and of the texts which humanism brings to light.[122] An influential early text which expresses its opposition to astrology in this mode is Pico's *Disputationes contra astrologiam divinatricem* of 1496.[123] The arguments for and against engagement in intellectual enquiry by doctors are both made: on the one hand, it is not for men, limited as they are to seeing things in their own conceptual terms and through their own imperfect sense perception, to claim knowledge over the world about them; on the other, as they were born with the desire to know nature[124] and, through nature, God, He must have intended them to know, even if their knowledge cannot be complete or perfect. The medical profession finds itself caught here in an ideological trap: it has to accept dogmas imposed on it from above, but it is enjoined by the exercise of its discipline to doubt, to negate, to hesitate, to query, to engage with the singular and the exceptional, to seek for sufficient (rather than necessary) causes; doctors, of all the professions (so it seems to me), are, if not the most intellectually cautious, at least the least suggestible at this time.[125] It seems to me also inevitable that parts of the profession would resist vigorously the claims of theology to govern their minds on issues which were so closely involved with the practice of their art.

3.7 THE PROFESSIONAL DOCTOR

I am now in a position to offer an ideal-typical description of the professional doctor at this time. His duties are set out in various places: the

---

[122] Schmitt 1967: 15.

[123] Pico does not exempt doctors from his critique; other humanists allow for the usefulness of astrological knowledge for medicine and agriculture: see Copenhaver 1988.

[124] *Metaphysics*, i.1, 980 a 22.

[125] For some expressions of intellectual caution, see Cardano 1663: 3.398; Blum 1992: 53 (on Scotus's claim that our scientia is 'quoad nos'); Fonseca 1599: 1.73 (on the paradoxes of curiosity); Pittion 1987: 122.

summary in Hippocrates's *Epidemics* provides a useful starting point:

Declare the past, diagnose the present, foretell the future; practise these arts. As to diseases, make a habit of two things: to help, or at least to do no harm. The art has three factors, the disease, the patient and the physician. The physician is the servant of the art. The patient must cooperate with the physician in combating the disease.[126]

There are of course, much higher-minded accounts of the duties of doctors: the various versions of the Hippocratic oath, and the pseudo-Hippocratic *Precepts*, in which the love of the medical art is described in terms of philanthropy, are two of them.[127] Galen stressed also the more intellectual qualities of love of work and the spirit of enquiry.[128] But there are less exalted accounts also: these stress the need for 'cautelae' or shrewd behaviour among doctors, not only to preserve reputation but also to profit by the exercise of the profession.[129] The literature which deals with this is able to be construed in either high-minded or cynical ways, and the image of the doctor which emerges from it can be characterised either as the master of his profession, or its servant, as we shall see.[130]

3.7.1 Critiques

There are attacks on the profession which reflect the cynical appraisal of the doctor and his role. Among the best-known of these is that of Henricus

---

[126] Hippocrates, *Epidemics*, i.13. On this see Debus 1999. Also Hippocrates, *De flatibus* (on the sympathy of doctors for patients' pain).

[127] Rütten 1996; these texts may be syncretised with Platonic and Old Testament texts and the Apocrypha (Ecclesiasticus 38:1–15); see Alonso 1598: 8; Victorius 1598: A3r. The *degré zéro* of medicine is of course the healthy human being who has no need either of regimen or of doctors, as Celsus points out in *De medicina*, i.1: 'sanus homo qui et bene valet et suae spontis est, nullis obligare se legibus debet, ac neque medico neque iatralipta egere', cited by Lommius 1558: 1 and Cornarius (in Mikkeli 1999: 92–3). This is properly an issue in hygiene (the part of medicine which deals with 'res non naturales'); Cardosus 1620: 3–8 produces a quaestio on this topic (whether an 'ars conservatrix' is necessary), citing Hippocrates, *Aphorisms*, i.5, ii.50, *Airs, waters, places*, Celsus, and Galen, *De sanitate tuenda*, i, K 6.1ff. as those who negate the proposition, pointing out also that neither peasants nor animals have recourse to doctors: only those of noble birth do. *Econtra* (i.e. the winning side of the argument) he produces another set of loci (including the *Ars parva* and *De sanitate tuenda*, vi.6, K 6.381ff.) to demonstrate the need for the medical art. See also Mikkeli 1999. Another line on the redundancy of learned medicine is taken by Agrippa (cited by Siraisi 1990b: 226–7), who points out that trained physicians know less about cures than village healers.

[128] *De locis affectis*, iii.7, K 3.167. Lloyd 1988: 41 argues that Galen was led to argue that the body had an influence on the soul in order to enhance the status of the medical profession, which could help bring about the balancing of the individual's crasis.

[129] On the medieval background, see McVaugh 1997.

[130] Linden 1999 and French 1993 for these two possible interpretations. See also Siraisi 1999: 361 (quoting Cardano on medicine being both good for wealth and good for humanity).

Agrippa von Nettesheim in his *De incertitudine et vanitate scientiarum omnium et artium* of 1528, whose satirical (and possibly ironical) demolition is inspired, as is the rest of the work, by Christian anti-intellectualism.[131] It is worth citing here Pagel's résumé of his arguments in full:

The uncertainty of medical knowledge is primarily revealed by the lack of unanimity among the investigators in quite fundamental matters, such as the process of development. There prevails the same jealousy among the schools as among the systems of philosophy. Hippocrates refers the causes of disease to the pneuma, Herophilus to the humours, Erasistratus to the arterial blood, Asclepiades to the pores, Alcmaeon ascribes them to the lack of excess of physical energy, Diocles to inequality of the elements composing the body and to the air, Strato to excess and indigestibility of food. Medical practice is built upon absolutely erroneous experiments, and hence patients frequently suffer more from the physician and remedy than from the disease itself. The best physician is he whom the apothecary, who shares his fees, recommends. Magnificent garments, stained fingertips, a foreign origin or even only a difference of faith, a boldly lying tongue and the continual prescription of drugs create authority, renown and influence. The physician observes the patient with gravity, inspects the urine, feels the pulse, looks at the tongue, examines the chest, tests the excretions, asks questions concerning the customary diet and other intimate details, as though, by such means, he could weigh the elements and the humours of the body and bring them into equilibrium. Then, with great solemnity, he prescribes the medicine. Mild illnesses he protracts as long as possible, suggesting ridiculous measures which will be agreeable to the patient, such as water dripping into a basin as a cure for insomnia. If the illness is severe and the outlook doubtful or hopeless, he prescribes a special routine, orders unusual things, forbidding the usual, finds fault with whatever has been given to the patient, threatens death, promises life, and demands a high fee. If death occurs, it is the result of a pulmonary oedema or some other incurable condition, or no doubt, is due to the disobedience of the patient or the carelessness of the nurses, or it may even be a colleague or the apothecary who is responsible. Aesculapius himself was a rogue, the offspring of an incestuous marriage. In fact, physicians are the greatest criminals, the most quarrelsome, envious, and deceitful of men. One physician will never approve of the prescriptions of another. They are always dirty, because for the sake of gain they roam around privies and their home is in the filth of men. Cato was right when he forbade all physicians to reside in Rome. They fall into three categories: the very learned who lose all their patients, the illiterate who cure them, even those who have been given up, and a third class whose rich patients alone recover, while peasants and common people suffer greatly.[132]

Agrippa concludes his declamation by declaring the ignorance of learned doctors of the nature of the cures they impose and contrasting this with

[131] On the possibly irony of this work see Vickers 1968: 188.
[132] Pagel 1985: 121–3.

the homely skills of village healers. There are a number of issues here which recur throughout the discussion of medical ethics and practice in the Renaissance: the fee, which is associated here with the greed of the doctor, is also discussed in terms of the medieval categories of remuneration;[133] the protectionism of the guild, mainly directed against unlicensed practitioners, which is fiercely denounced by Paracelsus, but enshrined in many municipal and College statutes;[134] the nature of the art, and its relationship to successful practice; the self-glorification of the profession; the relationship with the patient; prognosis; and professional prudence (or cynical self-protection).

3.7.2 Cautela: treatment and cure

According to Taurellus, the three factors which bring doctors fame are 'the happy outcome of their treatments, the secure knowledge of disease, and the true prediction of its future course'.[135] The first of these factors relates to the much-quoted dictum 'natura medicatrix morborum, medicus autem minister', which has been discussed above (3.2.3). The last is most glorious if a recovery is correctly predicted against the expectations of those attending the patient.[136] All three factors provide material for the energetic counter-claims to Agrippa written by a host of learned doctors whose mutual praise and, more especially, self-praise contributed to the rise of medical prosopography (see above 2.2.3). Galen had, of course, set the standard of self-advertisement through his

---

[133] García Ballester 1993a; the loci classici of categories of payment are Plato, *Republic*, 340 c and Aristotle, *Politics*, i.3, 1258 a 10ff., which is systematised by Albertus Magnus and Aquinas in the Middle Ages. On the relationship between money-making and the medical art, see Siraisi 1999: 361, quoting Cardano 1663: 6.1–4: 'si enim nomen seu divitias aut amicos parare velis, disciplina nulla melius aut uberius praestare potest'; see also Linden 1999: 32 (on 'humane' remuneration); Temkin 1973: 130 (citing Paracelsus on the greed of doctors); but as Henri de Mondeville pointed out much earlier, patients do not think they are receiving anything of value unless they pay for it (from which it follows that the more they pay, the greater value they attribute to the goods (see García Ballester 1993b: 51).

[134] E.g. the Laws and Statutes of the Senate of Nuremberg, viii, cited in Hagecius ab Hagek 1596: 37: the imposition of a ten-guilder fine on any of the following found practising without permission: 'Tyriacks kraemern, Zauberchern, Alchymisten, Distillatorn, Verdorben handwerckern, Juden Schwarzkuenstlern, auch allen Weibern, so der kranken zu warten unnd sich zu rhuemen pflegen also hetten sie der Doctors kunst und ertzney erlernet'. See also French 1994: 133–8.

[135] Taurellus 1581: 1: 'felix curarum successus, certa morbi cognitio, vera futurorum praedictio'; cf. Liddel 1604: ddir on the three advantages of 'praesagia' being to gain the trust of the patient, to apply a better therapeutic regime, and in cases where death is predicted, to avoid calumny and blame for the outcome.

[136] Fonseca in Jacchinus 1615: 187: 'gloriosum profecto est, et pene divinum si praeter omnem vulgi expectationem hominem sanandum praedicas'.

spectacular cures, especially in the *De locis affectis*; a Renaissance emulator is Cardano (*De mirabilibus operibus in arte medica per ipsum factis*, 1557); it is not clear whether Paracelsus's insistence on the 'lumen naturae' which operates through a given individual is also a version of this (see below 5.3.5). Certainly, it seems to have been thought that the ability to explain extraordinary particulars makes the exegete himself extraordinary.[137] There is a paradox here, which is perceptible in some of these writings: the performer of the cure proclaims an art which is both outside himself and greater than he; and yet as the performer of that art, he expresses his self-confidence in his own ability which is seen to be the dominant factor in the cure. It is plausible to argue that this is one of the features of medical thought of the time that distinguishes it most clearly from the claims made after the advent of the new (mechanical, experimental) knowledge of the seventeenth century;[138] but it also related to the more mundane point that all medicine is in part a skill, a 'peritia', that cannot be simply acquired through the teaching of a method.[139]

3.7.3 Cautela: patient–doctor relations

The patient-doctor relationship is an area which attracts comment and generates advice. This is seen to be one of the 'res non naturales', in so far as it relates to the 'passiones animi'; ideally, mutual confidence should characterise it.[140] The relationship should both reflect the authority of the doctor, and allow him to be modest about his claims to knowledge.[141] At issue is not only the doctor's use of language (while he may be amusing, he must abstain from all attempts at persuasion which could be construed as self-interest; and he must express himself in the terms of art, even if he needs to explain such terms to those present), but also his dress and appearance, and his physical location in the sickroom (neither in the dark out of sight of the patient, nor at his head, but in front of him). Detailed instructions are given on how to take medical histories; this task is best entrusted to doctors who already know the patient, to prevent the sort

---

[137] See Daston and Park 1998: 170 (on della Porta and Cardano); cf. the Paracelsian 'göttlicher Arzt' cited in Goldammer 1991: 92–5.

[138] There may even be a hint of the mentality of magic or the magus here: the location of the skill in the performer makes it easier to explain any failure (through the intervention of other factors, or the imperfect performance of the ritual). Cf. Grafton 1999: 328 on the 'confirmation bias' in astrological prediction.

[139] Rondelet 1586: 591.

[140] García Ballester 1993b: 51 (citing Henri de Mondeville). See also 7.4.

[141] Liddel 1628: 511–12.

of mistake referred to by Sennert, where an ill-favoured individual born with a sharp nose, hollow ears and sunken temples is taken to be on the verge of death (these being classic signs of imminent demise) by a doctor who is not aware that such is his usual appearance when in good health.[142]

Skill in diagnosis and prognosis is also an index of correct medical practice. Both Hippocrates and Galen have important advice to offer on this topic:

> If a physician discover and declare [unaided] by the side of his patients the present, the past and the future, and fill the gaps in the account given by the sick, he will be the more believed to understand the cases, so that men will confidently entrust themselves to him for treatment.[143]

Hippocrates also says that a doctor should be prepared to seek second opinions; Galen, for his part, stresses that the good physician must be able to say more than the layman could about the future course of the disease.[144] Correct prognosis makes a doctor into a public oracle and maintains his authority with the patient;[145] this is a skill based on a 'naturalis coniectandi facultas' which is shared with chiromancy and other conjectural sciences (see below 8.8).[146] There are several issues involved in prediction: will the patient survive? will the illness last a long time? will it end in a crisis? if so, of what sort, and on which day?[147] This wide range of questions calls for caution in making prognoses. The doctor may fail to predict a death, and be accused of undue inactivity; or

---

[142] Castro 1614: 248–51 (on telling jokes); Lemosius 1598: 17v (citing Celsus, *De medicina*, vi.3, on position relative to patient); Campilongo 1601:)(8r (a dichotomous table illustrating Capivaccius's technique of taking a medical history); Sennert 1650: 1.449 (the case of a patient having 'nares acutas, oculos cavos, tempora collapsa', where 'non mors mox praedicanda est': see also Galen, *In Hippocratis de officina medici*, K 18b.648, and Cardano 1663: 8.595, quoted by Siraisi 1997: 137). While rhetoric is forbidden in respect of persuasion, it is needed for effective communication: Vallesius 1606: 279 (iv, preface: on the authority of Galen). Patients can of course also affect themselves, as some doctors point out: Horst 1574 writes a treatise on autogenic disease which arises from various wrong ethical and habitual behaviour on the part of patients; also Ferrier 1574: 220–1 (on beneficial autosuggestion). See also García Ballester 1993b: 42–3 (citing Arnau de Vilanova's four requirements of doctors: intellectual knowledge, openness to all information available, expression of judgements 'secundum artem medicam' and communication of these in an appropriate form to others).

[143] Hippocrates, *Prognosis*, i.

[144] Vega 1571: 900, citing *Praecepta*, viii, and Galen, *De difficultate respirationis*, iii.1, K 7.888–9. Galen, it was remembered in the Renaissance, boasted never to have made a prognostic mistake: Cardano 1568: 619 (xliii): 'Galenus gloriatur nunquam in praedicendo aberrasse'.

[145] Varanda 1620: 6 ('instar oraculi').

[146] Liddel 1628: 596–600; Peucer 1553: 614 (on 'naturalis coniectandi facultas' derived from experientia); Silvaticus 1601: 83 (on the habitus of conjecture); Albertus 1615: B5–6.

[147] Cardano 1568: 590 (iii.39).

he may misdiagnose on the basis of an erroneous prediction. A number of pieces of advice are offered to prevent this happening. Celsus had already proffered guidance on how to protect one's reputation in prognosticating; Arnau de Vilanova offers very practical guidance to doctors on this matter;[148] Zerbi develops this further, and suggests that all predictions should be made only after a number of prior conditions have been clearly met (the doctor must be good; the patient must obey him; his nursing care must be exemplary; and even then, the unexpected can happen). Cardano, who correctly states that the only way to avoid all error is never to engage in prognosis, suggests that no attempt should be made to treat an illness where failure is obvious; Argenterio produces one quasi-mathematical rule for getting prognosis right (cited below, 5.2.2), but he also suggests that in cases of uncertainty, one should wait, as time will always show.[149] There is an ethical (and theological) problem in the prognosis of death: should a patient be deceived into believing in his own recovery for his peace of mind? What is of interest in all this writing on the topic of prognosis is the stress laid on the avoidance of error, which is a marked feature of other aspects of medical discourse (see below 5.4).[150]

Much of the advice offered in the tradition of counselling known as cautelae sounds much more cynical. Don't dispute in front of the laity, because it reduces your authority as a profession; don't begin by discussing fees; appear reasonably affluent, and live in a big house (or your patients won't think that you are successful); avoid treating the princely, the violent and the young; impress your patient by picking up clues from accidental signs in the sick room, in a Sherlock Holmesian way; don't write down your diagnoses and prognoses, and be sure to make

---

[148] Arnau de Vilanova 1585: 1711 (advising caution with gossipy attendants, attention to the life cycle of illnesses and to the sequential administration of treatments; care over the positioning of the patient's bed; preparedness for contingencies and rare events; and suggesting the right mode of behaviour when more than one doctor is present).

[149] Cardano 1568: 4 (on Galen's anecdote about the advantages of remaining silent in *De praenotione*, vi–vii, K 19.497–511); *ibid.*, 619 (iv.43); Siraisi 1997: 28 (all on the need to avoid treating incurable diseases, for fear that the doctor will be blamed for the ensuing death); *ibid.*, 144; Argenterio 1610: 1779–81.

[150] Campilongo 1601:)(8v (Jessenius quoting Celsus, *De medicina*, v.26 on the method of predicting which saves the doctor's reputation); Alonso 1598: 8; Alpini 1601: 4; French 1993: 88 ('the model for Zerbi is Galen's highly conditional judgement that a patient will escape the disease if he has a good doctor, is himself obedient, has diligent servants well prepared with all external necessities and if nothing unexpected happens'); Galen, *In prorrhetica* (also implicit in Hippocrates, *Aphorisms*, i.1), cited by Cocus 1601: A4v (ms addition); Scholze 1589: 3; Edwardes 1532: 12v (on caution in predicting death); Jacchinus 1563: 3; Valleriola 1577: 402–7 (on whether or not to deceive a patient about his condition).

them ambiguous; prescribe expensive medicines; keep your dignity and gravity at all times.[151] All these points are found in Zerbi, but it would be unfair to say that this is all Zerbi's *cautelae* are; he also stresses the Hippocratic precepts and oath, and the priest-like role of the doctor.[152]

3.8 CONCLUSION: THE DOCTOR AS MASTER AND SERVANT OF HIS ART

In the end, the doctor turns out to be both the master and the servant of medicine. Its dignity as a learned discipline, and its association with restrictive practices predispose him to claim authority over knowledge of disease, of past, present and future, of the patient, of nature itself. This case had had to be argued from the very beginnings of Greek medicine: the Hippocratic *On ancient medicine* had made the case for the physician who both was a rational exponent of his art and also relied on his experience to be able to draw correct inferences from the differing states of the body. Plato discusses in several places the claims of medicine, or uses it as an analogy.[153] The issue of mastery emerges clearly in these discussions; it comes as no surprise that Montaigne, that shrewd reader of ancient texts, points this out and discusses it in his *Essais*:

L'expérience est proprement sur son fumier au subject de la medecine, où la raison luy quitte toute la place. Tibere disoit que quiconque avoit vescu vingt ans se debvoit respondre des choses qui luy estoyent nuisibles ou salutaires, et se sçavoir conduire sans medecine. (C) Et le pouvoit avoir apprins de Socrates, lequel, conseillant à ses disciples, soigneusement et comme un tres principale estude, l'estude de leur santé, adjoustoit qu'il estoit malaisé qu'un homme d'entendement, prenant garde à ses exercices, à son boire et à son manger, ne discernast mieux que tout medecin ce qui luy estoit bon ou mauvais. (B) Si faict la medecine profession d'avoir tousjours l'experience pour touche de son operation. Ainsi Platon avoit raison de dire que pour estre vray medecin, il seroit necessaire quie celuy qui l'entreprendroit eust passé par toutes les maladies qu'il veut guarir et par tous les accidens et circonstances dequoy il doit juger. C'est raison qu'ils prennent la verole s'ils la veulent sçavoir penser.[154]

---

[151] Siraisi 1997: 38, 54; Nutton 1993a; Barton 1994 (on the parallel between Galen and Sherlock Holmes); also Daston and Park 1998: 170 (on the reputation derived from explaining the extraordinary).

[152] French 1993; also Hippocrates, *Precepts*, iv, vi.

[153] E.g. *Laws*, 857 c–e.

[154] Montaigne 1965: 1079 (iii.13); Starobinski 1982: 194; *Phaedrus*, 270 b–d; *Republic*, iii; also Xenophon, *History*, iv.7; Cardano 1663: 8.231 (the paradox of the commentator); Schleiner 1995: 207–8; Bono 1995: 89 (quoting Fernel).

No doctor would wish to follow this logic, and suffer all the ills he himself might have to treat: so his therapeutic claims must rest upon his experience and observation of the sufferings of others and the rational deductions which he makes from them. But these very claims, and their attendant effects, lead him to be the easy target of satire for any of the failings that can undermine his authority: ignorance, arrogance, pretension, exclusiveness, deceit, greed. It is no wonder that both Molière and Oscar Wilde had such a field day at his expense.

CHAPTER 4

The arts course: grammar, logic and dialectics

I am neither a superstitious man, nor a lover of fables, but a student
of the truth.

(Ferrier)[1]

4.1 INTRODUCTION

I am not setting out in the following chapters to give a comprehensive
survey of Renaissance instruments of thought; my focus is on those instruments which are found in the sections on logic included by teachers
of medicine in their courses.[2] The relationship of this chapter to chapter
7 (and of the section on signs in this chapter to chapter 8) is approximately
one of 'form' to 'content' of argument;[3] I shall concentrate here more on
how doctors thought rather than what they thought. In beginning this
study with chapters on the transmission of medical knowledge and the
nature of its institutions, I have already placed the argumentative structures employed by physicians in one of the contexts in which they were
produced; although I am here separating the form of argument from
its content as far as this is possible, I do not wish to prejudge the issue
whether this form makes any contribution to the content's sense and significance. Since, however, contemporaries clearly distinguish the modes

---

[1] Ferrier 1574: 221: 'Neque...superstitiosus homo sum, neque fabularum amans, sed veritatis
studiosus'.

[2] Prominent among these are those of da Monte 1587, Argenterio 1610, Capivaccius 1603,
Campilongo 1601, and Liddel 1628.

[3] These terms are usually met in the context of literary studies, and the division they imply is
now seen as wrongly conceived, in that it fails to take into account that the form (the genre)
itself contributes to the content, and that its constraints and properties convey meaning as
well as the words which make up the text: see White 1987. More recently, titles in the history
of science such as *Science incarnate* (Lawrence and Shapin 1998) have drawn the attention of
scholars to a similar division – that between scientific theories and the role of social factors in
their formulation, or 'truth and narrative', which has given rise to heated debates: see Jardine
and Frasca-Spada 1997.

of these arguments from what they are about, it seems appropriate in
the first instance to follow their practice in this, and to comment in the
postscript on the semantic and rhetorical consequences of the choice of
argumentative modes.

As Edward Grant has pointed out, the emergence of universities as
institutions independent from faculties of theology or local bishops is
connected with the development of the arts course, whose core by the
end of the Middle Ages consisted in the trivium of grammar, logic and
rhetoric on the model of Paris.[4] This came in due course to embrace elements of the quadrivium, notably mathematics, and to include elements
of natural philosophy, based on the *Libri naturales* of Aristotle. For the
higher faculty of law, the arts course was propedeutic in that in it were
taught the arts of grammar and logic on which jurisprudential reasoning
and practice depended; for the higher faculty of medicine, the arts course
both underpinned its logical structure and inculcated the knowledge of
the world in which the university-trained doctor was destined to work.
This was a changing world; I have already indicated that there was an
awareness of how far its confines had expanded by the second half of the
sixteenth century. It is not clear whether it was also thought that new (or
newly recovered) rational tools and procedures were becoming available
to contribute to this expansion, or whether there was a general assumption both that man's senses marked the limits of his knowledge, and that
Aristotelian logic provided all the conceptual apparatus to which man
could aspire.[5]

For doctors, there existed another source of logic and method: the
'membra disiecta' of Galen's own lost *De demonstratione*, which Jakob
Schegk (1511–87) among others tried to reconstruct.[6] Many texts by
Galen contain reference to, and use of, his logical theories, which
incorporated some elements of post-Aristotelian logic and inference;
the methodology they evince became thereby something eclectic and

---

[4] Grant 1996; Hale and Highfield 1965: 28 argue that Paris was the model for all Europe through
its statutes. See also French 1994: 10; Ridder-Symoens 1996; Schmitt 1985: 4–5.

[5] See Simon Grynaeus's comment on geometry in his introduction to the Greek text of
Euclid of 1533, quoted by Schmitt and Skinner 1988: 782; also Siraisi 1990a: 178; Jardine
1974: 26–7.

[6] Schegk 1564; Champier 1516b; L'Alemant 1549; Cardano 1663: 1.293–308 (*De dialectica*); Viottus
1560: e1v, e4v–5v (who makes the connection with the reconstruction of Galen's lost work clear,
and refers also to *De constitutione artis medicae*, K 1.244–304, *De placitis Hippocratis et Platonis*, ii,
K 5.211–84; *De temperamentis*, ii, K 1.572–645; *De semine*, K 4.512–651; and *Methodus medendi*, ii,
K 10.78–156). Other works at this time with similar titles (e.g. Foxius Morzillus 1556) declare
that their inspiration has been the rise of studies in dialectic, which has caused demonstration
to be neglected or misconstrued.

peculiar to that discipline.[7] At the same time, developments in dialectics in the late fifteenth and early sixteenth centuries influenced medical studies in a way which might be compared to the influence which the zoological teachings of Aristotle had on anatomical studies.[8] This reaction increased rather than reduced the complexity of medical reasoning. Although the principle of elegance (in the shape of Ockham's razor) is sometimes evoked, as we shall see, it remains true that doctors were committed to a complex form of argument in which division plays a particularly important role. They also remained in touch with contemporary developments in logical teaching (notably in Padua), which are reflected in the sections on logic included in their lecture courses;[9] and from the beginning of the century, they were involved in debates among themselves about the correct understanding of Aristotle and Galen on this topic.[10]

University teachers of medicine who included logic in their courses (in nearly every case, these were Italians or Italian-trained)[11] did not all order their material in the same way, although all were agreed on the superiority of scientific over endoxical argument, and the superiority of both of these over practical reasoning. The particular uptake of medical discourse from the arts course is marked both by an aspiration to rigour and certainty, and by the pursuit of more makeshift ways of weighing factors against each other, of reaching decisions about evidence and of justifying them. Although, as shall be seen, demonstrative logic is not as representative of medical procedures as are lesser forms of argument, it is necessary here to give a brief account of it to make clear both how these are interrelated, and how odd are the claims pressed by doctors on behalf of the certainty and rigour of their art's precepts. University teachers of medicine (who in some cases, such as that of Schegk and Aubéry, are also, or have also been, teachers of logic) make fairly frequent reference to the higher forms of logic; its presence in their manuals will be indicated in the footnotes. For convenience's sake, these chapters will follow the ordering of the Organon – grammar, categories, demonstrative logic, dialectics, topics

---

[7] Bartolettus 1619: 297 says that *Methodus medendi*, i.4, K 10.30–9 shows that Galen's demonstrative method is the same as that of Aristotle; other treatments of logical issues are found in *De differentiis pulsuum* and the *Ars parva*.

[8] Ashworth 1988; Cunningham 1997.

[9] Mikkeli 1992: 44ff.; an example is afforded by Capivaccius 1603: 1004–51 (*De differentiis doctrinarum, logicis, philosophis, atque medicis pernecessaria*, first published as a separate treatise at Padua in 1562).

[10] Gilbert 1960.

[11] See the remarks made above (1.5.1) on the different styles of Padua and Montpellier.

and rhetoric (here incompletely represented as argument from signs, analogy, exempla, induction and loci), sophistical reasoning – before turning to aspects of medical reasoning that are peculiar to it: the use of mathematics, the input of sensory information, the relative validity of reasoning, experientia and authority; the issue of method.[12] I shall refer throughout my account to the contrasting uptake of the arts course by law as a means of characterising that of medicine.[13] In discussing these topics, I shall cite Aristotle and Galen as Renaissance doctors did: that is, as though they were their contemporaries. When parts of the corpus of both writers were included in sixteenth-century texts, it was done not in an antiquarian spirit but to incorporate them organically into the argument.

4.2 LINGUISTIC ISSUES

Unlike jurists, doctors make no claim that the language arts are particularly necessary to their discipline: we have noted already (3.7) that the use of rhetorical persuasion or reliance on argumentation *in utramque partem* was forbidden to them: 'patients are cured by medication, not eloquence', as Pietro Castelli puts it.[14] Although some doctors write as scholars on rhetoric (Gerardus Bucoldianus, Johannes Sinapius, Schegk) and many engage in liminary versifying, the term 'grammaticus', when applied to an individual or to a school, is one of abuse. Argenterio makes this plain by alluding to a German colleague derisively as the 'grammaticus tubingensis', and by accusing the members of 'the most outstanding academy in the world' (presumably Paris) of being 'grammarians rather than physicians' because of their emphasis on Greek philology and Latin rhetoric.[15]

[12] Cf. Ashworth 1988: 82–3 (giving Fonseca's slightly different order of chapters in his *Institutiones dialecticae*); Velsius 1543: 20 gives as the sequence 'demonstrativum seu scientificum; dialecticum seu topicum; rhetoricum; adulterinum seu sophisticum'.

[13] For further details about the discourse of law see Maclean 1992.

[14] Schmitt 1985: 14 (citing Pietro Castelli's *De optimo medico*): 'non eloquentia sed medicamentis curantur aegri'; cf. Albertus 1615: 3–5; da Monte 1587: 14 (both condemning the use of sophistical argument and rhetoric). For Galen's rejection of dialectics, see *De locis affectis*, i.6, K 8.56 and *De differentiis pulsuum*, iv.17, K 7.73 quoted by García Ballester 1981: 35; but see also Kusukawa 1997: 420 (on Sebastian Montuus's use of the genre of 'dialexis', a practice of arguing from both sides in the pursuit of truth).

[15] Siraisi 1990a: 169 (citing Argenterio 1592: 1.7). The German in question must be either Schegk or Fuchs. But this does not mean that physicians were not concerned with 'bene dicere' as opposed to persuasion in their consultation with patients: on this see Argenterio 1606–7: 1.270–1 ('De consultandi ratione, ch. xii: de probandi pronuntiandique ratione in consultationibus') where he deplores the perverse or ambitious doctors who speak to their patients and their attendants 'ad apparatum, ad ostentationem, vel ad victoriam', and recommends doctors

4.2.1 Res et verba

Although there is such a thing as knowledge without discourse (this is skill or 'peritia' derived from the senses prior to any linguistic formulation), 'scientia' proper is taken to be 'cum discursu': discourse being here both speech and logical construction ('logos', 'logismos', 'ratiocinatio').[16] But to suggest from this, as their detractors do, that rational doctors ('dogmatici') are more concerned with words than things is an unwarranted although persistent accusation.[17] Whereas it was alleged that jurists construct reality out of words, in spite of their claim to be committed to referential meaning, doctors insist that things determine names.[18] 'Knowledge does not create its own objects, but depends for its existence on the existence of things themselves', says Victor Trincavellus (1496–1563), commenting on Galen's *De differentiis febrium*;[19] 'as things are in their being, so are they to be taken in our knowledge of them', declares David Crusius, quoting Zabarella.[20] Sennert associates this with the Protagorean claim made famous by Nicholas of Cusa that our mind is the measure of all things: 'things are the measure of our knowledge, not the other way round; nor is it the case that things are in a certain way of being because we know them in a certain way, but rather because they are in a certain way of being we must know them in that way, if we want truly to know them'.[21] Words are the clothing of things: 'words should

to speak 'ad decorum, utilitatemque aegri, cum summa modestia, et humanitate, non tremula voce, non stridenti, sed firma et moderata, cum quadam gravitate: ex quibus rebus medicae artis antiqua fama et authoritas apud omnes retinentur'.

[16] Capivaccius 1603: 144 (citing Galen, *De officina medici*); and below (5.3.4 on operative knowledge, and 8.7 on indication, although an intellective function is claimed for the latter operation).

[17] Siraisi 1990b: 223 (citing Agrippa).

[18] See above, 3.5.1, esp. note 96.

[19] *In primum Galeni librum de differentiis febrium explanatio*, in *Opera omnia*, Lyon, 1586, 7D, quoted by Lonie 1981: 24; see also Galen, *Ad Thrasybulum*, K 5.867–8.

[20] Crusius 1615: 13: 'qualiter res in essendo taliter se habent in cognoscendo' (quoting Zabarella, *De naturae constitutione*, v); he quotes also Vives, *De anima et vita*, ii, making a similar point: 'cognitio velut imago quaedam rerum in animo expressa tanquam in speculo'.

[21] 'Res enim mensurant cognitionem nostram, non contra; neque quia nos ita cogitamus, res ita se habent, sed quia sic se habent, ita eas cognoscimus, cum recte cognoscimus': Sennert 1676: 179 quoted by Eckart 1992: 157; I have been unable to locate this quotation in other editions. The argument is still used against the alleged error of modern linguistic semiologists; see McGinn 2000: 62: 'we categorize objects by means of their shapes and sizes, for example, but objects have their shapes and sizes independently of the words we use'. For the opposite view, see Nicholas of Cusa 1983: 172: 'sic omnis rei mensura vel terminus ex mente est; et ligna et lapides certam mensuram et terminos habent praeter mentem nostram, sed ex mente increata, a qua rerum omnis terminus descendit'; Montaigne 1965: 410a (ii.10): 'ce que j'opine [des choses], c'est aussi pour declarer la mesure de ma veuë, non la mesure des choses'; Bacon 1878: 210–11 (*Novum organum*, i.41), stressing that sense perception as well as the mind imposes measures on man.

fit things as clothes fit the body'; words are made for things, not things for words.[22] There are several Galenic loci which make the same point; names are instruments, and all concentration on them in themselves is to be avoided.[23] There are as many definitions as there are things, since definitions belong to the order of words, not things; so disputes over words are largely vain, and it doesn't matter, for example, in speaking of the contrary of health, whether you say 'insalubre', 'aegrotabile' or 'aegrum' or refer to an 'aegrilatilis valetudo'.[24]

But the exactly contradictory claims can also be found in Galen and his followers. The master avers that error can be avoided if words are grasped in their correct meaning;[25] the pupil da Monte declares that the 'definitio nominis' is prior to the 'definitio rei'. It is in the nature of human knowledge to distinguish the way we know something (through a word, for example) from what we know; a rule of use and mention is here invoked.[26] According to da Monte, here quoting Aristotle, it is absurd to seek simultaneously for knowledge and for the means of obtaining it. He deduces this view from both *Metaphysics*, ii.3 (995 a 12–14) and from *Physics*, i.1 (134 b 12–14), where the name *qua* brute indication of a thing comes before its definition and the determination of its properties; thus all men call both parents 'mother' until they learn to distinguish mother from father. This is a recognition that linguistic

---

[22] Cardano 1565: 146r (i.6.6): 'debent verba, ut vestes corporibus, sic illa rebus convenire'; also Cardano 1663: 1.123: 'verba propter res ipsas facta esse, non res propter verba'; Silvaticus 1601: 22, quoting Clement of Alexandria, *Stromata*, i: 'dictio vestis in corpore, res autem sunt carnes et nervi. Non oportet ergo maiorem vestis, quam salutis corporis curam gerere.'

[23] See Hankinson 1994 for an excellent survey of Galenic loci on the conventionality of language, the correct use of names, and naming and natural kinds. He concludes (187) that 'Galen's philosophy of language turns out to be part of his epistemological and metaphysical realism.'

[24] Silvaticus 1601: 22 cites *In Hippocratis prognosticum*, ii. 39, K 18b.166–8; *Methodus medendi*, ii. 1, K 10.81–4; *De differentiis pulsuum*, i.1, K 8.711. See also *De differentiis symptomatum*, i, K 7.46–7, quoted by Siraisi forthcoming as 'plurimi omnem suam vitam de nominibus altercando conterunt'; *De usu partium corporis*, vi.1, K 3.464–5, quoted below, note 200; *De differentiis pulsuum*, ii, K 8.567; *De optima corporis nostri constitutione*, K 4.738, quoted by Joutsivuo 1999: 42; *Methodus medendi*, i.7, K 10.50 (on the interchangeability of 'constitutio', 'habitus', 'natura', 'dispositio', and 'affectio'); Joutsivuo 1999: 98 (on the dispute over the neutrum as a 'quaestio [inutilis] de nomine'); *Methodus medendi*, xi.12, K 10.770; Arrizabalaga 1998: 25 citing Francesc Argilagues's evocation in the *Articella* of Galen, *In aphorismos*, ii.22, K 17b.503 and *Ars parva*, iii, K 313–14 and Averroes on Aristotle's indifference towards terminology.

[25] *De complexionibus*, i.5, K 1.534–6.

[26] Da Monte 1587: 229: 'definitio nominis seu notionalis rei definitionem antecedit': cf. Mikkeli 1992: 86 (against this position); *ibid.*, 101: 'Aristoteles bene dixit, absurdum est simul et scientiam, et modum sciendi quaerere'; cf. Siraisi 1997: 103 (on Cardano's image of the eye observing itself and its parts).

notation or names are necessary for all rational activity or 'iudicium', called by Guidus Antonius Albanesius a 'cognitio discursiva'.[27] This does not make names into causes, merely into the signs of the mind's movements ('notae passionum animi'). They are imposed on things by convention in accordance with the Aristotelian doctrine in the first chapter of the *De interpretatione*; they are however only correlatively linked to their objects as 'signum' is to 'signatum'.[28] In this respect, they have a crucial role to play in the identification of such things as new illnesses and newly discovered plants, even though they are only arbitrarily related to the thing.[29] The discussion of the name 'rhabarbarus' in Leoniceno and Manardo, for example, is about the referent of a word defined historically (that to which Pliny was referring).[30] The role that names play makes it important that they should not be used redundantly, for fear of creating unnecessary distinctions of fact or theory.[31] Their conventionality opens up also the possibility of the vapidity of which the users of such terms as 'virtus dormitiva' in respect of opium were to be accused in the following century.[32] The further risk that neologisms can lead to terminological ambiguity or obscurity is one of the factors which motivate scholars to produce lexica at this time and to enquire into the foundations of hermeneutical method.[33] But all disciplines need terms of art, and medicine is, according to Guinther von Andernach, deficient in them; so that new names have to be created, even though they are

---

[27] Albanesius 1649: 7.

[28] *De interpretatione*, i, 16 a 4ff.; Capivaccius 1603: 12: 'teste Aristotele in principio de interpretatione, ubi dicit, voces esse notas passionum animi, non tamen esse causas passionum in animo'; Silvaticus 1601: 247: 'in his quae nomine carent, quemque suo arbitrio iis nomen imponere Galenus permisit' (referring to Galen, *De differentiis febrium*, i.2). The linguistic sign shares with other kinds of signs the function of representing something to the mind through the senses (the Augustinian locus 'quod seipsum sensui et praeter se aliquid animo repraesentat' is repeated in this regard by Goclenius 1613: 1045). What the linguistic sign represents (a thing, or a concept) and how it is articulated with other signs will be examined below, 5.1, 8.9.1.

[29] Siraisi forthcoming (quoting Galen, *Aliquot opera*, Basle, 1549, 58–9); Cardano 1663: 3.357f.

[30] Towaide 2000; Fuchs 1530: ii–viii (on Leoniceno and Manardo); Silvaticus 1601:21: 'nullus quidem hoc negabit qui sciat rebus imposita esse nomina ut cognoscantur, utque dicebat Averroes lib. 4 de sapientia comment. 11 sicuti diversa idem significare possunt, ita, et multa unum'; Hieronymus 1995: 98 (on German names for plants).

[31] Cardano 1583: 124–5 (on the distinctions between 'lethargus', 'gravido' and 'caro').

[32] Molière, *Le Malade imaginaire*, intermède iii; it is suggested that he was inspired in this by texts such as Claude Gellé, *L'Anatomie française* of 1630: 'le pouls vient de la faculté pulsifique, la pulsifique de la faculté vitale, et la faculté vitale de la présence de l'âme'; see Jouanny in Molière 1962: 880.

[33] See Draut 1625a: 907, 929 (listing lexica, including those by Brunfels 1534, Foesius 1588 and Gorris 1601); Galen, *De differentiis pulsuum*, iii on using metaphors if the comparison can be shown to be useful.

decried.[34] Doctors therefore both cling to a paraphrastic theory of nomination, according to which any formula will do if its referential force is sufficient, and slip at the same time towards the fixing of names for pedagogical and disciplinary reasons.[35] The practice of using words not just as terms of art but as a means of obfuscation, which is associated with the 'primi philosophi', the 'hermetici' and practitioners of 'prisca philosophia', and more recently with natural magicians, is not however condoned by medical writers.[36]

4.2.2 Excursus: William Harvey

Many of these issues of language arise in an important text written at the end of our period by William Harvey, the *Exercitationes de generatione animalium*, published in 1651, but almost certainly written some twenty years before.[37] The relevant passage from the Preface is worth quoting in full:

> Whoever entereth this new and unfrequented path, and inquires for truth in the vast volume of *Nature*, by Anatomical dissections, and experiments, he meets with such a croud of observations, and those too in such exotick shapes, that to unfould to others the mysteries himself hath discovered, will be more toyl, then the finding of them out: for many things occur which have yet no name; such is *the plenty of things, and the dearth of words*.[38] So that if a man should cloath them in Metaphors, and express his new inventions by old words, and such as are in use: the Reader could no more understand them, then canting: and would never be able to comprehend the business, since he never saw it.

---

[34] Guinther von Andernach quoted by Durling 1961: 239–40; Joutsivuo 1999: 139 (on 'insalubre' and 'aegrum' becoming technically distinguished); also Dorn 1584 (Paracelsus's lexicon); Bartolettus 1619: 259–60 and Wolf 1620: A4v (on Paracelsus's abuse of language); also Kuhn 1996.

[35] Galen, *Methodus medendi*, ii.1, K 10.81; for other loci which discuss names see Hankinson 1994. On medical terminology in earlier periods, see Mackinney 1938.

[36] Bono 1995: 93, referring to Fernel 1610a: 2.5 (*De abditis rerum causis*, preface): 'primorum philosophorum mos fuit, quaecunque divina attigissent, tanquam mysteria contegere, aut integumentis quibusdam et involucris implicata enuntiare, seu imperitiae multitudinis offensionem veriti, seu quia haec tam abstrusa si nullo negotio intelligerentur, probatam iri minime sperarent. Quocirca anno adhinc vigesimo odoratus quippiam subdivini nomine in medendi arte penitus obvelatum latere, quod nondum satis pateret, coepi illius studio et amore incitatus quid esset investigare'; Maclean 1984: 234–7; Siraisi 2000: 25–6, quoting Gabriel Naudé on Paracelsus's language.

[37] Whitteridge 1981: xix–xxv; Webster 1967.

[38] See *De sophisticis elenchis*, i, 165 a 10ff.: on names and a quantity of terms as finite, and things infinite in number. See also Maclean 1992: 127–8 quoting Cicero, *Pro Caecina*, xvii.51, on the consequence that the same expression and the single name must necessarily signify a number of things and must give rise to problems of polysemy and homonymy.

And then again to mint up new and fictitious terms, would rather cast a mist, then enlighten. For so he must needs express things unknown: and the Reader would be more afflicted to unriddle the *words*, then to understand the *matter*. And therefore *Aristotle* by unexperimented persons is thought obscure: And this perhaps was the reason, why *Fabricius ab Aquapendente* chose rather to describe the Fabrick of the Chicken in the Egge by *tables* then *words*.

Therefore be not offended, Courteous Reader, if in setting out the *History of an Egge*, and in the description of *the Generation of a Chicken*, I make use of a new method, and sometimes of unusual terms.[39]

This is a complex text, which at first sets out two apparently unacceptable strategies (old words invested with new meaning; neologisms) as solutions to the problem under discussion, next suggests one solution (a new notation through the use of tables) and ends up with one of the two unacceptable strategies (the use of unusual terms) reinforced with a 'new method', namely to incite readers to confirm the meaning of terms themselves by repeating Harvey's experiments, and thus make sense of his new coinages by seeing for themselves.[40] But Harvey's actual practice in the text is rather different: there he takes words with newly reformed meanings (for example 'contagion', whose meaning Fracastoro had modified in his work *De morbis contagiosis* of 1546) and uses them analogically to express a relationship (between semen and ovum, efficient cause and material cause) for which no existing terminology was available to him.[41]

---

[39] Harvey 1653: ℙ 8; Harvey 1766: 1.179–80: 'Qui novum hoc et inusitatum iter ingreditur, et ex ingenii naturae volumine, per dissectiones anatomicas ac experimenta, veritatem inquirit; ei tanta observatorum copia, tamque peregrina facie sese offert; ut a se inventa et observata explicare aliis ac describere difficilius possit, quam ipsimet eadem invenire laboriosum fuerat: adeo multa occurrunt, quae nomina desiderant; tantaque est rerum foecunditas, et verborum egestas. Quod si per metaphoras ea explicare, et antiquis atque usitatis vocabulis conceptus suos de nuper repertis exprimeret; ea lector haud melius, quam aenigmata, intelligeret; remque ipsam, haud visam, neutiquam assequeretur. Novis autem factisque appellationibus usus, sententiae suae non tam facem adhibere, quam nubem offundere videretur. Scilicet ignotum per ignotius exponeret: majoremque operam lector verborum interpretationi, quam rerum ipsarum intellectui impenderet. Ideoque rerum inexpertis Aristoteles multis in locis obscurus creditur: et fortassis ob hanc causam, Fabricius ab Aquapendente fabricam pulli in ovo picturis potius ostendere, quam verbis explicare maluit. Quare, lector benevole, ne aegre feras, si in exornanda ovi historia, et generationis pulli descriptione, nova methodo et verbis aliquando insolitis usus fuerim.'

[40] Harvey himself also adopts new substantival forms such as to 'τò inesse' which he tried to disambiguate: *ibid.*, 2.603: 'quoniam vero τò inesse forsan aequivocum est, et res *simul esse* multifariam dicuntur; ideo dicimus et asserimus speciem futuri pulli et formam immaterialem esse *aliquo modo* causam praegnationis sive foecunditatis uteri...'; on his adaptation of the Aristotle passage in the Preface see Schmitt 1984b. On the use of diagrams to convey medical theory, already well established as a practice in the Middle Ages, see below, 5.2.1.

[41] See Pagel 1986: 4.501, on Harvey's use of 'anima' to mean 'the natural function in blood, blood which acts as the material substratum necessary for the appropriate effect to be obtained

The terms used by Harvey in this way are not given sense by opposition, as would be the case in a Saussurean system, but by definition
and analogy; in other words, he does not do what Thomas Kuhn says
that scientists in a given paradigm do, which is to show the meaning
by using the terms;[42] rather, he uses a separate language to explicate
them. He also speculates about their relationship as tokens to a type or
'eidēs', using the analogy with painting offered by Seneca (*Epistulae*, 58).
The 'eidēs' are for him both 'praecognita' (cognitive data) and 'formae
informantes', i.e. a version of spiritus or souls; they are not altogether neoplatonist pre-existing mental objects, but, like the foetuses about which
he is writing, conceptions consisting of a material and a vital component.
His adaptation of the Aristotelian model is undertaken, it seems to me,
to give prominence to the role played by (clear and distinct) sense-events
(individual acts of seeing) as opposed to the (to us) obscure and confused
universals of which they are tokens.[43] This is a tendentious reading of the
commentary tradition on the relevant passages of Aristotle referred to
by Harvey elsewhere the Preface ('confused' is normally associated with
sense impressions, not universals: see below 4.3), but one which betrays
one of Harvey's major concerns: to establish the absolute primacy of
the senses over mental acts. It has a paradoxical outcome, in that the
existence of a vital force undetectable by the senses is predicated on an
act of non-observation.[44]

in physical life': Fabricius's choice of tables as a means of description to which Harvey refers
is taken up a little later in the century by Robert Hooke in his *Micrographia* of 1665; there he
points out the discoveries due to the microscope, and comments on the problem of words in a
different way (1665: a2v): 'It seems not improbable, but that by these helps (instruments such
as the microscope) the subtelty of the composition of Bodies, the structure of their parts, the
various texture of their matter, the instruments and manner of their inward motions, and all
the other possible appearance of things, may come to be more fully discovered: all of which the
antient <u>Peripateticks</u> were content to comprehend in two general and (unless further explain'd)
useless words of Matter and Form. From whence there may arise many admirable advantages
towards the increase of the <u>Operative</u> and <u>Mechanick</u> knowledge, to which this Age seems so
much inclined, because we may perhaps be inabled to discern all the secret workings of Nature
almost in the same manner as we do those that are the productions of Art, and art managed
by Wheels, and Engines and Springs, that were devised by human Wit.'
42 Kuhn 1970: 43–51.
43 On praecognita and 'notiora natura' or 'a nobis', see below 4.3 and 7.1. For other views of
Harvey on linguistic issues, see Bono 1995: 85–122 and Bates 1998.
44 This is an outcome of 'occult qualities' which had been remarked upon by others, e.g. Montaigne 1965: 589–90 (ii.12): 'Que sçait-on si le genre humain faict une sottise pareille, à faute
de quelque sens, et que par ce defaut la plus part du visage des choses nous soit caché? Que
sçait-on si les difficultez que nous trouvons en plusieurs ouvrages de nature viennent de là?
Et si plusieurs effects des animaux qui excedent nostre capacité, sont produits par la faculté
de quelque sens que nous ayons à dire? Et si aucuns d'entre eux ont une vie plus pleine par
ce moyen et entiere que la nostre? . . . Les proprietez que nous appellons occultes en plusieurs
choses, comme à l'aimant d'attirer le feu, n'est-il pas vraysemblable qu'il y a des facultez

4.2.3 Words as signs: modi significandi

The 'modi significandi' of medical signs are treated as though they constitute linguistic relations to things, either in the mode of proper or common nouns.[45] Proper names, like completely individual characteristics, have no power of communication: a passage in the *Physiognomica* attributed to Aristotle (ii, 806 b 22) states that 'if anyone were to pick out the individual characteristics of each animal, he would not be able to explain of what these are the signs'.[46] So signs have to be specific or generic to be of use to the doctor: 'if there is such a thing as a "simple" disease, it does not partake of the logic of the sign', as Campilongo puts it;[47] a world in which all things were individually named would have no 'discursus' at all.[48] Every act of diagnosis is therefore cognate to a receiver hearing a sentence in a natural language; even if that sentence had never been uttered before, the fact that its constituents are known to the hearer in their common signification makes possible its comprehensibility in the individual circumstances of the utterance.[49]

4.2.4 Words with power

Words can be claimed to have powers beyond conventional nomination as in Paracelsian doctrine, according to which words are things, or in

sensitives en nature, propres à les juger et les appercevoir, et que le defaut de telles facultez nous apporte l'ignorance de la vraye essence des choses?'

45 Argenterio 1610: 148: 'quaedam [signa] significare ut communia, quaedam ut propria, quaedam ut immediata: alia vero ut mediata, nonnulla suapte natura, alia vero aliorum ratione, et quo quaedam ita significent, ut magnam vim in significando habeant, alia vero parvam, aut incertam obtineant. Sumuntur enim hae omnes differentiae a significandi modo et ratione'; Capivaccius 1603: 9–12 (on the correlative relationship between signum and signatum); Silvaticus 1601: 21; Heath 1971.

46 Fontanus 1611: 34 paraphrases this passage as follows: 'ex propriis autem signis nullo pacto quicquam inferre potest'. See below 5.1.

47 Campilongo 1601: 19v: 'si fuerit affectus simplex praeter naturam non habet rationem indicantis', citing (loosely) Galen, *Ad Thrasybulum*, xxv–xxvi, K 5.851–2.

48 Foucault 1966: 112 makes this point, a version of which is found in Lodovicus 1540: a6v, cited by Meinel 1992: 23 (as the number of human beings equals the number of occult qualities because 'proprietates' derive from unique combinations of humours, the 'singular' is 'unknowable'; see below 5.1.5). But if everything was a common noun, meaninglessness is also in prospect: 'non omnia significant omnia', as Argenterio 1610: 1688 puts it, citing *Rhetoric to Alexander*, xii, 1406 b 33f.

49 A similar point is made by Zabarella 1586–7:) (6r–v, in the preface to his *Opera logica*: having argued (against linguistic purists) that philosophers can use coined Latin words because meaning ('res') and clarity are the highest priority, he goes on to point out that it is a feature of Greek philosophical writing that meaning resides as much in collocations and in syntax as in bare terms; and that it does not follow that where any text is grammatically at its most simple, it is least obscure (he cites here the example of Aristotle).

cabbalistic discourse, in which words are seen as the bark covering the sap of invisible arcane knowledge,[50] or in incantations, which are much used in popular medicine. The efficacy of these, together with other objects of virtue such as amulets or inscriptions, is denied on the whole by rational doctors, using standard Aristotelian arguments about the conventionality of language.[51] An important text on this subject is that of Thomas Erastus (1524–83). In a polemical anti-Paracelsian text, he directs his attacks against those who, like Ficino, Pomponazzi and Auger Ferrier, claim that characters, images, amulets and verbal formulae have inherent force which can be harnessed for healing purposes. His argument is a very Aristotelian defence of the conventionality and arbitrary nature of linguistic signs, accompanied by a clear adherence to mentalism; it is somewhat unfair in respect of Ferrier, who had only said that the reason for the efficacy of such cures was to be sought in the 'vis animi' of the patient, whose belief in the remedy allows it to work.[52]

---

[50] Béhar 1996; Pittion 1987: 122ff.; Vigenère 1586: 115v, 164r (citing Romans 1:20).

[51] Gentilcore 1993; also Ottosson 1984: 267; Biesius 1573: 95–7 ('characteres et verba non habere vim talem, qualem magi pollicentur'); Scribonius 1584: 89; Siraisi 1997: 163–4 (on Cardano and Pomponazzi).

[52] Erastus 1572: 1.169–70: 'verba partim sunt naturalia, partim artificialia, sicut Imagines. Equidem materia verborum, ut imaginum, naturalis est, nempe vox cuius materia est sonus. Forma autem est articulatio certa . . . Et quemadmodum Imago repraesentat rem aliquam, sic et verba (si modo non sint barbara et ignota) animi sensa significant. Significant autem non natura, sed ex pacto conventoque hominum.' A number of arguments follow, including the claim that since the deaf cannot speak by nature, words must be artificial. This view is accompanied by a clear mentalism: 'cogitationes, qui a nobis natura insunt, eaedem sunt apud omnes'. 'Signa naturalia' do exist however in the form of animal communication: *ibid.*, 173. For the attack on Ferrier, see *ibid.*, 179: 'verbis et characteribus vim adimit quidem, sed in Doctis et Intelligentiam habentibus'. This is a misrepresentation of Ferrier's point in his discussion of 'homerica medicatio' (the use of amulets, characters and incantations on the authority of respected ancient authors), where he avers that although loath to controvert the experience of trustworthy authorities who have witnessed it ('nam ijs quae sensibus exposita sunt contravenire, sani hominis non est: Doctorum vero experimenta infirmare, temerarium'), one can offer a different explanation: 'tu vero (dices) qui haec inculcas, quid sentis? Dicam libere. Neque enim superstitiosus homo sum, neque fabularum amans, sed veritatis studiosus. In quam cum toto animo, ac studio omni incumberem, prodigiosus quoque has curationes attingere volui, ne qua parte in artis operibus deficerem. Deprehendi itaque curationis huius eventum non e caracteribus, non ex carmine promanare. Sed tanta est vis animi nostri, ut si quid honesti sibi persuaserit, atque in ea persuasione firmiter perseverarit, idipsum quod concepit agat, et potenter operetur: modo alterius in quem agit animi non habeat repugnantem neque differentem. Nam si etiam fidentem et coadiuvantem habuerit, citius quod intenditur perficitur. Si neque fidentem, neque diffidentem nihilominus vis animi agentis operabitur. [Ferrier here points out that a 'praecantator' can get rid of toothache by singing, but if the patient doesn't believe in the singer, it won't work.] Non sunt ergo carmina, non sunt caracteres qui talia possunt, sed vis animi confidentis, et cum patiente concordis, ut doctissime a poeta dictum sit:

> Nos habitat, non tartara, sed nec sydera caeli
> Spiritus in nobis qui viget illa facit.

4.2.5 Styles of writing

A last aspect of names and grammar is style. It is worth mentioning that Hippocrates and Galen represent in some (but not in all) eyes two extremes of this: Hippocrates, as aphoristic, terse, substantial; a writer having 'a compressed verbal style and concise subtlety'; Galen whose excessive 'asiatic exuberance' is seen, by Argenterio at least, as ill-ordered and confusing: 'he explains many things in a variety of ways, which confuse those of less subtle minds, and he does not seem to keep to his premisses ('principia') once he has stated them'.[53] Arnau de Vilanova was an early enthusiast for aphoristic writing;[54] at the beginning of the sixteenth century, Victorius sees the alternative styles as excess and defect and recommends to those who write commentaries a happy medium between them, not one of rhetorical elegance but of veridicity and economy: having expressed the wish that 'the slender words of Hippocrates be relieved by greater richness ('uberius excipiantur') and that the verbose documents of Galen be bound together with greater brevity ('brevius colligantur'), he continues:

In these lucubrations I wanted to gather only the flowers of truth, and did not set out to affect concinnate and polished figures of speech; lest by making no more than sonorous noise without content, I should omit through ignorance a hidden nucleus of truth. Wherever the truth of philosophy is extracted from precepts and made deeper, there we need least of all the coloured

Verum confidentia illa, ac firma persuasio comparatur indoctis animis per opinionem quam de caracteribus et sacris verbis conceperunt. Doctis et rerum intelligentiam habentibus, nihil opus est externis, sed cognita vi animi, per eam miracula edere possunt . . . Indoctis ergo animus, hoc est suae potestatis et naturae inscius, per externa illa confirmatus, morbos curare poterit. Doctus vero, et sibi constans, solo verbo sanabit: aut ut simul indoctum animum afficiat, externa quoque assumet, non solum quae vulgo probata dicuntur, verumetiam alia quoque a se inventa, vel quaecunque illi ad manum, aut in mentem prompte venerint': Ferrier 1574: 221–2. I am grateful to Constance Blackwell for giving me the reference to Erastus's text. See also Pomponazzi 1567: 51 (on autosuggestion); *ibid.*, 84–93 (on the power of words, characters and talismans to cure). Horst 1585 is a book on the prayers suitable for doctors preparing to engage on their task of healing, and does not include incantatory material.

53 Argenterio 1610: † 4: 'verborum pressa proprietas, concisa subtilitas'; 'ubertas asiatica'; 'multa varie explicat, quibus rudiores confunduntur et semel posita principia perpetuo servare non videtur'; Temkin 1973: 152; Velsius 1543: 56; Albertus 1615: F4v (quoting Argenterio, above); ironically Galen, the author of several million words, declares himself to be in favour of aphoristic style, and demands in his commentaries that doctors write 'exacte, breviter, aperte': see Heurnius 1637: 17.

54 Arnau de Vilanova 1585: 1700: he says that the following three features are necessary in an aphorism: 'quod sit sententia vera, vel semper, ut quando est de necessariis, vel ut plurimum, quando est de contingentibus: secundum est, ut superfluitate careat, et in his consistit integritas aphorismi: tertium ad manifestationem veritatis eius, et ad doctrinae certitudinem est utile, ut causam dicti explicet, vel insinuet . . .'

allurements of speaking. The matter in hand spurns decoration, and is content
to be taught.[55]

It is notable that in some traditions of law there is an express preference
for presentation in axioms and aphorisms, because 'they leave the wit of
man more free to turn and toss, and make use of what is delivered to
more severall purposes and applications'.[56] Even if some of the 'severall purposes' alluded to here, which include adversarial argument, are
firmly eschewed by doctors, the juristic practice of deriving legal norms
from tersely expressed rules and laws finds a parallel in the medieval
praise of the aphoristic form by Arnau de Vilanova, and later, after 1560,
in the Hippocratic revival, in which the presentation of medical theory
through cases and aphorisms is seen to embody precepts and exemplify
the true Hippocratic method.[57] Presentation of such precepts through
the medium of aphorisms does not entail the elaboration of a complete
system; only those precepts which need to be cited in the context of the
aphorism need be alleged. In this, the recommendation by doctors of
aphoristic discourse prefigures some developments in the natural philosophy of the seventeenth century, in which local explanations are put
forward for phenomena, and no attempt is made to link these to a broader
system of thought.

4.3 DEMONSTRATIVE LOGIC

I turn now from grammar to categories and scientific demonstration.
A necessary condition of scientific discourse is the limit imposed on
predicability by the ten predicaments or categories: substance, quantity,
quality, relation, time, place, position, possession, acting, being acted
upon. This does not mean that all that is knowable is confined to the ten
predicaments as though these had the force of Kantian categories; we
can, if not know, then at least conceive of, prime matter, or infinity, or
impossible objects, which lie beyond the categories;[58] it entails only that
the intellect's ability to discourse about objects is so confined. This is the

---

55 Victorius 1598: a2v: 'ut gracilia Hippocratis verba uberius excipiantur, et verbosa Galeni
     documenta brevius colligantur'; 'in iis [lucubrationibus] solum veritatis flores decerpere volui,
     et non concinnitatas dictionis expolitae figuras affectare constitui: ne vacuo tantum verborum
     strepitu personans, occlusum veritatis nucleum ignarus omittam. Ubi philosophiae praeceptis
     veritas altius effoditur, ibi fucatis dicendi lenociniis minime indigemus. Ornari res ipsa negat,
     contenta doceri.' The last sentence is paradoxically a hexameter.
56 Daston and Park 1998: 229 (quoting Bacon, *Elements of common law*, London, 1630, B3r: composed
     1596/7 as *Maxims of the law*). See also Vickers 1968: 60–95.
57 Nutton 1989.
58 See *Physics*, iii.8, 208 a 15f.; *De interpretatione*, i, 16 a 17f.; *Categories*, iv, 1 b 25ff.

account given in several medical logics;[59] debates involving the categories which are relevant here are principally those concerning definition of terms of art, such as illness (see below, 7.5).

I have already touched upon scientific demonstration in discussing the debate about the status of medicine as an art or as a science (above 3.2). Descartes, it will be remembered, planned to work on medicine to see whether 'il y a moyen de trouver une médecine qui soit fondée en démonstrations infaillibles'.[60] He clearly thought that Galen's claim to have achieved this (in the lost work *De demonstratione*) was unwarranted. When Jakob Schegk tried to reconstitute this work in 1564, he ended up by writing something very closely calqued on the *Posterior analytics*, a work which at Padua was recognised to be particularly suitable for use by doctors,[61] and which is certainly in tune with their thoroughgoing realism; for how to reveal the 'res ipsae' is claimed to be the aim *simpliciter* of the methodical doctrine of doctors.[62] But demonstration in its highest form is more associated with the syllogistic procedures of the first figure set out in the *Prior analytics*, and with a hierarchy of disciplines which Zabarella determined in relation to causal knowledge, subject matter and elegance (as represented by the smallest number of premises).[63] The highest discipline in this account is metaphysics, followed by physics, psychology, mathematics and logic (looked upon in this instance not as an instrument but as a science); an art such as law or medicine falls below these.[64]

This hierarchy is sometimes linked by medical writers to the question of certainty and truth. Wolf repeats the topos (from Galen's *De locis affectis*,

---

[59] Galen, *Methodus medendi*, ii.7, K 10.126–56; ix.9, K 10.634–5; Champier 1516b; da Monte 1587: 1–19; Capivaccius 1603: 1003–51.

[60] Descartes 1996: 1.106 (letter to Mersenne dated January 1630).

[61] Cf. L'Alemant 1549, whose *Ars parva* resembles dialectics; Viottus 1560; Kusukawa 1999: 170 (on Schegk); Cardano 1663: 1.301–4; Jardine 1974: 24 says that the *Posterior analytics* was not always part of the arts course, but it seems to have been taught at Northern Italy: Wallace 1988: 212–13; and it was certainly taught in Freiburg: Ott and Fletcher 1964: 82. Galen's *De demonstratione* was perhaps known to Averroes (see Nutton 1981: 19, citing Strohmeier); but there is no indication of this fact being known in the Renaissance.

[62] Capivaccius 1603: 1009; the aim 'secundum quid' is the 'modus docendi'. On 'simpliciter' versus 'secundum quid' (sometimes 'ut nunc') see *De sophisticis elenchis*, iv, 166 b 20–7; Joutsivuo 1999: 127.

[63] Mikkeli 1992: 36; Schegk 1579b: A2r makes the connection between science and demonstration clear: 'omnis scientia propter ἀποδείξεις dicitur θεωρητική'.

[64] *Nicomachean ethics*, i.3, 1094 b 12–27; Wildenbergius 1585; Olivieri 1983b. On arts and sciences: Hollerius 1582: 3r; Blair 1997: 41; Aquinas, *In Boethium de trinitate*, 1 ad 9; Maclean 1992: 22–3; Velsius 1543: 20; Magirus 1603: 580 (commenting on the views of Melanchthon). Capivaccius's title of his 1562 treatise (*De differentiis doctrinarum logicis, philosophis atque medicis*) implies a hierarchy of disciplines.

i.1, K 8.18–19) that there are three levels of knowing: 'certissimae notae', 'indubitatae indices' and 'exquisita notitia' together constitute the highest level, which can be called scientific knowledge; 'artificiosa quaedam coniectura' or inference guided by art the second, and 'pura ignorantia' the third.[65] The 'indubitatae indices' include the products of 'experientia' (that which constitutes a common body of knowledge derived from the senses),[66] which can be presupposed or 'pre-known' ('praecognita'), as is pointed out in *Physics*, ii.1 (193 a 4ff.): 'it is patent that many things corresponding to our definitions do actually exist: and to set about proving the obvious from the unobvious betrays confusion of mind as to what is self-evident and what is not'.[67] It is clear here that the objective, extramental certainty of logical procedures ('exquisita notitia') has become conjoined not only with sensory information but with the psychological state of certainty, as it has in the related Thomist threefold scheme of knowledge (*Summa theologiae*, 1a 2ae 112.5): 'per revelationem'; 'per seipsum' or 'certitudinaliter'; and 'per aliqua signa' or 'coniecturaliter'. Aquinas's knowledge 'per revelationem' manifestly belongs to a domain above medicine and natural philosophy;[68] his middle category conjoins 'indemonstrativa universalia principia' with 'conclusiones demonstrativae', certainty with logic. These principles of knowledge can be described as criteria, as by Melanchthon, whose rather different triad is 'experientia universalis' (aisthēsis), 'notita principiorum' (prolēpsis) and 'intellectus ordo in syllogismo' (gnōsis).[69] The partially psychological

---

[65] Wolf 1620: A2v: 'est enim inter exactam notitiam, atque puram ignorantiam quodammodo media: ad quam rem inprimis confert Anatomicae doctrina, ex qua universi corporis dispositionem et quidem: qualis sit cuiuslibet partis essentia, deinde actio, usus, situs et communis sive societas, quam cum aliis habet, edocemur'; Cachetus 1612: 758; Bartolettus 1619: 247.

[66] See Dear 1987; Dear 1990; Dear 1995.

[67] 'Praecognita' in this sense fall into the category of statements, which, according to Aristotle (*Topics*, i.1, 100 b 30f.) are 'things . . . true and primary which command belief through themselves and not through anything else; for regarding the first principles of science it is unnecessary to ask any further question as to "why" but each principle should of itself command belief'; see also Kessler 1995: 303. Biesius 1573: 158r refers to 'certa demonstratio' as 'omnibus nota principia demonstrationum omnium, quae axiomata vocant: ut totum esse quavis sua parte, de rebus omnibus affirmationem vel negationem esse veram'; he further glosses 'certa' as 'quae sensu bene constituto ab omnibus percipiuntur'. For others, all doctrine, including doctrine in the order of the intelligible, is said to be derived from 'praeexistens cognitio'; 'omne iudicium sumi ex aliquo praecognito, sive id sit sensibile sive intelligibile': Goclenius 1613 s.v. praecognitio. On the error of demonstrating what is self-evident, see Galen, *De optima secta*, i–ii, K 1.106–10.

[68] Magirus 1603: 583–4 refers (after Melanchthon 1834–60: 13.151) to revelation as 'patefactio divina', which is found in the decalogue and in the 'vox Evangelii'.

[69] Melanchthon 1834–60: 13.150–1, followed by Victorinus Strigelius, *In Philippi Melanchthonis libellum de anima notae*, Leipzig, 1590 (on whom see Kusukawa 1999: 130–1) and Magirus 1603: 581–2. Melanchthon attributes these criteria to the Stoics.

notion of certainty to which these theories relate is consistent with a correspondence theory of truth ('adaequatio rei et intellectus') or an attenuated version of this, in which the adequation is with sense impressions, not with 'res'.[70] The thoroughgoing sense epistemology of Aristotelians, expressed in the tag 'nihil in intellectu quod non prius in sensu',[71] is related not only to the formation of universal terms by a quasi-inductive process (*Posterior analytics*, ii.19) but also to the development of metaphysical notions derived by necessary reasoning from sense data, although in many cases they come to 'precede' such data in terms of logical priority. I do not need to go further into this area;[72] it is however relevant to both the problems raised by those, such as Lutherans, for whom medicine is involved with theological issues,[73] and to certain issues that all doctors face, such as defining what 'indicatio' is, since 'indicatio' refers to the relationship of sense data to the processes of intellection (below 8.7).

The correlate of criteria in terms of content are 'praecognita', which are the products of 'praecognitio'. The Aristotelian doctrine is to be found at the beginning of the *Posterior analytics* (i.1, 71 a 12ff.), where 'praecognitio' is divided into (i) prior knowledge of fact, (ii) prior knowledge of the meaning of a term, and (iii) prior knowledge of both; and all such prior knowledge is distinguished from the actualisation of potential knowledge, which is what occurs when we engage in reasoning.

---

[70] The problem of the psychological or mind-independent status of such criteria is discussed in the Renaissance: see e.g. Grawerus 1619: 17 (on the distinction between the 'veritas objecti' and a double notion of correspondence): 'adaequatio notionum in intellectu cum rebus et orationum cum notionibus, ita ut oratio consentiat cum notionibus animi, notio animi cum re ipsa extra animum vere existente'; Martini 1593: B4v (arguing that philosophy is a 'mentis habitus' not 'extra mentem'): 'si nullus sit homo capax artis, et per consequens nulla hominis mente ars, ubi tuae artes habitabunt? An apud ideas Platonicas? Vel in Utopia simul cum vestra philosophia? Ut si nullus sit sutor in rerum natura ubi erit ars sutoria?' See also Aquinas, *De veritate*, 2.1 ad 4 (on scientia as either 'in deo' or a 'habitus conclusionis'); Maclean 1992: 74 (on Scaliger); Leijenhorst forthcoming (on Toletus's assertion, followed by Case, that truth is causally in things *qua* objects, instrumentally in propositions *qua* signs, and formally in minds *qua* terms); Eckart 1992: 156 (on Sennert); Herberger 1981: 93–4 (quoting Galen, *De optima secta*, ii, K 1.108–10); see also Keckermann 1614: 1596–1600.

[71] On the origin of this see Cranefield 1970; it is quoted by Capivaccius 1603: 282.

[72] Mikkeli 1992: 102–3; for the connection with induction (*Prior analytics*, ii.27) and 'prior by nature' and 'prior to us', see 4.3.5.

[73] The theological dimension to this doctrine is its link with the Fall and the corruption of man's capacity of knowledge, preventing him from seeing things 'per se' and reducing him to the perception of hidden things through the shaky inferences of conjecture; above, 3.6.5, and Kusukawa 1995a: 94–5. For Lutherans, the Fall corrupted men's knowledge of the first two of Melanchthon's criteria, causing them to misread signs, to fail to see the true dogmas of natural philosophy, and to be reduced in their perception of hidden things ('occulta et involuta') to conjecture. These views are not of course unique to Lutherans.

'Praecognitio' is often linked to the principles of any discipline, which are 'neither derived from anything else, nor from each other, but from which all else is derived'.[74] Such 'praecognita' are usually said to be specific to disciplines: those of physics are supplied by metaphysics and are necessary; those of medicine are supplied by natural philosophy, and have the same status; but the 'praecognita' specific to medicine (health) may be no more than endoxical (see below 7.1ff.).[75]

According to *Posterior analytics*, ii.1 (89 b 23ff.), there are four questions relevant to logic: fact ('to hoti: an sit'); cause ('to dioti: cur sit'); existence ('ei esti; quod sit') and essence ('ti estin: quid sit').[76] These are reproduced by medical logicians in ways to show their relevance to medicine.[77] The questions 'quia' and 'propter quid' are however principally concerned with composites (of subject and predicate) and therefore demonstration: I shall return to them below. Before that, it is pertinent to point out what other rules or laws of demonstrative logic are invoked frequently in the adaptation of the arts course to medical pedagogy.

4.3.1 *Identity and difference*

There is the law of identity and non-contradiction, invoked to achieve thematic coherence (predication is 'in respect of one and the same thing, to itself and according to itself, in the same manner and time').[78] There is also the square of contraries which is a test of non-contradiction, and a mode of proof *per impossibile* (fig. 4.1). Demonstration *per contradictionem* or *per impossibile* is afforded by this square (by reading of the diagonals);

---

74 Sennert 1650: 1.7: 'neque ex aliis sunt, neque ex se mutuo, sed ex quibus omnia': Aristotle, *Physics*, i.5, 188 a 27–8; Galen, *Methodus medendi*, i.4, K 10.33–4.

75 'Praecognitio' is a word with different senses according to discipline: in medicine it can mean both prognosis and prior knowledge of theory, in physics it can indicate the presuppositions taken over from the superior discipline metaphysics (form, matter, privation; act and potency, etc.): Ingolstetter 1596: A1; Lemosius 1598: 1r.

76 See Vasoli 1968: 132ff. (on Giorgio Valla's reduction of these four questions to 'coniectura', 'definitio' and 'consecutio'); Blair 1997: 62 (referring to Francis Bacon's reduction of 'cur sit' to 'an sit', which is found also in Schegk 1579b: A4r); also Blair 1999: 180.

77 Capivaccius 1603: 1024; Clementinus 1535: 1 (applying the questions to fevers; 'utrum febris sit, quid sit febris, quare illud accidens inest suo subjecto (quare Socrates febricitat) quia (assignamus causam: Socrates habet calorem nocivum, accensum in corde, inflammationem corporis)'.

78 Sanctorius 1630: 743 (xi.6): 'respectu unius et eiusdem, ad idem et secundum idem, eodem modo et eodem tempore'; Sanctorius *ibid.*, 69 (i.21) and *passim* also refers to the three laws of predication ('kata pantos', 'kath'auto', 'katholou prōton'): see *Posterior analytics*, i.4, 73 a 21ff.

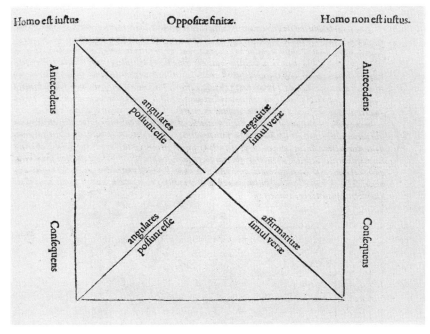

Figure 4.1. Jacopo Zabarella, *Opera logica*, [Heidelberg,] 1586–7, vol. 5, p. 33. The four propositions are: top left: 'every man is just'; top right: 'no man is just'; bottom left (not illustrated): 'not every man is not just'; bottom right (not illustrated): 'every man is not just'

this has its importance, if only by contradistinction, in medical discourse, whose contradictories are not always susceptible to such treatment, as we shall see. The diagram also is adapted for other logical purposes, such as the demonstration of the relations between middle terms, as in the diagram by Claude Aubéry (fig. 4.2).[79] This diagram contains the relationship in logic which Sanctorius claims is the most important for diagnosis, namely universal negation in the second figure ('negans univer[alis] in sec[unda] figura'); it is also adapted for specific medical purposes (see below 4.4, esp. note 120).

Opposition between terms is by contradiction (here in the sense of affirmation or negation), privation and possession, correlation and

---

[79] Aubéry 1584: 327. The practice of using contentious theological propositions as examples seems to stem from Melanchthon. For medieval parallels for various of these figures, see Murdoch 1984: 50, 64–5. On Aubéry see Zanier 1983: 112.

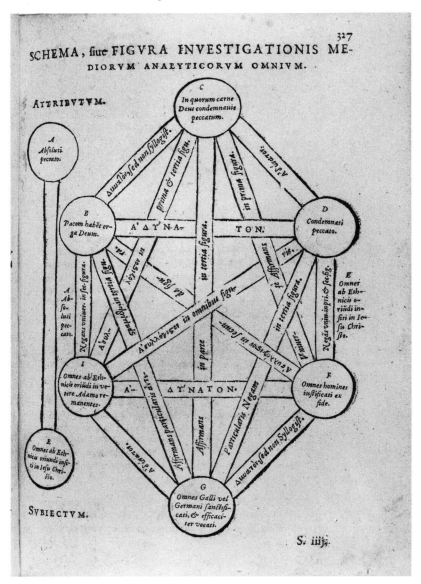

Figure 4.2. Claude Aubéry, *Organon, id est, instrumentum doctrinarum omnium in duas partes divisum, Nempe, in analyticum eruditionis modum, et dialecticam, sive methodum disputandi in utramque partem*, Morges, 1548 (AA 119(1) Art), p. 327

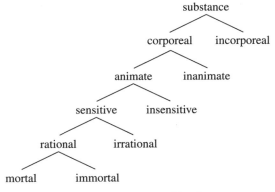

Figure 4.3a. The tree of Porphyry

contrariety, which may be immediate (as in odd/even) or mediate (as in black/[grey]/white). Contraries are defined in Aristotle's *Categories* and *Metaphysics* and in two Galenic loci as 'things furthest apart from each other in the same genus'. This doctrine is reproduced entire in some medical logic courses.[80]

4.3.2 Porphyry's tree: division and definition

Division and definition are interdependent. Division is a technique of relating terms and separating 'genera generalissima' from 'genera subalterna' and 'species' best exemplified by Porphyry's tree (fig. 4.3).[81] We may note here that for the division to be scientific, the differentiae (corporeal/incorporeal, animate/inanimate, etc.) must be thematically appropriate and in the correct order (one could not, for example, insert 'high/low' or 'soft/hard' before 'corporeal/incorporeal'), both petition of principles and over-division must be avoided, and there can be no remainder; the division of the term must be perfect and necessary. Porphyry's tree is able to supply the scientific definitions of stone (corporeal, inanimate substance), plant (corporeal, animate, insensitive substance), animal (corporeal, animate, sensitive, irrational, substance) and man (corporeal, animate, sensitive, rational, mortal, substance). In these

---

[80] *Categories*, x, 11 b 15ff.; *Metaphysics*, 1055 a 5ff., 1018 a 30; *Methodus medendi*, i.7, K 10.50, xi.12, K 10.770; Capivaccius 1603: 1036–7; Sanctorius 1630: 743 (xi.12): 'contraria sunt duae formae extremae in eodem genere.'
[81] Boethius; *In categories*, PL 64.169–70. Champier 1516b: v uses this diagram.

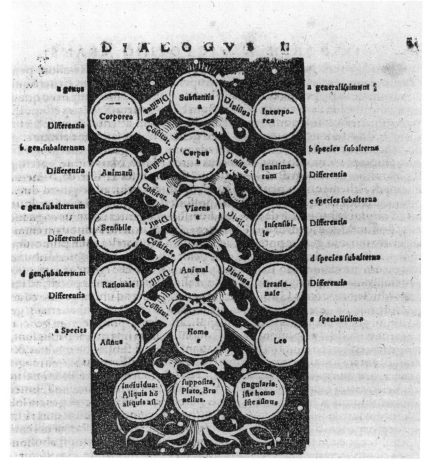

Figure 4.3b. The tree of Porphyry: Boethius, *Opera*, Basle, 1570, p. 25

definitions, it is to be noted that not only the genus inheres in the species, but the species in the genus.[82]

In the *Physics*, as we have already noted, Aristotle relates division to a heuristic process (children call both parents 'mother' before distinguishing mother and father), and in the *De anima*, iii.6 (430 a 26ff.),

[82] Wear 1973: 170, quoting Sanctorius 1630: 797–9 (xii.6). See also *ibid.*, 795, 802 (xii.60) on all individuals in universals, and universals in all individuals.

he identifies one of the functions of the agent intellect as division and combination to the end of producing (true) knowledge; but in the *Posterior analytics*, the 'via divisiva' is said not to inform us about anything which we did not already know; if used by itself it merely leads to a petition of principles.[83] It is associated with a version of Ockham's razor; because the 'methodus divisiva' is a 'brevissima via', 'we must not increase the number of entities unnecessarily'.[84] It is also the major source of error when misapplied: Galen declares that 'all errors in medicine arise from bad division'.[85] But as a 'via' or method it is none the less described as 'divine' on the authority of Plato,[86] and is said to be the mother of demonstration and definition,[87] of which there are two sorts: nominal ('quid nominis') and real ('quid rei').[88] The latter is the more scientific, and consists in formal statements of quiddity by genus, species, proprium, and differentia; to this list 'accidens' is sometimes added.[89] But there are many examples of the use of nominal definition, which gives rise to the characteristic subtle distinctions (also employing the predicaments) for which all disciplines based on the trivium are famous.[90]

---

83 *Posterior analytics*, i.3, 72 b 5ff.; Sanctorius 1630: 25–9 (i.7: 'ostenditur non posse per viam divisivam occultum aliquem affectum inveniri'); see also below 4.3.3.

84 Da Monte 1587: 23: 'quia methodus divisiva est brevissima via, non debemus entia sine necessitate multiplicare'; Aristotle, *Physics*, i.6, 189 a 15f.; Galen, *Methodus medendi*, v, K 10.305ff.; *Ad Glauconem*, i, K 11.1–6; Ferdinandus 1611: 15: 'in hac rerum universitate non sunt infinita multiplicanda entia absque necessitate'; he also provides a quotation from Horace as a version of the razor (*Satires*, i.1, lines 107–8: 'est modus in rebus, sunt certi denique fines / quos ultra, citra nequit consistere rectum'). See also Nutton 1990b: 211 (on da Monte's objection to Fracastoro's notion of contagion because it postulated another layer of hypothetical entia); Jardine 1974: 27 (on whether new things can be learned from principles, citing Lee 1935: 122–3).

85 *Ad Glauconem*, i, K 11.1–6; Argenterio 1610: 2.24; Capivaccius 1593: 4r.

86 Da Monte 1587: 5–14, 95.

87 *Ibid.*, 231; *Metaphysics*, vii.12, 1037 b 30ff.

88 *Posterior analytics*, ii.7–10, esp. 92 a 26–7; da Monte 1587: 229.

89 Galen, *De differentiis pulsuum*, iv.2, K 8.699–720; Capivaccius 1603: 1031 (citing Averroes); da Monte 1587: 230 (defining proprium as 'quod cum re ipsa convertitur'). On the need for convertibility, see Maclean 1992: 107; on the distinction between proprium and accidens, see Jardine 1974: 20–1: it is proper of Royal Mail vans to be red, i.e., an invariable feature, but one which could be otherwise; it is an accident (a contingent attribute) of a handkerchief to be red. *Topics*, ii, 108 b 34ff. and v, 128 b 34ff. offers a more complete taxonomy of accidents and properties.

90 Two subtle examples are to be found in Lonie 1981: 22, who cites Sennert's distinction between 'calidum innatum' and 'caliditas' (as substance from quality); and Horst 1629: 6, distinguishing between privation and positive difference: 'formale morbi non consistit in privatione, sed in positiva disconvenientia qualitatum constitutioni sanae contraria'.

4.3.3 Syllogistic

I turn now to syllogistic demonstration.[91] Its figures and the means employed to reduce one to another are taken for granted by doctors at this time.[92] The figures can be represented diagrammatically; an example is afforded by Giambattista della Porta's application of the technique (which Panizza asserts is Byzantine in origin) to *Prior analytics*, ii.27 (70 b: cited below 5.1.1): see fig. 4.4.[93] This figure is, as we shall see, adapted for the specific purposes of medical discourse.

---

[91] It is slightly puzzling that modal logic and consequentiae, which are part of demonstrative logic, are rarely alleged by doctors. Silvaticus 1601: 21–2 is unusual at this time in linking possible and rare events. On consequentiae (hypothetical syllogisms), see below, 4.4.

[92] I offer here a brief account of syllogistic logic (following closely Panizza 1999: 35, whose account is based on Peter of Spain's *Summulae logicales*), as background to the examples of syllogisms given below. The formal syllogism is made up of three propositions: two Premisses (Major and Minor) and a Conclusion. Each Premiss has a Subject and a Predicate, also known as 'Terms'. The 'Middle Term' is the Subject or Predicate that is repeated twice in the Premisses, thereby serving as a link; it is eliminated in the Conclusion (e.g. 'all men are animals; all animals are mortal; therefore all men are mortal'). The Subject of the Conclusion is known as the 'Minor Term' and the Premiss in which it appears as the 'Minor Premiss'; the Predicate of the Conclusion is known as the 'Major Term' and appears as the Major Premiss. There are four possible types of proposition, knowns as 'moods': universal affirmative ('all . . . are . . .') (mood A), universal negative ('all . . . are not . . .') (mood E), particular affirmative ('some . . . are . . .') (mood I), particular negative ('some . . . are not . . .') (mood O). There are (for our purposes) three figures of the syllogism; they are distinguished by the position of the Middle Term. In the first figure, which is taken to be strongest, the Middle Term is the Subject in the Major premise, and the Predicate in the minor (as in the example 'all men are animals . . .' above); the Conclusion can take any of the four moods in this figure. In the second figure, the Middle Term is Predicate in both Major and Minor Premisses; all valid Conclusions in this figure are negative; a fallacious kind of second figure leading to an affirmative Conclusion is referred to in medical literature because it reflects what rational doctors take to be the reasoning of empirics (the 'fallacia consequentiae'): Sanctorius 1630: 27 (i.7): 'argumentum ex duabus affirmativis in secunda figura non sequitur'. In the third figure, it is Subject in both; all the Conclusions of this figure are particular. Some, but not all, types of syllogism in the second and third figure can be reduced to the first figure. The letters A, E, I, O (designating the moods) are used in the following mnemonic verse which records the complete scheme of figures and moods of the syllogism:

> Barbara Celarent Darii Ferio Baralipton
> Celantes Dabitis Fapesmo Frisesomorum
> Cesare Camestres Festino Baroco Daralipti
> Felapton Disamis Datisi Bocardo Ferison.

'Camestres', for example, describes a syllogism in which the Major Premiss is universal affirmative and both the Minor Premiss and the Conclusion are universal negative (see below, note 120). In subsequent examples in the text, where they need to be identified for reasons of clarity, M is used to designate Middle Term; S, Subject; P, Predicate.

[93] Porta 1593: 58; Panizza 1999. The syllogism can be transcribed as follows, the terms being strong (A), having large extremities (B), and lion (C):

everything having large extremities is strong	(all B is A)
all lions have large extremities	(all C is B)
all lions are strong	(all C is A)

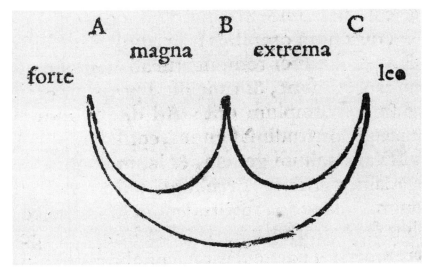

Figure 4.4. Giambattista della Porta, *Physiognomia*, Hanau, 1593, p. 58

4.3.4 Causes

The first figure, the most scientific form of syllogism, has a cause as its middle term. This is not simply an efficient or proximate cause, but any of the Aristotelian quartet, all of which are translatable into medical terms (see below chapter 7): material (members, spirits, humours and elements), efficient (the six non-naturals), formal (complexions, virtues, compositions), and final (the functionality of the human body).[94] Of these, the final cause has particular importance in medicine; but it is not the only cause adduced, as we shall see (below 4.4.4). Allegation of these causes may generate great complexity of argument.[95] Without allegation of cause, medicine is reduced from a rational art to an empirical practice.[96]

Porta adds to the Minor 'and some animals' (and hence also to the conclusion): this to demonstrate that the attribute of large extremities can have signifying force in individual animals belonging to other genera.

[94] Ottosson 1984: 72, quoting Avicenna, *Canon*, i.1.

[95] According to García Ballester 1993b: 39, the complexity of argument is seen as an attractive feature of the discipline in the Middle Ages.

[96] Horst 1629: 25 points out that Galen omitted 'morbi totius substantiae' from his treatise *De morborum differentiis* because the cause was not known.

4.3.5 *The demonstrative sign*

It is possible for a sign (tekmērion) to be the middle term of a necessary demonstration ('upwards' from cause to effect), even though a sign is usually conceived of as an effect, not a cause. Such necessary signs must be convertible; they may be either proper signs (of a given cause) or common signs 'collected together into syndromes',[97] where the syndrome operates as does a perfect induction, by which a property of a subject can be inferred from knowledge of the whole class. In *Prior analytics*, ii.23 (68 b 15ff.), where the rules for inductive reasoning are set out, the example given is the class of mule, horse and man, all of whom are long-lived: from the lack of bile in one member of the class, it can be inferred that all its members have no bile. This is not induction in the modern sense of the accumulation of particulars; such 'enumerative' induction, which is described as imperfect, belongs to rhetoric rather than logic, where it is called a paradigm (see below, 5.1.5).[98] The argument from sign is strictly speaking more a Platonic than an Aristotelian argument, as in it universals are taken to be prior to particulars, allowing a tekmērion to override the distinction upheld elsewhere in Aristotle between that which is 'better known by nature' and that which is 'better known to us'.[99] The latter is known initially through the senses (so, in medical terms, the signs of health are better known to us than its causes); the former is a universal which is derived from the accumulation of sensory particulars.[100] But in the order of knowledge, universals are better known to us than the particulars of sensory experience.[101] This is not a straightforward claim, as it appears to render valid only positive terms which can be derived from sensory experience, and to exclude such notions as vacuum, infinity and privation.[102] What is in question here is both the method of discovery

---

[97] L'Alemant 1549: 29–30, quoted below, 5.1.1.

[98] Sanctorius 1630: 771–804 (xii.2–6) writes at great length on this subject; see also Wear 1973: 152–75.

[99] *Physics*, i.1, 184 a 16–21; *Metaphysics*, i.2, 982 a 25. See also Morrison 1997; Jardine 1974: 34, 45.

[100] *Posterior analytics*, ii.19, 100 a 10ff. (on the formation of universals); Mikkeli 1992: 96 (citing Zabarella's view that universals are thus the furthest from sense); see also da Monte 1587: 229; Mikkeli 1992: 143n. The alternative view is the Platonic view of reminiscence, on which see *Meno*, 70 a ff. (rendered by Ramus 1569: 1.293 as 'there is no discovery, because if we do not know, we will not recognise what we have found, and if we know in fact, then we have no reason to enquire' ('inventionem nullam esse quia si nescimus, etiam inventum non agnoscemus: si vero scimus, frustra quaerimus').

[101] According to Bruyère 1984: 173, 128–30, Ramus disputes this.

[102] Schmitt 1969: 101 (citing Zabarella); French 1994: 56–7 (on Ramus's denial of the vacuum, refuted by Magirus and Case); see also below, 5.3.3–4, for the argument that the senses can tell us of unseen states of the body (antiperistasis and countersensory information).

of universal terms of science and the method of presentation of the results of such enquiry.[103]

4.3.6 'Quia' and 'propter quid': regressus

This brings me to the question of regressus, and the distinction between demonstration 'to hoti' and 'to dioti', or 'quia' and 'propter quid': the former known as 'via resolutiva' or 'via analytica', the latter as the 'via compositiva' or 'via synthetica'; the former starting from facts, effects, signs, all in the order of the senses, the latter having as its middle term a cause or intelligible explanatory proposition which is in nearly all cases not evident to sense;[104] the former being a process of discovery, the latter a process of teaching; the former being appropriate for arts, the latter for sciences; the former being a movement a posteriori (or downwards), as it were from roof to foundations; the latter being a movement a priori (or upwards), as it were from foundations to roof.[105]

The procedure known as 'regressus' is that which ensures the passage from 'demonstratio quia' to 'demonstratio propter quid.' As Jardine describes it, it is a passage from observation (with a 'confused' knowledge of an effect) through induction and demonstration to the accidental knowledge of cause: this is then turned into absolute knowledge by a process of 'negotiatio' or 'consideratio' and the 'demonstratio quia' becomes an absolute knowledge of the effect from the cause in the order of 'propter quid', these transitions altering the nature of both division and definition

---

[103] E.g. Vigenère 1586: 100v (quoting Geber): 'compositionem rei aliqui scire non potest, qui destructionem seu resolutionem illius ignoraverit'; Morrison 1997: 16–19 (on Galen, *Ars parva*, i, K 1.305).

[104] *Posterior analytics*, i.13, 75 a 14; *Metaphysics*, i.1, 981 a 30; Burnett and Mendelsohn 1997: 56ff., on Averroes's division of demonstration into 'signi' (quia), 'causae' (propter quid) and 'simpliciter' (cause and existence: 'potissima'); Ottosson 1984: 113 (on the confusion about this topic which was sorted out in the Middle Ages); Wear 1973: 199–201; Wear 1981: 238, suggesting that Leoniceno's interpretation of the resolutive order as the progression not from effect to cause but from purpose to art is 'a primitive move towards a free standing science'; Jardine 1988: 688 (on Nifo); Capivaccius 1603: 1017–22, 1038–9 (attacking Leoniceno, da Monte and Zimara); Aubéry 1585: 16; Mikkeli 1992: 86 (on Zabarella); Gilbert 1960 (for a general account).

[105] The Boethian topos of the house is in the *De divisione*, PL 64.876–7; it is cited by Thriverus 1592: 3; see also Wear 1981: 241. A relevant Aristotelian locus is *Nicomachean ethics*, iii.3, 1112 b 18–20 (the first link in the chain of causes being the last in the order of discovery). There is a third order, 'a definitione', which begins in the middle and is appropriate for mnemonic purposes: da Monte 1587: 230; Capivaccius 1603: 1004ff. writes variously against Argenterio, Leoniceno and da Monte, and denounces the confusion of art as purpose and art as method; Gilbert 1960; Mikkeli 1992: 179. See also Jokissus 1562: viii (on the ordering of cause, body and sign (the 'ratio scientiae'), sign, body and cause (the 'ratio artis seu sensus') and body, sign and cause (the 'ratio artis et scientiae') as in Galen, *Ars parva*).

in the process.[106] The standard example given is the following (in the first figure):[107]

'demonstratio quia'
Major	non-twinkling things are near	M + P
Minor (effect)	planets are non-twinkling things	S + M
Conclusion (cause)	planets are near	S + P

'demonstratio propter quid'
Major	what is near is non-twinkling	M + P
Minor (cause)	planets are near	S + M
Conclusion	planets do not twinkle	S + P

It has been argued (most famously by Randall) that regressus is a forerunner of scientific method; but this claim has recently been attacked.[108] The dispute is not directly relevant here, but the procedure is, as it marks to some degree the distinction between natural philosophy and medicine (which, according to some, takes its praecognita and hence its causes from natural philosophy), and to some degree that between the theoretical and practical parts of medicine (above 3.1).

4.4 ART AND DIALECTICS

From the arena of 'scientific' demonstration, we now pass to that less elevated practice more often associated with arts: that is, dialectics; it is described also as 'artificiosa coniectura', as we have seen (4.3). The syllogistic rules may remain the same, but the premisses are only 'probable.' The conclusions to be derived from these lower orders of demonstration are correspondingly degraded: verisimilitude, probability in its various senses (conclusions true for the most part, true on the balance of the evidence, approved opinions, credibility, approximations, frequency judgements), finally sophistical reasoning, all of which are relevant to both medical theory and medical practice.[109] This sphere includes both

---

[106] *Posterior analytics*, i.2, 71 b 9–12; *Physics*, i.1, 184 a 10 for confused (in the sense of compounded) knowledge; Ottosson 1984: 113 and Mikkeli 1992: 98–9 (both quoting Pietro d'Abano); Capivaccius 1603: 1025; Aubéry 1585: 40 treats the two modes 'quia' and 'propter quid' as reciprocal: 'oportet enim in demonstationem hoti perfectam signorum enumerationem adhibere, nempe eiusmodi, ut cum causa dioti, et effectu ipso sit reciproca. Neque vero aliter colligenda sunt signa quam quo modo colliguntur *Antecedentia* et *Consequentia*, ad medium analyticum constituendum' (the 'demonstratio signi' is an Averroistic term); Horst 1609: 9 (on the passage from imperfect knowledge to perfect knowledge via 'cognitio confusa'); Jardine 1988.

[107] *Posterior analytics*, i.13, 78 a 22ff.; Kuhn 1997: 321; Jardine 1974: 55–6.

[108] Randall 1961; Jardine 1988.

[109] See Demonet 2001: 20 (quoting Scipion Dupleix) for a contemporary text linking these terms.

topics and those parts of rhetoric whose procedures are not necessarily linked to argument *in utramque partem*: persuasive (forensic) argument is prohibited; doctors may however engage in the dialectical assessment of evidence by looking at more than one construction of it ('dialexis'). They are enjoined moreover to use logic only in the service of truth, that is, for decision-making and for inference from evidence. Although the use of the term 'topica' would be appropriate in the terms of Aristotle's book on the subject,[110] it is very rarely invoked partly because it already exists as a medical term of art (a 'topicum' is treatment by local application), partly because the term dialectics (which is often taken to be its synonym)[111] had come, as the correlate of 'naturalis ratio', to be associated with a new intellectual position in the Renaissance, that of Agricola, Melanchthon, Ramus and their followers who answer the quaestio 'whether dialectics can treat of all subjects?' in the affirmative.[112] Against this view, there are those who argue in what seems to be a non-consilient way that different disciplines, and different parts of the same discipline, require different standards of proof: physics requires necessity, but zoology is less demanding.[113] Aristotle's (and Galen's) classification of arts as either speculative (metaphysics, mathematics and physics), operative or factive is implicitly in accord with this view.[114]

---

[110] *Topics*, i.1, 100 a 31: 'reasoning is dialectical which reasons from generally accepted opinions'; *ibid.*, i.2, 101 a 35f., referring to raising difficulties on both sides (of an argument), and to the usefulness of topics *inter alia* for scientific discourse. Cf. Montuus's use of 'dialexis' to mean the production of arguments to be weighed against each other rather than in competition with another orator: 1537: a2r: 'ea autem est argumentorum ad aliquid probandum vel improbandum comparatio'; see also Perfetti 1999a: 459 quoting Pomponazzi on the possibility of the coexistence of various opinions.

[111] E.g. Velsius 1543: 20; Crellius 1621: 602; Argenterio 1610: 15, who distinguishes necessary demonstration from 'probable' or 'dialectical' syllogisms and 'apparentia' or sophisms: 'probable' has here the sense given to it in *Topics*, i.1, 100 b 22f.: 'generally accepted . . . commending itself to all or to the majority of the wise'.

[112] Galen, *De differentiis pulsuum*, iii.6, K 8.682–3; Cardano 1565: 50v (i.3.1): 'dialectica an medico necessaria', citing Galen, *Ars parva*, K 1.306; *De sectis*, K 1.64–5; *De simplicium medicamentorum temperamentis ac facultatibus*, ii, K 11.459–60 and Averroes, *In metaphysica*, ii.15: 'dialectica [generalis] docet regulas communes omnibus scientiis'. Goclenius 1599: 9 (on 'an dialectica disputet de omni ente' against Scaliger 1592: 15–16 (i.3), who answers in the negative): 'dialectica tradit modum disputandi et docendi de quavis propositione; fabricat instrumenta [sc. definitionem, divisionem, argumentationem] ad docendi modos Analyticum et Syntheticum'; Jardine 1974: 26–7; Bruyère 1984: 269; Mikkeli 1992: 60–1; Blair 1997: 83; Mack 1990. See also below 5.3.5 on lumen naturale and its relationship to natural reason; and Zabarella 1586–7: 1.11 (*De natura logicae*, xii).

[113] Cardano 1565: 50v (i.3.1, on 'dialectica particularis'); Liddel 1624: 9 ('ordo veritatem in singulis artium partibus et theorematibus respicit'); Herberger 1981: 15–1; Siraisi 1997: 103–4 (on Cardano's discovery of the forty-four rules of true dialectic).

[114] *Nicomachean ethics*, vi.4, 1140 a 1–24; *Metaphysics*, i.1, 981 a 13f.; Galen, *Ad Thrasybulum*, xx, K 5.860–4; pseudo-Galen, *Definitiones medicae* (cited by Ottosson 1984: 69); Argenterio 1610: 38–9

A new claim is made by Cardano (citing Galen as his authority) that the right form of reasoning for medicine is in a geometrical mode, beginning with axioms, which are not however given the status of scientific principles.[115] In speaking of physiology, Fernel compares these to geometrical postulates, but claims that they are none the less 'the most solid foundations'.[116] As Quintilian had pointed out of such axioms, 'things that are plausible are confirmed and refuted in the same way as things in the order of truth'.[117] In this sense dialectics is an operative art: it uses the premisses it inherits from other disciplines and the higher processes of argument for its own instrumental purposes.[118] It deals in inference, and translates its results into syllogistic or enthymematic form.[119] As reasoning in medicine begins usually from effects and moves to causes, and requires the elimination of inferences as much as their establishment in a causal form, the relevant syllogistic forms belong to the second figure; and of these, that known by the mnemonic camestres is said by Sanctorius to be the most pertinent of all, because it can be reduced to the first figure and can provide information about individual subjects (which otherwise cannot appear in a demonstrative syllogism) *per negationem*.[120] Moreover, as an art, medicine is devoted to utility; its purpose is not

(reducing logic, rhetoric and grammar to the status of 'peritia'; see also Perfetti 1999a: 441 on medicine as a 'peritia', a view derived from *Nicomachean ethics*, i.3, 1094 b 27–1095 a 2 and *Politics*, iii.11, 1281 b 40–2); Horst 1621: 4–5; Wallace 1988: 210 (citing Toletus); Siraisi 1997: 103–4 (on Cardano).

[115] Cardano 1565: 50v; Cardano 1663: 5.206 (cited by Grafton and Siraisi 1999: 45) claims that of all arts, medicine is the most certain (because of its ability to predict the future); also Canziani 1988: 218–19 (quoting the claim in the introduction to the *Metoposcopia* that all disciplines and arts dealing with corruptible things depend on 'ut plurimum' or 'magna ex parte' logic: see below note 124). Cf. Agricola, *De inventione dialectica*, ii.6; Jardine 1974: 28.

[116] Fernel 1610b: 49: 'firmissima artis medicae fundamenta iactavimus, dum descripta humani corporis confectione, omnes eius particulas singillatim ob oculis proposuimus: quarum cognitio si sensuum fide atque constantia firmabitur, vim quodammodo iam adipiscitur aut communium evidentiumque notionum, aut earum quas Geometrae non demonstrare sed postulare solent ut sibi concedantur, ex quibus posthac aditus ad demonstrationem facilis patebit'. Cf. the very different medieval use by Gordon 1574: 984 of the adjective 'geometrical': '[medicus rationalis] operetur secundum artem, et in hoc condemnatur omnis ars augurandi, sicut est ars geometrica, suspendendi herbas ad collum, omnia empirica, sorticinia, fascina, et alia quam plurima quae non est bonum revelare propter abutentes, qui, conscientia neglecta, utuntur magicis . . .'.

[117] *Institutio oratoria*, xii.1.45: 'non aliter autem veri similia quam vera et confirmantur et refelluntur'.

[118] Agricola, *De inventione dialectica*, ii.7 (on dialectics borrowing its principles from metaphysics); Stump 1988: 281n.; Liddel 1628: 3 (on medicine's debt to other disciplines).

[119] On enthymemes, see below 5.1.1.

[120] Zabarella's example of camestres is:

all men are animals
no stone is an animal
therefore no man is a stone

knowledge *per se*, but a practical end, and to achieve this it may employ a practical syllogism (one which has as either minor or major proposition a purpose or command), often presented in the form of an enthymeme; in medical discourse the missing premiss is always either 'contraria contrariis curantur' or 'similia similibus conservantur', and determines the appropriate therapy, as we shall see (8.7).[121] An even looser form of the enthymeme is a sort of free association similar to that by which Argenterio characterises the relationship of the sign to its signifier; Aubéry calls this a 'physiognomonic syllogism' and gives as an example: 'coltsfoot is associated with pulmonary congestion; therefore pulmonary congestion is associated with coltsfoot'.[122] This form of reasoning is strongly

The conversion of this to the first figure (celarent) reads:

no animal is a stone
<u>all men are animals</u>
therefore no man is a stone

Cf. the comment of Campilongo 1601: 8v: 'media inter contraria per negationem perspicua redduntur et exprimuntur'. See also Sanctorius 1630: 801 (xii.6): 'praeterea per subiecta, quae sunt causae remotae, non perveniemus ad universale, qui ex subiectis solum colligimus conclusionem negativam in secunda figura in camestres . . . si vero a causa remota bonam velimus colligere conclusionem, oportet, ut semper sit negativa, et semper reducatur ad illum modum, qui dicitur camestres, quia ex puris affirmativis in secunda figura nihil colligitur'. A similar point is made by Caselius 1580: A3: 'in hoc collocatio medij termini convenit cum secunda figura, ut ille sit praedicatum in utraque propositionum praemissarum, tam in maiore, quam in minore. Enthymema est. Crito anhelat: febricitat igitur. Medius terminus est . . . anhelare: maior, febricitans: minor, homo quispiam. Inter syllogismus sic habeat. Febricitantes anhelant: Crito anhelat: Crito igitur febricitat. Facile hoc solvi potest, etiamsi verum sit, quando anhelant et alii, qui minime febricitat. Insuper etsi hic syllogismus in forma est secundae figurae: in modo certe nullo est. Non enim ipsa recepti syllogismum per omnia affirmativum: neque aliter, nisi negative concludit. Quare hoc signum ἀσυλλόγιστη est.' The use of third figure is similarly rejected by Caselius, *ibid.*, and Sanctorius 1630: 895 (xiv.10). See also Cardano 1663: 1.149, 307 (on Ptolemy's mode of dialetic).

[121] Liddel 1628: 607–8 argues that this is the case when a rational doctor proceeds from the signs to what they signify without explicit reasoning, though the procedure can be reduced to explicit argument: 'hic modus procedendi ab indicantibus ad indicata sine expressa ratiocinatione fit, et tamen ad expressum reduci poterit. Ea ratiocinatio syllogismus factivus est, cuius tota vis ex duobus principiis dependet: contraria contrariis curantur, similia similibus conservantur. Assumptio fit ex indicationibus, conclusio ex indicatis. Proinde ipsa indicatio sive processus ab indicante ad indicatum est Enthymema compositum ex antecedente indicante et consequente indicato: veluti, Plato febricitat, ergo est refrigerandus.' It is debated at the time whether the enthymeme belongs to logic or rhetoric: See Demonet forthcoming.

[122] Aubéry 1585: 15: 'si null[um] signum praetermissum sit ex illis quae observata sunt, tum *Hominis* morbi, tum etiam *Foeminae* sive externo remedio inesse licebit syllogismus syllogismum Physiognomicum conficere quo intelligamus hunc morbum esse huius remedij, et hoc remedium esse huius morbi: verbi gratia, Tussilaginem [coltsfoot] esse obstructionis pulmonum: et obstructionem pulmonum esse Tussilaginis. Sed Regis maximi opus est, efficere ut multi docti viri, Physiognomicae Anatomes restituendae gratia, instituant συζήτησις [joint enquiry] et in ea praestantissima doctrina sedulam seriamque operam ponant.' This is similar to the practical syllogism, but has no purposive or jussive element.

reminiscent of the hypothetical syllogism ('if smoke, then fire') about which Aubéry also writes.[123]

Dialectics yields less certainty both because of the nature of its subject matter and its mode of argument. Nature, as we shall see (7.2–3), is capable of being 'other than it is for the most part' and is governed by laws which have no more than regularity 'for the most part'; things may occur by chance, and of chance there is no knowledge, only intimations of the most limited kind.[124] Reasoning about nature may therefore only yield 'certitudo probabilis' – an oxymoron to the modern ear – in the human mind, which according to Melanchthon is not vouchsafed knowledge of substance but only accidents.[125] Dialectical principles and logical procedures are endoxical as opposed to demonstrative: they are based on opinion, even if this opinion is sanctioned by the best procedures and assumptions of which the fallen human mind is capable.[126] Both certainty and truth become expressible as comparatives: 'verius', 'certius'.[127]

There are those who like Ramus are more sanguine about the potentialities of the human being, and who claim more than this. The 'naturalis ratio' in which opinions reside and which processes them is in some way guaranteed by the divine mind, and can aspire to higher truth. He seems to have had few disciples in medical circles, which are on the whole less

[123] Aubéry 1584: 151; see also Demonet 2001: 16–21, where the relationship between potency and consequentiae is also examined.

[124] The loci which speak of 'hos epi to polu' ('ut plurimum'; 'ut in pluribus'; 'magna ex parte') are: Metaphysics, v, 1026 b 27ff.; vi.2, 1027 a 12 (the accidental as 'what is capable of being otherwise than as it for the most part is'); ix.8.4, 1064 b 32; Prior analytics, i.13, 32 b 1–24; Posterior analytics, i.8, 75 b 24–5; i.30, 87 b 19–20 (on there being no demonstration of the fortuitous); see also Biesius 1573: 16; Sennert 1650: 1.14 (on an accident producing a substance); Canziani 1988: 218–19; Meinel 1992: 26; Kusukawa 1993: 40 (on Melanchthon's view of chance); Mignucci 1981. Cicero, De inventione, i.57 offers a very different treatment of 'for the most part' propositions, designed to eliminate their uncertainty by 'ratiocinatio'.

[125] Kusukawa 1997: 423 (quoting Melanchthon 1834–60: 13.528ff.); Metaphysics, vi.2, 1027 a 12; Galen, De placitis Hippocratis et Platonis, ix.9, K 5.791–805; Aquinas, Contra Gentiles, iii.99.9; Maclean 1999b: 307 (citing Aquinas, Summa Theologiae, 1 a 79 on the mind's accidental knowledge of itself). 'Certitudo probabilis' is used by Albertus Magnus: see Kantola 1994: 181; see also Magirus 1603: 511; De interpretatione, ix, 19 a 18–23.

[126] Libavius 1594: 100 points out that any judgement can only be as certain as its 'praecognita'; Bylebyl 1991: 184 cites da Monte as averring that the art of medicine is too long to be encompassed in any one lifetime; see also Galen, De differentiis pulsuum, iii, K 8.636–7 cited by Heurnius 1637: 17.

[127] Liddel 1628 passim is particularly rich in examples of such comparatives (on which see also below, note 134). See also Maclean 1996: 24–7 (citing Fonseca 1599: 1.785–817 on the hierarchy of truth and verisimilitude).

positive about natural reason.[128] Jean Sturm, the logician and teacher of Ramus, wrote to one of his correspondents that medical demonstration was less persuasive than that of demonstrative logic; and at about the same time, Valleriola points out that many different approaches to truth need to be adopted in medicine because man is an imperfect, changeable, variable, blind animal faced with an art of great length whose content is continually changing: 'in this earthly prison, we strive laboriously after this truth, through the exercise of the best disciplines and arts, through the contemplation of studies, through assiduity, through wakeful care, through the explanation of difficulties and the clarification of the texts of authorities'.[129]

It is pertinent however here to point out that Valleriola also makes the claim that 'the precepts of the medical art are of the order of eternal and necessary truth';[130] this seems contradictory, and calls for some comment here. The claim could simply be motivated by the need to defend the scientific status, and hence the dignity, of medicine (see above 3.2); it could also relate as a claim only to precepts, which are prescriptive and not compromised by the physician's encounter with the variability of patients and conditions.[131] But similar, if not greater, claims are found in the writings of practici such as Jacobus Hollerius, who avers that 'art is the understanding or doctrine drawn from true, certain, universal and mutually consistent precepts directed to a single end', bringing together what Lorraine Daston has called the four 'epistemological virtues' of

---

[128] Crusius 1615 is an exception. Paracelsus's natural light is of a different order: see below 5.3.5. Arnau de Vilanova 2000: 183 cites Romans 12:3 as a divine ordinance not to know more than is necessary for the practice of the art ('non plus sapere quam oportet'). Hawenreuter in Zabarella 1597:): (4r points out that Ramus's major error lay in his introduction of issues of place and time into logic.

[129] Backus 1989: 250 (quoting Sturm's letter to Leonard Stertel of 1565); Valleriola 1577: 131–2: 'in hoc terreno carcere tamen ad illam (veritatem) nitamur labore, exercitatione optimarum disciplinarum atque artium, contemplatione studiorum, assiduitate, vigili, cura rerum difficilium explanatione, et authorum illustratione'. Cardano 1565: 83r (i.3.20) classifies arts as 'certa per se' (arithmetic), 'certa per se, coniecturalis in exercitatione' (medicine and agriculture) and 'coniecturalis per se et in exercitatione' (divination): for the link of medicine and agriculture, see Cicero, *De divinatione*, i.112, and Ptolemy, *Tetrabiblos*, i.2.4. Argenterio 1610: 15 proposes the use of all modes of proof, because anything that might give access to the truth (he lists 'sensus, intellectus, resolutiva, compositiva, definitiva, divisiva, doctrina, resolutio, compositio, divisio, syllogismus demonstrativus, dialecticus, sophisticus, enthymeme, inductio, exemplum, epilogismus. Quibus addi possunt analogismus, experientia, authoritas, testimoniumque illorum quos vera tradidisse arbitramur') is worth trying.

[130] Valleriola 1577: 558: '[praecepta medicae] artis [sunt] perpetuae et necessariae veritatis'.

[131] Herberger 1981: 223, 182 (on precepts as prescriptive and not requiring encounter with reality; and on dogma as 'doctrina per os sapientium promulgata').

truth, certainty, objectivity (*qua* universality) and coherence, and linking them to the goal-directedness of art.[132]

These claims do not seem easy to reconcile either with Galen's and Celsus's description of medicine as 'coniecturalis ars' which is used contingently to determine the remedies appropriate to individual cases, or with Galen's admission elsewhere that medicine is an operative art related to the practical intellect.[133] For these authorities, it is not paradoxical to refer to 'more universal principles' ('universaliora principia') that are not 'perpetuae veritatis', and to invoke a correspondingly weaker form of argument from the majority of cases which is set out in *Posterior analytics*, ii.12 (96 a 8–19) (see below 5.2.3).[134] This form of argument has several consequences. While it is said that nature avoids the infinite and that everything in the sublunary world is finite because that world itself is finite, in practice the properties of individua *qua* individua are infinite, or if not infinite, too many to be counted; and nature, if not infinite, is yet imperfect and subject both to the necessity and vagaries of becoming and to the indeterminacy of matter.[135] Art

---

[132] Hollerius 1582: 3r: 'ars est compraehensio seu doctrina ex praeceptionibus veris, certis, universalibus, consentientibus inter se et ad unum finem'; Daston 2000. See also Herberger 1981: 236–7 (quoting da Monte's claim that the dogmas of medicine are preferable to those of law not only because they are not tyrannical (i.e. prescriptive), but also because they use the most sure reasoning, not fallacious experience: 'non experimentis fallacibus sed rationibus firmissimis utitur'); cf. Cardano 1663: 8.211–12, opposing this view on the authority of Hippocrates: 'at vero quae non ordinibus constat, partim quidem et quo ad nos, et quo ad nostram scientiam, effugit nomen ipsum scientiae, et coniecturalis vocatur, qualis quae in unoquoque est eorum, tamen scientia est apud meliores nobis quae extenditur ad singulas gentes non solum, sed etiam homines singulos, et singulas operationes, et casus fortuitos. Sed ista sunt comprehensa rationibus infinitis . . . et horum infinitorum ea scientia est apud incorporea, ex qua fatum et causae naturalium et singulorum et tempora et modi et eventus, de quibus nec coniectura est nedum scientia. Ergo de hac neque loquitur Hippocrates, sed de priore de qua apud nos per ordines coniectura est.' Albanesius 1649: 7 also gives a less exalted definition of art: 'habitus intellectus conceptus ex variis memoriis eorundem eventuum in operationibus, directus ad simile operandum'.

[133] Valleriola 1577: 558, claiming that Galen's definition of medicine as an 'ars coniecturalis' applies only to the 'ars factiva' of medicine (the 'actio et edentium opera'); see also *De constitutione artis medica*; *Ad Thrasybulum*; *Ars parva*; Kessler 1994b: 25 (quoting Salutati); Siraisi 1990b: 223 (quoting Agrippa).

[134] For the mathematical consequences of arguing from propositions true for the most part, see below, 5.2.1; cf. *Rhetoric*, 1356 b 16–18; 1357 a 30–7 (things capable of being different from what they are); according to Arnau de Vilanova 1585: 1700 'vera' means 'ut plurimum de contingentibus' and 'de necessariis' in respect of 'scientia'. It is possible that 'universalior' in some contexts might mean no more than 'somewhat universal', but its comparative sense is also found: e.g. Capivaccius 1603: 1040: 'in divisione progressus est ab universalibus ad minus universalia'.

[135] Ingolstetterus 1596: 31: 'natura in omnibus semper finem quaerit et vitare solet infinitum' (citing *De generatione animalium*, i.1); one of the Aristotelian definitions of infinity refers to the practically limitless field of knowledge which the arts have to cover: *Physics*, iii. 3–8, 202 b 30ff.;

in the case of medicine is indeed the 'de infinitis finita doctrina'.[136] This means that as well as gaps in knowledge, there will be residues of evidence not used; Galen refers to redundant information in diagnosis; others to the 'res eventu rarissimae' which do not fall under the art of medicine and are often banished to separate treatises dealing with mirabilia and extraordinary cases.[137] Moreover, the categories and rules of the art of medicine will accommodate exceptions: Emericus cites a 'universalis regula' which is followed in his text by the word 'praeterquam', and a list of cases not falling under the rule. And he is not alone.[138] There can moreover be no absolute rule for the practice of the medical art.[139] Bacon's call in the *Novum organum* for a deeper rule to explain exceptions is indeed hostile to medical science on this point, although he shows elsewhere more sympathy with

---

Metaphysics, xi.10, 1006 a 35ff.; *De caelo*, i.5–7, 217 b 1ff.; iii.4, 302 b 10ff.; Suterus 1584: 27; da Monte 1587: 949: 'individuorum proprietates infinitae sunt'; Ferdinandus 1611: 15, quoted above, note 84; Melanchthon 1550: α3v: 'Deus . . . varietatem pene infinitam effectionum in elementis et mixtis includ[it] certis metis.' Some ancient sources are *Metaphysics*, v. 19, 1024 b 32ff.; viii.3, 1043 b 29ff.; *Theaetetus*, 201 d; *Sophist*, 251 b; Sextus Empiricus, *Hypotyposes*, ii.15. 204: 'particulars are infinite and indefinite'. The threat of the infinite is clear in Schegk 1579 b: B2r: 'medicina scientia est . . . omnium, nisi mutilam artem esse velimus. Et non omnium etiam quatenus singularia quaedam, et τό δέτι existunt, nisi infinitorum scientiam esse libeat dicere: sed omnium, quatenus καθόλου et τοῖόν δέτι ὄντα sunt. Quare faciendum nobis est, et omni conatu in id incumbendum, ut Duce methodo, et Comite experientia, sine claudicatione in operibus artis, quam foelicissime versari valeamus.' On the irreducibility of art (in this case of astrology as well as medicine) to certainty because of its subject matter see Cardano 1578: 120: 'ex adiacentibus provenit, hisque quae nequaquam ex arte sunt minui potest diligentia, atque solertia, non autem tolli . . . ex materiae mobilitate, mistioneque ac propria dispositione, tum astrorum non exquisita cum praecedentibus configurationibus similitudine nulla ex parte tolli potest, sed manet'. He goes on to claim that the only vices of the art of medicine which can be eliminated are human moral ones (negligence, avarice, ambition); Heurnius 1637: 21 (citing Celsus): 'est perpetuum in Medicina quod fieri debet, non tamen perpetuum est quod sequi conveniat. Siquidem multa latent in corpore ignota medico'; Blair 1997: 141 (citing Bodin).

[136] Maclean 1992: 73 (from Porphyry); cf. Boethius, *In categorias*, i, PL 64.161, quoted by Herberger 1981: 177: 'rerum ergo diversarum indeterminatam infinitamque multitudinem, decem praedicamentorum paucissima numerositate concludit, ut ea quae infinita sub scientia cadere non poterant, decem propriis generibus diffinita scientiae comprehensione claudantur'. For Arnau de Vilanova forthcoming, 'ars' 'stricte' is 'ratio directiva operis cuiuslibet ad finem per debita media' and 'large' is 'collectio regularum [sive] praeceptorum ad unum finem tendentium'. This part of the text does not seem to have been printed in the Renaissance editions. A reference to art as the finite doctrine of infinites is found in Pietro d'Abano 1548: 5v (iii).

[137] *Methodus medendi*, ii.3, K 10.92–3; Blair 1997: 37 (on Lemnius); Wierus 1567; Silvaticus 1601: 27.

[138] Emericus 1552: S1r; also Melanchthon 1834–60: 13.195 (on medicine as an 'ars magna ex parte'); Argenterio 1610: 1779–81; Campilongo 1601: 9v (exceptions to 'contraria contrariis' rule); Blair 1997: 45 (citing Bodin).

[139] Vallesius 1610: 348 (vii.16): 'praeceptum practicum perpetuum esse non videatur'; there are not even stable categories of health: da Monte 1556: 189, cited by Joutsivuo 1999: 115: 'nam nullus est homo, qui habeat sanitatem, ut alius'.

the practical requirement of an art to grasp the diversity of the natural world.[140]

The consequence of these features – redundancy and exception – is that there is an imprecision about the frontiers of knowledge both within and outside the art; both in its sensory sources, and in the intelligible data it draws from them: as Cardano implies in his brief discussion of symptoms, causes and diseases, if knowledge is in fact finite then not knowing everything leads to imperfect categories; if it is infinite in nature (through combinations of individual properties and future contingency) then the categories (the ten predicables, making infinity finite) provide the only access to it: we are back to the 'de infinitis finita doctrina',[141] a 'looser' area of knowledge ('scientia latiori sensu') in which all the logical tools – signs, contraries, genera – are correspondingly less rigorous.[142] The list of 'dialectical questions' is also longer and less rigorous than that of scientific demonstration (above 4.3); it begins with the same two ('an sit, quid sit'), but then passes on to 'what species and parts, what causes, what effects, what cognates and similarities, what things opposing, what testimonies and examples.'[143] In respect of 'pugnantia', it is pertinent to note here a feature of medical reasoning which arises from its involvement with complex oppositions. To cure an illness is to combat

---

[140] Daston and Park 1998: 227–8, citing Bacon 1878: 433–5 (*Novum organum*, ii.28); cf. Bacon 2000: 98.

[141] Cardano 1583: 1: 'cum tria sint praeter naturam, symptoma *plerunque* notius est, morbus autem causa semper, ideo dubium relinquitur an a morbo, an a symptomate incipiendum. Et causarum externae *persaepe* notiores sunt speciebus morbi, non tamen causae dici possunt, nisi morbus adsit: proper hoc morbo iam supposito, de causis agere licebit: non solum ad cognitionem specierum eius, sed etiam quandoque generis *plerunque* autem, et aliarum causarum, velut antecedentium et coniunctarum...' (my italics). See also Boethius, *In categorias*, i, PL 64.161, cited above, note 136.

[142] For declaration of loose use of technical words (contrarium, similitudo, signum, scientia, symptoma, natura) see Gemma 1575: 218–19: 'multo latius hoc nomen accipi medicis quam philosophicis'; Valleriola 1577: 240–1: 'latius accepto vocabulo'; Campilongo 1601: 12r: 'signum latius nomen quam in logicis'; Sylvius 1539: 7: 'scientia latiori sensu'; Liddel 1628: 226–8 (on symptom); da Monte 1587: 355 (on nature). These doctors refer to a number of much quoted Galenic loci (from *De methodo medendi*, i.7, K 10.49–63; *De constitutione artis medicinae*, K 1.244–304; *De compositione medicamentorum*, viii, K 13.116–26). On ancient sources of argument of laxity (with special reference to Celsus), see von Staden 1998.

[143] This is the list given by Valerius in his *Anacephaleosis*, reproduced by Voet and Voet-Grisolle 1980–3: 5.fig. 50: 'octo fere locis seu quaestionibus explicatur simplicis thematis natura, quae sunt: an sit, quid sit, quae species et partes, quae caussae, qui effectus, vires et officia, quae cognata et similia, quae pugnantia, quae testimonia et exempla'. Kusukawa 1999: 136 (on Ramus, Melanchthon, and the 'inveniendi organon' listed as: 'an sit, quid sit, quibus caussis partibus constet, unum an multa, quae partes, quae comparatio partium, quae officia, quae affinia, quae contraria'); Jardine 1974: 39; also Scribonius 1584: 69: 'essentia morborum e definitionibus et distributionibus cognita, quamprimum e causis, subjectis, adjunctis, aliorumque argumentorum generibus'.

it with a contrary; but the doctor is also enjoined not to harm the patient by the prescription of an inappropriate remedy; and he is equally duty-bound both to conserve health actively, and not damage it with wrong hygienic recommendations.[144] Contraries of two sorts therefore arise in the administration of treatment; a parallel complication is found in the assessment of evidence from signs in the form of contradictory, absent, negative or falsifying evidence ('testimonia et exempla'), as we shall see (5.1); and in both cases, this complicates the process of reaching conclusions and making decisions.

4.4.1 Identity and difference

For comparison's sake, I shall examine dialectics in the sequence followed above for scientific demonstration, beginning with identity, difference and contraries. These operative concepts are now taken explicitly from Aristotle's *Topics* rather than his *Analytics*, as can be seen from the following quotation from John Cotta:

> It is a chief pointe on all learning truly to discerne between differing similitudes and like differences... Many accidents commonly fall out seeming alike, yet have no affinity: and againe in shew the same, yet indeed contrarie. Contraries have oft in many things likenesses, and likeness contrarieties easily deceiving the unwitting and unlearned.

He goes on to show that the similarities and differences of diseases have 'intricate ambiguities', quoting Galen: 'similarities do not only deceive the vulgar but even sometimes learned doctors'.[145] Contradictions are therefore not easy to resolve; both 'similitudo' and 'contrarietas' are to be taken in a very broad sense ('latius accepto vocabulo').[146] The term 'contrary' equally 'is taken in a much broader sense than it is among philosophers'; this means that we are not speaking of contraria 'proprie et vere', and that as a consequence there can be elements of difference

---

[144] Hippocrates, *Praecepta*, i: 'iuva aut ne noceas'.

[145] Cotta 1612: 17: he cites 'Arist de Top. unum est de principiis humanae sapientiae rerum differentium similitudines et similium differentias rite dignoscere'; see *Topics*, i.2, 101 a 36ff.; i.8, 108 a 37ff.; also Galen, *In aphorismos*, iv.2, K 17b.659: 'similitudines non modo vulgares sed etiam medicos eruditos aliquando decipiunt'; cf. Montaigne 1965: 1070 (iii.13) citing St Augustine; Schmitt 1969: 95 (citing Zabarella).

[146] Heurnius 1637: 9, 21 (on the difficulty of distinguishing similia and dissimilia). Cf. Otto 1992: 60–1 (discussing the categories of similarity ('convenientia secundum formam essentialem, secundum analogiam, per quandam cognationem, per proportionem') in Micraelus's *Lexicon philosophicum*); see also Agricola 1967: 34–41 (i.6), on identity and difference in respect of genus, species and accident.

within the same genus (which also becomes a 'latius nomen').[147] Galen recognises this himself by defining 'generally' as both 'what happens always' and 'what happens for the most part' in his *Ars medica*.[148]

Contraries, which in scientific demonstration are maximally different, now become 'those things which are largely different in the same genre'.[149] It is hardly surprising that Valleriola admits that the term is taken in a much broader sense than it is among philosophers. The major contraries cited in medicine (notably health – sickness) are contraria mediata;[150] this is unlike law, in which the contrarium immediatum is the norm. In writing about the condition of neutrality which is the mediate state between health and sickness in 1539, Sylvius lists all of the following versions of mediacy: not altogether healthy nor altogether sick; not more healthy than sick; between healthy and sick; partly healthy, partly sick; sometimes healthy, sometimes sick.[151] Contraries can even change over time, and turn into their opposite.[152] This loosening of logic is found also

---

[147] Valleriola 1577: 240–1, referring to *Physics*, i.6, esp. 189 b 10–11; see also *Historia animalium*, vii, 588 b 4–17 and the 'scala naturae' of *De partibus animalium*, iv.5, 681 a 12.

[148] *Ars parva*, i, K 1.308; on which see Joutsivuo 1999: 118–19.

[149] Campilongo 1601: 42v, citing Galen, *De compositione medicamentorum secundum locos*, viii.6, K 13.190–1: 'cum res inter se multum distant, contraria appellantur'; cf. Cardano 1570: 50: 'praesupponunt in omnibus, quod contraria sint contrariorum affectuum causae: non possumus autem dicere quod omnino: quoniam ambo sunt media duorum aliorum contrariorum'. An important discussion of contraria, in connexion with the axiom 'contraria contrariis curantur', is found in *Methodus medendi*, xi.12, K 10.767–72; Lacuna 1551: 919–20 gives the following precis of it: 'at vero contraria dicuntur, quae sub uno eodemque genere, plurimum inter se dissident. Si autem in illo genere quod mediocre est, hoc est medium inter duo extrema, intellexeris, infinitam quandam contrariarum rerum multitudine, quae maioris minorisque ratione inter se dissideant, ex eo invenies. Non enim in corporum modo qualitate, verumetiam in quantitate, eiusmodi contrarietatem invenias: quam utique Aristoteles non contrarietatem, sed oppositionem nominat. Verum Hippocrati, omnia id genus contrariorum habent appellationem; sicuti etiam Platoni, qui ex contrariis esse dicit generationes. Contemnere tamen nomina oportet, minime autem scientiam rerum. Cuius non ignarus Hippocrates, ait: Medicina appositio est, et detractio: deficientium quidem appositio, redundantium autem detractio. Porro deficiunt, redundantur nonnulla, quidem in quantitate, quaedam autem in qualitate.' The coming together of nominal, logical and quantitative issues here is striking (see above, 4.2, and below, 5.2).

[150] Thriverus 1592: 5 argues that it is the engagement of doctors with empirical evidence that leads them to prefer to see health and sickness as a mediate rather than immediate contrary. 'Contrarium' is also a term of art with a specific sense in medicine: Lacuna 1551: 919–20, paraphrasing *Methodus medendi*, xi.12, K 10.767–72, cited in the previous note; Liddel 1628: 605: 'vocabulo contrarii hic [viz. in methodo curativa], non solum intelliguntur, quae manifestis facultatibus inter se pugnant sed etiam quae occulta facultate et specifica forma; praeterea privantia, et tam ea, quae ex accidenti et potentia talia sunt, quam per se actu'.

[151] Sylvius 1539a: c1r. Another example which illustrates the inadequacy of the contrary is sex difference: see Maclean 1980: 34–46; on overlapping classes, see *De generatione animalium*, ii.1, 732 b 15; see also 7.6.1.

[152] Sanctorius 1630: 361–72 (iv.5): 'corpus in varias, et aliquando contrarias naturas mutari posse'.

in references to qualities, which signify not only both positively or absolutely but also negatively;[153] and in references to immediate contraries, allowing Liddel for example to insert a middle term between natural and non-natural.[154] Even medical *similia* and *contraria* (i.e. the preservatives and remedies of the maxims 'similia similibus conservantur' and, 'contraria contrariis curantur') are said to obey the same loose logic.[155]

4.4.2 Latitude of forms

A further consequence of this is that what constitutes the mediate contrary is also made a looser category, sometimes in contradiction of the doctrine of substantial forms, which would seem to determine in a fixed way the nature of any physical object. Both Aristotelian and Galenic loci speak of change as occurring through the medium:[156] this change presupposes a continuity which comes to be known as the 'latitudo formarum'. This involves the distinctions 'simpliciter' (haplos) and 'ut nunc' (en to nun), potency and act, and the four qualities described in *Categories*, viii (8 b 25f.) (state and condition, natural capacity, affective qualities and shape or form).[157] Latitude of forms is a doctrine particularly pertinent to medicine: 'for medicine is the knowledge of everything in degrees, from the smallest to the largest', as da Monte says.[158] If there were no latitude, then medicine would turn into a doctrine of perpetual pathology, which Galen recognised as a fallacy.[159] This whole issue has been pellucidly set out by Timo Joutsivuo in respect of the concepts of health and neutrum, and will be examined in detail below (7.4.3), together with its diagrammatic representation (5.2.1); I have tried elsewhere to show how it arises in the context of the distinction of sex.[160] The logical issues are here closely entwined with such ontological problems as whether the passage from 'salubritas' to 'insalubritas' is continuous, or gradual through degrees (a 'medium transitus'); whether the middle term between health

---

[153] Thriverus 1592: 15 and Collado 1615: 9ff. (on 'frigiditas' as both a relative term and a quality).
[154] Liddel 1628: 558–79.
[155] Valleriola 1577: 240–1 (on Galen, *De constitutione artis medicae*).
[156] Aristotle, *Physics*, iii.1, 200 b 29–201 a 9; Galen, *De sectis*, K 1.64–105.
[157] Waldungus 1611.
[158] Da Monte 1556: 151, quoted by Joutsivuo 1999: 117n: 'est enim medicina scientia omnium in latitudine, et a primo gradu ad ultimum: sive enim latitudo fuerit in ipsa sanitate, sive in morbo, sive in neutralitate, semper medicina est scientia horum omnium graduum'; cf. Torrigiano and Gentile da Foligno in Torrigiano 1557: 25v, 26v.
[159] *Ars parva*, K 1.317 (on the false doctrine that human beings are perpetually ill to some degree); cf. 7.4.3, on the problem of the perfect constitution and the canon of Polykleitos.
[160] Joutsivuo 1999: 70ff.; Maclean 1980: 34–46.

and sickness participates in both extremes, or excludes both extremes
(a 'medium formae' or 'medium in genere'); whether an overlap is possible; whether the latitude of health refers only negatively to resistance
to disease; whether it refers both negatively and positively (to degrees of
health), and whether the neutrum which is perceptible to sense (such as
stomach pains, headaches, a bitter taste in the mouth) does not exist in
the order of the intelligible (and hence of truth).[161]

4.4.3 Division and definition

Division and definition undergo the same loosening. The standard discussion of endoxical division is found in Aristotle *Topics*, i.4 (102 a 1ff.) and
in a number of Boethius's topical works, notably the possibly spurious
De divisione and the *De topicis differentiis*, which (to judge from the format and
number of surviving editions) were textbooks in early sixteenth-century
Paris. Boethius specifically stresses the usefulness of 'divisio bimembris'
or simple disjunction,[162] but concedes also that there are other forms
of classification. The *De divisione* breaks division into four classes: genus
into species (e.g. animals into rational and irrational animals); whole into
parts (also known as enumeration: e.g. house into roof, walls and foundations); polysemic words or propositions into single senses (which in the
scholastic system becomes the 'sic distinguitur' by which contradictions
are resolved by appeal to *ratio, ordo, modus*, etc.); and finally the species
of 'divisio secundum accidens', which is itself divided into three classes
(subjects divided by accidents (e.g. some men are black, some white);
accidents divided by subject (things desired are desired either by the
body or by the soul); and accidents divided by accidents (some white
things are solid (pearls), others liquid (milk)).[163] This last is particularly

---

[161] Joutsivuo 1999; Vallesius 1606: 8 (i.4: 'de qualitatibus contrariis in eadem substantia'); cf. also
Categories, 12 a 10–12; *De generatione animalium*, ii.1, 733 a 34ff.; the analogy with shades of colour
in Galen, *De sanitate tuenda*, i, K 6.14; Blair 1999: 139ff. (on Bodin); below 7.4.3.

[162] See *In Porphyrium*, i.9, PL 64.79–81; *De divisione*, PL 64.877; Sanctorius 1630: 734 (xi.3); 420
(v.2): 'omne divisio melius et commodius docet, si (ut ait Boetius) ad bimembrem reducatur';
Ong 1974: 199; Jensen 2000: 196, who points out that this recommendation conflicts with
De partibus animalium, i.3, 643 b 9ff., which itself would appear to be a refutation of the Platonic
doctrine of *Sophist*, 212 c.

[163] On the Renaissance doctrine of endoxical division, see Maclean 2001. In Valerius 1573, both
'divisio' and 'definitio' are subjected to distinction by 'res et nomen'; and Boethius's categories
of 'divisio' are distributed between 'divisio nominis ambigui' and 'divisio rei' (that is, 'divisio
generis in species', 'totius in partes', 'subjecti in accidentia', 'accidentis in subjecta', 'accidentis
in accidentia'). Boethius also uses division to categorise 'res': *In categorias*, i PL 64.169–170; before
him, Cicero, *Topica*, v.26, distinguishes in a similar way between things that are ('quae sunt')
and things such as we perceive them ('quae intelliguntur').

relevant to medicine, as the attempts to distinguish between cause, illness and symptom (also referred to as 'accidens') reveal (see below, 7.5.2).

Endoxical divisions begin, like Porphyry's tree, with the 'genus generalissimum' and end with the 'species infima', but unlike it, they can progress not by necessary and sequential steps but by ungrounded dissimilarity/similarity decisions; that is to say, there may be no causal knowledge of the objects divided, and hence, no adequate account (in Aristotelian terms) of their identity and difference. Endoxical division may be heuristic in nature; as such, it constitutes a method or 'via divisiva'.[164] It belongs to art, not science, and accommodates judgements of plausibility and marginal cases. For all that, it is subject to error and falsification, as Galen points out.[165] Like Ramist dichotomies, it is pedagogically useful;[166] it can be, but does not have to be, exhaustive; but although less rigorous than Porphyry's tree, it cannot accommodate exceptions in the same synoptic table. It calls to mind Aristotle's comments on provisional taxonomy in his various treatises on animals;[167] especially the passage from the *De partibus animalium*, i.3 (643 b 9ff.), which marks the point at which division breaks down altogether:

Each of these groups [of birds and of fishes] is marked off by many differentiae, not by means of a dichotomy. By dichotomy, either these groups cannot be arrived at at all (because the same group falls under several divisions and contrary groups under the same division), or else there will be one differentia only, and this either singly or in combination will constitute the ultimate species [i.e. this procedure will never completely represent any actual group or species: 644 a 6ff.].

One commentator (Niccolò Leonico Tomeo) points out moreover that zoology is limited in its claim to truth because it deals with things that happen for the most part, and with things which are 'nobis notiora'.[168] It is tempting to see this and Aristotle's passage on division as influential in medical thinking, but there is little direct evidence of this: if most doctors concede the first point, only Argenterio and Cardano, to my

---

[164] Capivaccius 1603: 1035 points out that there is no division of the 'via divisiva' (another way of saying, presumably, that there is no rule for the application of a rule).

[165] See Galen, *Ad Glauconem*, i.1, K 11.4–5, quoted by Argenterio 1592: 2.24: 'omnes errores qui in medicina nascuntur, ex malis divisionibus provenire'.

[166] Gilbert 1960: 104–5 (quoting Manardo).

[167] See *De partibus animalium*, i.3, 643 b 9ff.; also *De generatione animalium*, ii.1, 732 a 1ff.; *Historia animalium*, i.6, 491 a 4ff.

[168] Quoted by Perfetti 1999b: 313.

knowledge, refer to the latter.[169] The best indication of the influence of this and other issues of taxonomy found in zoology and botany is to be found in the pioneering work undertaken in these spheres by doctors such as Fuchs, Rondelet and Aldrovandi and natural philosophers such as Andrea Cesalpino (1524/5–1603). Although among writers on education, only Ramus recommends that Aristotle's zoological works be read,[170] they were frequently printed in the sixteenth century, and there is some indication that they were taught in natural philosophy courses; and there are also a few commentaries; the most remarkable of these is the manuscript in the Ambrosiana entitled 'Selecta ex Aristotel[is] histor[ia] de animalibus et partibus', to which Stefano Perfetti has kindly drawn my attention. This concentrates almost exclusively on the issue of division, and the unsatisfactory nature both of a Porphyrian 'divisio bimembris' and a division by privation or accidents.[171] Cesalpino also writes in an original way on the issue of plant classification, with reference not only to the loci cited above but also *Metaphysics*, vii.12 (1037 b 8–1038 a 36). As Kristian Jensen has shown, he attacks the solution proposed by Fuchs, rejects the notion of a single ultimate differentia (that which finally defines a species) for the purposes of classifying composite substances, and envisages the possibility of one plant belonging to several genera. He also shows himself to be aware of the need for any classification to be able to deal with as yet undiscovered plants.[172]

The possible inclusion of accidents in division, which is touched upon in the chapter of the *Metaphysics* discussed by Cesalpino, gives rise to a problem for Renaissance taxonomists; Fuchs seems to have believed that it was possible to categorise plants by including accidental features related to their life cycle, and using these accidents in a differential description designed to eliminate other species until a single species could be identified with certainty.[173] This approach to definition, which is also employed by Rondelet, may be derived from the Boethian distinction between

---

[169] Argenterio 1610: 1463: 'quantum enim difficile sit bene dividere, docet Arist. *initio Operis de partibus animalium*, tantoque profecto difficilior nobis est dividendi ratio: quid nemo hactenus ex antiquis scriptoribus enim satis explicare sit conatus'; Cardano 1663: 9.487; Siraisi 1987a: 327; Furlanus 1574: 16, 27–65 (commenting on the problems of taxonomy); Cunningham 1985: 195–9; also Jardine 1997: 205–6 (on Zabarella and Piccolomini recommending *De partibus animalium* for medicine and physiology).

[170] Cranz and Schmitt 1984: 201 (listing thirty-nine separate printings of the Latin text); Perfetti 1999b; Kusukawa 1999: 132; also the evidence of disputed quaestiones in Bodley MS Rawl. D 274 (Liber Ioannis Daij Londiniensis, 1589).

[171] MS Milano B Ambr. N 26 Sup, esp. 2v, 4v, 8r, 13r.

[172] Jensen 2000.

[173] Kusukawa forthcoming a.

separable and inseparable accidents,[174] yet it conflicts with *Posterior analytics*, i.6 (75 a 20), where it is stated that accidents do not admit of demonstrative knowledge, and *Metaphysics*, v.30 (1025 a 14ff.), where the nature of an accident is discussed.[175] It also has implications for the relationship between illnesses and their symptoms, which, as has been said, were known in the Middle Ages and later as 'accidentia' (see below 7.5.2, 8.2.2).[176]

The term 'divisio' (of genus into species) is sometimes distinguished from 'partitio' (of wholes into parts), as it is by Cicero (*Topica*, v.28). 'Partitio' is usually taken to be potentially exhaustive, but Cicero allows for instances which are imperfect or incomplete.[177] 'Partitio' is sometimes distinguished in turn from 'enumeratio', which can also be an open class. Quintilian's term for this is 'anacephaleosis', which he defines both as 'a summing up', and as a 'division into headings'.[178] The term is used in both senses in the Renaissance, and indeed many of the tree diagrams provided in medical books are no more than a synoptic table of chapters grouped by subject matter; an example of this is afforded by Capivaccius's account of fevers.[179]

In medical writing division appears in a number of guises. Da Monte, who quotes the full Boethian list as pertinent to the art, recognises two orders of division: 'essentialis' (or 'speculativa'), and 'accidentalis' (or 'activa vel factiva').[180] For him and for others, division is a method (like resolution and composition); the 'via divisiva' defines the best doctor, and

---

[174] Rondelet 1554–5; Boethius, *In Porphyrium*, ii, PL 64.51. Jensen 2000: 188–9 points out that Fuchs claims to have derived his view of definition from genus and inseparable accidents (in conflict with *De partibus animalium*, I, 644 b 7ff.) from Agricola, possibly 1967: 62–5 (i.11) ('de adiacentibus').

[175] See *De partibus animalium*, i.3, 643 b 9–644 a 11; also Sennert 1650: 1.14.

[176] Stupanus 1614: 591, who translates 'oikeia symptomata' as 'propria accidentia'. Demonet forthcoming quotes Fuchs as preferring to translate 'symptoma' by 'casus' because he associates the word 'accidens' with methodist doctors.

[177] See also *Topica*, v.28f., vii.31, and viii.33 ('non est vitiosum in re infinita praetermittere aliquid'); and Nörr 1972: 20ff.

[178] See Goyet 1996: 553–6, quoting Melanchthon; Quintilian, *Institutio oratoria*, vi.1.1.

[179] Capivaccius 1603: 1003–5; cf. Liddel 1628: 228ff. (symptoms grouped by the ordering of Galen, *De differentis symptomatum*, iii, K 7.55–62). Schmitt 1983a: 58 has an illustration of anacephaleosis as a table of chapters (of the *Physics*). For other manifestations of interest in the doctrine of division and partition see Vickers 1968: 30–59.

[180] Da Monte 1587: 101: 'divisio multiplex est, alia essentialis, alia accidentalis'; but cf. *ibid.*, 6 on 'divisio multiplex': 'divisio continui in suas partes quantitativas vel proportionales, generis in species, vocis in sua significata, compositi in sua componenta, in potentiam et actum, subjectum in sua accidentia, divisio artificialis [id est] progressus ab universalibus ad minus universale, et rursus a minus universali, in partes adhuc minus universales quousque ad particulares ventum fuerit, et tandem ad individuas, ut amplius fieri divisio non possit'; the 'divisio artificialis' is the appropriate mode for doctors, as it reaches the individual to be treated; *ibid.*, 230 (repeating

is apparently subjected to the same rules as scientific division.[181] It is subject to reality and inductive knowledge, and derives from what is known; it cannot create similarity and difference.[182] Galen's definition of illness in his *Methodus medendi* (i.3, K 10.25–6) is an example of division into infimae species; but as the parallel works of Fuchs (1537a) and Sylvius (1539a) show, different trees can be created for signs, indicating simultaneously the pedagogical usefulness of the tree diagram and its non-necessary nature. I have already mentioned the use of dichotomies associated with Ramus; it is clear that both in typographical and in pedagogical usage, doctors, grammarians and philosophers preceded him in this practice, and that they owe nothing in the later part of the century to his own Platonic unitary theory of dialectics.[183] Whereas some lawyers could benefit from his method and style of presentation, doctors are too committed to a non-consilient approach to learning and to a non-monotonic logic to be able to make use of it, unless for synoptic diagrams of chapters (anacephaleoses).[184]

I turn now to dialectical definition. Its scientific equivalent (see above 4.3.2), whether nominal or real, is characterised by convertibility, and is principally class-inclusive in character. Doctors are principally concerned with real definitions which cite just genus and differentiae (which define by class-exclusion).[185] Galen himself used differentiae extensively, as is witnessed by the title of certain of his treatises on pulses, illnesses, and symptoms. His own loose categories of medical definition are given

Boethius); Campilongo 1601: 18v (citing the claim in *Ad Glauconem*, i.1, K 11.4–5 that division (of health from disease) defines the best doctor).

[181] Da Monte 1587: 6; cf. also 14, where he compares the 'ars dividendi' to induction, and says that 'usus divisionis maxime facit ad omnes artes et actiones, quae circa particularia versantur'; Capivaccius 1603: 1036ff.; also Gilbert 1960: 104–6.

[182] *Prior analytics*, i.31, 46 b 36–40; Averroes, *Colliget*, i.1; Campilongo 1601: 16r: 'ea quae divisione inveniuntur, quae ad cognitionem similis et dissimilis spectant, adiuncta esse'. Yet in *De placitis Hippocratis et Platonis*, ix, K 5.720ff., Galen says that division is based on similarity/dissimiliarity decisions and that there are three sorts of division: genus to species; whether same or different; what is same and different. See also, on the relationship of division to reality, Herberger 1981: 91; Crusius 1615: 106: 'divisionem rerum admittit natura, ratio comprobat[,] auctoritas stabilit'. Crusius allows for the possibility of a 'divisionis novitas' (Fracastoro's doctrine of contagion), provided that it has been empirically tested. The question whether or not new things can be discovered by division is not clearly settled in Aristotle: see Jardine 1974: 24 (quoting Lee).

[183] Maclean 2001.

[184] On the lawyers' use of dichotomies, see Maclean 1992: 38–43. An ancephaleosis of Capivaccius's method of interrogating patients is produced by Campilongo 1601: 8r.

[185] Argenterio 1610: 930; for the parallel legal interest in definitions, which are predominantly nominal in character, see Maclean 1992: 104–14.

in *De differentiis pulsuum*, iv.2: they are 'the exposition of what a name means; reference to a feature of a thing; a close definition of a thing; the pure doctrine of the thing'.[186] These do not go uncriticised in the Renaissance. Capivaccius attacks him for his alleged confusion of species and differentiae and for attempting real definition by form rather than by effect.[187] Capivaccius himself prefers Averroes's division of real definition into two classes: 'formaliter' and 'effective', the latter being scientifically less demanding than the former,[188] as it can accommodate the claim that 'some things change their essence in generation, mutation and alteration; some things retain their substance'.[189] This means in effect that definition can be of a combination of genus and accident, as it frequently is in plant classification in the Renaissance.[190] Accidents are acknowledged to pose problems (see *Topics*, i.5, 102 b), and it is recognised that there is no 'scientia' of the accident.[191] This is similar to the looseness found in Aristotelian zoological enquiry already mentioned, in which animal groups are distinguished by many differentiae which cannot be reduced to a tree or a dichotomy, and are furthermore 'more or less' of a kind (see below 5.2.3).[192] Some categories can even be mixed, such as zoophytes and sexually ambiguous beings.[193] Like lawyers, doctors (and among them those who engage in botanical and zoological studies) have recourse in the end to descriptions rather than definition proper.[194] In modern terminology, one might describe some of their classes as polythetic.[195]

---

[186] Cardano 1565: 118v (i.5.8): 'quid nomen significet exponens'; 'aliquid attingit de re'; 'multo melius explicat rem'; 'puram rem docet': see also Valleriola 1577: 176–7 on Galen's method and use of definition.

[187] Capivaccius 1603: 1005.

[188] *Ibid.*, 1031.

[189] *Methodus medendi*, ii.3, K 10.88.

[190] Ottosson 1984: 202; Kusukawa 1997: 422–3.

[191] *Posterior analytics*, i.4, 75 a 20ff.; *Metaphysics*, v.30, 1025 a 14ff.

[192] *De partibus animalium*, i.2, 642 b 10ff.; i.4, 644 a 15; Rondelet 1554–5: 1.3: 'differentiae nomen hic latius patere, cum enim verae differentiae in tanta penuria, antiquorum Philosophorum exemplo ad alias nobis confugiendum fuit' (with references to Theophrastus, *De plantis* and Aristotle's 'vis' in *Historia animalium*, i.1).

[193] Daston and Park 1998: 56 (on zoophytes in the medieval period); Montuus 1537: 165–6; Cardano 1663: 8.152, 204, 210 (on custom and region affecting sexual difference); Campilongo 1610: 17r–v (on modes of differentiae); Liceti 1634; Maclean 1980: 39 (citing Bauhin).

[194] Capivaccius 1603: 1026 (a reference to 'definitionem seu descriptionem'); for legal parallels, see Maclean 1992: 97, 108–11. Description is associated with visual representation: see Quintilian, *Institutio oratoria*, ix.1.40; Cicero, *De oratore*, iii.43.202; Mack 1990: 151.

[195] Needham 1975; an example of such a class is provided by Sanctorius 1630: 741–2, quoted below, ch. 8, note 108.

4.4.4 Causes

We may finally turn in this chapter to causes. Scientific demonstration is by its definition causal: 'scire est rem per causas cognoscere', as the maxim has it;[196] it is grounded in the doctrine of the four causes. Medicine has a more pragmatic interest in causes, which need to be distinguished from symptoms and illnesses and attributed either to the patient and his nature or to the environment.[197] There is a specific Galenic doctrine of causes derived from his treatise *De causis procatarcticis*, as we shall see (7.5.4) which distinguishes between 'causa continens' (usually rendered as 'sustaining', 'internal', 'material', 'remote', or 'occult') and 'causa procatarctica' ('preliminary', 'external', 'material', 'proximate', 'efficient'); this gives rise to a debate in the Renaissance about their meaning, range and combination. Among the formal questions asked is whether illnesses can have an infinite number of causes which would render them in Aristotelian terms unknowable.[198] Argenterio gives to cause the meaning of precondition attributed to the term by Cicero;[199] it is striking that he makes no reference to modal logic or the logic of consequence, which would have been useful to his account of medical etiology. Instead, he reconstitutes out of the Galenic corpus a doctrine of eight rather than four causes: the Aristotelian quartet of formal, material, efficient and final, together with subjective, instrumental, catalytic, and necessary but external. These extra four are linked respectively to the idiosyncratic nature of subjects (all individuals are differently configured), the functionality of organs and spirits, the need to account for the efficacy of composed medicines, and the influence of 'res non naturales' (below, 7.4).[200] It is easy to see that such a range would make the distinction of cause and quality difficult when dealing with such topics as

---

[196] Sennert 1676: 109, quoted by Eckart 1992: 147.

[197] Galen, *Methodus medendi*, i.7, K 10.50 (on nothing occurring without a cause); Campilongo 1601: 2r; Cardano 1583: 1. Torrigiano 1557: 26v has a two-term incomplete matrix for causes based on weakness/frequency: the three classes he gives are 'debiles frequenter occurrentes'; 'medicores communiter occurrentes'; 'potentissimae raro occurrentes.'

[198] Vallesius 1606: 171ff. (iv.1–2).

[199] Argenterio 1610: 1491: 'quae quidem perfectionis nihil addit rei, qua fit, ab illis tamen, quae conferunt, seiungi non potest: vel ut brevius dicam, causa huiusmodi est, sine qua res fieri nequit'); see Cicero, *Topica*, xxv.

[200] Argenterio 1610: 1493: the eight are 'quid faciat rem esse [formalis]; a quo [efficiens]; ex quo materialis; in quo (subiectivus); cuius gratia (finalis); per quod (instrumentalis); sine qua non; cum qua melius, facilius res peragitur'; see also *De usu partium corporis*, vi, K 3.464–5: 'nos autem ne futiliter de nominibus concertare videamur, concedentes plura esse causarum genera, primum quidem, ac potissimum, cuius causa aliquid sit; secundum vero a quo sit, tertium ex quo, quarto propter quid, et quintum si uis secundum quod fit, ad singula genera respondere ipsos de omnibus?'; Argenterio 1610: 929 citing *De causis procatarcticis*'s list as 'formam rei,

contagion, even if it permits an answer to be given to problems relating to objective reality.[201] Such proliferation of causes is also a feature of natural philosophy; in Melanchthon's *Initia doctrinae physicae* there are more than ten types of efficient cause alone listed.[202] The possible existence of occult causes (especially astrological ones) – again a disputed topic – also makes it difficult for cause straightforwardly to be the middle term of a syllogism, even if cause is only understood in a loose sense.[203] The profusion of causes in medicine contrasts with the claim made by advocates (who use the four causes for pedagogical reasons) that they mainly rely on two in the practice of their profession (final and efficient); and the claim made after 1630 that science should concern itself with only one (the efficient).[204]

As we have seen, the parallels between demonstrative logic and dialectics are explicit in the manuals of university teachers of medicine; this is surprising insofar as the scientific and rational status of medicine is affirmed, but then concessions are made about the nature of the propositions, logical processes and causality which are employed in medical reasoning. The differences between this and apodictic logic even go beyond the distinction made in *Topics*, i.1 between demonstration and dialectics. Both the degree of certainty of the propositions, divisions and definitions is weakened, and the processes by which they are used to generate conclusions and inferences are less rigorous. As we shall see, this loosening of the structures of thought which are found acceptable is found also in the other parts of the arts course – inference from signs, analogy, induction, argument from example – which are the subject of the next chapter.

---

efficiens, materiam subiectam, finem, instrumentum, cum quibus, sine quibus'; *De usu partium corporis*, vi.12, K 3.464–5, cited by Moraux 1981: 99 as final, agent, material, instrumental, organic, and formal; cf. Blair 1997: 63.

[201] On this aspect of contagion, see Nutton 1990b: 205.

[202] Melanchthon 1581: 216ff.: his sources include Galen and Plato. See also Valerius 1573 and Velcurio 1553.

[203] Copenhaver 1992; Stump 1982: 284; Keil 1992: 175; on cause being identical with effect (symptom or sign), see below 7.5.2–3.

[204] Coras 1591: 25 (distinguishing the interests of lawyers from physicians and philosophers); Bacon 1878: 339–40 (*Novum organum*, ii.2), who admits only efficient and material causes, because 'the final cause corrupts rather than advances the sciences except such as have to do with human action'; Argenterio 1610: 1489–95. Both medicine and the law refer also to remote and proximate causes. See also, on the comparison of the two faculties, Maclean 2000b, where the point about the different senses of 'regulariter' and 'generaliter' (allowing no exceptions in law, but admitting them in medicine) is also made: see, for examples in medical discourse, Silvaticus 1601: 374 and Horst 1629: 131.

CHAPTER 5

The arts course: signs, induction, mathematics, experientia

5.1 SIGNS

In the second part of this review of the art course, I pass to instruments of thought which in some cases are less exalted and in others more specialised. Because of its importance in diagnosis and prognosis, sign theory is a particular concern to university teachers of medicine, as are analogy (in identifying illnesses and treatments) and induction (in reasoning from limited data). In different ways, issues of quantification (of humours and doses), of probability (of one construction of evidence against another), and empirical knowledge (including that acquired indirectly through the experience of others) also arise. I shall look at these issues in turn.

It is pertinent first to consider the doctrine of signs, which, together with topical argument and the theory of forensic oratory, was enriched after the discovery in the early fifteenth century of certain rhetorical works by Cicero and Quintilian.[1] Elements of the earlier doctrine of signs inherited by the Renaissance have already been alluded to: in respect of logic, both the 'tekmērion' as the middle term of a necessary demonstration and the Averroistic 'demonstratio signi' (see above 4.3.5–6); in respect of the linguistic sign (see 4.2.1 and 4.2.3), Augustine's definition of the sign as 'that which reveals both itself to the senses and something beyond itself to the mind',[2] and his distinction between natural and intentional signs. The former of these possess no signifying intention, such as smoke as a sign of fire, or the tracks of an animal, or signs of emotion on the face; the latter are the intentional expressions of living beings of their thoughts and feelings.[3] From this, the doctrine of the 'signum reale'

---

[1] See Murphy 1974: 358–60; Kennedy 1980: 195–219.
[2] *Principia dialectica*, v, PL 32.1410: 'signum est et quod seipsum sensui et praeter se aliquid animo ostendit'.
[3] *De doctrina christiana*, ii. 1.2–3, PL 34.1.36–7: 'signorum igitur alia sunt naturalia, alia data. Naturalia sunt quae sine voluntate atque ullo appetitu significandi, praeter se aliquid aliud

as opposed to the 'signum doctrinale' is derived, and the sign is associated with inferential reasoning both in the form of the demonstration 'quia' (above, 4.3.6) and the hypothetical syllogism or consequence ('if smoke, then fire', which is not distinguished in medieval logic from 'smoke, therefore fire').[4] In medicine, where the sign is also known as 'nota', 'indicium', 'connotans' and 'indicans', it is recognised to be, according to a formula with which we are now familiar, a 'latius nomen quam in logicis'.[5] Argenterio says it is broader because it is latent and plural;[6] but it is also broader because it belongs to Aristotelian language theory, to syllogistic and Stoic logic, to the conjectural arts and to rhetoric. It will be helpful first to set out the relevant parts of the Aristotelian doctrine before considering the debate among Renaissance doctors about the status of the sign and their uptake of the sign theory of the Stoics.

5.1.1 Aristotelian signs

Signs appear in a number of Aristotelian contexts.[7] We have already met the designation of the linguistic sign (the name) in the *De interpretatione*, i (16 a 4ff.) as bearing no more than a conventional relationship to that which it signifies (above 4.2.1). In *Prior analytics*, ii.2 (70 a 5ff.), a general term ('sēmeion') is introduced, and distinguished from a probability ('eikos'):

A probability is not the same as a sign. The former is a generally accepted premiss; for that which people know to happen or not to happen, or to be or not to be, usually in a particular way, is a probability, e.g. that the envious are malevolent or that those who are loved are affectionate. A sign, however, means a demonstrative premiss which is necessary or generally accepted. That which coexists with something else, or before or after whose happening something else has happened, is a sign of that something's having happened or being.

Aristotle goes on to discuss enthymemes which are syllogisms involving 'eikota' and 'sēmeia', consisting only in a proposition and a conclusion,

---

ex se cognosci faciunt . . . Data vero signa sunt, quae sibi quaeque viventibus invicem dant ad demonstrandos, quantum possunt, motus animi sui, vel sensa, aut intellecta quaelibet.'

[4] See Boh 1982: 307–8; Goclenius 1613: 1045–9; Ashworth 1990a (who illustrates its involvement in debates about natural, conventional and customary signification, and the distinction between 'facere cognoscere' and 'exprimere'); Meier-Oeser 1997; Singh Gill and Manetti 1999–2000; Demonet 2001; and Demonet forthcoming, who quotes Paré as associating 'indicium' with 'indicatio', which is unusual at this time. Manetti 1987: 57ff. points out that 'nota' is used by Boethius to translate both 'sēmeion' and 'symbolon'.

[5] Campilongo 1601: 12r; Sennert 1650: 1.448; Varanda 1620: 16 (on 'indicans' and its cognates).

[6] Argenterio 1610: 1677.

[7] Weidmann 1989.

and shows that there are three ways of including signs in syllogisms which correspond to the three figures of the syllogism. As a sign is singular, the syllogisms derived from it have a limited validity, and indeed are only valid if they are in the first figure (darii):

> All who have milk are pregnant
> This woman has milk
> _____
> Therefore she is pregnant.

In the third figure (moods I-I-A), the argument is clearly fallacious:

> Pittacus is good
> Pittacus is wise
> _____
> Therefore all wise men are good

The same applies to this less obviously fallacious version (moods A-I-I):

> All who are pregnant are sallow
> This woman is sallow
> _____
> Therefore this woman is pregnant.[8]

These Aristotelian examples are cited by doctors and by those writing as natural philosophers.[9] Frölich calls the sign in the example cited above a 'rhetorical', as opposed to 'logical', sign; the fallacy with which it is

---

[8] On the weakness of syllogistic of signs see Alonso 1598: 26 (on the fourth figure, on which see also Zabarella 1586–7: 41–53); Sanctorius 1630: 723ff. (xi, xii *passim*). The fallacy of the Pittacus example is that the conclusion is universal; the fallacy of the sallowness example is that the Minor Premiss would have to be negative to generate a true conclusion. On this see Caselius 1580: A3–4: 'enthymemata igitur τεκμηριωδή quoniam hic proceditur ab universali ad singulare, referuntur ad primam figuram, in qua medius terminus est in maiore subjectum, praedicatum in minore. Enthymema est: lac habere: maior, uterum gerere: minor mulier, de qua dicitur. Sic igitur syllogismus integer. Lac habentes, uterum gerunt: glycerium lac habet: glycerium igitur uterum gerit.' This is fallacious 'cum non legitima sit connexio'; as are the examples he gives of the other figures of the syllogism: 'in hoc collocatio medij termini convenit cum secunda figura, ut ille sit praedicatum in utraque propositionum praemissarum, tam in maiore, quam in minore. Enthymema est. Crito anhelat: febricitat igitur. Medius terminus est . . . anhelare: maior, febricitans: minor, homo quispiam . . . syllogismus sic habeat. Febricitantes anhelant: Crito anhelat: Crito igitur febricitat. Facile hoc solvi potest, etiamsi verum sit, quando anhelant et alii, qui minime febricitant. Insuper esti hic syllogismus in forma est secundae figurae: in modo certe nullo est. Non enim ipsa recepit syllogismum per omnia affirmativum: neque aliter, nisi negative concludit. Quare hoc signum ἀσυλλόγιστη est. Sic etiam tertium, quod procedit a particulari ad universale. Ex hoc ductum enthymema respondet syllogismo tertiae figurae, ubi medius terminus est subjectum, et in maiore et minore propositione. Exempli gratia. Socrates est iustus: sapientes igitur sunt iusti. Medius terminus est [Socrates] [Caselius in fact writes 'Pittacus' here, thinking of the Aristotelian example]; maior, iustum esse: minor sapientem esse. Sit syllogismus. Socrates est iustus: Socrates est sapiens: sunt ergo sapientes iusti. Solvitur hoc facillime, etiamsi verum sit: tum, quam instantiam dare in proclivi est, tum quia nihil colligitur ex meris particularibus, nedum ex meris singularibus.' See also Burnyeat 1982.

[9] E.g. Chiaramonte 1625: 1–6; Campilongo 1601: 71r; Sanctorius 1630: 99–104 (i.29).

associated is the fallacy of the consequent (if all A is B, then all B is A: see *De sophisticis elenchis*, vii, 169 b 7f.); it is the one most to be avoided in medicine.[10] To extricate themselves from this fallacy, logicians have, according to Donald Morrison (citing Philoponus), to be Platonists (i.e. to take universals to be prior to particulars) and hence to unite 'prior in nature' with 'prior to us'.[11] Otherwise the paralogisms in *De sophisticis elenchis*(167 b 10ff.) apply: not only the fallacy of the man being hot having a fever, but also the paralogism (associated with a syndrome of signs) of a well-dressed man roaming the streets at night being the adulterer (see below 5.2.2; 8.4.1).

A further discussion in *Prior analytics*, ii.27 (70 b 12ff.) relates signs to physiognomy:

[Supposing that] one grants that body and soul change together in all natural affections . . . and also that there is one sign of one affection, and that we can recognise the affection and the sign proper to each class of creatures, we shall be able to judge character from physical appearance . . . in the first figure, provided that the middle term is convertible with the first extreme, but is wider in extension than the third term and not convertible with it: e.g. if A stands for courage, B for large extremities and C for lion. Then B applies to all of that to which C applies, and also to others, whereas A applies to all that to which B applies, and to no more, but is convertible with B. Otherwise there will not be one sign of one affection.[12]

These passages may be linked to discussion of signs in rhetoric: *Rhetoric to Alexander*, xii (1430 b 30ff.) develops some of the distinctions mentioned above:

One thing is a sign of another — not any casual thing of any other casual thing, nor everything whatever of everything whatever, but only a thing that normally precedes or accompanies or follows a thing. Something happening may be a sign not only of something happening but also of something not happening, and something that has not happened may be a sign not only that something is not a fact but also that something is a fact. A sign may produce either opinion of full knowledge; the best kind of sign is one that produces

---

[10] See also Quintilian, *Institutio oratoria*, v.9.5–7 (a legal context); v.8.6; v.10.11; Frölich 1612: A2r; for a medical example of its use, see da Monte 1583: 1.107: 'habet [iuvenis] bubones, ergo laborat morbo gallico non sequitur, sicut a nullo signo alio solo argui potest, quia semper committetur fallacia consequentis'.

[11] Morrison 1997: 10: 'Since Aristotle holds that universals are posterior in nature to particulars, he would not agree that "tekmeriodic proof" – from posteriors to priors – could cover reasoning from particular to general. What permits Philoponus to include induction as a variety of tekmeriodic proof is his Neoplatonic belief that universals are prior to particulars.' Philoponus's commentary on the *Posterior analytics* was well known in the Renaissance, being published in Paris in 1544, and in Venice in 1553, 1559 and 1560.

[12] See above 4.3.3, fig. 4.4, for Giambattista della Porta's diagrammatic representation of this.

knowledge, but one that causes an extremely probable opinion is the second best kind.[13]

Here mention is made not only of a hierarchy of certainty, to which I shall return, but also the possibility of signs bearing negative information, and of absence or omission being possibly a sign of something positive.

The term 'eikos', used for probability in the passage cited above, is used in *Rhetoric*, i.2 (1356 b 1ff.) to mean sign and is described as a 'protasis endoxos', a likely or probable sign which occurs only generally ('hōs epi polu': 'ut multum', 'ut plurimum', 'magna ex parte'); that is to say, even if generally accepted as having a certain sense, it is capable of having a different one. It is linked to a discussion of enthymeme, analogy and induction. Quintilian also refers to eikos and gives eikota three meanings: what usually happens (a judgement of frequency); what is highly probable ('propensius'); and that against which nothing can be said. These meanings do not include the modal sense (what is possibly the case) or a mathematical sense (what is approximately the case) which we might expect to be mentioned in this context.[14]

A third Greek term for sign is tekmērion: in Aristotle (and according to some doctors, Hippocrates), a widely quoted distinction is made between tekmēria, which are necessary and can be used in the construction of a syllogism of the first figure, and sēmeia which, being no more than 'probable', cannot. Galen records this distinction in a much quoted discussion in his *In prognostica*, iii.39 (K 18b.306–13), in which he associates the former term with demonstration and certainty, and the latter with 'probability' and empirical observation.[15]

---

[13] Alonso 1598: 21 uses this passage to argue that there can be no inference from particular signs, and no demonstration from common signs; see also Fontanus 1611: 34.

[14] Quintilian, *Institutio oratoria*, v.10.16; also v.8.6ff.; v.9.5–12. Sylvius 1539a: 25 refers to this text. Demonet 2001: 26–9 points out that there is another, even weaker, sign cited by Quintilian in this passage, of which the example given is 'non esse virginem Atalantam, quia cum iuvenibus per silvas vagetur'; the context in which this sign arises is (illicitly) persuasive argument, and I have not seen it cited by doctors.

[15] Caselius 1580: A1–4 is a diagrammatic representation of this doctrine and a clear exposition of *Rhetoric*, i.2 in the light of other relevant Aristotelian texts: he makes the point first that the enthymeme deals principally with contingency not necessity; he defines its propositions as 'verisimiles' ('quod enim plerumque sciunt; aut fieri aut non fieri; aut esse aut non esse') and its subject matter as 'res [quae] se aliter habere possunt'. He then examines enthymemes in the different figures of the syllogism and distinguishes tekmeriodic from semeiotic enthymemes: See above, note 8. See also Montefusco 1998: 10–12; Horst 1609: 131 (on the distinction of sēmeion and tekmērion); cf. Vega 1571: 1197–8 (on Hippocrates, *Prognosis*, iii.39): 'certae coniecturae sive tecmeria semper eadem indicant, et semper talia sunt qualia indicantur; signa tamen salutis quae signa sunt non tamen tecmeria, semper talia indicant; verum non semper talia fiunt, qualia indicantur. Accidentia vero decretoria, neque semper talia indicant, neque semper talia fiunt, a qualia indicantur'; Donatius 1591: 32; Lemosius 1598: 39–42. Liddel 1628: 511ff.; Argenterio 1606–7: 1.101, cited below, note 27. Campilongo 1601: 70v produces a minor out

Signs appear elsewhere in the Aristotelian corpus, with consequences for medical science. In the *De divinatione per somnum*, i (462 b 27ff.) and ii (463 b 23ff.) it is pointed out that they may be empty of content, or may provide no information about causes, or may be insignificant if overtaken by signs of more powerful causes.[16] And in the *Physiognomica*, which is a doctrine 'wholly located in the discernment of sensory signs',[17] a number of distinctions and theoretical points about signs are made, including the general rule that one sign is not sufficient to show a cause, but that a number of signs consistent with each other are required. The distinction between proper and common signs is upheld; the latter are only acceptable, according to Chiaramonte, in the second figure of the syllogism.[18] It is also argued both that there can be no inference from a proper sign (see above, 4.2.3), and that there can be no (scientific) demonstration from a single ('common') sign, as the text of the *Physiognomica* points out (ii, 806 b 37ff.):

Generally speaking, it is foolish to puts one's faith in any one of the signs; but when one finds several of the signs in agreement in one individual, one would probably have more justification for believing the inference true.

Giambattista della Porta quotes this text and expands on it:[19] he also makes the negative point about the proper sign:

Nor are proper signs of any use, for proper signs are proper of nothing other than that one thing, and correspond to nothing else, and signify their proper

---

of four symptoms – all *sēmeia* – when taken together: 'et quoniam in prima figura praedicatur medius de minore et subjicitur maiori extremitati, veluti videtur ex Aristotele in signis demonstrativis, dicere possumus, omnes habens lac peperit, haec autem mulier habet lac. Ergo peperit. Habere lac est signum seu terminus medius, quo hanc mulierem peperisse indicatur. In demonstrativis exemplum erit huiusmodi. Omnis homo habens dolorem lateris, tussim, febrem, difficilem respirationem, patitur pleuritidem. Hic homo habet haec symptomata. Ergo detinetur pleuritide. His enim quatuor symptomatibus, tamquam termino medio, demonstrat hunc patientem esse pleuriticum.'

[16] Alonso 1598: 24–5: 'signa aliqua sunt quae null[o]s affectus eorum quos signabant consequantur, adveniente superiori causa, quasi diceret propter hanc rationem signa significantia futura fiunt incerta, quia habent causas potentes impedire effectus nondum ad extra productos, sed solum in suis causis latitantes' but he adds 'ex communibus demonstrativis signis decet fidem praestare ad cognoscendum morbum generice, non vero hunc specifice'.

[17] Fontanus 1611: 34: 'physiognomia tota sita in signis sensibilibus dignoscendis'. According to Demonet 2001: 24, both Agricola and Ramus refer to the physiognomonic sign as 'coniectura animi'.

[18] Chiaramonte 1625: 6.

[19] Porta 1593: 55 points out that this applies to common signs only, and adds a confirmation of the point from a Galenic source: 'uni signorum credere fatuum esse, scilicet communium: sed plura circa unum convenientia pensiculanda esse, et plura testimonia ad unum accommodanda, ut ex iis mox securius iudicium proferatur. Quod est etiam a Galeno confirmatum, qui Physiognomos multum errare crederet, quod uni signorum credant, nisi proprium signum id fuerit.' See also Galen, *De placitis Hippocratis et Platonis*, v.5, K 4.257 (the error of Posidonius). Cf. Fontanus

passion; and if they were to correspond to anything else, they would not be proper signs, and as no affect is proper to the animals from which we practise physiognomy, there would not be a peculiar sign either.[20]

Other points of doctrine in the *Physiognomica* decree that signs can demonstrate *a negativo* or *a contrario*;[21] that they can be both innate and acquired, and permanent and labile; that the same sign can indicate quite different mores, and can indicate an accidental not a substantial feature.[22] L'Alemant's summary of Aristotelian doctrine is as follows:

There are [three] sorts of demonstrations from signs. The first is inferred, when a cause unknown to us is proved from a manifest effect, as in this case: as often as these symptoms are seen, namely difficulty of breathing, a stabbing pain in the side and persistent fever, there will be inflammation of the intercostal membrane; but pleurisy has these symptoms; therefore pleurisy is an inflammation of the intercostal membrane. The second sort infers an effect hidden from us from a sign. Whenever stiffness follows on from an ardent fever, it causes the fever to go away. But when the bile inflaming the skin is evacuated through sweat, stiffness occurs. Therefore when the bile inflaming the skin is evacuated through sweat, the ardent fever goes away. The third sort assumes a remote cause, as in this example: anything which is troubled by melancholy is an animal; a plant is not an animal; therefore a plant is not troubled by melancholy.[23]

1611: 34: 'signa autem sunt aut propria aut communia, quae a Galeno dicuntur propria vel inseparabilia. Siquidem ex communibus signis suas textuerit ratiocinationes aliquis, non erit demonstrativa argumentatio. Nam demonstratio ex propriis et necessariis constat ex Aristotele lib 1 de demonstr. Neque certe rationi consonum est, si cervo cum cane aliquod signum est commune, illud magis significare mores cervi quam canis: ut enim propria signa aliquid peculiare denotant, ita communia commune, quae Physiognomo nullo modo commoda esse possunt.'

20 Porta 1593: 26–7: 'neque [propria signa] quoque ad rem faciunt; nam propria signa nulli propria, nisi cui propria sunt, nullique competunt, propriamque passionem ostendunt; et si alteri competerent, propria signa non essent, et cum affectus nullus proprius sit animalium, ex quibus physiognomoniam exercemus, nullum etiam signum peculiare erit'. Part of his refutation of Plato's view is that 'si homo universum corpus alicui prorsus animali consimile habuerit, iisdem etiam moribus et affectibus, quibus illud, afficeretur'.

21 *Ibid.*, 38–9: 'quod etiam per signa a contrario sumpta mores diiudicare possimus'. Cf. *Physiognomica*, ii, 807 a 31f., 807 b 5f. (the contrasting features of the brave man and the coward). See also *Prior analytics*, i.46, 51 b 1ff., on deriving negative conclusions.

22 Fontanus 1611 : 31f.; cf Melanchthon 1547: R7v.

23 L'Alemant 1549: 29–30: 'demonstratio signi duplex [!sic] est. Prima connectitur, quando per effectum manifestum causa nobis incognita probatur: ut, quotiescumque hae visa fuerint, nempe spirandi difficultas, lateris dolor pungens, assidua febris, erit inflammatio membranae succingentis costas. Sed pleuritis illa habet, igitur pleuritis est inflammatio membranae succingentis costas. Secunda ex signo effectum nobis occultum concludit. Quandocumque rigor febri ardenti succedit eadem solvit. Sed cum bilis ad cutem impetum faciens, per sudorem vacuatur, fit rigor. Ergo cum bilis ad cutem impetum faciens per sudorem vacuatur, febris ardens solvitur. Tertia causam remotam assumit, ut quicquid melancholia vexatur est animal. Planta non est animal, igitur planta non vexatur melancholia.'

We can see here three medical examples, including the standard medical example of a syndrome of signs (see below 8.4.1) accommodated to syllogistic structures.

These Aristotelian texts generate both areas of agreement and clear differences of opinion among Renaissance doctors. It is also universally accepted that construing signs involves a passage from the known to the unknown, which, in the case of a posteriori reasoning, is a conjectural passage.[24] But whether the sign is sensory or intelligible in nature, whether it is a pre-rational datum, or a middle term, or the minor proposition of a syllogism are matters of debate. This is still of particular interest, as some elements of the debate recur in present-day disagreements between analytic philosophers and linguistic semiologists such as Umberto Eco. In reviewing the latter's work, Colin McGinn asks, 'what non-trivial theory can be derived from treating human languages and measle spots as both instances of interpretable signs?' and claims that 'the perceptual recognition of signs and other objects is not itself a process of semiotic inference'.[25] This position may be compared with that of Argenterio, who adopts a very radical stance. For him signs fall into two classes: things which signify something and things which indicate that something should be done:[26] the second is the indication, which will be examined below (8.7). Of the first, he says that he sees no need to make a distinction between sēmeion and tekmērion; he believes that the broader sense given to sign absolves him from distinguishing not only between necessary and probable signs, but also between modes of signification, whether by effect or in any other way. For him to signify is tacitly to indicate one thing by another; this tacit admonition occurs through the comparison of the signifer with the signified, which is simultaneously grasped by the intellect without an express act of reasoning. There is no inference involved; the sign is a substitute for its signified, as is smoke of fire (a standard example, given a new use here).[27] This is

---

[24] Capivaccius 1603: 9 ('nam a noto ad ignotam procedimus').

[25] McGinn 2000: 65.

[26] Argenterio 1610: 1677.

[27] Argenterio 1606–7: 1.101: 'porro sive signa, sive indicia, vel notas, vel alio verbo voces, quod rem occultam declarat nihil referre velim. Non enim inter haec nomina eam differentiam agnoscimus, quam Graeci ponunt inter σημεῖον et τεκμήριον quod sicilicet, hoc necessarium sit indicium, illud vero non necessarium existat. Atque illud etiam ignorari nolim, latius a nobis signi nomen sumi quam ab Aristot. capiatur. Ille enim tantummodo ab effectis signa sumi docet. Nos vero quicquid potest aliquid eorum quae in corpore nostro fiunt significare, nomine signi donamus. Porro significare est tacite admonere unum ab alio: fit autem tacita haec admonitio ex comparatione rei significandi cum significata, simul enim a[t]que facta est huiusmodi comparatio, deprehendit intellectus quod quaerebat: qua ratione ex fumo significare

consistent with the claim that signs simply stand for something else, as do tavern signs.[28] A substitutive sign of this kind is a particular discovered by sense; Vega says that it is what is submitted to sense, leading us to the knowledge of something hidden from our senses, as pallor indicates the excess of bile in the body; Fernel describes the sign as something evident to our senses which accompanies something hidden from them; Lucius declares that it can indicate both the latent and the manifest ('apparens').[29]

But signs can also be described as mental objects, whether propositions discovered by reason or middle terms in a syllogism. Capivaccius is responsible for the prevalent definition of the sign as proposition:

Therefore the medical sign is a proposition, produced by the intellect from some sensory object or objects, revealing a posteriori something in the medical art which was unknown. From this it follows that every sign is to be sought either

ignem dicimus. Nam quum notum sit effectus a suis causis nasci, non mirum est si uno cognito aliud protinus animus concipit, id quod est significare, quapropter eadem re utimur ad significandum, indicandum, et demonstrandum, nam ex causa morbi relata ad ea quae facienda sunt in aegrotis elicitur indicatio, ex eadem confecto syllogismo fit demonstratio ad symptomata morborum probanda, quum autem affectionem aliquam cognoscere volumus absque expressa ratiocinatione causa huiusmodi signum sit. Omnia ergo haec probant ex uno diversa, prout ad diversa referuntur.' Cf. da Monte 1587: 50 (i.56) for a different use of the smoke–fire example. Argenterio's is an adaptation of the Conciliator's doctrine that signs are immediate to sense and mediate to prognostication: Pietro d'Abano 1548: 123v (lxxviii): 'signum [est] correlativum. Duplex fore ipsius significatum unum nempe immediatum: cum quo praesentaliter existit ut tactum quod dicitur offerens se sensui. Aliud mediatum, in intellectu signum prognosticorum dictum.'

28 Demonet 1995: 107 (referring to a wide range of Renaissance sources); Demonet 1994: 16–18 (citing Clichtove and Caesarius, on things as signifiers and on language signs ('signum suppositionum' vs. 'signum instrumentale' or 'manifestum'); Maclean 1992: 99 (on things as signifiers). Demonet forthcoming cites Roger Bacon's *De signis* and Ockham as the sources of the example of the tavern sign, and in Demonent 2001: 12, Caesarius's definition of the 'signum reale' is given as 'quae neque vox est, neque scriptura, neque conceptus [est], praeter se ips[u]m tamen est alicujus significativ[um], ut iris signum est pluviae, et circulus ad tabernam suspensus signum est vini venalis, id est, vini quod illic venditur'.

29 Vega 1571: 900: 'signum est quod sensui subiicitur, ducens nos in cognitionem alicuius rei sensui occultae ut color pallidus qui bilis redundantiam in corpore ostendit'; this is repeated by Alonso 1598: 21, who adds the following reference to Aristotle, *Rhetorica ad Alexandrum*, xii, 1430 b 30f.: 'signum est alterius ad aliud non quodvis cuiusque, neque omnis omne, sed quod aut ante fiunt, aut in ipso negotio, aut post fieri consueverit'. Fernel 1610b: 1.209 (ii.7): 'quicquid igitur sensibus nostris obvium, aliud quippiam latens et occultum comitatur, id illius est signum'; quoted by Frölich 1612: A2v, and refuted by Campilongo 1601: 12v; Lucius 1597: 63 (citing *Aphorisms*, iii.87); see also Gavassetius 1586: 45: 'signum [esse] affectionem quandam corporis sensibus manifestam, quae affectum praeter naturam sensibus latentem, et occultum comitatur. Quod autem occultum est, praesens est aut futurum.' Weckerus 1576: 264 gives a similar definition ('signum sensui oblatum in rei obscurae ducit cognitionem'), but goes on to divide the hidden sources of the sign into essential (through form, matter, the elements, qualities and physiology) and accidental (the non-naturals).

from what preceded the thing signified, or followed it; therefore, from the cause or from the effect.[30]

He here characterises medical signs (or rather their forms) as belonging to the order of the intellect (which is their efficient cause), and links their use with the Aristotelian doctrine of enthymeme.[31] At the same time however he stresses their necessary reference to objects perceived by the senses. In other passages, he derives from two Aristotelian loci (*De interpretatione*, i, 16 a 3f.; *Posterior analytics*, i.6, 75 a 28ff.) three distinct ways of looking at signs: the first involves looking at them either a priori (which can be done either by seeing the sign as a 'causa essendi' [simpliciter] or 'causa inferendi' [secundum quid]);[32] or a posteriori (as in the case of words which are signs of the passions of the soul); this latter mode can only be determined by inference. The second way involves looking at them formally (signifier and signified thereby become correlative, and are of the same nature); the third 'fundamentally', in the cases where the signified is posterior to the sign. His purpose here is to demonstrate that there are as many modes of sign as there are of things signified.[33] Although this division appears in the writings of others and has the warrant of Galen, one may sense here a particularly Paduan predilection for scholastic logic, which leads to the slightly surprising allegation of a premonitory sign as a cause.[34]

---

[30] Capivaccius 1603: 282: 'Signum ergo medicum est propositio, producta ab intellectu, non sine obiectis sensibilibus, ostendens a posteriori ignotum in arte medica. Hinc sequitur quod omne signum petendum sit, ab eo quod vel praecedit, vel sequitur signatum: quare vel a causa vel ab effectu.'

[31] See *Rhetoric*, ii.25, 1403 a 12ff.: 'signs (sēmeia) and enthymemes based on signs, even if true, may be refuted . . . for it is clear from the [*Prior*] *Analytics* (ii.27) that no sign can furnish a logical conclusion . . . But necessary signs (tekmēria) and the enthymemes derived from them cannot be refuted on the ground of not furnishing a logical conclusion, as is clear from *Analytics*; the only thing that remains is to prove that the thing alleged is non-existent.'

[32] Cf. Campilongo 1601: 12v: 'causa saepe accipit rationem signi, et ideo ex aere califaciente, a cibis calidis, exercitu valido aliis eiusmodi [i.e. non-naturals] in cognitionem ardentis febris devenire consuevimus'.

[33] Capivaccius 1603: 9: 'quotuplex erit signatum, tot erunt et signa'.

[34] Liddel 1628: 512 makes this a little more comprehensible: 'medicis vero signum est propositio in mente producta a certis sensuum obiectis, vel ex rebus manifestis demonstrans ignotum aliquod in arte medica. Cognoscitur enim signatum ex signo demonstratione "hoti" ab effectu, vel a causa remota. Quare omne signum nobis notum erit, et semper petendum vel ab effectu, qui consequitur signatum; vel a causa evidenti, quae praecedit.' See also Chiaramonte 1625: 3 who uses the example of man the rational animal whose property is to laugh, and says that a sign can be (1) a cause of an effect, as in the case of a man signified as rational which is the cause of his laughing; (2) an effect of a cause, as in the case of a man laughing which is caused by his rationality; (3) an effect of an effect, as in the case of two effects of rationality

Campilongo, although in some matters a declared disciple of
Capivaccius, adopts a third position, which is to define the sign as a
middle term and not a whole proposition. In the passage in which he
speaks of non-prognostic signs, he cites the Aristotelian example from
Prior analytics, ii.27 (the pregnant woman having milk) and the standard
Galenic example of the four signs of pleurisy, which taken together are
'like a middle term' ('tamquam termin[us] medi[us]'), and then adds an
appendix to his work justifying this claim against some unnamed opponents, who presumably include followers of Argenterio and Capivaccius.
He engages in a technical logical and exegetical exercise both to save the
text of Aristotle from inconsistency, and to establish that it is not correct
to conclude from various loci that the Stagirite claims the sign to be a
proposition; and finishes with a defence of the dual nature of signs as
sensory and intelligible.[35] His position is modified in this last respect by
Horst, who calls a sign 'a certain mental concept, by which something
in the operation of the medical art which is unknown is derived from

(laughter, the ability to learn) which are mutually derived from rationality. The sign always
leads to the signatum, and can do so in various ways 'a priori, sive a posteriori, sive a simili':
Campilongo 1601: 13r, citing Galen, *Ars parva,* viii, K 1.329: the sense of 'a posteriori' and 'a
simili' here is clear: knowledge is obtained 'a priori' of a signatum in that it is itself an antecedent
cause.

35 The text which causes most difficulty is *Prior analytics,* ii.27, 70 b 1–8; see Campilongo 1601:
70–1, 92–3: 'Statuunt hi [the objectors] malam esse propositionem: quod probant hac ratione.
Enthymema constat ex propositione, ut dixit Arist. 2 Rhet 26. Enthymema constat ex signo.
Ergo signum est propositio, ut habet Arist. 2 Prior. 33. Verum nullo modo signum potest dici
propositio. Quare signum neque affirmat, neque negat, neque est universale, neque particulare:
et praedicatur de maiori extremo, subjiciturque minori, et constituit primam figuram; et praedicatur de utroque extremo, et constituit secundam; et subjicitur utrique et constituit tertiam, ut
docuit Arist. Prior. 34 et cum eo Avenroës in comm. Sed propositio neque praedicatur, neque
subjicitur alicui extremo. Ergo signum non est propositio. Ratio aliorum nihil concludit. Quare
deficit: quoniam est a simpliciter tali ad secundum quid. Neque enim est verum simpliciter:
omne, ex quo constat enthymema, esse propositionem. Nam constat quoque ex terminis. Et
si haec illatio esset simpliciter vera, posset facile addi illatio; sed enthymema constat ex signo:
et ita posset concludi, ergo signum est propositio. Ad Aristotelem vero dicentem signum esse
propositionem respondemus, sique Aristotelem aliorumque sententiam tuemur, dicentes: posse
capi signum vel secundum se, vel in ratiocinio. Primo modo non est propositio, sed medium, quo
indicatur signatum. Secundo modo est propositio, et dici quoque potest totum argumentum;
veluti quoque definitio secundum se non est propositio, in demonstratione vero est propositio,
ab ipsa demonstratione solo situ differens. Propterea Aristoteles capiens signum, ut est in ratiocinio, non solum dixit esse propositionem, sed cap 29 Secundi prior. Et cum eo Avenroës
in comm. statuit signum simile esse Syllogismo: quemadmodum exemplum simile esse induc-
tioni. Et in cap. 33 et cum eo Avenroës in comm. statuit signum esse vel ex probabilibus, vel ex
necessariis, et consequenter totum esse argumentum. Captum igitur signum secundum se, est
medium a dogmaticis inventum, secus scilicet, aut ratione. Nonnulla signa sunt inventa tantum
sensu [Campilongo later gives the example of 'aër calidus']; coctio ventriculi imminuta, qua[e]
denotat temperiem frigidam, non est inventa, nisi ratione et quamvis sit inventa ratione, non
tamen sine sensibus inventa est.' The last point (that signs are derived both from the senses and
reason) is supported by a reference to Galen, *In Hippocratis de officina medici,* ii, K 18b.719–815.

existing knowledge'.[36] Part of the issue here is the status of indications, on which some doctors such as Argenterio and some faculties such as Montpellier place great weight, and which others (mainly Paduans) reduce in importance. In showing the role of the sign in the syllogism, the latter declare their explicit adherence to Aristotelian logic. The former, by concentrating on indications, stress the performative nature of the medical art. Among the medical logicians, therefore, there is a clear difference of opinion about the nature of the sign, whether proposition (conjunction of subject and predicate) or just middle term.

5.1.2 Stoic signs: epilogism and analogism

As well as in Aristotle, signs play a role in Stoic thought, which is mediated to the Renaissance in the work of Galen, who makes frequent reference to it. Signification is stressed in the pseudo-Galenic definition of signs as 'all those things which signify something, or all those symptoms (accidentia) which reveal something unknown and hidden'.[37] In his work may be found the same Aristotelian distinctions between tekmēria (which demonstrate in a necessary way) and sēmeia (which are not necessary, and which only signify 'ut plurimum'),[38] and between proper (inseparable, in Galen's terms) and common (separable) signs; this latter distinction is extended by Cardano through combinatory logic to encompass signs which are proper and inseparable, proper and not inseparable, not proper and inseparable, and neither proper nor inseparable.[39] The most important part of Stoic sign theory concerns the distinction between analogism and epilogism; the former (rejected by empirics) being an inference from an indicative sign which is unverifiable by experience, and which uses sensory phenomena to infer hidden conditions of the body; the latter, being an inference from a commemorative or hypomnestic (associative) sign, which is observed in conjunction with what it signifies,

---

[36] Horst 1609: 131 'signum [est] quasi rei alicuius significativum et generaliter loquendo Medicis nihil est aliud, quam conceptus quidam mentalis, quo ignotum quiddam ex noto in operatione Medica colligitur.'

[37] Sennert 1650: 1.447, citing pseudo-Galen, *Definitiones medicae*, K 19.394: 'omnia ea quae rem aliquam significant: seu omnia accidentia, quae rem ignotam et occultam patefaciunt'.

[38] Peucer 1553: 204r, citing Galen, *In Prognostica*, iii, K 18b.306–13: 'τεκμήρια rem unam atque eandem sua natura perpetuo necessario que citra aliquam ambiguitatem demonstrant, nec fortuitis notantur observationibus, sed ratione logica firmaque et demonstrativa consequentia ex veris causis, aut effectibus certo cognitis colliguntur, σήμεια contra nec necessario, nec perpetuo, sed ut plurimum eadem rem indicant: et constant ac nituntur consentientis experientiae argumentis'; see also Cardano 1568: 4.

[39] 1583: 47–8; but also see below 8.3.2.

as is smoke with fire. This latter is accepted by empirics, who declare this
to be verifiable empirically and able to be stored in the memory. The
distinction clearly separates empirics from rational doctors who argue
that just as geometry can show that there are only three types of triangle
(this not being a matter of experience), so also the rational doctor can
interpret combinations of signs beyond recalled individual cases.[40] As
diseases have many manifestations, memory alone cannot lead to their
identification, but rather a judgement about a range of symptoms and
their strength and power. What is in question for rational doctors is not
simple similarity but relevant or dominant similarity, used as a logical or
interpretational tool.[41]

Epilogism allows you to say that something is so from its effect ('quod
ita sit ab effectu'); but analogism can answer the question why it is causally
so ('cur ita sit a causis').[42] This reading of the distinction (by Cardano in
the middle of the century) is somewhat different from that undertaken
earlier by da Monte, for whom analogism is a 'sort of relation of the
particular to the universal, permitting of a particular conclusion which
takes the form that the major is a universal proposition, and an individual
the subject of the minor'; and epilogism 'a comparison of like with like,
which is proper to empirics in the same way that analogism is proper to
[rational] doctors'.[43] Da Monte here allows transgressively the middle
term to be a particular, which he extends to the empirical individual.[44]
After Cardano, Sanctorius rejects both analogism and epilogism on the
authority of another Galenic text (*Methodus medendi*, ii. 6–7, K 10.115–56)
and stresses the role of demonstrative division.[45] His chapter
on this topic (xi.2) is entitled 'Demonstration drawn from Aristotle
and Galen that remedies can be investigated only by the method of division and never by experientia or analogism'.[46] For Sanctorius, particulars

---

[40] Galen, *De sectis*, v, K 1.75–9. Sedley 1982 denies the Stoic origin of this doctrine.
[41] See Hankinson 1995: 74, citing the disagreement recorded in *De sectis*, v, K 1.71ff. between
rational doctors and empirics over how remedies are discovered; Fernel 1610b: 1.208 (ii.7) (on
medical art being conjectural because internal disease can only be known through signs).
[42] Cardano 1568: 18 (i.10) citing *inter alia* Galen, *In Hippocratis de victu in acutis*, xliv, K 15.508–10;
De sectis, v, K 1.75–9.
[43] Da Monte 1587: 26–7, 233: 'relatio quaedam particularis ad universale et concludit particulare,
et fit demonstratio a signo' which 'ab universali particularia concludit ita, ut maior sit universalis, individuum vero minoris subjectum. Epilogismus comparatio est similis ad simile, estque
empiricorum proprius ut medicorum analogismus.' See above, ch. 4 note 180.
[44] See Sanctorius 1630: 795 (xii.6): 'praedicata in propositionibus naturalibus non possunt esse
particularia'.
[45] *Ibid.*, 733 (xi.3): he calls this 'indicatio', which is defined as 'dividenda generalissima in subalterna
eiusdem generis, et haec in specifica'.
[46] *Ibid.*, 726–32 (xi.2): 'ostenditur ex Aristotele et Galeno in methodo per solam indicationem
perquiri posse remedia et nequaquam per experientiam et analogismum'.

cannot belong to the sphere of knowledge; what is relevant is the cause or 'indicans', not similarities in the affected parts, diseases or palliatives ('iuvantia'), and he uses paralogism (the fallacious forms of the syllogism) to demonstrate the failings of unconvertible particular propositions.[47] Campilongo extends the discussion to the activity of the mind in accepting data; for him commemorative signs lead us to the knowledge of the disease, in which the intellect acquiesces; whereas there are signs of things which lead us to knowledge in which the intellect does not acquiesce; such counter-intuition has a role to play in indication (see below, 8.7).[48] The smudging of the line between the order of the objective and the order of the psychological (subjective) is here again detectable.

There are other aspects of post-Aristotelian sign theory which are picked up by doctors; one of these is the developed version of the distinction between the common ('koinon','commune','separabile') and proper ('idion','proprium','inseparabile') sign, found in Sextus Empiricus and Galen; another is Cicero's and Quintilian's discussion of signs and enthymemes and the signs peculiar to weather, dream interpretation and other conjectural arts.[49] In the end, a hybrid doctrine is evolved by which the medical art is admitted to be 'defective in those parts which concern signs, more or less completely conjectural and hardly necessary or demonstrative at all'.[50] This defect arises from the enthymematic, inductive aspect of medical semiotics; it is merely resolutive in that it is inductive and proceeds through sensory knowledge; it suffers the vice of 'magna ex parte' logic, and consists in the 'artificiosa coniectura' which Galen places between 'exacta notitia' and 'omnifaria ignorantia' (above, 4.3). The certain enthymemic reasoning using the necessary or unambiguous sign seems to be an asymptote, as there seem to be no single

---

[47] See above, note 8, and *ibid.*, 501–2 (vi.1), attacking Argenterio for arguments from proportion and similarity as well as analogism. For fallacious forms of second figure, see above, 4.3.3.

[48] Campilongo 1601: 10v, 19v: 'signa memorativa nos deducunt in cognitionem affectus, in qua intellectus acquiescit'; 'quamvis dixerit Hipp 1 de off. med. in princip. res praeter naturam et secundum naturam maximis et facilimis signis agnoscendas esse: dicimus tamen res praeter naturam et natura in genere facilimis quidem signis notas fieri, non autem maximis . . . signa rerum praeter naturam et natura deducunt nos in cognitionem quandam, in qua non acquiescit intellectus'; cf. *De interpretatione*, iii, 16 b 19: 'he who speaks [names] establishes an understanding, and he who hears them rests'; and Maclean 1992: 161–2.

[49] The Galenic loci have been cited above; Sextus Empiricus, *Contra mathematicos*, ii.152–4; Cicero, *De inventione*, i.48; *Partitiones oratoriae*, 34; *Rhetorica ad Herennium*, 11.2.3; Quintilian, *Institutio oratoria*, v.9.8–15.

[50] Silvaticus 1601: 83: 'defectuosa dici ars potest medica, quae in his quae ad signa attinent, tota fere est conjecturalis et minime necessaria, sive demonstrativa'; Cardano 1663: 5.602; Chiaramonte 1625: 1.

pathognomonic signs which are cited in these manuals (below, 8.4).[51]
Sanctorius insists that we must have a 'convertibilis cognitio' of any diagnostic conclusion, and that in nearly all cases ('fere semper') this will
come from a syndrome of signs. The example he offers of this is pleurisy
(for which he invokes a greater syndrome of signs than any other source).
It is not clear whether he is arguing that all of these signs need to be
present, or whether they constitute a polythetic class;[52] but he does concede that there is a fault in the logic of the syndrome of signs unless each
sign is convertible with the disease, which, as they are common signs,
they will not be.[53] So his 'infallible [diagnostic] science' of 'six sources of
information, no more, no less', is not infallible, by his own admission:

For the rest, as common signs are more or less infinite in number, we have only
agreed to include those which succeed the antecedent and subsequent causes,
which we can carry over into our six sources.[54]

The claim that six is a sufficient number is a mathematical, not a logical claim (he calls it at one point an 'argument from the enumeration
of a sufficient number of parts');[55] it is symptomatic of the movement towards computation which is examined below (5.2). For his part,
Liddel introduces such words and formulae as 'magna ex parte', 'pauca

---

[51] Bartolettus 1619: 247–8; Sextus Empiricus, *Contra mathematicos*, i.179; Frölich 1612: B4r says that
pathognomonic signs are 'vel plura simul et junctim concurrunt vel unum duntaxat', but gives
an example (pleurisy) only of the former.

[52] Sanctorius 1630: 33–4: 'quia omnis morbus ferme est compositus, ideo per plura signa fere
semper in cognitionem venimus'; cf. Needham 1975 (on polythesis).

[53] Sanctorius 1630: 84 (i.24) (on the four common signs of pleurisy): 'error logicus committitur,
quia quatuor signa pathognomica universaliter sumpta constituunt argumentum a positione
consequentis ad positionem antecedentis, veluti si homo, est animal, sed est animal, ergo est
homo, quod non valet, est enim in secunda figura ex duabus aff. et multis modis peccat, ut
alibi ostendimus, est dolor lateris, tussis, difficultas spirandi, et febris acuta, ergo pleuritis, non
valet nisi sic fiant convertibiles termini, est dolor lateris pungitivus, ergo pleuritis: et caetera
limitentur, et coarctentur signa propria, ut infra, si velimus inferre consequentias'. What follows
is a table showing in two cases (pleuritis and inflammation of the liver) that more than four
signs are needed; Sanctorius argues that his six 'fontes' are all necessary, and 'quod vero nec
plures, nec pauciores esse possint fontes; a quibus signa communia possunt in hunc usum colligi,
talis ingruit necessitas' (*ibid.*, 45 (i.9)). Elsewhere (*ibid.*, 422 (v.2)), he confirms that signs must be
convertible, and they can be either syndromes of proper or common signs, on the authority of
both Aristotle and Galen; but proper signs are said to be very rare, 'ideo methodum certam de
signis propriis tradere non possumus, cum de illis, quae non sunt semper, nulla Methodus, vel
scientia detur': *ibid.*, 30 (i.8). Cf. above, note 15 (Campilongo 1601: 70v).

[54] Sanctorius 1630: 34 (i.9): 'caeterum cum signa communia sint propemodum infinita nos illa
amplecti dumtaxat constituimus, quae immediate insequuntur causas antecedentes et subse-
quentes; quae ad sex fontes hos transferre possumus' (the edition of 1631 reads: 'quae in vim
propriorum subrogari et scientiam infallibilem in animos conferre potuerunt'). Sanctorius claims
that his aim is to expurgate contingency and 'probabilitas' from diagnosis as Aristotle had done
in the *Physics* (ibid., 427 (v.2)).

[55] *Ibid.*, 533 (vi.6): 'argumentum ex sufficienti partium enumeratione'.

sunt . . . quae . . . ' and 'plerumque' at various points of his text to allow for exceptions, which indicates, I believe, the same trend.[56]

Others claim even less than 'being right for the most part' for the semiotic arts. Cardano has this to say about the chance element in dream interpretation in comparison to therapy:

We must enquire whether there is an art [of dream interpretation]. If the question is directed at dreams in general, there is absolutely no such art; but if it is directed at those dreams which are unambiguous ('evidens') and perfect, the greater part of which take effect, there will be an art and a scientia of them. Most are true, and there is some information about them; just as there is no scientia about getting better, because many people are cured by chance, but there is a certain art and logic ('ratio') about those cures which come about through medicine.[57]

Other sources show that there can be no science based on accidental signs, and that signs can be mixed or inconsistent over time, or indicative of contrary things, or change into the indication of an opposite (see below 8.5), or be plural and variable, conveying no fixed relationship between external factors on which to ground a valid inference from one to the other.[58] They may also be so rare as not to be easily known to the doctor, or to be applicable only in a percentage of cases.[59] Semiology in this guise is no more than an approximate doctrine because the 'causae concurrentes' of signs as effects may arise from different systems of cause (that is, be non-consilient), be remote from observational knowledge and the senses, and be processed by a human mind which varies over time and place in how much it knows (i.e. those things which constitute its 'praecognita').[60] The strong influence of sceptical argument may be felt here: but also the sturdy reliance on a finite art which manages these

---

[56] Liddel 1628: 511–600.

[57] Cardano 1663: 5.704, quoted by Siraisi 1997: 177: 'Ergo videndum, an sit aliqua ars. Et certe si ad totum genus somniorum res haec referatur, ars omnino nulla est. Sed si ad evidentia et perfecta, quorum maxima pars sortitur effectum, erit de illis ars atque scientia: plurima enim horum vera sunt, taliumque aliqua notitia; veluti sanationum nulla est scientia: quoniam plurimi casu sanantur: sanationum autem quae a medicina fiunt, ars aliqua est, et certa ratio.' This translation is a little different from that of Siraisi.

[58] See e.g. Kusukawa 1997: 420, 422 (quoting Montuus); *Physiognomica*, ii, 807 a 25–6 (on contradictory signs); Sylvius 1539a: 41 offers a practical example of the complexity of evidence: 'nulla actio laeditur, nisi pars actionis causa effectrix laedatur idiopatheia, vel sympatheia, protopatheia, vel deuteropatheia, vel duobus, vel tribus, vel omnibus modis simul, sed diversis rationibus'.

[59] Argenterio 1610: 1780.

[60] Gemma 1575: 1.133 (on the signification of the conjunction of planets): 'haec saepe . . . significationis obscurissimae causam nobis abscondit, vel si scire permiserit, id tantum aut adiuncta hypothesi, vel subnotione penitus generali. Verum caelestis influxus in meteoris, significationes secundum naturae leges, saepe certissimas habet; et si ex multiplicitate systematis

problems, and which persists from the Middle Ages to the Renaissance. The subtlety of the medieval view is worth recording here. The Galen of the *Isagoge Joannitii* and Haly's commentary on the *Ars parva* divided signs into substantial signs, immediate accidental signs, and mediate accidental signs: the first are absolutely true, and can be verified by experience; the second have all the appearance of truth, and the last are no more than often reliable.[61] We shall return to these gradations (which are to be found in other ancient sources, such as Theophrastus's treatise on weather) when we come to consider the question of probability (5.2.2). Haly's tables of signs leave room however for a trial of argumentative strength in which the outcome is decided not on necessities but on likelihoods.[62] Persuasion, banished ab initio from medicine, finds its way back by this devious route.

5.1.3 *The locus 'a signis et circumstantiis'*

A final element of sign theory is derived from the topical locus 'a signis et circumstantiis'. This involves all the aspects of sign theory above, together with a consideration of the variables indicated by the term 'circumstantiae', which is found in both law and medicine.[63] Both faculties have to grapple with the problem of the infinite variability of their subject matter and the need to make this intelligible and to classify individual cases under given rules; in both this is done by appeal to a set of contextualising questions. For law these consist in but six (who? what? where? when? why? with whose help?);[64] these are the variables through which the identification of the criminal act is accomplished; they apply also to natural philosophy and to medicine. Celsus refers to circumstances as variables which prevent the formulation of certain rules in

---

propterque distantiam naturarum agentium a sensibus nostris, intellectusque infirmitatem, particularium locorum, et temporum, et magnitudinum praecognitio prope sit impossibilis.'

[61] Haly, *In artem parvam*, cited by Ottosson 1984: 204: 'signa corporum sanorum tria sunt, unum eorum est assumptum ex eo, quod in eis est in diffinitione eorum substantiae, et ista signa sunt necessariae verificationis. Et secunda sumpta sunt ex operationibus membrorum, et ista item sunt apparentis veritatis. Et tertia sunt sumpta ex accidentibus consequentibus ab eo, quod in eis est in diffinitione substantiae eorum, consequentibus iterum ab operationibus, et ista multitoties sunt veridica.'

[62] See Burnyeat 1982: 202 for Aristotelian sources.

[63] Liddel 1628: 11; they are called 'coindicantia' by Argenterio 1610: 928 and 'adiacentia' by Cardano 1578: 120, possibly after Agricola 1967: 62–5 (i. 11).

[64] Quintilian, *Institutio oratoria*, v.10.104 and Boethius, *De differentiis topicis*, iv, PL 64.1205; both cite these ('quis? quid? ubi? quando? quomodo? quibus auxiliis?'): see also Maclean 1992: 81.

medicine;[65] Galen's equivalent discussion concerns what comes to be called the rule of relation ('pros ti') according to which all states of bodies are relative to themselves and the conditions surrounding them.[66] There can be as many as twenty-two factors of these kinds in respect of diagnosis. The following is Sanctorius's list in his *Methodi vitandorum errorum* of 1630: the nature of the patient, his or her age, the season of the year, the location, the present constitution of the patient, his or her strength, habits, practice of life, usual occupation, the illness, its cause, place, symptoms, its relation to similar illnesses, its course and nature, how full the patient is (of peccant humours), the appearance of the major parts of his or her body, his or her pulse, mental state, and factors aggravating or alleviating his or her condition.[67] These affect also treatment, which according to Campilongo is governed, as well as by environmental and non-natural considerations, by the following questions: what should be done? with what? how much of it? how administered? when? in what order?[68]

---

[65] *De medicina*, iii.4.7: 'Nihil autem horum utique perpetuum est . . . Refert enim qualis morbus sit quale corpus quale caelum quae aetas, quod tempus anni; minimeque in rebus inter se multum differentibus perpetuum esse praeceptum temporis potest.'

[66] Justus 1618: N3r invokes this rule, which is implicit throughout Galen, and expressed in various loci, including *Ars parva*, ii, K 1.310; see also Temkin 1973: 104ff. This makes Galenism a relativist doctrine, without reducing its commitment to reality.

[67] Sanctorius 1630: 791 (xii.5), citing Galen, *Ad Glauconem*, ii.1–2, K 11.71–84: 'natura aegrotantis, aetas, tempus anni, regio, praesens constitutio, robur, habitus, consuetudo, solitum exercitium, morbus, causa, locus, symptomata, morbi similes, mos, motus, repletio, figurae partium, pulsuum motus, animi mores, iuvantia, laedentia'. Sanctorius also records two of the 'carmina [quae] vagantur per scholas', i.e. student mnemonic verses based on Avicenna, *Canon*, i.4; the first reads:

> Ars, aetas, regio, virtus, complexio, forma,
> Mos, et symptoma, repletio, tempus, et usus,
> Et, bene si numerus, figuram addere debes.

Cf. Maclean 1992: 104 (a legal mnemonic verse); Hippocrates, *Aphorisms*, i.2 (cited by Sanctorius) and *Epidemics*, i.23: 'the following were the circumstances attending the diseases from which I framed my judgements, learning from the common nature of all and the particular nature of the individual, from the disease, from the patient, the regimen prescribed and the prescriber – for these to make a diagnosis more favourable or less: from the constitution, both as a whole and with respect to the parts, of the weather and of each region; from the custom, mode of life, practices and ages of each patient; from talk, manner, silence, thoughts, sleep or absence of sleep, the nature and time of dreams, pluckings, scratchings, tears; from the exacerbations, stools, urine, sputa, vomit, the antecedents and consequents of each member in the succession of diseases, and the abscessions to a fatal issue or a crisis, sweat, rigor, chill, cough, sneezes, hiccoughs, breathing, belchings, flatulence, silent or noisy, haemorrhages, and haemorrhoids. From these things we must consider what the consequents also will be.' This list is usually reduced to a small number of primary signs: see e.g. Wolf 1620: A2r, citing Galen, *De locis affectis*, vi, K 8.377ff.; Campilongo 1601: 49–50; Bylebyl 1991: 171 (on Altomare).

[68] Campilongo 1601: 10v; Sanctorius 1630: 806 (xiii.1), citing Galen, *In Hippocratis de morbis vulgaribus*, vi.32.

5.1.4 Analogy and the locus 'a simili'

Associated with sign theory are analogy, induction, probability, quantification and the treatment of the singulars of experience. I shall look at these issues in turn. The 'argumentum a simili' is discussed principally in Aristotle's *Topics*, although analogy does figure in the *Prior analytics*, ii.24, 68 b 38ff.;[69] it is also discussed by Galen in the *De optimo methodo docendi*, K 1.40–52 (how to draw inferences from one set of circumstances to another) and in the *De sectis*, K 1.87–92 in relation to empirical practice.[70] It is part also of a rational doctor's intellectual armoury.[71] But it is clearly seen as problematic. It is subject to a four-term scale implying a fifth (always similar / for the most part similar / similar half the time / rarely similar / (implicitly) never similar) which exposes its uncertainty in terms of frequency rather than logic.[72] The same scale also poses the question of dissimilarity as a method of elimination or falsification, and of neutrality (what Quintilian refers to as 'that against which nothing can be said [by not being dissimilar]': *Institutio oratoria*, v.10.16). It requires exact knowledge of that with which the *comparatio* is being made, and it requires moreover for that act of comparison to have been frequently engaged in; it cannot reveal anything that was not known already.[73] Yet it is claimed to possess a heuristic value, especially in respect of comparative anatomy.[74] Sextus Empiricus points out that analogy cannot compare all the properties of the things to be compared;[75] it is weak as a basis for truth in the sense of adequation or correspondence.[76] Its conjectural

[69] Capivaccius 1603: 96v: 'quando fit transitus ab uno vel pluribus particularibus ad aliud simile'.
[70] See also *De differentiis pulsuum*, iii.6, K 8.670–85 on induction and analogy; Campilongo 1601: 13r, citing Galen's recommendation of 'signa per simili et dissimili' in *In Hippocratis de officina medici*; Agricola 1967: 6–9 (i.2); Siraisi 1997: 27–8 (citing Cardano).
[71] Campilongo 1601: 15r (identifying it with analogism, as does Ferrier 1592: 19); Liddel 1628: 10 attributing the form of argument to the empirics: 'nam uni medico impossibile videtur in omnibus aegris concursum signorum observare. Quia autem evenerunt saepe affectus incogniti, quorum explorata illis non erant remedia, instrumentum excogitarunt, transitum ad similia.'
[72] Hankinson 1995: 65; Galen, *Subfiguratio empirica*, ii.6 (specifying only four of the terms, omitting 'never similar'): Galen 1556a: 1.32r–v.
[73] Galen, *De placitis Hippocratis et Platonis*, ix, K 5.791–805; Campilongo 1601: 40r: 'nam quid potest aliquis rerum ignorata veritate similitudinem eius quod ignorat vel parvam vel magnam in aliis discernere potest? Nequaquam potest.' On similitude as source of irreducible error, see Cardano 1578: 120: 'ex materiae mobilitate, mistioneque ac propria dispositione, tum astrorum non exquisita cum praecedentibus configurationibus similitudine nulla ex parte tolli potest, sed manet', quoted above, ch. 4, note 132.
[74] Wear 1973: 87–8 (Ulmus's use of analogy between similar bodily structures having similar functions). The correspondence theory of hermetic philosophy operates in this way: see Vickers 1988b.
[75] Sextus Empiricus, *Hypotyposes*, ii.204.
[76] Galen *De locis affectis*, iv.2, K 8.298.

nature reveals an area where even the experienced doctor can make mistakes, as Jacchinus points out; a fact demonstrated by the disagreement of learned doctors around the same bedside about the diagnosis and treatment of the case in question.[77] As Lemosius declares, the art of medicine needs to get 'similitudines' right to achieve its aim of minimising error.[78] These cautionary remarks, which have echoes in law, show how wrong the Foucauldian characterisation of Renaissance thinking, and especially its doctrine of 'similitudo', is.[79]

5.1.5 Induction, particulars and singulars

Ancient induction, avers Bacon in the *Advancement of learning*, was 'vicious and incompetent, no more than conjecture';[80] as he famously claims, 'in the process of exclusion are laid the foundations of induction, which however is not completed till it arrives at the Affirmative';[81] his proposal to include particulars of 'nature erring' in a new history of nature (see below 7.4-6) is equally famous. He was not however the first to attempt to reconfigure the ancient 'vicious' theory, which is characterised by the passage from singular to universal as opposed to universal to singular (deduction) or singular to singular (exemplarity).[82] It has various elements important for medicine. The account Aristotle gives in *Posterior analytics*, ii.19 of the production of universals resembles an inductive process in a negative form: fleeing impressions stop and form an 'army': this is the only form of induction explicitly accepted as legitimate by Sanctorius.[83] I have already referred to the perfect induction of *Prior analytics*, ii.23 (above 4.4.3); 'enumerative' induction in the modern sense of the

---

[77] Jacchinus 1563: 5: 'nemo tamen sibi persuadeat aequalem semper esse agnitionis certitudinem, quin potius multum distant inter se . . . etiam praestantes medicos inter se dissidere' (he quotes an example).

[78] Lemosius 1598: 19r: 'minime errare'; he attributes to Plato, *Republic*, i the following advice: 'primum debet ille, qui alios fallere, a nullo falli vult, similitudinem rerum optime tenere'.

[79] Foucault 1966: 32–59; Otto 1992: 89–91; Maclean 1998a.

[80] Bacon 2000: 109; before him, Vives had warned against premature generalisation; see Noreña 1970: 286–7.

[81] Bacon 1878: 395–6 (*Novum organum*, ii.19); see also Daston and Park 1998: 221–3.

[82] E.g. Cesalpino 1588: 363–5, who suggests that induction (relying on similitudo and convenientia) is the path to derive universals from singulars: division (relying on dissimilitudo and differentia) places singulars in species, and definition (relying on propria and substantia) resolves species into elements.

[83] Wear 1973: 171, quoting Sanctorius 1630: 802 (xii.6): 'non tamen negamus inductionem, vel experimenta conferre posse ad cognoscendum universale, quia ut dicit Boetius in praedicamentis, experientia est exemplorum collectio, post quam collectionem intellectus proprio lumine excitatur ad separandam naturam universalem ab individuali; tota enim natura universalis est in quolibet individuo, ut saepe visis individuis, saepe quoque intellectus offeratur universale'.

accumulation of particulars is discussed in the *Rhetoric* (1393 a 22ff.), where it is called a paradigm. What is seen as important is the persuasive force of relevant similarity, not the accumulation of particulars;[84] in law, this can take a number of forms: parity, equality, equivalence, equity. These terms are of great importance for jurists. One of the definitions of equity is 'the equivalence of things, which requires the same laws to be applied in the same cases';[85] the equivalent in medical discourse would seem to be the looser form of taxonomy found in the zoological works inspired by Aristotle (see 4.4.3). The analysis of resemblances between instances, based on substantial and not fortuitous points of comparison, shows the availability to generations before Bacon of the very tool which is seen by him to be the hallmark of his new natural philosophy. Imperfect induction can be used to establish the existence of something, but most commonly to achieve empirical inferences of the kind: cassia cured Socrates's cold: therefore it will cure Plato's cold; or guaiac wood has cured Italians and Frenchmen of syphilis: therefore it will cure Germans. These, as we have seen, are condemned as fallacies of the consequent (above 5.1.1). It is for all these problems – its paralogism, its non-scientific status, its reliance on sensory information, its potential circularity (nothing new can be discovered from it) and its toleration of similarity rather than identity – that Sanctorius is led to denounce it in theses ringing terms:

When experience shall be collected from particulars, it will not be conclusive because out of pure particulars nothing follows. Nor should you object that experience is not collected from two particulars but from many; because we will reply that if you gather it from a thousand, you will not be able to infer a universal conclusion or rather if you induce through a thousand million, still you will not be able to derive a universal conclusion, since any universal species whatsoever subsumes infinite particulars.[86]

This could have been written any time from the late Middle Ages onwards, after the already mentioned recovery of the dialectical and topical

---

[84] Fludd 1631: 113: 'according to the old maxime, unum vel aliud exemplum non probat argumentum'.

[85] Maclean 1992: 175: 'rerum convenientia, quae in paribus causis paria iura desiderat'.

[86] Sanctorius 1630: 795 (xii.6), quoted by Wear 1981: 253: 'quando experimentum colligitur a particularibus, non concludet, quia ex puris particularibus nihil sequitur. Neque obiicias, quod experientia non ex duobus particuliaribus, sed a pluribus colligitur: quia respondemus, quod si ex mille eam colligere, non posses universalem conclusionem inferre; quini modo si per milliona millia induceres adhuc non posses conclusionem universalem haurire; quoniam quaelibet species universalis sub se continet infinita particularia.' The same point is made by the lawyer Jean de Coras: see Herberger 1981: 250–1.

texts of Cicero and Quintilian; but it is not clear whether Sanctorius's other pronouncements about induction could have been made that early. Elsewhere, he admits that 'induction gives sufficient proof' and calls it an 'instrumental doctrine' which gives rise to knowledge when combined with memory.[87] In this he overcomes the division between sensory experience and intellection: as he does ten years later in his statement in his *Statica medica* that 'eyes and hands can feel truth'.[88] The fact that the same author can espouse two contradictory positions in this way is clear mark of a transition in attitudes towards induction.

I come now to particulars, singulars, and universals. The issue for doctors is clearly set out in a much quoted passage from Aristotle's *Metaphysics* (i.1, 980 b 14–24):

Experience is the knowledge of particulars, but not of universals... It is not man the physician cures except incidentally, but Callias or Socrates or some other person similarly named, who is incidentally a man as well. So if a man has theory without experience, and knows the universals, but does not know the particular contained within it, he will fail in his treatment: for it is the particular that must be treated.[89]

Galen also argues that knowledge of the individual and of the common form are different modes of knowledge.[90] But the same author is credited with the view that the specific is the object of the medical art, and not the particular: 'the proper nature of all individuals cannot be said or written nor conceived at all by the mind... medicine is the scientia "of what kind" ('scientia qualium'), that is, the scientia of species, not individuals'.[91] The way out of this apparent impasse is to argue that every particular contains its total universal nature, which is grasped by the intellect; or more precisely the practical intellect, which is more closely

---

[87] Sanctorius 1630: 258 (iii.2) has the chapter title as 'probatur inductione, morbos constitui in esse specifico a differentiis partium nostri corporis specificis'; but the edition of the following year has the title beginning 'probatur inductione sufficientissima...'. Herberger 1981: 302–3 argues that Conring is the first to bring new induction into medicine.

[88] Sanctorius 1642: †4r: 'veritatem ipsam sinceram et puram... non solum animo et intellectu percipiunt [omnes], sed oculis etiam, ac ipsis quasi manibus palpent'.

[89] Sennert 1650: 1.261; Rondelet 1586: 584.

[90] *Methodus medendi*, ii.7, K 10.148–9 (on Dion and Theon having distinct cases of fever); *De constitutione artis medicae*, in Valleriola 1577: 278–80.

[91] Campilongo 1601: 7r: 'Galenus [*Methodus medendi*, iii.7, K 10.131–40] scribit: naturam propriam omnium individuorum nec dici nec scribi nec omnino mente concipi posse: ut idem [*Ars parva*, ii, K 1.309–313] dicebat: medicinam esse scientiam qualium, id est scientiam specierum, non autem individuorum'; Fernel 1610b: 1.208 (ii.7): 'nulla est singulorum scientia'.

related to sensory perception.[92] It is even doubted whether God knows singulars in the intellective order of knowledge.[93] The division between knowledge of sensory particulars and intellective knowledge of species also marks that between rhetoric and logic, and that between examples and species. Thomists and strict Aristotelians had denied that there is a path from individual cases to scientific knowledge; the republication of Hippocrates's *Epidemics* in the Renaissance on the other hand added impetus to an approach to knowledge through individual cases.[94] The imperfect inductions of Aristotle's zoology mentioned above (4.4.3) may also have had an influence in this domain. A grave difficulty is generally acknowledged; the properties of individuals are to all intents and purposes infinite (see above, 4.4.1); the possible combinations are therefore also infinite, and cannot be known perfectly by a combination of reason and sense experience.[95] Fracastoro even thought that diseases were infinite in number and that each had a specific form; but like da Monte, he seems to identify 'ultimae species' (or 'infimae species') with individua. This may appear to be the same as the position of Paracelsus, for whom each individuum was wholly peculiar and for whom there were as many diseases as patients;[96] it is however less radical, as Fracastoro espouses the Galenic theory of idiosyncrasy which permits an identification of individual cases as unique combinations of the four humours without the claim having to be made that an exact knowledge is possessed of them.[97]

---

[92] *De anima*, iii.7, 431 b 5–18; Aquinas, *Summa theologiae*, 1a 79.11; 1a 86.1; Herberger 1981: 210ff.; Mikkeli 1992: 166 (on medical treatments being not universal *per se*, but only illustrating universals in particulars); Cardano 1565: 21v (i.2.1) (on art presupposing knowledge of the individual in three modes: 'singularis comprehensio et dicitur sensus; singularium plurimum et est experimentum ut in memoria colligitur; universalium prout ad singularia comparabantur, et sunt artis vel prudentiae habitus'). Siraisi 1997: 57 records Cardano's proposal that Galen's medical doctrine should be reformed by being based on particulars. There seems to be no discussion by doctors of Scotus's 'haecceitas' although it is once mentioned (apparently belonging to the same paradigm as 'forma') by Sanctorius 1630: 27 (i.7). See also above, note 83.

[93] Siraisi 1997: 66 (citing Cardano on this point).

[94] Crisciani 1996b: 7; Siraisi 1997: 128.

[95] Da Monte 1587: 949: 'individuorum proprietates infinitae sunt'; *Metaphysics*, iii.3, 999 a 24ff.; Arnau de Vilanova 1585: 48, cited by Pagel 1935: 112–13; Herberger 1981: 218–19 (on D 28.2.39.2 and legal discussion of the point).

[96] Pagel 1935: 105ff.

[97] Nutton 1990b: 217; da Monte 1587: 229; Sanctorius 1630: 739–42 (xi.4). In his *De pulsibus ad tyrones*, ix, K 8.463, Galen explicitly recommends that the individuality of a patient be approached through a judgement of similarity (tautotēs) and communality (koinon), which is not inconsistent with traditional forms of epistemology: see García Ballester 1981: 21–3.

5.2 BEYOND LOGIC: GEOMETRY, PROPORTION, QUANTITY

5.2.1 Mathematics

We now come to the input of mathematics into medical theory, and to the related questions of arithmetic and quantification, ratio and proportion, geometrical argument and diagrams, and probability. Mathematics (consisting in arithmetic, geometry, astrology and music)[98] had an established place in the quadrivium of the medieval arts course; its application to medicine is demonstrated in such textbooks as the *Articella*, which include treatises on weights and measures, and in studies of proportion and ratio such as those of the medieval Oxford calculators which Italian doctors among others caused to be revived at the beginning of our period.[99] In the sixteenth century, it was a vigorously debated subject; there is a well-documented discussion of the certainty of mathematics, concerning its status in respect to the logical adequacy of its proofs, in which some natural philosophers and doctors (notably Cardano) take part.[100] It will come therefore as no surprise that it was prescribed for doctors by most Renaissance pedagogical writers;[101] this prescription is often specifically linked to Galen's geometrical (axiomatic) method whose operations are the constitution of objects from elements, the comparison of existing objects and their reduction into their constitutive elements.[102]

[98] The term 'mathematicus' can designate an astrologer. Stars are indices of regularity in physical causation, and Ptolemaic astrology is in this respect mathematical in a modern sense. Grafton and Siraisi 1999: 33 claim that astrology is a quantified art insofar as 'the positions of the ascendant and the planets and the laying out of the houses of the horoscope are quantitative data'. Music is not recommended for study by medical students, although it has a part to play in therapy: see Horden 2000; Camerarius 1626–30: 267ff. (iv.14–15). See also above, 3.6.

[99] See Polcastris n.d.; Victorius 1506; Achillinus 1515; Swineshead 1520 (ed. Trincavellus); Burnett 1999: 16; Schmitt 1983c: 227 claims that after 1550 the Greek commentators supplant the calculators as sources of mathematical discussion. Bradwardine's treatises on proportions and the latitude of forms were prescribed reading in the mid-fourteenth-century Freiburg University statutes: see Ott and Fletcher 1964: 46.

[100] Henry 1997: 21 identified the four new factors in the study of mathematics as the editions of ancient Greek texts, the weakening of Aristotelian physics, the activity of mathematicians outside the universities, and the rise in the status of practitioners, especially those employed in courts. On disputes, see Jardine 1988: 693–7; Dear 1987: 161–3 (on the competing discourses of mathematics and physics); Mancosu 1996: 153 (on logic and mathematics); Herberger 1981: 260ff. (on mathematics in law).

[101] E.g. Castellanus 1555: 9v–11r; Valleriola 1577: 114 (citing Galen, *De constitutione artis medicae*): 'est namque Arithmetica in id medico necessaria, ut morborum tempora decretorios dies, morborum initia (quae sine numerandi peritia scire neutiquam possunt) deprehendere ac numerando discernere queat'.

[102] *Ibid.*, 176–7 (referring to 'demonstratio, definitio, communes conceptiones, postulata'); on geometry in Galen, *Methodus medendi*, i.4, K 10.34–5; *De cuiusque animi peccatorum cognitione atque medela*, v,

Associated with mathematics are diagrams, that is, abstract quantified spatial representations. There is a modern debate about the contribution of technical innovations in illustration in the Renaissance (most notably perspective) to the scientific revolution: this is only relevant here insofar as some participants in this debate argue for the importance of diagrammatic symbolisation of mental abstractions above those, like perspective, which are still representations of the real world, and see the former as a step on the path to full algebraic notation of geometry.[103] Not all Renaissance thinkers were persuaded of their usefulness: Argenterio describes the diagrams of Manardo and Akakia reproduced below as 'vain and false tables and figures';[104] but I shall argue here that they were related to the uptake of doctors from the arts course insofar as well-known logical diagrams reproduced above (4.3.3) were adapted by them for their own purposes.

It is often said that Galenic medicine is qualitative in nature, a 'scientia qualium' (above 5.1.5);[105] but there is a serious input of quantification in it also. The warning in *Philebus*, 55–6 that 'all that would be left for us (without the science of measurement) would be to conjecture and to drill the perception by practice and experience' seems to be taken seriously by Galen and his followers.[106] Quantification is even enjoined upon doctors by Holy Writ.[107] It was moreover ordained that every medical man should be able to calculate the time and period of the

K 5.80–93 ('declaratio verae methodi per exempla mathematica, ac adversus eos qui ab ea deficiebant'; the examples are mainly drawn from architecture); Cardano 1663: 3.346 (ic); Pittion 1987: 120 (quoting Fernel); also Severinus 1571: 2 (on 'mos geometricus' and its application to Paracelsian doctrine). Otto 1992: 98–9; Kessler 1995: 298–301; cf. Hobbes, *Leviathan*, i.4, on geometry as 'the onlie science that it hath pleased God hitherto to bestow on mankind'. Interesting points about ancient debates concerning Galen are made by Hankinson 1995: 69 and Burnyeat 1982: 230, who suggests that there is a relationship between Epicureans as atomists who engage in inferential and combinatory operations on the one hand, and Stoics as providentialists on the other, for whom the visible and invisible are connected in an organic unity governed by divine reason.

[103] This debate is usually traced back to Panofsky 1924–5; it is associated with the name of Edgerton 1980 and 1985; on his thesis, see Mahoney 1985; Franklin 2000; Kemp 2000, who records at 17–18 the view of Michael Mästlin that astronomy was incomprehensible without a diagram, and at 21 Vesalius's view that pictures and formulae were insufficient of themselves to obtain an understanding of anatomy, and concludes at 46 that 'the relationship between illustration and visualisation seems quite different in the various sciences'.

[104] Argenterio 1610: 250–1: 'vanas et falsas tabulas et figuras'.

[105] Campilongo 1601: 7r; Wear 1995a: 161.

[106] García Ballester 1981: 20; the quotation continues 'with the additional use of the powers of guessing which are commonly called arts and acquire their efficacy by practice and toil'.

[107] Wisdom 11:20: 'thou hast ordered all things by measure, number, weight', quoted by Vigenère 1586: 133v ('omnia in numero ponderis et mensura disposuisti'); see also Wallis 1995: 121, citing Isidore of Seville.

day, and the passage of the seasons, because they are a factor in the changes which bodies undergo.[108] In humoral theory, there is clearly an element of qualitative medicine present: but the variables involved cause this also to be subject to quantification.[109] The coming together of quality and quantity in Galenic medicine is perceptible in such texts as *Methodus medendi*, xi.12, K 10.771–2,[110] and the following, taken from a commentary on Galen's *De sanitate tuenda*: 'being more or less is a property of quality; health is a quality; therefore we may correctly say that the quality of health is more or less of something'.[111] The question 'quantum', together with 'quomodo' and 'quando', separates rational doctors from empirics.[112] But as well as being a source of information, the answer to 'quantum' can also be a source of error, as Gemma points out: 'the principal error in all disciplines lies hidden in the computation of quantity; for God reserves for his arcane knowledge alone the measures and weights of all things'.[113]

The reasons for this become clear when the literature on medical quantification is examined. This concerns combinatory calculations for the most part: the technique can be used to create a taxonomy of a whole field, as Aristotle points out in *Politics*, iv.3 (1290 b 25–38):

If we wanted to obtain a classification of animals, we should first define the properties necessarily belonging to every animal (for instance some of the sense

[108] Thorndike 1923–58: 4.141f. (on Paris); Westman 1993: 2 (on the duties of the holder of the chair of mathematics at Bologna).

[109] Durling 1961: 289 records the Renaissance editions of Galen's *De ponderibus*. There are treatises on doses, weights and measures and proportions in the *Articella*. A greater number of monographs are brought together in a series of composite volumes on the science of doses, beginning in 1556 and culminating in Meietus 1584. The non-ontological theory of illness (see below 7.5) leads to disease not being submitted to the same degree of measurement as the treatment: see Rondelet 1586: 584: 'non enim curatur morbus, sed hic morbus: non curatur in homine, sed in Callia et Socrate ob subiectum particulare quod individua quadam proprietate dotatum est. Morbus alius non est in specie, sed in magnitudine, vehementia, parvitate, remissione, aut in plus aut minus periclitando. Ob hoc non solum in curandis morbis contrarietatem remediorum invenire oportet, sed et iustam quantitatem, quae a morbi magnitudine, tempore, loco, et consuetudine indicatur'; it is the 'particularis morbi proprietas' which enables the 'inventio iustae quantitatis remediorum'.

[110] See above, ch. 4, note 149.

[111] Joutsivuo 1999: 115, quoting Jacobus Bordingus, *Enarrationes in vi libros Galeni de sanitate tuenda*; Rostock, 1605, 29: 'qualitatis proprium est suscipere magis et minus. Omnis sanitas est qualitas. Sanum igitur magis minusve aliquid recte dicemus.'

[112] Campilongo 1601: 7r; Wear 1973: 155–66 discusses Sanctorius's claim that medicine is a conjectural art because of the computation of quantity in diseases, of power in remedies, and the understanding of their constitution, and his development of instruments; on which see also de Renzi forthcoming (quoting Sanctorius on the 'certitudo mathematica' provided by his pulsilogium).

[113] Gemma 1575: 194–5: 'omnium disciplinarum error praecipuus in terra aestimanda quantitate sepultus latet. Deus enim soli arcanae scientiae suae . . . rerum mensuras et pondera servat.'

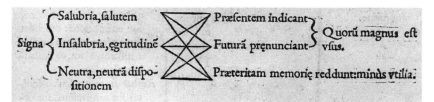

Figure 5.1. Jacobus Sylvius (Jacques Dubois), *Methodus sex librorum Galeni in differentiis et causis morborum et symptomatum in tabellas sex ordine suo coniecta paulo fusius, ne brevitas obscura lectorem remoretur et fallat. De signis omnibus medicis, hoc est, salubribus, insalubribus, et neutris, commentarius omnino necessarius medico futuro*, Paris, 1539, p. 25 (C 2 4 Med(3)).
The diagram translates as follows:

signs	healthy, health		of the present indicate:	these are of great use
	morbid, disease		of the future predict:	these are of great use
	neutral, a neutral disposition		of the past call to mind:	these are less useful

organs, and the machinery for masticating and for receiving food . . .). And if there were only so many necessary parts, but there were different varieties of these (I mean for instance various kinds of mouth and stomach and sensory organs . . .), the number of possible combinations of these variations will necessarily produce a variety of kinds of animals . . . so that when all the possible combinations of these are taken they will all produce animal species, and there will be as many species of animal as there are of the necessary parts.

This technique can be applied in various ways. At the simplest level, it can used to represent exhaustively various kinds of medical data; Sylvius's use of it relates temporal signs to health, neutrality and sickness (see fig. 5.1).[114] Capivaccius lists the problems of conjunctions of illnesses, causes and symptoms in the same way.[115] Manardo goes further, and adapts the square of contraries to represent not only all the possible combinations of temperaments (combinations of cold and hot and wet and dry are cleverly excluded) but also inserts a mediate point to represent the absolutely temperate body: see fig. 5.2.[116]

This adaptation of the square of contraries (which has precedents in the medieval period) shows the appropriation for their own use by doctors of the logical instruments at their disposal.

[114] Sylvius 1539a: CIr. Combinatories are connected to Lullism: see Risse 1964: 541; Rossi 1960.

[115] Capivaccius 1603: 15 (not in diagrammatic form, and not exhaustive); Manardo 1536: 57–8, 63 offers other examples (the three meanings of 'neutrum' plotted against causes, bodies, and signs and modes in relation to time; the nine combinations of temperaments).

[116] *Ibid.*, 63; Aubéry 1584: 327 (fig. 4.2 above); cf. Zabarella 1586–7: 5.33 (fig. 4.1). Cf. also Murdoch 1984: 67 (lxiv) (Oresme's adaptation of the square of oppositions for the purposes of natural philosophy).

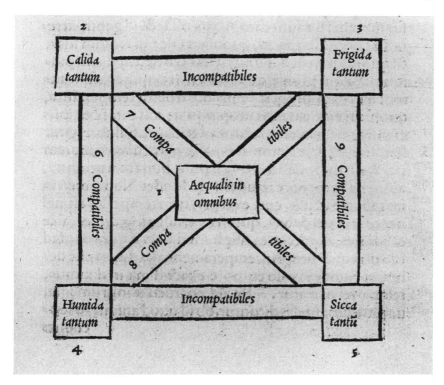

Figure 5.2. Giovanni Manardo, *In primum Artis parvae Galeni librum commentaria*, Basle, 1536 (4to M 15(1) Med), p. 63

As we have seen, it is a feature of medical thinking to take into account many circumstantiae or variables, and, over time, the numbers of variables taken into consideration increases. Cardano worked out in the middle years of the century that to take into account astronomical, environmental and physiological variables in diagnosis and prognosis would mean taking 2,936 (later recalculated as 3,194) equiprobable outcomes into consideration, and even then there would be exceptions, whose possible occurrence undermines the usefulness of exhaustive calculation and makes clear the need to generate workable rules.[117] The most controlled version of these accounts of variables is that of Johannes Hasler, who sets out in his *De logistica medica* of 1578 the data concerning the elements of remedies in a table with seven factors ('materia crassa', 'frigidum',

[117] Siraisi 1997: 131; Cardano 1578: 120; 1663: 8.19, 9.36.

'calidum', 'siccum', 'humidum', 'internae partes', 'morborum species')
and divides the variables into nine classes (including the individual's
temperament (in respect of age, time of year, latitude and the physician's
touch in determining the temperature of the patient), to arrive at medicinal compounds and weights.[118] He brings together in the same table
disease and idiosyncrasy; according to Siraisi, this collocation represents
a departure from Galenic therapeutic method.[119]

Around 1600, Sanctorius went further, and attempted to compute
the number of combinations of two, three and four peccant humours
in animals (of which there were, according to him, 165 in all), having
subtracted impossible combinations. He came to the figure of 80,084
possible equiprobable mixtures of up to four (out of 165) peccant humours; the prospect that doctors would have to master such an array of
variables is used by him to justify his more practical method for avoiding
errors in diagnosis. He employs in fact a wrong method to obtain the
result, and is consequently woefully short of the real figure;[120] but this
may not in fact be of great importance; whatever the outcome, the figure
is 'pene infinitus', and a demonstration of the need for a method which
brings the calculation into the realm of finite art.

Proportion is another area of mathematics which is enjoined on all
doctors in computing dosology and in determining health ('aequalitas'),
temperament and humours.[121] Its study is, according to Crombie and

---

[118] Hasler 1578.

[119] Siraisi 1987a: 374–6, who associates the move from the rebalancing of humours to the treatment
of disease to Sanctorius.

[120] Sanctorius 1630: 630–9 (vii.9). He calculates correctly by the use of addition the combination
of two peccant humours (13,530) but wrongly the combinations of three and four peccant
humours out of the possible 165 (13,530 + 13,366 + 13,203 = 40,099); he subtracts impossible
combinations (fifty-seven) and multiplies by two to cover intrinsic and extrinsic cases. His answer
is reached by
$$2[^{165}C_2 + {}^{164}C_2 + {}^{163}C_2 - 57]$$
where ^nC_r is the modern notation for the number of selections that can be made, r at a time,
from n objects, regardless of any different arrangements which can then be made (thus abc, acb,
bca count as one selection only). The correct answer is given by
$$2[^{165}C_2 + {}^{165}C_3 + {}^{165}C_4 - 57]$$
By this calculation the answer to Sanctorius's sum is twice 30, 521, 425 less 114. I am grateful to
Peter Corlett and Edward Catmur for information and calculations. Vigenère 1586: 42 has a
cabbalistic nightmare version of this – the number of combinations of the twenty-two letters
of the Hebrew alphabet – which is commendably close to the right answer (3.4034×10^{29} as
opposed to 3.4143×10^{29}).

[121] 'In accordance with nature' is described as 'well-proportioned' ('aequalis') in *Ars parva*,
K 1.381. See also Valleriola 1577: 240–1, citing Galen, *Ars parva*, K 1.309–10; *Methodus medendi*, iii,
K 10.157–231: 'si enim decem numeris discessio ad calidum facta sit, decem numeris ad frigidum
deducere corpus oportet'. For a weak rule of thumb see Diocles of Carystus 1572: 7r: 'in omnibus signis et malis quae hactenus proposuimus infantibus quidem et iunioribus, clementiora
medicamenta, grandioribus vero et natu maioribus, validiora ac efficaciora exhibere conveniet'.

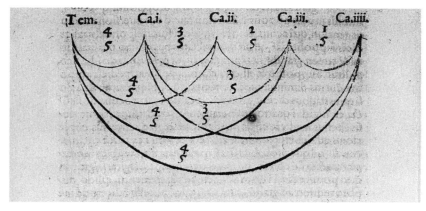

Figure 5.3. Laurentius Maiolus, *De gradibus medicinarum*, Venice, 1497 (Auct R 2 3 VI), sig. D3v

others, a feature of the medieval period; the development by Arnau de Vilanova of the work of the Arab philosopher Al Kindi was particularly important; there was a resurgence of interest in the topic at the end of the fifteenth century, when much work was done on dosology and on the degree, number, and virtue or strength of materia medica.[122] Underlying the calculations on the basis of these variables is Al Kindi's theory of proportions, which Arnau de Vilanova takes to be $x{:}x$; $x{:}2x$; $x{:}4x$; $x{:}8x$; $x{:}16x$, and which later writers understand as $x{:}x$; $x{:}x{+}1$; $x{:}x{+}2$; $x{:}2x$; $x{:}2x{+}2$.[123] The diagram used to represent these was an adaptation of the syllogistic geometrical diagram we have met before (above, 4.3.3 and fig. 4.4): see fig. 5.3.[124] In this representation of 1497 by Maiolus, the work of Arnau on degrees and of Al Kindi on musical proportions is critically examined through the use of an increasingly complex series of such abstract figures.

Even more ambitious use of diagrams can be found in relation to the latitude of health (above 4.4.2, below 7.4.3). In the medieval period, this was represented as an equilateral triangle segmented by vertical lines,

---

[122] According to Iliffe 1998: 357, 340, Crombie claims also that the Renaissance humanists replaced (good) medical quantification with (bad) qualitative precision and logical certainty; see also Clulee 1971; Müller-Jahnke 1992: 91ff. As the first degree of qualities is insensible, its calculation cannot be based on empirical evidence.

[123] McVaugh 1990; Meietus 1584: 237, 291–2 (Rondelet); Burnett 1999.

[124] Maiolus 1497: D3v. Boethius 1492: 16v has a similar diagram which represents no more than a set of combinations. The degrees of qualities are made complex by the fact that the first degree is not preceptible to sense according to some texts: see Arnau de Vilanova 1975: 54–5 (commentary of McVaugh).

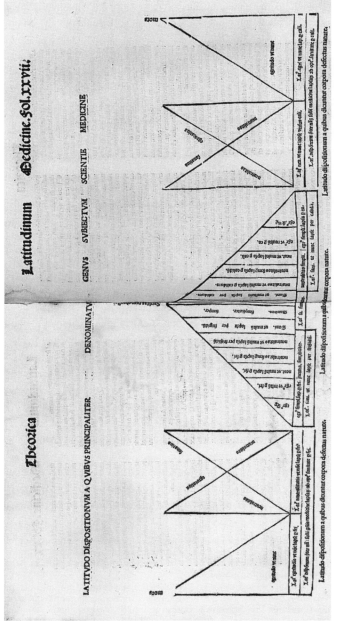

Figure 5.4. Benedictus Victorius (Faventinus), *Opus theorice latitudinum medicine ad libros tegni Galeni*, Bologna, 1516, fos. 26v–27r

with a point representing perfect health, and the sloping sides representing the declension into illness through various degrees; a fifteenth-century illustration of this type has been reproduced by Ottosson.[125] As in the case of proportions, the illustration could be used to represent the differences between (increasingly complex) theories. An example of this is found in the 1557 edition of Pietro Torrigiano's commentary on the *Ars parva*, in which two diagrams set out his interpretation of the latitude of health, and an accompanying commentary explains both what the diagrams represent spatially and how they illustrate the differences of opinion between Torrigiano and Gentile da Foligno.[126] This had previously been done by Victorius in 1516; his composite diagram (the culmination of three such figures) is spread across two pages – see fig. 5.4.[127] The penultimate section of this diagram on both wings has a sliding scale ('neutralitas aegrotativa'; 'neutralitas sanativa') which represents the 'latitudo ut nunc' between health and sickness, with the four corners of the diagram reduced to these mediate contraries. The additions to the medieval model suggest an ambition to represent visually not only qualities but relative quantities and even change over time;[128] they also ape the square of contraries, and translate the diagonals of this into temporal sequences of degrees.[129] It is interesting to note that Victorius has attempted to overcome the difficulty posed by Galen's acceptance of two meanings of the word 'generally' (either 'always' or 'frequently').[130]

Akakia tries two different techniques to take this further. In the first, he adds in both combinatories (the lines joining the points) and directionality (the black dots and circles): see fig. 5.5.[131] In a second representation, he turns the degrees of latitude of health into trapezia, which become the visual icons for different degrees of

---

[125] Ottosson 1984: 176–7. See also Murdoch 1984: 160 (cxlv)

[126] Rota in Torrigiano 1557: 26r: 'illud vero in commune omnibus dispositum, non lineis, sed areis, ideo significari, ut nullum extare corpus existimetur quod sub eodem aut huc aut illuc ad diversa loca continue revolvi, aut in eiusdem spaciis assidue fluctuare; lineasque omnes corporum spacia circumscribere, et eorum vias indicare; ac traversas quidem varias habituum latitudines, in altum vero erectas, quantum in suo quippe habitu profecerit, demonstrare, praeter appendices, ornatus gratiam tantummodo apportantes: causarum praeterea, signorum, ac corporum ab una dispositione ad aliam, artis beneficio traductorum, in eandem figurae designationem cum istis venire, nominibus tantum immutatis . . .'. These remarks could also apply to the figures taken from Akakia 1549 (figs. 5.5 and 5.6).

[127] Victorius 1516: 26–7.

[128] Jokissus 1562 must have been accompanied by a diagram which unfortunately does not survive with the text in the British Library copy.

[129] Joutsivuo 1999: 133–4 suggests that Oddo degli Oddi's circular representation (which he reproduces) is more successful than that of Victorius.

[130] *Ars parva*, K 1.308. See below, ch. 7 note 133.

[131] Akakia 1549: 60.

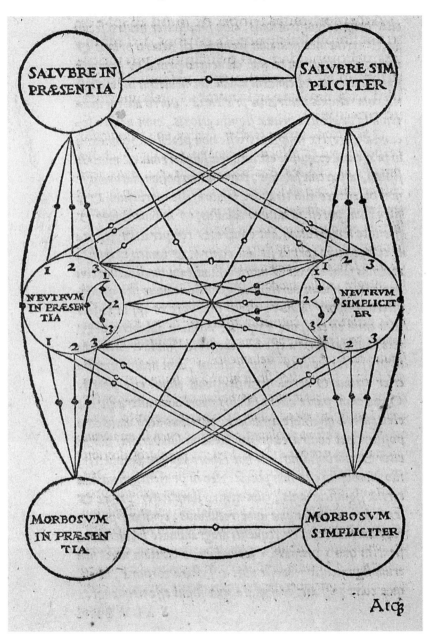

Figure 5.5. Martin Akakia, *Claudii Galeni ars medica quae et ars parva,*
Venice, 1549 (Byw N 2 23), p. 60

health: see fig. 5.6.[132] The interest in diagrams evinced by these writers is not just, I would suggest, inspired by the desire to clarify complex theories, although this is a stated aim;[133] it reflects also the presence of protomathematical as opposed to logical thinking in medicine at this time involving a quantification of predicates, and is an indication of the residues of arts course training in the writing of doctors. But to go beyond this and claim that doctors were fully fledged quantifiers of their art would clearly be wrong. That they had to quantify both the degree of severity of an illness and the dosage of the recommended treatment is clear; but it would seem that the application of the rules of quantification is subsequent to the act of judgement known as an indication (see below 8.7), and hence is a *post hoc* justification of such acts rather than the producers of them.

5.2.2 Probability

A related issue is that of probability, which arises naturally from quantification, combination, proportionality and degree. As is well known, it is difficult in all contexts to attribute precise meanings to the terms 'probabilitas' and 'verisimilitudo' at this time. On the one hand they represent the 'endoxa', or judgements made on the best available authority; as Aristotle declares in *Topics*, i.1, 100 b 18ff., that 'generally accepted opinions ('endoxa') . . . are those which commend themselves to all or to the majority or to the wise – that is to all of the wise or to the majority or to the most famous and distinguished of them'.[134] It is often the case, in both medical writing and law, that 'probabilius', 'certius', 'credibilius', 'verisimilius' or even 'verius' means 'having better support from trusted sources'.[135] But from Hippocrates onwards, other versions of imperfect or uncertain truth values are found in the literature of medicine and natural philosophy: relative frequency, dominance, some presence of error, inexactness, approximation, arguments from suspicion and

---

[132] *Ibid.*, 84.

[133] *Ibid.*, p. 83: 'quod [doctrinam] ut clarius intelligamus, sequentem formulam subiecimus'; cf. Sylvius 1539a: A5r: 'quapropter semeioticen hanc in Hippocratis et Galeni libris passim ita dispersam, ut paucis hactenus usui magno fuerit, ea methodo in tabellas coniecimus, ut iam possit etiam medocriter doctis, cum opus erit, in usum venire'.

[134] See Herberger 1981: 177–82 on the medieval reception of this in law, with respect to art and dogma.

[135] Cicero, *Disputationes tusculanae*, ii.1.5; Wear 1973: 140 (citing Vesalius); Daston and Park 1998: 142; Maclean 1992: 76, 92; Siraisi 1987a: 299 (quoting Giacomo da Forlì). See Glucker 1995 on 'pithanon' ('probabile' as the effect of an argument) and 'eikota' (individual arguments which are persuasive) as terms lying behind the Ciceronian usage which would have been known to Renaissance doctors.

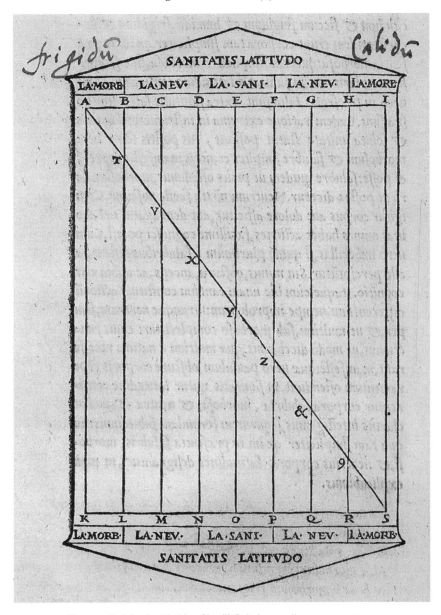

Figure 5.6. Martin Akakia, *Claudii Galeni ars medica quae et ars parva*,
Venice, 1549 (Byw N 2 23), p. 84

presumption; in other words, forms of deductive or non-deductive inference from complex evidence which take into account its incompleteness.[136] A quotation from Hippocrates's *Epidemics* (i.11) reveals some of these modes of thinking:

> In all dangerous cases you should be on the watch for all favourable coctions of the evacuations from all parts, or for fair and critical abscessions. Coctions signify nearness of crisis and sure recovery of health, but crude and unconcocted evacuations, which change into bad abscessions, denote absence of crisis, pain, prolonged illness, death, or a return of the same symptoms. But it is by consideration of the other signs that one must decide which of these results is the most likely.

This expression of prognostic probability is far from the only judgement of likelihood in Hippocrates;[137] and the question of relative probability is found in other works, such as Aristotle's *Physiognomica*, Theophrastus's *De ventis*, and in Celsus's *De medicina*.[138] Galen also refers to the 'gradus certitudinis' of dogmas; this phrase is used also in the Renaissance to describe the hierarchy of disciplines (see above 4.3); in law it is used to describe the degrees of presumption.[139] Galen's usage is connected

---

[136] The limit of this field may be taken to be chance, which is taken to be unknowable and unquantifiable at this time: see Hacking 1990. On suspicion, see below ch. 8, note 189.

[137] E.g. *Aphorisms*, iii.19: 'all diseases occur in all seasons but some are more apt to occur and to be aggravated in certain seasons'. Cf. Herberger 1981: 281, citing Cardano 1663: 6.316: 'inter experimenta potiora decet eligere'.

[138] *Physiognomica*, ii, 806 b 38: 'generally speaking it is foolish to put one's faith in any one of the signs: but when one finds several of the signs in agreement in one individual, one could probably have more justification for believing the inference'; see also Baldus 1621: 41(v): 'qua ratione in iudicando procedatur, quibus signis maior quibus minor fides sit adhibenda'; Theophrastus, *De ventis*, xv, where signs of rain are graded from the most unmistakeable ('manifestissimum') to the least certain; on which see Bonaventura 1593: 225, who shows that this point is understood but not developed: 'sunt enim signa de ortu sumpta multo meliora, id est certiora . . . et maiores res praemonia, quoniam a robustiori principio desumuntur'; Celsus, *De medicina*, Proemium, uses such words as 'multo saepius', 'potissimum', 'magis verisimile', and 'proxima veri'; ii.6.16–19 refers to a degree of acceptable error (0.001%) in construing signs: 'illa tamen moderatius subiciam, coniecturalem artem esse medicinam, rationemque coniecturae talem esse, ut, cum saepius aliquando responderit, interdum tamen fallat. Non si quid itaque vix in millesimo corpore aliquando decipit, id notam non habet, cum per innumerabiles homines respondeat . . . Neque id evitare humana imbecillitas in tanta varietate corporum potest. Sed tamen medicinae fides est, quae multo saepius perque multo plures aegros prodest.'

[139] *De placitis Hippocratis et Platonis*, x, K 5.777, quoted by Herberger 1981: 84; Cicero, *De inventione*, i.46 ('probabile autem est id quod fere solet fieri aut quod in opinione positum est aut quod habet in se ad haec quandam similitudinem, sive id falsum est sive verum'); Herberger 1981: 150, quoting Victorinus on the association of probability with the sublunary world: 'omnia quae in mundo aguntur, argumenta probabilia persuadere'; Gammaro 1584: 18.248v ('in principiis scientiarum est reperire triplicem gradum certitudinis'). The phrase 'gradus certitudinis' is also found in Bacon 1878: 175 (*Novum organum*, 'distributio operis'). For legal uses see Grotius, *De iure pacis et belli*, ii.16 and Specht 1998: 60 (on Leibniz).

to a process of elimination of possibilities or of noting the absence of
contrary evidence rather than a positive quantification of probability.[140]
Similar principles can be derived also from Aristotle's *Physiognomica*.[141]
Al Kindi's work on weather forecasting (the *De mutatione temporum*), which
contains judgements of probability, was also known in the Middle Ages,
and republished in the sixteenth century.[142]

Inexactness can be inherent in the object of study (as it is in nature
as a plural, infinite or imperfect phenomenon: see below 7.2), it can be
subjective (inherent in the limited capacity of the sense or intellect to
measure reality); it may reside in the imperfection of the method. These
are identified as problems by Cardano and Gemma.[143] No formal mathematical reasoning is engaged in, but by an act of *bricolage* a judgement
is reached about the strength of the evidence for a given conclusion.
This is derived from the combination of pieces of evidence, the use of
examples through analogy or induction, and the procedure to be adopted
when pieces of evidence conflict; that is, from the rough computation of
the relative strength of evidence of the same order. The problem posed
by discordant evidence leads to some kinds of evidence being preferred
to others according to a variety of criteria.[144] Some of these questions
are treated with great subtlety (but not mathematically) in law;[145] in
medicine, Argenterio provides an example of a quasi-quantified rule for
judging the relative strength of prognostic signs against their number:

If an equal number of signs are found, those which have the greater force determine the prediction; if the force of the signs is equal, then the greater number
offers the certain indication of what will happen; but if an equal number of
good and bad signs are mixed together, then an experienced medical practitioner, who has frequently engaged in prediction and will somehow recognise

[140] Herberger 1981: 84.
[141] See Baldus 1621: 41 (on *Physiognomica*, ii, 860 b 38ff.): 'noto autem ut aliquid certi decere
possumus, duo requiris, unum est, ut plura signa sint, qua idem testentur alterum est ut nullum
quod designat contrarium affectum, vel consequens, ad contrarium adsit, ut dico forte hunc
esse, primum quoniam habet magnas extremitates, latum pectus, pilosumque, os grande, carnem
duram, deinde quoniam in eodem non apparet quid quam eorum signorum, quod vel timorem
arguet, vel animi mollitiem, vel avaritiem, quae duo per se quidem non opponuntur fortitudini,
at comitari soleat tamen timiditatem'.
[142] Burnett 1999: Al Kindi's work was published in 1507 and 1540.
[143] Le Brun 1994; Gemma 1575: 200–1: prediction is only a 'probabilis ratio' because of 'particularium canonum multitudinem, inquisitionis difficultatem, sensus denique aut observationis
inopiam'.
[144] Baldus 1621: 41: 'quoniam autem capita et fontes sunt plures, rationabiliter poterat quaerere
aliquis: numquid omnes aequaliter ostendunt, an aliqui certiores sint alijs'.
[145] See Maclean 2000b.

the hidden powers of the eventual victor and what prevails in given diseases, is necessary, says Galen.[146]

The patient will not languish because the experienced doctor, unlike Buridan's ass, will always be 'somehow' inclined to one interpretation of the evidence over all others.

Frequency can also be found adduced in ancient medical texts:[147] as has been noted (5.1.4), there are said to be four (or five) levels of 'concursus' (always, for the most part, half the time, rarely: the implicit fifth is never). Death always ensues from a head wound, purgation occurs for the most part from scammony, death occurs in half the cases from a lesion to the dura mater, health is rarely restored in the case of a wound to the brain, and never in the case of a wound to the heart. These terms stand in determinate logical relations,[148] and suggest a distribution which, like that of Manardo illustrated above (fig. 5.2), might ape the logical square of contraries if the two diagonals were allowed to represent gradations rather than contradictories.

One can also find mathematicised forms of assessment, probability or prediction.[149] Cardano says that the prognoses of the best doctor are not one tenth in error, nor one twentieth, but one hundredth; 'the best' here is quantified as 99% accuracy.[150] Altomare attempts to establish probabilities in cases of patients suffering from more than one disease (and two sets of symptoms), without it being known whether one disease caused

---

[146] Argenterio 1610: 1780: 'quod si par numerus [signorum] reperiatur, quae maiorem vim habent, praedictionem attrahunt: quod si aequalis signorum vis fuerit, maior numerus certa praebet futuri indicia, at si bona malis permixta vi et numero paria videantur, exercitato in artis operibus viro opus est, inquit Galenus, qui ea saepenumero sit contemplatus, latentesque adhuc quodam modo vicentis vires, et quid in singulis morbis praevaleat, praenoverit'. Cf. Fonseca in Jacchinus 1615: 187: 'oportet coniecturam facere considerando non solum numerum signorum, sed vim et magnitudinem'. This is not a version of Galen's recommendation in *De differentiis pulsuum*, ii.7, K 8.612 first to typify the disease to determine its strength, on which see García Ballester 1981: 18–19, because determining its strength is a judgement of quality (*De constitutione artis medicae*, K 1.293–5; *De crisibus*, i.5, K 9.563–4; *Ad Glauconem*, i.11, K. 11.36–7: 'the magnitude of a disease cannot be described in words because it is derived from experience'). Cf. the use of guesswork to correct mistakes in *De locis affectis*, iii.4, K.8.145 and *De sanitate tuenda*, v.11, K. 6.365, on which see García Ballester 1981: 21.

[147] *Subfiguratio empirica*, ii, Galen 1556a: 1.32r–v.

[148] Hankinson 1995: 68.

[149] There is one medieval example of statistical reference to a population rather than an individual in Aquinas, *Contra gentiles*, 1.3.135 ('donors are not predictable individually, but are in a mass') which does not seem to have any echo in medical literature.

[150] Cardano 1568: 619 (iii.43): 'Galenus ... dicit, illum qui semel errat in viginti meliorem esse, quam qui in decem, et in centum aegris praestantiorem, quam in viginti, et in ducentis quam in centum.'

the other.[151] But all of this is very far from a mathematically quantified assessment of the following syllogism, based on *Posterior analytics*: most As are Bs; most Bs are Cs; therefore most As are Cs.[152]

After the recovery (around 1420) of the dialectical and topical texts of Quintilian, Cicero and Boethius, and (at a somewhat later date) the publication in Latin of the commentaries of Philoponus and Simplicius on Aristotelian logic, there were models available for quantified probabilistic judgements of a finite type derived from signs. These are collected together in Scipione Chiaramonte's book on physiognomy of 1625. There, the author gives the much-quoted example of the sign of pallor betokening a finite number of things (melancholy, fear, cold, anger, amorous passion),[153] and shows how a pallid individual can be interpreted as being increasingly likely to be suffering from one of these states by a process of elimination; if four could be eliminated this would allow one to be certain as to how to interpret the sign.[154] This logical process can also be transferred to cases of infinite probability, where the common signs of a condition can form a syndrome of signs which is persuasive.[155] If (in the standard example) a woman has breast milk, it may be the case

---

[151] Altomare 1559–60: 1–18; see also Daston and Park 1998: 144; Nutton 1990b: 211 on 'explanatory stasis' induced by a wide range of possibilities.

[152] Burnyeat 1994: 21. Aristotle, *Posterior analytics*, ii.12, 96 a 8–19 (on the analogy of the first figure, with 'most' ('hōs epi to polu') inserted before the terms of Major, Minor and Conclusion); cf. also *Prior analytics*, i.27, 43 b 35. This passage from 'all' to 'most' is found also in Galen, *Ars parva*, K 1.308.

[153] See *Physiognomica*, iv, 809 a 10 (pallor arising from fear and fatigue); Melanchthon 1547: r 7v ff. (pallor and indigestion); della Porta 1593: 12–13 has 'pallescentes' as 'meticulosos'; L'Alemant 1549: 29 (the pallid mathematician); Sanctorius 1630: 773 (xii.2) (pallor as a sign of the parturient woman).

[154] Chiaramonte 1625: 5–6: the sequence of reasoning runs as follows: the fully satisfactory case is of a sign as cause, in the first figure: whoever exposes his life for a friend truly loves him; Pylades exposed his life for Orestes; therefore Pylades truly loves Orestes. In the second figure, the sign cannot be used convertibly: whoever is afraid is pale; John is afraid; therefore he is pale; and it can even give rise to paralogisms: Hector is strong; Hector stutters; therefore all stutterers are strong. But the paralogism of the last example can be eliminated in the case of a perfect induction (i.e. one which covers every individual case, showing that Hector, Achilles and Samson, the only three men who can be called strong, all stutter); and there are ways of increasing the probability of the second case. Let us say that pallor is a sign of a person who is afraid, a person in love, a person who is cold, a person who is angry, and a person who is falling sick (and nothing else). The syllogism: 'pallor is a sign of fear; John is pallid; therefore John is afraid' 'lacks necessity' and only has 'refracted probability', according to Chiaramonte; but if you can show that John is not in love, is not afraid, is not cold and is not angry, with each successive demonstration 'a certain (and growing) degree of probability is reached' ('quod, si ostendatur, qui pallet, non amare, gradus aliquis accedit probabilitatis. Crescit autem, si neque aegrotare monstretur. Quod, si alia omnia membra; praeterquam timoris tollerentur, argumentum evaderet ex numeratione sufficienti partium'). This last phrase is used also by Sanctorius (see note 55 above).

[155] This point is made by Cardano 1578: 120, quoted above, ch. 4, note 135.

that she is pregnant; if she also has amenorrhea, bizarre appetites, frequent vomiting, lethargy, she is more likely to be pregnant.[156] Sometimes argument from multiple factors is said to be defective: as William Perkins points out in his diatribe against astrology, if you treat a patient from a pot of an unspecified number of herbs, then you cannot tell which was effective.[157]

Chiaramonte points out that there are univocal signs in the sense of *Prior analytics*, ii.27 (quoted above, 4.3.5) which yield certain conclusions; such signs are however rarely encountered, if at all, in medicine. Most signs are common or equivocal, and have to be conjoined with others to yield even probable information (e.g. wandering around at night is a sign of an adulterer, a thief, a sleepwalker, and no doubt other things; wearing fine clothes is a sign of an adulterer, a rich man, an actor, and no doubt other things; but wandering around at night in fine clothes is *more likely to be* a sign of an adulterer than of anything else).[158] This example is adapted by Chiaramonte from a sophism in the *De sophisticis elenchis* (167 b 10), and shows the proximity of this sort of reasoning to modes which were universally seen to be erroneous at this time. The same form of reasoning can be found in diagnostic writing.[159]

Probability therefore is a very complex area, closely allied not only to the assessment of the meaning of signs, but also to the distinctions perceptible in the field of terms used to designate it ('persaepe', like 'ut plurimum', means sometimes true, sometimes not, but more often true; 'verisimilis', 'verior' or 'credibilius' means plausible; 'probabilis' means supported by the best minds); it has a direct connection with the

---

[156] See above notes 137 and 141 (on the rule of the greater number). Sanctorius 1630: 94–116 (i.27–30) refutes this view at length.

[157] Chapman 1979: 281, quoting Perkins, *Four great lyes*, 1585, c6.

[158] Chiaramonte 1625: 5–6. In a sideways look at the law, Chiaramonte associates this conjunction of signs with the practice of extracting confessions from witnesses and the accused, and the signs given of mental perturbation during questioning (hesitation, growing pale, blushing); on this see Maclean 1992: 102–3.

[159] Da Monte 1583: 1.107: 'argumentum a signis consequentibus verisimilibus, et ubi multa signa concurrunt, suspicionem augent, licet certitudinem non faciant. Ita in hoc nobili iuvene [the subject of the consultation about a patient possibly suffering from syphilis] est suspicio accessisse aliquam infectionem primo ex bubonibus, et ulceribus pudendorum quae in omnibus solent contingere ante morbum gallicum licet non vertatur; ita ut non in omnibus qui bubones et ulcera pudendorum patiuntur, morbus gallicus consequatur. Accedit gravitas capitis prius non percepta, quae sequitur ad eum morbum et curavi multos, et credo Clariss. hos Doct. multos etiam vidisse qui nullum aliud symptoma habebant praeter dolorem capitis, et tamen laborabant morbo gallico. Praeterea in ulceribus est adustio et nigredo, quod si furunculi quos patitur, sedem etiam duram seu basim solidiorem haberent, augeretur magis suspicio, ita ut devenirem ad certiorem coniecturam. Hinc habeo magnam suspicionem ex omnibus simul additis de morbo gallico . . . '. On 'suspicio' defined in a legal context, see below, ch. 8, note 189.

field of variables recognised in various areas of medicine; it is even linked to metaphysics through the theory of the latitude of forms (4.4.2); and it has an intuitive connection to rationality through 'indicatio', as we shall see (8.7.2).

5.2.3 Plus aut minus: the locus 'a correlativis'

A final word should be devoted to the question of the phrase 'plus aut minus'.[160] The topical argument 'a correlativis' is a way of relating objects without stating absolute termini within which they exist;[161] it designates termini so as to allow what would otherwise be unquantifiable to be quantified.[162] This is the sense of 'more or less' in Plato's *Philebus* (14ff.); in Aristotle's zoology it can refer to variability of the propria of a species (e.g. the tolerated variation in the length of a leg or the hardness of a beak: *Historia animalium*, vii, 588 a 25); Galen refers to a 'ratio minoris maioris' in his discussion of medical contraries; Averroes alludes to it in respect of materia prima.[163] It is implicit in the definition of art as 'de infinitis finita doctrina'. The point at which this perception becomes directly associated with mathematisation is found in Kepler's *On the more certain fundamentals of astrology* of 1601:

Every variation arises from contraries, and the principal variation [arises from] principal contraries. Wishing to philosophise more sublimely, and more generally beyond geometry, Aristotle assumed in his *Metaphysics* the principal contrary was that of the Same and the Different. It seems to me that diversity arises in created things nowhere else than from matter, or because of matter; and where there is matter, there is geometry. Thus whereas Aristotle postulated a principal contrary without a middle between the Same and the Different, I find that in geometry that is philosophically examined, there is indeed a principal contrary, but with a middle: hence what was one term, Different to Aristotle, let us divide into two terms, More or Less.[164]

---

[160] Nicholas of Cusa, *De docta ignorantia*, ii.1, has a important use of 'plus aut minus' as termini in an infinite series.

[161] Maclean 1992: 80; cf. *Rhetoric*, i.2, 1358 a 10ff. (and Kneale 1962: 39) on more/less and induction.

[162] This can also be achieved by the dominance argument: an example is found in Valleriola 1577: 84–5 (the 'qualitas superans').

[163] *Methodus medendi*, xi.12, K 10.770–2, on which see above, ch. 4, note 149; Cardano 1663: 3.359: 'circumscriptos . . . habet [materia prima] limites magnitudinis et parvitatis, intro quos ceu quidam Proteus infinitos magnitudinis terminos subit'; Kessler 1994b: 47.

[164] Kepler 1941: 4.15: 'Variatio omnis a contrarietatibus est, et prima a primis. Primam contrarietatem ARISTOTELES in Metaphysicis recipit illam, quae est inter Idem et Aliud: volens supra Geometriam altius et generalius philosophari. Mihi Alteritas, in creatis nulla aliunde esse videtur, quam in materia, aut occasione materiae; at ubi materia, ibi Geometria. Itaque quam ARISTOTELES dixit primam contrarietatem sine medio, inter Idem et Aliud; eam ego in

What Kepler articulates here is the shift of the quantifier, which in the square of contraries is associated with the subject, to the predicate; a shift later suggested in the nineteenth century by Sir William Hamilton.[165] This insight had, I believe, already been intuited by Galen in the *Ars parva*, and by Galenic doctors with their peculiar uptake of the mediate contrary in respect of the latitude of forms (above 4.4.2 and below 7.4.3).

The central problem of this assertion of an intuitive awareness of quantification, as with all pre-mathematical probability, is this: are all apparent assessments of possible outcomes arising from unconscious inference, or ordinary language non-deductive reasoning about probabilities, no more than the grammatical possibilities given to Latin speakers by the existence of the comparative, by modals, and by words connoting truth, doubt, credibility, and the like? When in the index to Sanctorius's *Methodi vitandorum errorum* we find the phrase 'when there are several [competing] signs which are to be given the greater credence?' ('signa dum plura sint quibus magis sit credendum?'), does this betoken an awareness of a mathematically computable question (even if the formal means of answering it are not present) or rather an entirely different mind set based on aggregation of signs, or on proportional or 'magna ex parte' reasoning, all boosted with a little help from induction, analogy and elimination procedures or arguments *a negativo*? This problem is compounded by the indeterminate meaning of 'certitudo', which may designate a subjective state, or may indicate some sort of mind-independent criterion of reliability. The writing of doctors who were trained in mathematics, among them Cardano, Sanctorius and Liddel, suggests to me that they have an incipient awareness of the benefits of computability, but lack an agreed notation through which to communicate it to their contemporaries.

5.2.4 Sophisms

I come now to sophisms, which all agree should be eschewed by doctors; but as Cardano pithily puts it, 'ubi enim scientia, ibi etiam error'.[166] The

---

Geometricis, philsophice consideratis, invenio esse primam quidem contrarietatem, sed cum medio, sic quidem, ut quod ARISTOTELI fuit ALIUD, unus terminus, eum nos in PLUS et MINUS, duos terminos dirimamus.' I have used the translation of Mary Ann Rossi in *Proceedings of the American Philosophical Society*, 123 (1979), 93.

[165] Kneale 1962: 352–3; *ibid.*, 259 contains the suggestion that this shift was also thought of by William of Shyreswood.

[166] Cardano 1568: 653. He may be thinking of one of the three definitions of probable given in Sextus Empiricus, *Contra mathematicos*, ii.63 ('that which shares in truth and falsehood'; the other two being 'drawing us to assent, but true' and 'drawing us to assent, but false').

art of medicine, being in places at least ambiguous, plural, fragmentary, dialectical and even conjectural, cannot eliminate error from its processes of reasoning, because it may lurk in premisses, in the identification and interpretation of signs, or in the application of logic to the contingent circumstances and particulars of experience and human time. As Sanctorius points out, if Socrates has a cold and is cured by cassia, it does not follow that Plato needs cassia if he has a cold: he is composed of different humours, his style of life is different, the time of the year may not be the same, Plato may live in Germany and Socrates in Italy, Plato may be eighty years old and Socrates only thirty, and so on.[167] The logical fallacy referred to here is also that of failing to distinguish between 'simpliciter', which is invariant, and 'secundum quid', which implies adjustment by respect, time, place, or relation. Sophistry of this kind can not only seem absurd but also plausible, indeed even more plausible than truth itself in the case in which the best minds, who establish the 'probability' of a proposition, may all be wrong.[168] The specific weakness of medicine, an inferential art, lies, as has been said, in the error of the consequent: if A is B, then B is A; if an adulterer is a finely dressed nocturnal wanderer, then a finely dressed nocturnal wanderer is an adulterer.[169] The only solution to this, says Sanctorius, is to translate all syllogisms of the second figure into first-figure syllogisms of the order 'barbara'; which is in effect treating the Major as a genus and establishing a 'divisio' by the use of a causal middle term. But the logic of consequence, although not fully worked out,[170] can be used for inferential judgements of the kind doctors need to produce, even if this is open to the abuse noted by Sanctorius and that later noted by Bacon and Voltaire, namely that reliance on the doctrine of functionalism turns material causes into final ones (God invented noses to carry glasses).[171]

---

[167] Sanctorius 1630: 796–7 (xii.6).

[168] Pietro d'Abano (claiming that nothing prevents something false from being more 'probable' than something true), cited by Bylebyl 1985a: 230. See also Galen, *De differentiis pulsuum*, iii.6, K 8.670–85 (on non-scientific generalisations).

[169] *De sophisticis elenchis*, v, 167 b 1ff.; Sanctorius 1630: 5, 9–10, 27 (i. 2, 3, 7), referring to 'peccatum in forma syllogistica a positivi consequenti ad positivum antecedens'.

[170] Boh 1982: 300–1 has shown that the medieval logic of consequence does not distinguish between implication or conditional propositionality (if *p* then *q* where neither *p* not *q* is asserted), entailment (not *p* unless *q*: also without assertion of either *p* or *q*) and inference (*p* therefore *q*; an argument which is either valid or invalid). This would seem to hold for the Renaissance also.

[171] Bacon's example (2000: 87) is that of hairs around the eyes, which can either be described materially ('pilosity is incident to orifices of moisture') or finally ('the hairs are protection for the eyes'); see also Voltaire, *Candide*, i: 'Il est démontré, disait [Pangloss], que les choses ne peuvent être autrement: car tout étant fait pour une fin, tout est nécessairement pour la meilleure fin. Remarquez bien que les nez ont été faits pour porter des lunettes; aussi avons-nous des lunettes.'

5.3 AUTHORITY, REASON, EXPERIENCE

We come now to the most contested and decried forms of knowledge: argument from experience and argument from authority. The former of these relates to 'experientia' as that which is available to all through the senses; Montaigne famously refers to it in the context of the opening lines of Aristotle's *Metaphysics*:

[B] Il n'est desir plus naturel que le desir de connoissance. Nous essayons tous les moyens qui nous y peuvent amener. Quand la raison nous fault, nous employons l'experience

> [C] *Per varios usus artem experientia fecit:*
> *exemplo monstrante viam*

[B] qui est un moyen plus foible et moins digne; mais la verité est une chose si grande que nous ne devons desdaigner aucune entreprise qui nous y conduise.[172]

Of the rational arguments which have so far been the subject of this chapter, induction and analogy are closely associated with experience and example, and these are opposed to higher-order ratiocination on the one hand and argument from authority on the other.[173] Experientia is given various senses: that derived from *Metaphysics* to which Montaigne alludes is the 'universal habitus of the intellect of retaining in the memory something frequently repeated'; a second meaning denotes 'any observation made of sensibilia, excluding those drawn from experiment ('periculum')'; a third signifies 'the very exercise of the art'.[174]

5.3.1 Authority

Of the three orders of argument, the most decried is authority, and the most obviously weak recourse to authority is where sensory experience

---

[172] Montaigne 1965: 1065 (iii.13), citing *Metaphysics*, i.1, 980 a 22 ('all men naturally desire knowledge') and Manilius, *Astronomicon*, i.49. The truth he refers to here is the 'veritas objecti' (linked to the utility of art), not the 'adaequatio rei et intellectus' (linked to the speculation of science): see ch. 4, note 70, Porzio 1598: 170 (quoting Averroes, *In metaphysica*, ix: 'bonum esse in rebus, verum in mente'); Maclean 1996: 23–33.

[173] See Ottosson 1984: 208 (on quaestiones); Crusius 1615: 2v (on example, ratiocination and authority); Iliffe 1998: 336 records Crombie's claim that the argument from authority only became accepted in the late Middle Ages. Galen, *Methodus medendi*, ii.5, K 10.112 gives the three media of proof as demonstration, testimony and authority.

[174] Luca 1607: 3 (on the meaning of experience in *Aphorisms*, i.1): 'universalem intellectus habitum, eiusdem rei saepe memoria repetitae, quod artis principium dicitur'; 'aliquam in sensibilibus rebus factam observationem, in quibus non cadunt pericula'; 'ipsum exercendi actum praesertim in generosis auxiliis adhibendis, qui illegaliter factus valde periculosus existit'. Melanchthon 1834–60: 13.333 associates 'experientia' in astronomy and medicine with the epithets 'universalis aut certe regularis'.

contradicts the authority in question. In this regard there is an exemplary anecdote recorded by Sanctorius and repeated by Galileo: an Aristotelian is present at a dissection which shows by ocular demonstration that nerves originate in the brain and not in the heart (as Aristotle had claimed); he then confesses to the anatomist that he had made him see the matter so palpably and plainly that if Aristotle's text were not contrary to his ocular demonstration, and did not state clearly that nerves originate in the heart, he would be forced to admit that what he had seen was true.[175] This damning reference to Aristotelian authority, which is matched by the rhetorical topos of claiming to 'prefer to err with Galen (or Aristotle) than to be right with his detractors',[176] seems to consign argument from authority to complete rejection, notably by Paracelsians, but a word of caution should be added. In many cases, citing an authority is a short-hand way of citing the arguments and theories of that authority; this is how many Renaissance doctors (not to speak of the peripatetic Simplicio, who answers the Galilean anecdote about nerves in a perfectly sensible way) use citation.[177] Secondly, some experience can only be obtained

---

[175] Sanctorius 1630: 315 (iii.15); Galileo 1998: 116–17; see also Siraisi 1997: 101 (citing a similar anecdote relating to Cardano), Maclean 1980: 103 (citing Riolan). Perfetti 1999a: 458 cites Pomponazzi as decrying Aristotle for relying on reports about animals, but comparing this position to Christians not seeing Christ but believing in him (a reference to John 20:29).

[176] The locus classicus is in Cicero, *Disputationes tusculanae*, i.17.77: 'errare mehercule malo cum Platone . . . quam cum istis vera sentire': Altomare 1574: *2r: '[hoc opus] si qui pertinacia adducti aut malevolentia potius suffusi audeant contradicere sciant non mihi sed Galeno se contradicturos, quocum errasse malo, quam ad aliorum mentem recte sapere'; Riolan 1610: 134–5, cited by Brockliss 1993: 81: 'faverem peripateticis, nisi religioni christianae Platonicarum doctrina ex parte magis consentiret: malim errare cum ecclesia, quam cum philosophis bene sentire'; Barlandus 1532: BIV: 'malis [sc. Arnoldus Nootz] cum Avicenna tuo, ceu coelesti quodam Numine, male tum dicere, tum facere, quam cum alijs bene'; Riccoboni 1598: 99 (on the dispute between Augenio and Massaria); 'nimium et plus nimio in verba magistrorum iuraverit, ac eorum auctoritati nimis deditus videatur, cui responsioni solet respondere, se [Massaria] veritatis quidem causa id facere, sed male cum talibus videri errare, quam cum istis novatoribus vera sentire: qui enim istis videntur errare, meram esse veritatem'. The phrase has a theological application: see Lampert Auer, cited by Nischan 1994: 32: 'ego malo errare cum Concilio Tridentino quam sapio cum Confessione Augustana'. An equivalent sentiment is found in the sentence which Herberger 1981: 283 records du Chesne as claiming that Riolan wanted as the inscription above the portal of the Faculty of Medicine of Paris: 'medicorum titulo indigni iudicantur quicunque Hippocratem et Galenum quamvis probabiliter contradicunt'. See also Kühlmann 1992: 105 (quoting Croll). There may be here an allusion not only to the Ciceronian tag but also to the Psalms (83 [84]: 11): 'elegi abiectus esse in domo Dei mei magis quam habitare in tabernaculis peccatorum'.

[177] Simplicio in Galileo 1998: 117; Cardano 1663: 3.357; Crusius 1615: R3v; Ferdinandus 1611: 6; Castro 1614: 94–7; Mikkeli 1992: 174 (on Zabarella); cf. D 1.2.2.49; Pascal 1963: 357 (*De l'esprit géométrique et l'art de persuader*): 'Ceux qui ont l'esprit de discernement savent combien il y a de différence entre deux mots sembables, selon les lieux et les circonstances qui les accompagnent. Croira-t-on, en vérité, que deux personnes qui ont lu et appris par coeur le même livre le sachent également, si l'un le comprend en sorte qu'il en sache tous les principes, la force des

from the reports of others, which Cotta calls the 'eyes of experience'; it is acknowledged that doctors will not live long enough to accumulate all the experience which is available from such reports, and that they therefore need to supplement their own with them.[178] In this sense medicine is necessarily a textual discipline, and indeed remains so, in the area of 'empirical' remedies (i.e. ones which work without its being known why).[179] Finally it should be noted that both the authorities here cited – Galen and Aristotle – themselves caution against accepting statements by others as authoritative. Aristotle insists on the primacy of sense-perception and the secondary nature of unfounded assumptions and theory;[180] Galen's 'precept' is precisely to pay more attention to experience and theory than books.[181] A sequence of his successors – Alexander of Tralles, Rhazes and, in our period, Cardano and Argenterio – all point this out.[182] In fact there is a whole class of quotations from authorities disauthorising authority, including the proverb 'amicus Plato, magis amica veritas', and the maxims from Seneca and Horace which Daniel Sennert adapts and quotes in a cluster in his *De consensu*.[183] Attacks on authority may also take the form of 'paradoxa' or rehearsals of heterodox medical opinions.[184]

5.3.2 Reason and theory

While it is agreed that both reasoning and experience can trump authority, it is not always clear whether one of the first two has precedence

consequences, les réponses aux objections qu'on y peut faire, et toute l'économie de l'ouvrage: au lieu qu'en l'autre ce seraient des paroles mortes, et des semences qui, quoique pareilles à celles qui ont produit des arbres si fertiles, sont demeurées sèches et infructueuses dans l'esprit stérile qui les a reçues en vain?' cf. Maclean 1992: 87–8.

[178] Cotta 1612: 11–16; and above ch. 4, note 129. Blair 1997: 95 records the somewhat different point made by Lucien Febvre that, in the early modern world in which so much is not understood, almost no report can be rejected as unbelievable a priori.

[179] Thriverus 1592: 1; Brockliss 1993: 71 (quoting Fernel).

[180] *Physics*, viii.22, 253 a 32: 'to adopt the thesis that all things are at rest and (ruling sense-perception out of court) to attempt to prove it by reasoning, really amounts to paralysing intelligence itself, not only on the particular field in question, but universally'; see also Herberger 1981: 282 (quoting du Chesne).

[181] *In Hippocratis de morbis vulgaribus*, vi.2, quoted by García Ballester 1993b: 40: 'illos qui magis credunt auctoribus quam experientiae et rationibus esse temerarios'.

[182] Temkin 1973: 152, 118.

[183] See Guerlac 1978 (on 'amicus Plato'); Seneca, *De vita beata*, iii.2: 'aliorum quidem opiniones praeteribo, nam et enumerare illas longum est et coarguere. Nostram accipe', rendered here by Sennert 1676: 101 as: 'nos vero an omnes servi et mancipia alienarum opinionum nati sumus ?'; Horace, *Epistulae*, i.1.14: 'nullius in verba magistri iurare'; Eckart 1992: 156 (quoting Sennert 1676: 179); Papy 1999: 325 (quoting Thomas Fienus); also Camerarius 1626–30: 94–7 (ii.11).

[184] E.g. Platter 1625; see also Lonie 1981: 36.

over the other. They can be seen as equipollent and equally necessary
to the rational doctor:[185] this is the prevalent view. But some argue that
'experientia' is to be preferred to 'ratio'; others (including some influential medieval writers)[186] make the contrary case. 'Experientia' is said
to be 'magistrix rerum', 'der Wahrheit Mutter', and 'optimum philoso-
phandi principium';[187] but reason has also its role to play: 'reason will
be the commander in the domain of invention; but experience is its
master'.[188] 'Ratio' can even be considered above 'experientia', not only
by neoplatonists but also by those who, like Cardano, see that it is in reason that the origins of all taxonomy lies.[189] In this sense even Avicenna
prefers reason, in the guise of the 'truer' Aristotle, to experience in that
of the 'more manifest' Galen: truer in the sense of belonging to the
order of knowledge that is intellectual and unseen, as opposed to that
of the sensory information 'better known to us' (see above 4.3).[190] In
this sense too, Aristotle's stricture in *Meteorologica*, i.7 (344 a 5–7) applies:
'we consider that we have given a sufficiently rational explanation of
things inaccessible to observation if we have produced a theory that is
possible'.

There are risks in giving priority to sensory information; if the 'evidens
evidentia' is lent credence, then there is no way of reaching counter-
intuitive insights, not only about physical events such as antiperistasis but also about the calculation of dosages.[191] Evidentia is sensory,
and the Aristotelian theory of knowledge does not allow that (sensory)
particulars can yield conclusions.[192] Our senses are fallible; they can
only tell us about qualities, properties and accidents, not elemental substances; the inductive process which experience makes possible can only
lead to 'infinita particularia' about subjects; we need to know causes in

---

[185] Horst 1606: 13–14.
[186] E.g. Arnau de Vilanova 1585: 1679.
[187] Blair 1997: 96 (citing Bodin); Kühlmann 1992: 115 (citing Croll); Temkin 1973: 129 (citing
Paracelsus); Schmitt 1969: 86 (citing Agrippa); Keckermann 1614: 1801.
[188] Cardano 1663: 1.578, cited by Siraisi 1997: 27: 'pro inventione ratio dux erit, experimentum
autem magister'; Camerarius 1626–30: xx (i.50); Papy 1999: 323 (citing Fienus).
[189] Tuilier 1998: 389 (citing Ramus); Cardano 1565: 22ff. (i.2.3–4), making the point that only by
the use of reason can we recognise similia and imagine fictional cases for the testing of theories
or for teaching: see also 8.7.3.
[190] Siraisi 1987a: 317.
[191] Pittion 1987: 106–8; Schmitt 1969: 84; Horst 1621: 204–5; Vallesius 1606: 11 (i.5) (both on
antiperistasis); Maiolus 1497: 7v (on counter-intuitional proportions in dosage between degrees
of quality which 'mirabile videtur et prope modum incredibile'); Cardano 1663: 3.357 (on
subtlety).
[192] Sanctorius 1630: 795 (xii.6): 'praedicata in propositionibus naturalibus non possunt esse particularia . . . ex puris particularibus nihil sequitur'.

order to know *stricto sensu*.[193] In this sense Ferrier is able to amplify part of Hippocrates's first aphorism ('experimentum periculosum, iudicium difficile') and refer to the 'periculosum et *fallax* experimentum, iudicium hoc est ratio difficile sed *tutum*' (my italics).[194]

A final point to raise here is prompted by Valleriola's question whether doctors should be allowed to make up cases or should always rely on ones which have been reported by others. This raises the issue of thought experiments; Valleriola concludes that these mental constructs are one path to the 'rei essentia' which is true medical knowledge.[195] For this reason, for dogmatic physicians, both ratio and experientia are necessary, even in consultations.[196]

The danger of a false theory imposing itself on sensory data is clearly perceived, from Aristotle onwards.[197] Some, like Nicolas Oresme, had seen all natural-philosophical theories as provisional, and had claimed that 'there is no law which will not eventually need changing';[198] this being an insight derived from Aristotle's *Politics* and hence from the sphere of endoxical or practical knowledge. Pomponazzi ends his treatise on Incantations with an admission of the provisional nature of his conclusions, inspired by *Topics*, vi.14, 151 b 11f.[199] Various mid-century doctors (who cannot be expected to have known Oresme, but would have known *Physics*, ii.4) make the same point, especially after the publication of Vesalius's *Fabrica*, which was the clearest demonstration of the primacy of empirical evidence over argument and authority.[200] Before Vesalius, Berengario da Carpi had made a similar claim by restricting anatomy to 'anatomia sensibilis';[201] perhaps the most succinct formulation of this

---

[193] *Ibid.*, 799.

[194] Ferrier 1592: 17 (citing *inter alia* Galen, *De optima secta)*; Michael McVaugh has pointed out to me that 'fallax' appears in medieval translations of this aphorism, but my point is that it here reinforces 'periculosum', as does the addition of 'tutum' to 'difficile'.

[195] Valleriola 1577: 559: 'an medicus exempla ex se finget, an extrinsecus petat?'; cf. Galen, *Methodus medendi*, iii.1, K 10.157–62.

[196] Dodoens 1581: 20; Silvaticus 1601: 205; Herberger 1981: 28off. (citing Guinther von Andernach and Cardano). Dear 1995: 48 records the terms of art from astronomy in this regard ('phainomenon' is an appearance visible to everyone; 'observatio' is an act whereby a phenomenon becomes known through the senses; 'suppositio' is what must be accepted by a science and 'hypothesis' is what has to be constructed).

[197] Lloyd 1979: 200–25 (citing *Physics*, ii.4).

[198] Daston and Park 1998: 132; Sennert 1676: 179 quotes Seneca to this effect, as part of his argument that Paracelsian medicine should be taken seriously.

[199] Pomponazzi 1567: 325: 'nostrae responsiones tam diu teneant, donec meliores reperiantur'.

[200] But note that doubt has been cast on the purity of both the Vesalian discoveries and the illustrations used to convey them: see Straus and Temkin 1943; Saunders and O'Malley 1950.

[201] French 1985a; Wear 1995b: 267–8.

view is found in Pereira's *Novae veraeque medicinae, experimentis et evidentibus rationibus comprobatae, prima pars*:

> So enormous is the force of experience in discovering the truth that we must, when an apparent explanation ('ratio') is opposed to experience, place greater trust in the evidence of the senses ('experimentum') than the explanation, and search for a better one.[202]

Cardano goes further and suggests that the nature of medical epistemology makes doctors reliant on senses and not at all on truth.[203] Protestations of the primacy of *experientia* and *sensus* are even found in the writings of traditional doctors of the Galenic tradition such as Jean Riolan the Elder, who declares that 'it is stupid to refute the senses and experience with reason out of reverence for antiquity'.[204]

5.3.3 Experience and experiment

There are other points to be made here about experience: the first concerns the use of the terms 'experientia' and 'experimentum'. In some texts these seem to be interchangeable;[205] in others a distinction is made on which Peter Dear has written extensively. According to him, experience is something necessarily commonplace, confirming conclusions that were predictable according to the use of reason and validated by the authoritative structure into which they fitted. For Aristotelians, a finite empirical test or a particular observed event (experimentum) could not prove a universal truth.[206] There is another doctrine derived from Aristotle, *Posterior analytics*, ii.16 (100 a 3–9): 'sense-perception gives

---

[202] Pereira 1558: 11, cited by Lonie 1981: 42: 'adeo ingentem vim ad dignotionem veritatis experimenta habere, ut teneamur cum ratio apparens experimento adversatur, plus fidere experimento, quam rationi: cogamurque potiorem rationem, quam fuerit prior inquirere'. This view can be traced progressively back through Galen, *De morbis vulgaribus*, iv.2, Aristotle, *Physics*, viii.3 to pseudo-Hippocrates, *Praecepta*, i; cf. Pittion 1987: 112ff. (on Argenterio); Cardano 1568: 133 (ii.2–3): 'medicus debet credere evidentibus signis potius quam rationibus persuasivis, vel a priori'; Cardano 1663: 1.357: 'nulla [est] authoritas adversus experimenta scribentibus'; and Sherlock Holmes in Conan Doyle 1950: 50: 'at least my theory covers all the facts. When new facts come to our knowledge which cannot be covered by it, it will be time enough to reconsider it.'

[203] Cardano 1663: 6.415, quoted by Siraisi 1997: 51: 'cum igitur medicus sit sciens, et non purus artifex, et habeat operari circa subiectum suum, et subiectum non constet unquam sub uno affectu propter materiam: cogitur medicus solus inter omnes scientes diiudicare ex sensus, non ex rei veritate'.

[204] Cited by Maclean 1980: 103: 'stultum [est] ratione pugnare contra sensum et experientiam pro antiquitatis reverentia'; see also Arnau de Vilanova 1585: 1682 (on rhubarb).

[205] Gorris 1601 s.v.

[206] Daston and Park 1998: 237; Dear 1987; Dear 1990, Dear 1995.

rise to memory, and repeated memories of the same thing give rise to experience: because the memories, though numerically many, constitute a single experience'.[207] Whether the perceiver is active or passive in this process is not clear; he could instigate the process of repeating memories by a test ('periculum') or not.[208] Empirical evidence can be contradictory, and it has the drawback of taking the form of trial and error; this may however be the only path open to certain parts of medical practice (such as remedies for occult diseases), in which chance plays a part.[209] It is not a source of knowledge of causes, and it is not permanent or unrevisable.[210] It was thus important not to exaggerate its authority, and to submit it to rules.[211] Avicenna had already set down seven controls on medical experiment which reflect the logical strictures to which it had to be submitted: there had to be no accidental heat or cold present, only one disease in question, a test should be done for the contrary disease, the force and strength of the disease should be assessed, the time of any indication of its working should be noted, only the human body should be considered for its testing, and the results should be submitted to 'magna ex parte' logic, not apodictic demonstration.[212] An experiment, even in the sense of a test ('periculum'), is not a historical event which can be repeated by readers of it and be verified by them; it is principally a confirmation of an effect rather than a process of discovery. In this sense it is methodical: 'experiment is an instrumental doctrine by which we teach how to proceed from the known to the unknown'.[213] From seeing rhubarb purge bile in one man, then five, we can memorise this and

---

[207] Schmitt 1969: 93; Sanctorius 1630: 802 (xii.6); da Monte, cited by Mikkeli 1992: 145 (experientia as 'memoria multorum particularium'); also Cardano 1565: 21v (i.2.2), distinguishing on the authority of Galen, *Subfiguratio empirica*, experientia ('tota rei evidentis observatio') from experimentum ('multis sentiendi memoriis constare'); Schmitt 1969: 89. The connection of experience to analogism and epilogism is discussed above (5.1.2). Cf. the argument in Bacon that medicine began with experiment and then graduated to causes: 1878: 261–2 (*Novum organum*, i.74) quoting Celsus (incorrectly).

[208] Schmitt 1969: 114–15.

[209] Bylebyl 1985a: 238 (on contradictory information about the pulse, and the debate between Capivaccius and Bauhin); Ferdinandus 1621: 266 (on the chance discovery of the cure for tarantulism).

[210] Brockliss 1993: 70–2; Dear 1987: 142.

[211] Silvaticus 1601: 205; Eckart 1992: 154 (citing Sennert on need for many acts of observation, certainty of results and correct analysis); Ingolstetterus 1597: 105–6: 'ad cognitionem per experimentiam requirunt tria; 1. saepius animadvertisse effectum esse a caussa aliqua. 2. a sola hac, non alia conjuncta 3. non repugnante natura'.

[212] Avicenna 1608: 245–7 (*Canon*, ii.1.2).

[213] Henry 1997: 24; Capivaccius 1603: 1046: 'experimentum est doctrina instrumentalis qua docimur progredi a noto ad ignotum'. Schmitt 1969: 87 and Blair 1997: 105 cite 'periculum' and 'experimentum' as terms of art related to natural philosophy and alchemy: see also Agrimi and Crisciani 1990.

apply it. It is best of course to do this by autopsy (witnessing the event ourselves); but we must be prepared to accept the report ('historia') of others.[214] Again book-learning has a role restored to it, even if there is a rising demand for individual and personal experience.[215]

5.3.4 Sense epistemology

As is well known, there are many sceptical attacks on the reliability of sensory data. But medicine as a discipline has an interest in defending its validity as evidence, however limited. This is an inevitable effect of the Aristotelian doctrine 'nil in intellectu quod non prius in sensu', the concomitant claims derived from the *De anima*, iii.3 (428 a 13) that the senses cannot be wrong about sensations (the claim that one can only attribute the true/false distinction to intelligibilia and judgements of the intellect) and the doctrine of mental images set out in the *De divinatione per somnum*.[216] Touch, smell and sight have particular roles to play in medical practice, in taking the pulse and in other forms of examination.[217] In this the doctor is, as Sanctorius puts it, a 'sensatus philosophus' whose hands feel truth and who is able to conceive of ideas or forms of disease which are accessible to the senses.[218] There is some debate about

---

[214] Brockliss 1993: 73; Hankinson 1995: 68; Siraisi 1997: 196 gives two meanings for 'historia': the record of human experience, and the description of nature including specific cases. French 1994: 32 (on Vesalius); Daston and Park 1998: 230; Argenterio 1610: 15: 'experientia aliorum intendendum credendumque his, qui earum rerum naturam, et vim se perspectam habere referunt'.

[215] Siraisi 1997: 45; Temkin 1973: 152 suggests that Harvey's *Exercitationes de generatione animalium* of 1651 marks a watershed between traditional approaches and the use of the 'exercitatio anatomica' as the beginnings of a new practice. This question is involved to some degree with the question of secrets literature, and its articulation of a new concept of secularized experimentation, on which see Eamon 1994. An early medical example of this is afforded by Boderius 1555, who apparently tests the predictions of astrology by recording the horoscopes of patients at the beginning of illness and their outcomes, on which see Grafton and Siraisi forthcoming; see also their discussion of Cesare Ottato, *Opus tripartitum de crisi, de diebus criticis et de causis criticorum*, Venice, 1519, 7, adducing empirical evidence (the results of phlebotomy in hospitals) against the theory of critical days.

[216] *De divinatione per somnium*, 464 a 12; Aquinas, *Summa theologiae*, 1a 86.4 ad 3; *De anima*, ii.3, 427 b 10ff.; cf Schmitt 1967: 32ff. (on Giulio Castellani); Blair 1997: 98.

[217] On this see Castellanus 1555: 6r–9v.

[218] *De anima*, ii.9, 421 a 19; ii.11, 422 b 32–2; Gryllus 1566: β4v ('medicus autem [est] τεχνίτης αἰσθητικὸς'); Sanctorius 1642: † 4r, quoted above, note 88; Sanctorius 1630: 29 (i.7) (the doctor as 'sensatus philosophus'); Campilongo 1601: 52v: 'nonne per morbos Hippocrates [*Aphorisms*, i.12] intellexit formas seu ideas morborum: quam cum sint sensibiles, signa quoque suarum constitutionum dicuntur'; Kusukawa 1998: 134 (on Sylvius's claim against Vesalius that anatomy is not done with the eyes only but with the hands; and the demonstration of Sylvius's inconsistency on this point).

the hierarchy of ear and eye in this matter, and a curious silence about smell.[219] A connection may exist here with the traditions of alchemy, natural magic and the mechanical arts: what Hooke was to call 'operative knowledge'.[220]

5.3.5 The 'lumen naturae'

Paracelsians go further than this in their estimation of experience. For them 'experientia', the 'amica medicinae, parens et nutrix', recovers scientia from perceived objects by the use of 'natural reason'.[221] This is more than the 'naturalis lux' of human consciousness and conscience to which Melanchthon, Kepler and others refer.[222] The 'lumen naturae'or the 'lumen gratiae' is required to recognise the God-given information in the form of signatures, as Croll points out:

Two lights are known from which comes all perfect knowledge and besides which there is none. The light of grace gives birth to the true theologian, when accompanied by philosophy. The light of nature brings the philosopher into being, when accompanied by theology, which is the foundation of true wisdom.[223]

Sennert points out the risks of disciplinary anarchy in this:

They make up some light of nature and grace or other, with which they disguise the figments of their brain which cannot be proved by either reason or experience. If it is permitted for any new dogma to be brought forth free of all experience and reason, and that credence should be given to it by simple reference to the light of nature and of grace, the result will be that truth will

---

[219] Aristotle, *Metaphysics*, i.1, 982 a 23–4 (eye); Blair 1997: 99; Gryllus 1562: β4v: 'efficaciora vero argumenta sumuntur a gustu et tactu, a visu et odoratu infirmiora, ab auditu fere nulla'.

[220] Crisciani 1998; Daston and Park 1998: 223 (on Bacon); Hooke 1665: ix; Bennett 1998. Castellanus 1555: 13v–14r also connects natural magic to natural philosophy insofar as it deals with empirical repeatable effects whose causes are not known.

[221] Severinus 1571: 1–3r; Goldammer 1991: 54, 94, characterising Paracelsus's sense of natural reason as 'eine [von Gott stammende] anthropologische philosophisch-theologische Aussage für die "natürliche" Erkenntnisfähigkeit des Menschen', and pointing out that for Paracelsus, Christ was the source of all healing.

[222] Barker 1997: 359. The classical locus in Cicero, *Disputationes tusculanae*, i.1.

[223] Eckart 1992: 144 (quoting Croll, *Basilica chymica*, Frankfurt, 1609, 194): 'nota sunt dua lumina intra quae omnia, extraque nihil, et nulla perfecta rerum cognitio. Lumen gratiae verum Theologum gignit, non tamen sine Philosophia. Lumen naturae verum Philosophum efficit, non tamen sine Theologia, quae fundamentum est verae sapientiae'; the Paracelsian source is given in Hannaway 1975: 6–8: 'the father has set us in the light of nature, and the son in the eternal light (viz. of Grace). Therefore it is indispensable that we should know both.' See also Ashworth 1989.

be what it seems to be to anyone. No one can fail to see what confusion would come from this in every discipline.[224]

We may hear here the clear echo of the debate about the separation of medicine and theology (above 3.6) in which the line taken by Sennert is clearly a Paduan one. Not all who use the term give it the theological sense, however; some, like Friedrich Beurhusius, link it to a conception of natural reason consistent with the views of Melanchthon and Ramus (see above 4.4).[225]

In all this discussion of sensory experience and reason we may determine a sort of middle way as the path of the rational doctor, using senses, reason and experientia (in the form of written testimony of others) but using them as mutual correctives and complements in a way which strictly speaking is not consistent with the Aristotelian separation of the orders of sense and intellect, since one penetrates into the order of the other, in the form of indication and intuition into the order of sense (below 8.7), and in the form of the particulars of experience into the order of the intellect.[226] As the pseudo-Hippocratic *Praecepta* (i) have it:

One must attend in medical practice not primarily to plausible theories ('logismoi') but to experience combined with reason. For a theory is a composite of memory of things apprehended by sense perception.

5.4 PEDAGOGICAL METHOD AND THE METHOD OF DISCOVERY

I come finally to the question of method; how should the instruments for obtaining and handling knowledge be made to work in concert and in sequence? Method is that which defines the rational doctor: 'a doctor is scientific and rational insofar as he is methodical'.[227] Method is defined after Aristotle by doctors as a 'rational goal-directed habitus', a 'logical instrument teaching how to proceed from the known to the unknown in any discipline through the perfect knowledge of its theorems', or

---

[224] Eckart 1992: 145, quoting Sennert 1676: 194: 'nescio quod Lumen Naturae et Gratiae fingunt, quo sui cerebri figmenta, quae rationibus et experientia probare non possint, pallient. Quod si admittatur, cui libet pro libitu nova dogmata ab omni experienti et ratione aliena fingenti et illa ad Lumen naturae et Gratiae referenti fides habenda erit, et verum erit quod cuique videbitur. Ex quo quae omnium disciplinarum confusio oriri possit, nemo non videt.'

[225] *In P. Rami Dialecticae libros . . . quaestiones*, Dortmund, 1575, A8r, quoted by Kusukawa 1998: 139: 'est naturale lumen ratione utendi, inveniendo et iudicando, quo animus notitias rerum necessarias et universales non informatas a natura ipsa adfert, sed colligit facultate intelligentiae sibi, naturali et ingenerata'.

[226] Herberger 1981: 284ff.

[227] Bartolettus 1619: 295: 'medicus eatenus scientificus et rationalis quatenus est methodicus'.

'a universal way which is applicable to every individual case'.[228] So necessary is it to medical students that Christoph Heyll even bans those who are unmethodical from reading his methodically presented *Artificialis medicatio*.[229]

Ottosson, Gilbert, Edwards and Wear have already written at length on the contributions of Pietro d'Abano, Leoniceno, Manardo, da Monte, Capivaccius and Sanctorius to this field;[230] I do not need to cover the same ground in detail. It is sufficient to say that Galen's *Ars parva*, *De optimi docendi genere*, *Quod optimus medicus idem sit et philosophus*, *Methodus medendi* and *Ad Glauconem* contain most of the loci on which the discussion is based; indeed one late commentator (Fabritius Bartolettus (1576–1630)) even seems to believe that the *Methodus medendi* is the same as Galen's lost treatise *De demonstratione* (see above 4.1).[231] It is widely agreed that a different method applies to teaching and to discovery ('inventio'):[232] very broadly, teaching ascends from causes to effects (signs), whereas discovery descends from effects to causes. Galen puts this a slightly different way; practice begins with individuals, theory with universals.[233] We have already met this division before (4.3.5); it is that between the compositive and resolutive, and between 'things better known by nature' and 'things better known to us'.[234] As would be expected, a great

---

[228] Da Monte 1587: 231: 'habitus rationalis ad aliquem finem'; Campilongo 1601: 3v: 'bonus habitus intellectus'; Liddel 1628: 18: 'instrumentum logicum docens in disciplinis progredi a noto ad ignotum theorematum perfecte cognoscendorum gratia'; Capivaccius 1593: 1v, citing Galen, *Methodus medendi*, iv.4: 'viam universalem quae cuilibet individuo est applicabilis'. I have been unable to locate this quotation.

[229] Heyll 1534: 88: 'amethodos, et non diligentissimos prohibeo plane a librorum meorum lectione'.

[230] Gilbert 1960; Ottosson 1984; Edwards 1976; Wear 1981. See also Wightman 1964; Di Liscia, Kessler and Methuen 1997; Jardine 1974: 40–50 (on Willichius, Melanchthon, and on the confusions about Galen's three methods); Jardine 1997 (on the distinction between method and 'ordo' in the debate between Zabarella and Piccolomini). Ordo is defined by Jardine 1974: 29 as 'a method for laying out available material for clarity'.

[231] Bartolettus 1619: 299.

[232] Bylebyl 1991: 187 (on da Monte); Argenterio 1610: 499; Capivaccius 1603: 1047–9; Blair 1997: 99 (on Bodin).

[233] García Ballester 1981: 21–3, 29; but Galen also uses the technique of telling anecdotes (often about his own prowess) in *De locis affectis*; see also Lacuna 1551: 729, 533–4. A locus in Aristotle's *Metaphysics* (i.i.12, 981 b 8) implies that a grasp of theory has to be achieved before one can teach, which ability is a sign of acquired knowledge.

[234] Biesius 1558: 6v: 'verum cum diversa disciplinarum methodus sit, interdum enim ab effectis et compositis ad simplicia progredimur [ad] causas, hoc est ab ijs quae sensu percipiuntur, ad ea quae cognoscuntur intellectu, quod in artibus inveniendis et constituendis usu venire solet: interdum contra descendimus a superioribus ad inferiora, praecipue dum cognitas iam artes explicamus: nos hanc postremam potissimam methodum sequemur, a principijs enim communibus ordine progrediemur ad ea quae sensu cognoscuntur. Nonnunquam etiam a posterioribus et experimento cognitis causas inquiremus, semperque dogmaticos et rationales medicos imitabimur.'

deal is said about pedagogy. Some approaches are not recommended: these include instruction in argument *in utramque partem*, over-reliance on the commentaries of others, the 'quaestio' approach, certain modes of *accessus* to texts, and styles of writing judged by some as difficult, such as aphorisms.[235] Method is distinguished from 'ordo': the former is an instrument, the latter a descriptive class for the purposes of discovery (in the 'ordo resolutiva'), constitution (in the 'ordo compositiva'), and memorisation (in the 'ordo definitiva').[236] Clementinus links these orders to the questions set out in *Posterior analytics*, ii.1 (above 4.3) and derives from them 'inductive doctrine' (when we want to know of something 'utrum sit'), 'definitive doctrine' ('quid sit'), 'compositive doctrine' ('quia sit'), and finally resolutive doctrine ('propter quid sit'); the last two are slightly confusing because they relate to the question, not to the order of the syllogism (in which 'propter quid' corresponds to compositive and 'quia' to resolutive).[237] Definitive is also sometimes to be found described as divisive.[238] A confusion arises from Leoniceno's creation of four 'modi doctrinales' (definitive, demonstrative, divisive and resolutive) incorporating the 'doctrina ordinata' which is a means to an end, and separation of these from the three 'ordines' (compositiva, definitiva, resolutiva).[239] Capivaccius declares this schema to be an error and re-unites both Galen and Aristotle and orders and methods under the four headings 'definitive', 'demonstrative', 'divisive' and 'resolutive', which he discusses exhaustively;[240] Jokissus had earlier designated these as 'rationes', and distinguished between the 'ratio' appropriate to science, that appropriate to art and sensory data, and that which characterises

---

[235] Siraisi 1990a: 167–9, citing Argenterio 1606–7: 11–12, who attacks argument *in utramque partem*, accuses Sylvius and Akakia of relying too much on commentary, and deplores the 'quaestionaria doctrina' which is found in those who engage in textual reconciliation; Capivaccius 1603: 1049 (on the difficulty of teaching from aphorisms).

[236] Da Monte 1587: 1–19; Capivaccius 1603: 1047ff.; Campilongo 1601: 16v; Albertus 1615: B4r: 'Hippocrates Galenus [et] Celsus docent inventioni Methodum resolutivam inservire, constitutioni compositivam, memoriae divisam, veritati demonstrativam'; but cf. *ibid.*, 3v–5v offers a more eclectic account: for him, method is 'primo propositum in duas partes distribuatur [i.e. subject and attribute]; utrumque antecedentia, consequentia, repugnantia, causae, effectus, natura, accidentia inquirantur: utriusque cum alterius causa cum causa . . . se conferantur: ex ijsque et similibus argumenta deducantur, utentes Analyticis Topicisque Aristotelis: vel alphabetaria cabalistarum revolutione, quae infinitum propemodum copiam variam propositionum suppeditat'; Zabarella 1586–7: 1.68–135 (on confusion of 'ordo' and method in Averroes); see also Jardine 1974: 51 (on Schegk); Herberger 1981: 243 (on da Monte and Ehem).

[237] Clementinus 1535: 4; cf. Edwards 1976: 283ff., on Torrigiano's reversal of resolutive and compositive.

[238] Kuhn 1997: 334.

[239] Gilbert 1960.

[240] Capivaccius 1603: 1040–3.

Galenic practice;[241] Liddel renames divisive 'analytic' (which constitutes, for him, the easiest approach to a subject), and points out that different methods or orders are applied to different parts of medicine (compositive to physiology, resolutive to therapy).[242] In the method of discovery, there is a passage from the known to the unknown (which can be either something naturally unknown, or a middle term between something known to us and something naturally unknown to us); but in all cases the unknown is not previously unknown but only unknown in that context and known as a concept ('universaliter') to the intellect.[243] The same implicit claim that only 'praecognita' will be discovered is found in Sanctorius's *Methodi vitandorum errorum*, which is a (negatively conceived) syllogistically structured search for error in diagnosis, prognosis, choice of treatment, and manner of its administration.[244] The precise content of these 'praecognita' will however differ according to the nationality of the doctor, according to one writer.[245] I have only found one doctor who recommends a genuinely heuristic method (one which begins from difficult cases and derives theory from them), even though this approach is implied in many of the critiques of theory recorded above (4.4).[246] By 1560, a great deal of blurring of distinctions has occurred in the semantic field constituted by the word group 'methodus', 'ordo', 'ratio', 'modus'; although in some titles 'methodus' is used as a Ramist shibboleth, it seems that the word is used fairly loosely and freely by the end of the century.

5.5 CONCLUSIONS

Several conclusions suggest themselves after this survey of the uptake from the arts course. The first is its sophistication and inventiveness; I do not think that French is right to claim that 'there is a strong sense in which the height of medical reasoning reached by scholasticism before

---

[241] Jokissus 1562, cited above, ch. 4, note 105.

[242] Liddel 1628: 17–18; see also Edwards 1976: 303 on Zabarella's elimination of the definitive method and separation of the resolutive method (for practical disciplines) and the compositive (for speculative and theoretical sciences).

[243] Capivaccius 1603: 1022–5.

[244] Sanctorius 1630: 25–9 (i.7) (against the 'via divisiva'). He claims on the authority of Aristotle that only syllogisms can cause new knowledge to appear: 'nulla [est] via, quae adumbrata et caligine aliqua obruta in lucem efferat, quam syllogistica'.

[245] Albertus 1615: DIV–3v (on Italians, Germans and Poles); on Argenterio's critique of Paris, see Siraisi 1990a.

[246] Martinengius 1584: 68–95. One might also wish to link this discussion to the representation of information in alphabetical form, on which see Schmitt 1985: 276n; Nutton 1990a.

the Black Death was never again reached afterwards'.[247] In one sense this may be true; namely that the late fifteenth century had to recover certain materials, notably the mathematics of proportion, that seem to have fallen from view; but this revival of past insights and methods was accompanied by new departures inspired by dialectics, by mathematics and by innovative approaches to psychology; it was given an edge by strong referentialist claims in language. The second point to note is the great reliance placed in medical logic on the technique of division in its dialectical form. The 'via divisiva' is the means by which the rational doctor breaks down the composite and confusing reality with which he is faced, and proceeds to inferences about it. It is interesting to note the persistence of this approach to this day in such areas as differential diagnosis and even the employment of probability trees. The third conclusion is suggested by the comparison with the uptake by law, which reveals that for doctors their scientia, their signa, their causae, their contraria are all 'latior', and their divisions and definitions as no less lax; only in the area of analogy and the use of the 'locus a simili' can it be said that they impose stricter rules than the jurists. This would seem to suggest further that doctors might have been happy to retreat into a description of their discipline as a loose art; but such a suggestion is belied by their insistence on the scientific status of their discipline, even if they concede that it is also an art.

Such insistence may be sensed in nearly all the commentaries on Hippocrates's first aphorism, which refers specifically to the less than certain status of the profession's activities:

Life is short, the art long, opportunity fleeting, experiment treacherous, judgement difficult. The physician must be ready, not only to do his duty himself, but to secure the co-operation of the patient, of the attendants and of externals.

One might expect that this would give rise to a catalogue of the difficulties of practising the art, such as that given by Heurnius and alluded to in Liddel's general work on semiology by his qualification of many rules by limiting words such as 'fere', and 'ut plurimum'; but in fact some commentaries go the other way, and refer to the art (in the words of Hollerius, already quoted) as a 'doctrine drawn from true, certain, universal and mutually consistent precepts directed to a single end'.[248] Hollerius argues that although in its application, medicine may be conjectural,

---

[247] French in French, Arrizabalaga, Cunningham and García Ballesler 1998: 5.
[248] Heurnius 1637: 17ff.; Liddel 1628: 511–600; Hollerius 1582: 3r.

it has a scientific basis in its principia (the elements, the temperaments of the human body, the functions or spirits, the determination of illnesses, causes, symptoms and signs). Da Monte also refers to medicine being founded on 'rationes firmissimae', although he claims that these are not as tyrannical as the dogmas of law.[249] For these and other writers, although much of the doctrine is quite separate from the individual practitioners of it, there are none the less operations, of which 'indicatio' is the most notable (below 8.7), in which the practising doctor becomes the embodiment of the rationality of the doctrine, and the locus of its certainty. We encounter again the vexed problem of the frontier between objective and psychological truth.

Da Monte, Heurnius and Hollerius are all practici: why do they go to such lengths to defend the scientific status of medicine, something which seems on the evidence of this chapter to be patently indefensible? And why do so many of the university teachers referred to in this chapter include references to the most rigorous forms of demonstration in their manuals? First, I would suggest, to maintain the dignity of the profession against the lawyers by a dialectical use of the term 'certain'. Second, to retain the strong connection with Aristotelian physics, which has a scientific status; for medicine to be a liberal art, it must have a guaranteed basis in science. Third, I would venture to argue, to ward off the threat of unbridled empiricism, and specifically to control the use of analogy and induction. Fourth, to restrict the use of topical argument (more suited to the law court) in order to recognise simultaneously the primacy of the real over the verbal. These reasons taken as a group also help explain why many teaching manuals contain their own logical instruction although it could have been presupposed in medical students.

[249] Herberger 1981: 236–7.

CHAPTER 6

Interpreting medical texts

By the art of interpretation we are able to give meaning to the
impressions and thoughts of the mind and explain them to others.

(Ramus)[1]

6.1 AUTHORITY AND DISAUTHORISATION

Medicine as a body of knowledge, as a practice, and as a discipline draws
inferences about causes from effects of various kinds; this is a movement
from the outside, or surface, or posterior written record, to the inside,
or depth, or prior intention or meaning.[2] Some effects are recorded by
the senses, and interpreted by the intellect; these are the subject matter
of diagnosis and prognosis, and will be investigated in a later chapter.
Others come in textual form, and must be interpreted to extract their true
meaning; these are the subject matter of this chapter.[3] As we have seen,
there are better and less good roads to truth: the 'illustratio authorum',
by which their intentions and meanings are revealed, is one of the lesser
means we can employ to accede to it.[4] Galen brackets this together with
the act of consulting more experienced colleagues about diseases which
the physician had not yet encountered;[5] for him as for his Renaissance
readers, reading texts involves not only the exposure of the premises

[1] Ramus, *Schola dialecticae*, v. 1: 'Interpretari est ars qua possumus sensa, mentis et cogitata significare alteri et explicare.'

[2] See Cardano 1568: 2, 1663: 1.69–70, 105, 144, 147 for an association of these on the one
hand with 'prophetic' activities ('ex manifestis obscura cognoscere, ex obscuris manifesta, ex
praesentibus futura, ex mortuis iuvantia') and, on the other, with physiognomy, metoposcopy
and chiromancy, which are other conjectural arts drawing meaning from signs much as humans
do in reading texts and in engaging in prognosis and (illicitly) divination.

[3] There is discussion in the Renaissance of the narrative spoken to the doctor by patients or their
attendants (see below 8.6), but this is seen in terms of systematic interrogation from which data
rather than meaning has to be elicited.

[4] Valleriola 1577: 132 lists nine imperfect roads, of which this is one.

[5] *De locis affectis*, iii.5, K 8.147; García Ballester 1981: 34.

and arguments of texts written by others, but also the assessment of their account of events which cannot have been witnessed by the reader: what might be termed heteropsy. This sort of interpretation may involve a reductive strategy of selection and exclusion on the part of the interpreter, or it may lead to the conciliation of different sources of information.[6] It may, or may not, involve the interpreter's own experience of life or of his art. It may, or it may not, involve the translation of the parent text of the author into a new notation or language. In all these forms, it must acknowledge the fact that authority is looked upon as a weak form of argument, especially where sensory experience contradicts the text in question.

It is pertinent here to recall the exemplary anecdote quoted above (5.3.1) in which the Aristotelian who witnesses an anatomical demonstration disproving one of Aristotle's claims about the human body confesses that if Aristotle's text were not contrary to what he had seen, he would be forced to admit that what he had seen was true. There is, as I noted above, a rhetorical trope associated with this, that of claiming to 'prefer to err with Galen (or Aristotle) than to be right with his detractors'; but it would be incautious to see this as a sign of blind authoritarianism. Some sorts of information can only be obtained from the reports of others, which Cotta calls the 'eyes of experience'; no doctor will live long enough to accumulate first-hand all the experience which is available from such reports, and therefore all will need to supplement their own experience with them.[7] Such written accounts are furthermore 'the remedy of forgetfulness', both individually and collectively (see above 3.3.2). In this sense medicine is necessarily a textual discipline, and indeed remains so, in the area of rare medical conditions and empirical remedies.[8] Finally, the most widely cited authorities – Galen and Aristotle – themselves caution against accepting statements by others as authoritative, thereby disauthorising the authority of their works and so cutting the ground (whether consciously or not, is not clear)[9] from under their own feet (see above 5.3). 'Galen calls those who agree

---

[6] Papy 1999: 324 quotes Thomas Fienus (*De formatrice foetus liber*, Antwerp, 1620, 73–4) linking these two textual operations.

[7] Cotta 1612: 11–16; cf. the comment by Lucien Febvre recorded by Blair 1997: 95 that in a world in which so much is not understood, almost no report can be rejected as unbelievable a priori.

[8] Thriverus 1592: *4–6; Brockliss 1993: 71 (quoting Fernel).

[9] I would be inclined to argue that the relevant topos in Aristotle (*Physics*, viii.22, 253 a 32), and the manner of presentation of his solutions to the problems he perceives in the theories of his predecessors, indicate that he is prepared to see his own text undergo the same treatment; whereas the topos in Galen is difficult to square with his asseveration elsewhere that he never

[uncritically] with the writings of others slaves', proclaims Argenterio the anti-conciliator against Galen; 'let us be friends with Hippocrates, friends with Galen, even friends with Paracelsus; but let the authority of none of these be such that it becomes prejudicial to truth, who should be our friend above all others', writes Sennert, the last great conciliator.[10] Even if it is acknowledged that authors can be inconsistent with themselves, erroneous in fact and judgement, wrong in method and logically contradictory, they yet remain a path, albeit a reviled and uncertain path, to information; and they may have other, ideological, attractions, which is perhaps why conservative doctors of the stamp of Donato Altomare and Jean Riolan the Elder would prefer to be in error in their company than to be right in the company of their religiously unsound opponents.[11]

There are other, perfectly reasonable, grounds for relying on the word of authorities. One such ground is to argue that one is adhering not to their conclusions and dogmas but to their premises and logical procedures; this is the line adopted by the Aristotelian who tries to defend the reaction of his fellow-sectary in the anecdote recorded above. It may be that an authority has thought more about the subject in question and had more direct experience of it than his reader; this is the reason Fuchs gives for following Galen in his account of plants.[12] In choosing between an authority and other forms of evidence, a reasonable solution may be to steer a middle course between servile credulity and rash innovation: a course which Sennert recommends, one with which Harvey grapples in his preface to the *De generatione animalium* (above 4.2.2) and one on which a later writer, John Reynolds of Kings Norton, comments with particular clarity in his report of 1669 on a case of prodigious abstinence in Derbyshire which he sent to the Royal Society. Having listed many previous printed reports of similar cases, he addresses directly the question

failed to give a correct prognosis, and that others should trust his text even where it contradicts their own autopsy or direct medical experience (see above 3.7 and below 6.3.2).

[10] Argenterio 1610: †1r: 'Galenus servos vocat qui scriptoribus assentiuntur'; Eckart 1992: 153 (quoting Sennert 1676: 184r): 'amicus sit Hippocrates, amicus Galenus, imo amicus Paracelsus: sed nullius tanta sit auctoritas, ut veritati, quae prae omnibus nobis amica sit, praeiudicare debeat'.

[11] See above, 5.3.

[12] Fuchs, *De historia stirpium*, Basle, 1542, α6v, quoted by Kusukawa 1997: 413: 'cur autem Galeni sententia omnibus aliis sit praeferenda, nulla alia est ratio, quam quod is stirpium facultates partim certa quadam ratione et methodo, quam literis subinde mandavit, cognoverit, partim etiam experientia didicerit'; this reasoning may have induced Cardano to add accounts of his remarkable cures to his *De libris propriis* in 1557; and may have motivated writers such as Smetius 1611, Schenck 1609a and Donatius 1591 to publish.

of heteropsy:

That Uncharitableness [drops Blasphemy] which presumes to write *Falshood* upon all human Testimonies; they that assent to nothing, not confirmed by *Autopsia*, are unfit to converse in human Societies; for how can I expect that any Body should believe me, whilst I myself will believe no Body?'

But he then goes on to point out that 'as it is human Infidelity to disbelieve all such Reports, because some are false, so it is superstitious Charity to believe all, because some are true'. Unfortunately no very clear hermeneutic guidance is given here as to how one should avoid the Scylla of infidelity and the Charybdis of superstition;[13] earlier, as we shall see, no comprehensive method of dealing with the same problem is offered, although some thought is given to it, especially by Cardano, on whose reflections much of this chapter will be based.

The most common kind of authorities in the minds of Renaissance doctors are those represented by the 'sententiae antiquorum'. For Galen, the 'antiqui' included those writing as recently as one hundred years before him; but by 1500, the category excludes all who wrote in at least the preceding four hundred years.[14] The sense of reverence of the distant past, which is a marked feature of humanism and indeed of the Hippocratic movement of the middle of the century, is not characteristic of either Galen or of his predecessor Aristotle. The latter's destruction of the views of antecedent metaphysicians and psychologists in the opening books of his treatises on these topics bears witness if not to a progressivist then at least a revisionary notion of philosophical history; the former's occasional insistence on exposing the premises and logic of earlier medical writers also has the effect of dehistoricising philosophical debate while preserving a distinction between his own text and those of his predecessors, explicitly in favour of the former.[15] The inconsistency between ancient practice and Renaissance attitudes perceptible here is to be found in the writings of some humanist writers, notably Cardano. He not only evinces a sense of revelation through history, a belief that knowledge is accumulative, and a conviction even that the argumentation in ancient

[13] Reynolds 1745: 4.44: on which see Schaffer 1996. Reynolds's solution to this problem is to shift attention from the facts reported to the construction placed on them, and to disqualify explanations that rely either on the intervention of God in the world or on occult qualities by appealing to a version of Ockham's razor: 'beings are not to be multiplied without necessity'. In this he is following a by then hallowed path in denouncing those who see praternatural events as cosmic, political or religious signs or portents. See also Wear 1973: 290–1 (quoting Sennert).
[14] Campilongo 1601: 12v (citing Galen on 'sententia antiquorum'); Silvaticus 1601: 443–4 (citing Galen, *In Aphorismos*, vi.1, K 18a.1–2).
[15] Cardano says that he fails to do this when engaged in commentary: see below 6.4.1.

texts can be refined, but conjoins this paradoxically with the lionisation of Hippocrates as the founding father of medicine, whose works mark the end of the phase of empirical discovery and in whom is to be found all that is needed for the complete medical art.[16]

In what follows I shall first describe the *accessus ad auctores* and the Conciliator's mode of interpretation inherited from the Middle Ages; then survey Renaissance practice with regard to text, author and reader in turn, giving much space to Cardano, who reflects on these problems more than any other Renaissance doctor. As in the case of the preceding chapter, I shall end by a comparison with the practice of lawyers, and an indication of how the hermeneutics of Renaissance medicine relates to modern theories. It is worth pointing out that existing accounts of the history of hermeneutics rarely if ever give much place to the importance of medicine. But in one of the texts which are taken to be forerunners of hermeneutics (that of Michael Piccartus, which appeared in 1595 with the title *Oratio de optima ratione interpretandi*), there are frequent references to Galen as a model interpreter in the sense which Piccartus gives to that word.[17] Moreover, he does not mention the critique of Galen by Cardano in this respect, and his elaboration of a mode of interpretation which is intended to correct what he perceives as Galen's errors (see below, 6.4.1). One might be tempted to argue on the basis of such evidence that medical thinking in this area is at least as sophisticated as that of lawyers and theologians at this time.

6.1.1 'Accessus ad auctores'

The *accessus ad auctores* with which I begin is not of course limited to medical writing, although as Ottosson shows, there are examples of its use by expositors of medicine and natural philosophy: he cites Haly Ridwan's commentary on Galen's *Tegni* and Averroes's on the *Physics* of Aristotle. The former lists 'intentio', 'utilitas', 'ar[tis] excellentia', 'titulus', 'doctrine modus', 'ordo', 'auctoris et libri nomen', and 'libri divisio per partes et sermones' as the headings of *accessus*; the latter has a similar list, which includes also 'cui parti philosophiae [liber] supponatur'.[18]

---

16   Siraisi 1997: 58, 63; on Hippocrates marking the end of the phase of discovery, see Crisciani 1990: 120–5; Joutsivuo 1999: 46–7 (also above 1.4.1 on the expansion of the field of knowledge). It could be claimed that these two views can be made consistent if the pristine knowledge to be recovered is seen as bringing about an increase in knowledge.

17   Piccartus 1595: B1r, B2v, [B]3r–v; among the loci to which he refers are *In aphorismos*, iii, Proemium, K.17b.560–1; *In epidemica*, i, K.17a.7ff.; *De placitis Hippocratis et Platonis*, ix, 5.791–805.

18   See Ottosson 1984: 66–8. On the use of 'ordo' as a hermeneutic tool see Jardine 1997.

In the Renaissance, Giambattista da Monte adapts this method in his lectures on Rhazes to the new needs of his age by examining in turn seven points: how and by what general method to discover the subject; the significance of the name of the author; his motive for writing; his sect; his teaching method; the commentator's teaching method; the approach to be adopted by the pupil towards the teacher and the author in question.[19] These points include not only the mapping back of Rhazes on to the matrix of the three sects (above 3.3), but an acknowledgement that da Monte's teaching will be different in kind to that set out in the parent text, and that he as a teacher will need to tell his students how to approach both his teaching and the text. This stress on lecturing technique is not however universal: L'Alemant's preface to his commentary on Hippocrates's *Airs, waters, places* is less innovative:

We must do here what nearly all commentators are wont to do, that is, ask what title Hippocrates gave to this work; so that we may more easily understand his approach to his work, and the aim which it is very important to keep in mind in all genres of writing. Then we must discuss the utility of the work, whether it obeys the rules, to which part of medicine it should be assigned, and within what limits it should be ordered.[20]

Cardano uses this form of *accessus* in a more novel way in his autobiographical writings, as can be seen from this passage from the latter part of the 1562 edition of the *De libris propriis*:

The point of this book is for me to set out the arguments of my books, the logic, order and utility of their composition; principally these four points, but also as a consequence, the time, place and cause of my writing, what prompted me to write them, what benefit I derived from them, what sorts of errors arose in

[19] Da Monte 1556: 1–2: 'in primis ostendemus quo pacto et methodo invenire subjectum; de nomine Authoris aliqua dicemus notatu digna; tertio videbimus qua ratione fuerit Author impulsus ad libri compositionem, quarto quam sectam ex tribus imitatus fuerit, quinto quem ordinem servarverit in docendo, sexto quem ordinem nos servaturi sumus, qualem esse oportet discipulum tam ergo praeceptorem quam circa Authorem'. See also Mugnai Carrara 1999: 258–9 (on Manardo's use of *accessus*); Siraisi 2000: 10 on the importance of biography to *accessus*.

[20] L'Alemant 1557: 1: 'Cum omnes fere librorum interpretes facere consueverunt, hic quoque nobis faciendum, videndumque quo titulo hoc opus conscripserit Hippocrates: ut facilius consilium eius, et scopum quem in omni scripti genere maximopere tenere refert, intelligamus. Utilitas deinde quae sit, an legitimum sit opus, et ad quam medicinae partem referri debeat, quove circumscribatur ordine, dicendum.' On L'Alemant's acknowledged borrowings from Cardano, and the latter's reaction to them, see Siraisi 1997: 139. There are other versions of *accessus*: see French 1979 on anatomical *accessus*, which consists in a recital (*historia*) of the major organs, the action, function and purpose of parts of the body, observations of rarities and morbid conditions, solving problems in authors, and skill in dissection. It appears sometimes also in titles: see Joutsivuo 1999: 38 (citing Andreas Planer's *De utilitate libri Galeni Ars parva* of 1579); see also Siraisi 1999: 358–9 (on Cardano's use of *accessus* in respect to Avicenna and Vesalius).

them, how they were received, and what hindrances they suffered; what things excelled in this undertaking, and how many forms of argument, discussion and style there are.[21]

What Cardano sets out to reveal is both the context and evolution of his thought and the relationship of his most important writing to utility, and hence to the arts to which they belong.

6.1.2 Conciliation

The second mode of approaching the texts of medicine inherited from the Middle Ages was through conciliation, on the model of Pietro d'Abano's still utilised conciliation of Aristotle and Galen, which continued to be published in its original form until 1565 (see above, 2.4.1). Other texts practise a related mode of interpretation, in which the same quaestiones are considered but not necessarily resolved by conciliation; some of these were called 'contradicentia medica', others 'controversiae', or 'enarrationes', yet others 'verisimilia' (where textual emendation is the only solution under discussion).[22] The premiss underlying conciliation is that the authority of passages from different authors or the same author which appeared to be contradictory can be preserved by resolving the contradiction through the use of distinction.[23] The blame for the contradiction may be attributed squarely to the commentator, as Vallesius points out: 'there are no contradictions in what Galen says, only in the failings of its exposition'.[24] The conciliation may be applied to propositions, questions or loci;[25] this last mode contributes to the anthologizing of the text, as do epitomes (see below 6.4.2). It is effected by the distinction of polysemy ('distinctio nominis significationis': see above 4.4.3), or of genus, species and differentia, or of 'ordo', 'ratio', and 'functio'.[26] It is connected to translation and to what Argenterio calls the 'quaestionaria doctrina', as it is often structured by quaestiones.[27]

---

[21] Cardano 1663: 1.138: 'Hic finis est huius libri [*De libris propriis*], ut doceamus librorum nostrorum argumenta, rationem compositionis, ordinem ac utilitatem; atque haec principaliter, quae quatuor sunt: praeterea ex consequentia tempus, locum causamque scribendi, tum vero quae ratio sit conscribendi libros, qui fructus conscribenti, quot modis errare contingat, quam accepti fuerint libri, quae passi impedimenta; quae praecellerunt in hoc munere, quot genera argumentorum, tractationum, et stylus quam multiplex.'

[22] Cardano 1565; Aubéry 1585; Vallesius 1606; on verisimilia, see Draut 1625a: 1501–2.

[23] The sequence in Pietro d'Abano is principally: quod sic; quod non; dubitationes; resolutio.

[24] Vallesius 1606: 450–1: 'nam revera repugnans nihil est in Galeni assertionibus, sed quod enarratione indigent'.

[25] Capivaccius 1606: 17ff. applies conciliation to all three.

[26] See Siraisi 1987a: 229–37.

[27] Siraisi 1990a; Papy 1999: 324 (citing Fienus's quaestiones).

In the case of medicine, the problem of dealing with internal contradiction became acute after the publication of the much extended corpus of Hippocrates and Galen as well as other ancient medical authors in the Greek: lexical tools such as that of Brasavola revealed the extent of potential disagreements. Opponents of the conciliation technique, of whom the most outspoken is Argenterio, stress its reliance not only on faulty distinction, but on argument *in utramque partem* which in most contexts was forbidden to doctors (see above 4.2): as Theodorus Collado puts it, 'we cannot favour arguments *in utramque partem*; the truth does not support two contraries simultaneously'.[28] As an empirical discipline (at least in part), medicine cannot tolerate factual error or stipulate the truth of events in the way jurists can; this is a fortiori true of such parts of the discipline as anatomy. Conciliation, therefore, sins against the 'vis verborum' (whose purely referential nature must be preserved), the 'vis praeceptorum' or the rules of the art, and furthermore may lead to reality being misrepresented.[29] The last use I have found of Pietro d'Abano's *Conciliator* for teaching purposes is that by Gregor Horst in Giessen in the early years of the seventeenth century: it is respectful of the quaestio structure of the work, but in its additions it carefully transforms this into an account of recent controversies (such as that over the 'morbus totius substantiae': see below 7.5.7) in which one theory is preferred to the rest, and a conciliation does not take place at all.[30]

6.2 ISSUES OF TEXT

I pass now to the text, its language, and to the preparation of texts for the reader by edition, correction and translation. Many of the points made above about the relationship between res and verba in medicine (4.2.1) apply here also. Linguistic issues are not as extensive or as sophisticated as in the case of law, because doctors do not see the need to pay the same amount of attention to the historical sense of words, to proper and improper senses of words, to ambiguity and obscurity, or to the pragmatics and force of language; their concerns are more directly referential.[31] I know of only one locus in Galen (*De differentiis pulsuum*, iii, K 8.680–1) which discusses the use of metaphor as a means of elucidation

---

[28] Collado 1615: 3: 'nos utramque fovere partem non possumus: non enim duo simul sustinet contraria veritas' (citing du Laurens 1595 (i. 5)).
[29] Argenterio 1610: †2v.
[30] Horst 1621.
[31] On these issues in the law see Maclean 1992.

through comparison; against this, there are several which warn against getting too embroiled in discussions about words (see above, 4.2). The substance of discourse is known through conjecture (that is to say, it is grasped through signs, and is inferential in nature); it needs to be protected from having erroneous constructions placed upon it; and so due attention has to be given to the correct meaning of terms. As Argenterio points out in his critique of Galenists like Fuchs, meaning cannot be arbitrarily attributed to Galen's words.[32] The first text methodically to consider revising the meaning attributed to words in medical texts was Leoniceno's *De Plinii erroribus* of 1492. There Leoniceno distinguishes between errors which arise from a confusion of term and referent (one materia medica being confused with another, for example); errors which arise from different names being attributed to the same materia medica, leading to the assumption that more than one such substance exists; and errors which arise from the same name being applied to two different substances. An example of the last category is 'rhabarbarus' which is shown by Leoniceno to refer in Pliny not to the European but to the Indian genus; this correction made sense for the first time of the qualities and curative properties attributed to this plant by ancient authorities.[33] In Fuchs's *Errata* of 1530, a fourth version of referential error (together with these three) is given as the total ignorance of referent.[34] There are also words whose meaning changes over time; but they are not frequently encountered as they are in law; and the distinction between primary and secondary meaning, though occasionally met, is also not a prominent feature of textual discussion.[35] Leoniceno points rather to other forms of terminological error arising from mistranslation, misspelling, the multiplicity of languages being used in one text, and the confusion of words which resemble each other closely (such as 'cissus' and 'cisthus').

[32] Argenterio 1610: 230–1: 'cum ipsi medici sint et Galeni sectatores, debebant non ex suo arbitrio vocabulorum significationes effingere, sed ex solo Gal[eno] eas transcribere'.

[33] Nutton 1997b; Joutsivuo 1999: 24; Bylebyl 1985a; Mugnai Carrara 1999. On the previous puzzlement about the plant's properties, see Arnau de Vilanova 1585: 1682: 'Dioscorides, Galenus, et Avicenna, concorditer ponunt, quod rheubarbarum restringit ventrem, et confert dysenteriae et rupturis; etenim apud nos communis experientia invenit, quod laxat ventrem, et communiter Medici potius utuntur eo ad solvendum, quam ad restringendum'.

[34] Fuchs 1530: 5.

[35] Ottosson 1984: 205 (on 'significatio immediata' as opposed to 'mediata' or 'secundaria'). Somewhat later, the second generation of Paracelsians are keen in a similar way to establish stable senses of technical words in their discourse (as evinced by Adam von Bodenstein's addition to the 1566 edition of the *Opus chyrurgicum*: 'dazu denn auch jetzunder neuwlich kommen ein ausslegunge heimischer Paracelsischer Woerter'), but they do not dwell on these as problems of linguistics; Hieronymus 1995: 104ff. Those hostile to Paracelsianism accuse its adherents of 'abusing' words: Wolf 1620: A4v.

As one would expect from a humanist, the main perpetrators of these errors are said by Leoniceno to be medieval authors such as Albertus Magnus.[36]

6.2.1 Textual criticism

A different set of problems arose in the editing of texts by medical hellenists. Some of the manuscripts edited for the first time in this period were defective or contain illegible or unintelligible passages. The Renaissance genre of 'verisimilia' was devoted to making sense of these. The Greek Galen edition of 1525 generated some philological activity of this kind, which was not always uncontentious.[37] Correction may be, as here, corrections of a text; or it can be correction of fact or of consistency. A genre of such corrective publications grows up in the wake of Leoniceno, which helps promote the healthily critical attitude to all authority by the end of the century. Yet another form of correction at the textual level concerns the identification of spuria; Vives had already pointed to this problem:

> In ancient times grammarians who were erudite, diligent, and well versed in all kinds of author used to make judgements not only about sayings but also whole books . . . as to whether they were written by the person to whom they were ascribed . . . Now, because those good old grammarians have disappeared into obscurity and professors of the major arts have expelled grammar from their classrooms . . . not only inept and stupid words and opinions but also the most sordid and abject works are attributed to the most illustrious group of authors of the past. Aristotle, Plato, Origen, Cyprian, Augustine, Jerome, Boethius, Cicero and Seneca are blamed for writings they would never have dreamed of in their sleep; works unworthy not only of the genius and erudition of such men, but even of their Scythian or Chinese slaves, if they ever had them.[38]

---

[36] Towaide 2000.

[37] Vallesius 1606: 440–52 (on the 'locis manifeste pugnantibus' in Galen, some identified by Lacuna 1551); see also Joutsivuo 1999: 89 (on Leoniceno and new translations of Greek terms).

[38] Quoted by Noreña 1970: 159 (*De disciplinis*, Cologne, 1536, i.1.6): 'olim enim grammatici magna, et multa patenti eruditione, per omnia scriptorum genera diligenter versati, non dicta solum, verum etiam integros libros . . . censebant, essentne, cuius inscriberentur, auctoris . . . nunc vero, quia et grammatici se in tenebras quasdam prostini abdiderunt, et grammaticam professores maiorum artium contubernio suo expulerunt . . . idcirco non modo dicta, et sensa, inepta ac stulta, sed sordidissima quoque, et abiectissima opera genti ac familiae clarissimorum auctorum supponuntur: adscripta sunt Aristoteli, Platoni, Origeni, Cypriano, Hieronymo, Augustino, Boethio, Ciceroni, Senecae, quae ipsis numquam, ne per quietem quidem, in mentem venerunt, indigna quidem non solum tantis ingeniis, atque illa eruditione, sed etiam eorum servis, si quos habuerunt Scythas aut Seres . . .'

Cardano and others act on this critique in the sphere of medicine, and generate a set of rules for separating vera from spuria: the author's own testimony; the witness of contemporaries; the judgement of an expert; stylistic criteria (which are recognised to change over time and over genres).[39] Cardano himself, as well as others, ventures into the murky waters of the corpus Hippocraticum with a view to making a triage.[40]

6.2.2 Translation

Cardano it is also who produces rules for translation: these are very reminiscent of a number of humanist guides to the practice, notably those of Etienne Dolet and Joachim Périon:

> Moderation, to avoid forcing the text too far; a method for distinguishing parts of the text so that everywhere things are made clearer and in each part there is no error; exact grammatical exposition of the words of the text in the same language used by the author [here, Hippocrates]; in the particular sections, the inclusion of something witty or informative.[41]

Unlike Justinian, who specifically prescribes 'foot for foot' translation for jurists as a way of attempting to control the proliferation of interpretative activity,[42] Cardano disapproves of such mechanical literality and thinks that true translation is of the order characterised by the Horatian quotation: 'nec verbum verbo curabit reddere fidus interpres'.[43] It is worthy of note that the printed versions of the *Articella* contained not just one but several translations of major medical texts; one reason for this might be that different translations were in use in different schools, but the editors may also have believed that the collocation of these translations would help fix the sense of difficult passages in the texts.[44]

---

[39] Siraisi 1997: 126.

[40] Siraisi 1999: 348ff.

[41] 1570: 35: 'moderatio ne non nimis plura inculcet; ratio distinguendi partes ut dilucidior ubique habeatur atque hac in parte ferme culpa omni caret; ut verba ad unguem exposuerit grammaticus et in lingua eadem cum Hippocrate exercitatus; ut aliquid in singulis sectionibus salis aut intructus loco inspergat'; see also Worth 1988; also Jardine and Segonds 1999: 208–11 (on Périon); and in general Rener 1989: 88–142.

[42] Maclean 1992: 50–2 (citing D *De confirmatione digestorum* [*tanta*] §20).

[43] *Epistula ad Pisones (Ars poetica)*, 133–4; quoted by Cardano 1568: 15 and Barlandus in Galen 1533: A2–3. Against this Leoniceno preferred verbatim translation and transliteration; Joutsivuo 1999: 27. See also Durling 1961: 238–9, quoting Guinther von Andernach's criticism of the literal translations of Niccolò da Reggio, and his espousal of a translation technique includes both the literal and the adherence to the sense.

[44] See Arrizabalaga 1998.

6.3 AUTHORIAL ISSUES

I pass now from issues concerning the text to those concerning the author. One of these is connected with his moral character, which Cardano links to the principle of charity adopted by the interpreter in approaching texts: one has to believe that it is worthwhile to protect authors from unfair criticism, not only because of the truth of the texts in question but also because of their authors' commitment to them. The issue of the moral status of writers appears quite often in Renaissance polemic; it is implicit in much hostile criticism made for confessional reasons (above, 3.6). It is however conceded that one can be a good author (in the sense of producing sound intellectual doctrine) and have a bad character.[45]

Another issue is that of authorial or subjective meaning as opposed to the objective meaning of words. Galen himself shows his awareness of this issue in an anecdote he relates about the poet Parthenios in his *De sententiis medicorum*, in which the poet comes upon two grammarians who do not know him, and who are discussing the meaning of some of his verses; one who was espousing the meaning the author intended to give to them, the other who was advocating quite another sense, which he claims to Parthenios's face to have from the poet himself.[46] This text seems unfortunately not to have been known to Renaissance readers; but Galen's point here is one that he makes elsewhere, namely that deprived of their author, words as well as books 'habent sua fata'. In his *De libris propriis* and *De ordine librorum suorum*, which had been made newly accessible in Joannes Fichardus's Latin translation of 1531,[47] he discusses what measures might be taken by an author to guarantee the sense of his writings, and deals with topics such as style, intended readership, forms of misrepresentation (interpolation or false attribution, abridgement, alteration), the order of composition of works in a corpus, their contents, and the justification for writing commentaries of the works of others.

6.3.1 The 'ordo legendi libros'

The problems one may encounter in making sense of an author can in part be solved by the order in which one reads his texts; Galen himself offers one such ordering in the *Ars parva*, and another in the *De ordine*

---

[45] Siraisi 1999; 2000.
[46] Lightfoot 1999: 85–7.
[47] Galen 1531: 160–6.

librorum suorum.[48] Such autobiobibliography was imitated by at least one
prominent Renaissance physician as a means of fixing the sense of his
texts.[49] The order of [reading a given author's texts can also lead to the
exclusion of some of these from the corpus, and can have the effect of
creating different authors out of the same corpus of texts: this is the case
of Galen, for example. Depending on whether the *De diebus decretoriis*
is included, he becomes either an astrological doctor or an astrological
sceptic. Ordering suggests a pedagogical as well as thematic sequence,
beginning with the most accessible and ending with the most arcane or
most difficult; but it does not address the question about conflicts of sense
in the same author. Such contradiction can be treated logically, as in the
conciliation literature (6.1.2); this is the line taken by those who wish to
see no error in their favoured author, such as Vallesius or Altomare. But
if inconsistency is found, it has to be dealt with, and here a variety of possibilities emerge in the middle of the century.[50] Galen himself admitted
only to changing his mind on one topic (the order of creation of the organs
of a foetus);[51] but critics such as Argenterio and Lacuna find many more
inconsistencies than this. Because Galen wrote 'almost infinite volumes',
claims Argenterio, he must have made many statements without thinking them through.[52] Even his use of terms designating disease, passion,
action, disposition, 'affectus' can be shown to be inconsistent. The different pedagogical approaches he adopted in different works led to different
doctrines; he was negligent in composition of his works; what he said,
though copious and long-winded, was often incomplete.[53]

6.3.2 Internal contradiction and interauthorial contradiction

Those who want to salvage as much authority as possible from his writings
do so by a number of strategies. Some distinguish his early from his late

---

[48] Galen, *Ars parva*, K 1.407–12; Joutsivuo 1999: 18 (on the *Articella* and order of reading Galen,
referring to Iskandar 1976), 155 (on da Monte); Gentile da Foligno in *Articella* 1529: 155–6;
Arrizabalaga 1998: 32, 59; Sylvius 1539b; Siraisi 1997: 141 (on Cardano); Mugnai Carrara 1999:
258–9 (on da Monte's prefatory letters of 1541 and 1550 to the Giunti edition of Galen).

[49] Cardano followed him (and Erasmus) in this: see Maclean 1999a.

[50] It is interesting to note from the evidence of marginal notes that the practice of reading illustrated
books involves the conferring of one text with another, and not the conferring of the illustration
with the text: see Kusukawa forthcoming a.

[51] See *De substantia facultatum naturalium*: also the sequential entries in Brasavola's Index to Galen
(Brasavola 1556: 203: 'Galenus semper eadem de eisdem asserebat', referring to *Ad Thrasybulum*;
'Galenus mutavit sententiam pro melioribus', referring to *De antidotis*, i).

[52] Argenterio 1606–7: 2.1 '[Galenus] semel posita principia perpetuo servare non videtur'; Temkin
1973: 151–2.

[53] Siraisi 1990a; also Siraisi forthcoming.

writing, and attribute authority to the latter.[54] This is what Fernel does over a contradiction on intermittent fevers between *De crisibus*, ii and *De differentiis febrium*, ii. Fernel determines the former text to be the work of young Galen (on what evidence is not clear: in his *De libris propriis* Galen does not say in which order he wrote them, but this order seems to be implied by Gentile da Foligno in the *Articella*).[55] Silvaticus also accepts that Galen contradicts himself, although he allows Galen an escape clause by saying that sometimes he does not speak 'absolutely': that is to say, that he offered only plausible views on some occasions.[56] Sanctorius goes further than this and claims that in respect of astrology Galen was not seriously putting forward views, displacing thereby the epistemological problem of 'probabilitas' on to the moral ground of commitment.[57] Others suggest that a writer's authority can be preserved by imagining how he would have reacted if he had been exposed to relevant experience or knowledge: Sanctorius suggests in this way that Aristotle would not have made health and sickness an immediate contrary (see below 7.5) if he had been a practising doctor.[58] Others adopt the strategy of identifying spuria and dubia: the Galen Latin edition does this, and there is a great deal of writing in the second half of the century on the authenticity of parts of the Hippocratic corpus, which involves claiming 'Hippocrates' to be a name common to several authors to whom works can be separately attributed.[59] This activity effectively configures the author to the scholar's

---

[54] See above, p. 217.

[55] Fernel 1610a: 3.115 (*De abditis rerum causis*, ii.13 [Eudoxus]): 'Haec [statements about fever] sunt quae a Galeno iuvene pronunciata haud quaquam receperim: quandoquidem tum aetatis non aliam sedem humoribus quam venas designabat, in quibus vel illi putrescerent, vel illinc in corporis habitum irrumperent. Caeterum aetate et rerum observatione iam maturior, secundo de differentiis febrium anxie admodum causam investigans intermittentium, et cur hae circuitione quadam repetant, aliam his originem aliumque fomitem instituit'; see also Lonie 1981: 32.

[56] Silvaticus 1601: 298: 'Galenum manifeste seipsum refutasse.'

[57] Wear 1981: 256, quoting Sanctorius, *Commentaria in 1 Fen i*, Venice, 1626, 79: 'illum librum esse factum propter curiosos'. The Galenic authority for this is *De diebus decretoriis*, K 9.934: 'illum tertium librum invito scripsisse, id est precibus quorundam amicorum', to which Sanctorius adds: 'scilicet curiosorum, non ut fidem aliquam his nugis, sed ut aliquid auribus stultorum daret'.

[58] See Joutsivuo 1999: 104 (quoting Sanctorius, *Commentaria in artem medicinalem Galeni*, Venice, 1630, 85b–c: 'Verum, si Aristoteles egisset de arte medica sine dubio sanitatem divisisset in sanitatem firmam et lubricam, si voluisset scientifice, et ex arte medicinam docere'). Cf. Maclean 1992: 144ff. (on recreating the sense of a legislator by imagining him in the (new) circumstances in which his law is to be interpreted).

[59] Nutton 1989; Siraisi 1999; 1997: 126 (referring to Girolamo Mercuriale, *Censura Hippocratis*, Basle, 1584), 135; Ulmus 1603. Cardano 1663: 6.337, cited by Grafton and Siraisi forthcoming, describes the *De diebus decretoriis* as so puerile that it cannot be by Galen; see also Joutsivuo 1999: 83, 88n.

taste, and is a demonstration of the mastery of the interpreter of the
parent text of which he declares himself to be the servant.

6.3.3 Contradiction with experience

It is also possible for an author to contradict the experience of a reader
(that is, to be measured against an empirical criterion). Galen shrewdly
parries this line of attack by suggesting that although readers might find
a counter-example in their own experience to his text, his conclusions
are not necessarily threatened, as he based them not on one but on many
examples.[60] The most common clash is not that between textual claims
and individual experience but that between statements, evidence and
arguments produced by various authors, of which there are too many:
'infinita est scribentium turba', as Vives points out.[61] If laborious conciliation is not adopted as a strategy in such cases, then the real 'inimicitas'
between texts has to be confronted.[62] One solution to this is to adopt different authorities for different disciplines; this had been recommended
by Albertus Magnus.[63] In this way Galen and Hippocrates can offer
solutions which are authoritative in the conjectural and instrumental art
of medicine, and Aristotle in the science of natural philosophy. We might
compare this to the 'Papinian rule' of the lawyers, who have a means of
resolving an ambiguity by identifying an authority who is to be followed
in the last instance.[64] Sanctorius affords an example of this in medicine
by alleging that in doubtful cases of this kind, Aristotle is to be taken as the
final arbiter.[65] Sometimes another rule, also familiar to jurists from the
Theodosian code, is invoked; namely, that one should accept the majority view on any issue, as does Valleriola in respect of the controversy over
causes (below, 7.5.4).[66] Sometimes a hierarchy of authorities is established by the principle that either the most ancient, or the most recent is
to be accorded the most credence:[67] by the former of these rules, Vesalius

---

[60] *De anatomicis administrationibus*, i.ii, K 2.278–9.

[61] Noreña 1970: 154; Maclean 1992: 32 (on trusting one authority only).

[62] Siraisi 1990a: 168–9 (quoting Argenterio 1610: †2v).

[63] García Ballester 1995: 147 (citing Albertus Magnus, *Super 2 Sent 27* on following Aristotle in natural philosophy and Galen and Hippocrates in medicine).

[64] Maclean 1992: 58, 93, 118.

[65] Siraisi 1987a: 269 (citing Sanctorius, *Commentaria in ii Canonis*, Venice, 1646, 162–4); see also Joutsivuo 1999: 80–1.

[66] Theodosian Code, 1.4.1; Valleriola 1577: 379–80, asking how can Fuchs alone be right in his view if Sylvius, Fernel, Akakia, Thriverus, Argenterio, da Monte, Arabs and yet others are all agreed on another.

[67] Rogerius 1584: 1.387v (xxvi); Noreña 1970: 155 (citing Vives's refutation of the proposition that 'the older the author, the more credit he has').

is trumped by Galen according to Sylvius, as is Fernel (in the latter case not only in conclusions but also in argument); by the latter, Riolan the Elder, although a traditionalist, is able to follow Falloppia rather than Galen.[68]

6.4 ISSUES OF READERS AND READING

I come now to the theories or methods of interpretation based on methods of reading. These are not as extensive or as sophisticated as in the case of law. Like the author, the reader has to be endowed with intelligence and moral goodness; those who misread are, according to Altomare and Cardano, either stupid or malicious; they are referring here to a topos from Aristotle's *Rhetoric* (ii.1, 1378 a).[69] The moral quality of reader and author is therefore a mode of successfully conveying the sense of a text through the principle of charity ('scribere/legere in bonam partem').[70] Sometimes general advice is given on how to read, as well as in what order: Cardano recommends that one should begin by marking off the useless or redundant passages (so that one can skip them the second time round) and the obscure ones (to be studied at length at a later date) and concentrate on the 'continuitas sermonis' (by which I take him to mean the broad context of a sentence, paragraph and argument); in this way error can be avoided.[71] Some authors comment on the way to produce and use indexes, and the usefulness to the reader of tables and diagrams is noted.[72] Some evidence of how this advice is taken up may be derived from the marginalia left behind by contemporary readers. These may be minimal (a few underlinings, the provision of chapter headings, rubrics indicating topics), or more copious, reflecting in some cases the humanist practices of identifying quotations and extracting

---

[68] Temkin 1973: 142; Bylebyl 1985a: 234 (citing Riolan).

[69] Altomare 1574: *2r ('quod [hoc opus] si qui pertinacia adducti, aut malevolentia potius suffusi, audeant contradicere, sciant non mihi sed Galeno se contradicturos, qui cum errasse malo, quam ad aliorum mentem recte sapere'); also the title of Cardano's *Actio prima* of 1559, where he identifies the critics of his *De subtilitate* as either 'stulti' or 'malitiosi'. There is a milder version in Crusius 1615: 188, who in defending Paracelsus refers to the 'legentis inhabilitas'. The full title of Dannhauer's hermeneutic treatise of 1630 is *Idea boni interpretis et malitiosi calumniatoris, quae obscuritate dispulsa, verum sensum a falso discernere in omnibus auctorum scriptis ac orationibus docet, et plene respondit ad quaestionem unde scis hunc esse sensum et non alium.*

[70] Maclean 1998b: 181–2 (on Rabelais and the principle of charity).

[71] Cardano 1568: 462 (ii.74), quoted below, note 94; Siraisi 1997: 53 (citing Cardano 1663: 1.31).

[72] Kusukawa 1998: 133–6; but Argenterio calls them 'vanas et falsas tabulas et figuras': 1606–7: 250–1, and Cesalpino thinks that words are better than pictures to express the differentiae of plants: Jensen 2000: 194.

loci, in others supplying evidence for or against an argument, and giving additional bibliographical data.[73]

6.4.1 Commentary

Most attention is paid to modes of approaching and writing commentaries. For long, Galen was seen as a model in this genre, so much so that a diligent Renaissance editor went to the trouble of forging one of his missing Hippocratic commentaries.[74] As one might expect, the advice not to read commentaries at all and to return to the original text is not infrequently found; Pomponazzi pointed out to his pupils that many commentaries are hindrances rather than aids to the understanding of a text, and Girolamo Borro's seventh cause of human ignorance in his treatise *Multae sunt nostrarum ignorationum causae* of the late sixteenth century arises from the neglect of the [parent] text and the erroneous pursuit of the expositions of it by others.[75] Borro also notes however that it is commentators themselves who denounce commentary; indeed, it seems that the practice of 'enarratio', 'expositio' and 'explanatio' was an unavoidable by-product of both scholastic and humanist culture.

Among the first to reflect on commentary in the medieval period was Arnau de Vilanova (in respect of Hippocrates's *Aphorisms*), who writes as follows about it:

The complete exposition of any aphorism or text consists in three things: the first is to explain the mind or intention of the author; the second is to show the truth of what he said; and the third is to reveal the usefulness of the text. The first is done by interpreting the significant words which the author uses in expressing his thoughts; the second by a lucid consideration of the signified things of which he speaks; and the third is achieved by appropriate application of his text to the practice of the art in which he is instructing his listeners. The first two are accomplished by forming propositions ('sententiando') and construing the text itself; the third is added to fill out the brevity of the aphorism or text. It is however useful to know that in expounding or dealing with an aphorism in these ways, the

---

73 Sherman 1995: 53–78.
74 Siraisi 2000: 9; also Grafton and Siraisi forthcoming, citing Cardano 1663: 5.93–4.
75 Perfetti 1999b: 301 (quoting Pomponazzi). Girolamo Borro's seventh cause reads: 'de negligentia textuum scripsit Averroes tertio de anima commentatione contra Avicennam et contra semetipsum, dum dixit, "quod fecit istum hominem errare et nos etiam longo tempore fuit, quia moderni dimittunt libros Aristotelis et considerant libros expositorum"'; quoted in Schmitt 1976a: 475. Borro's awareness of the self-destructive nature of the criticism by Averroes of others is noteworthy. Siraisi forthcoming argues that Fernel, in constructing his textbook of medicine along novel lines, was effectively doing away with a commentary and thereby creating the space for new topics such as celestial spiritus and 'morbi totius substantiae'.

expositor is not permitted to exceed what is in the logic of any statement in the aphorism, or to interpret extensively its words; its terms have prescribed limits beyond which one should not extrapolate the text. The force and logic of the aphorism or text reveal these limits: the force of the text is known from its subject matter, the logic from its form or style. The expositor should extend his interpretation only so far as is sanctioned by these two elements [matter and form].[76]

What Arnau sets out here is a sequence of procedures – the 'subtilitas intelligendi', 'subtilitas explicandi' and 'subtilitas applicandi' which is usually attributed to J. J. Rambach writing more than four centuries later.[77] Arnaus's practice includes syllogistic reduction; this is found also in Italy, where there were later recognised schools of commentary, the 'via Gentilis', and the 'via plusquam commentatoris'. Gentile da Foligno, the eponymous practitioner of the former, was known as the 'speculator' because of his 'subtilissimae quaestiones' and Thomistic analysis of the logic underlying the text;[78] the 'plusquam commentator', Pietro Torrigiano, does not recognise the limits placed on interpretation by Arnau, but freely admits to his use of the parent text as an excuse to expand not just on the 'brevitas aphorismi' but on the doctrine itself, thereby arrogating to himself his sobriquet:

And because we have not only set out to comment on Galen's meaning ('mentem') but have also strayed to other matters which are of use to doctors, we have called this exposition a 'plusquam commentum'.[79]

---

[76] Arnau de Vilanova 1585: 1677: 'Perfecta expositio cuiuslibet aphorismi, et cuiuslibet documenti consistit in tribus: quorum unum est mentem, vel intentionem auctoris explicare; secundum est dictorum eius veritatem ostendere; tertium est utilitatem documenti manifestare. Primum fit per interpretationem vocum significantium, quibus auctor utitur in exprimendo conceptum suum; secundum per claram considerationem rerum significatarum, de quibus idem loquitur; tertium fit per congruam applicationem eius documenti ad exercitium artis, in quo imbuit auditores. Duo prima complentur sententiando, et literam construendo, tertium autem post haec duo subiungitur ad supplendam brevitatem aphorismi, vel documenti. Est tamen utile sciendum, quod in exponendo, vel tractando aphorismum praedictis modis, non licet expositori, quantum est de ratione declarationis aphorismi, quemlibet excedere, vel prolongare sermones suos; sed praefixi sunt ei termini, ultra quos procedere non oportet sua documenta. Illos autem terminos indicat vis et ratio aphorismi, vel documenti: vis documenti cognoscitur ex materia, de qua loquitur; ratio ex forma, vel modo docendi. Unde quanta ista duo tolerant, tantum debet extendi expositio.'

[77] J. J. Rambach, *Institutiones hermeneuticae sacrae* (Jena, 1743); see also Gadamer 1962: 290–1: 'man unterschied eine subtilitas intelligendi, das Verstehen, von einer subtilitas explicandi, dem Auslegen, und im Pietismus fügte man dem als drittes Glied die subtilitas applicandi, das Anwenden, hinzu (z.B. bei J. J. Rambach)'.

[78] See Torrigiano 1557: 2211–40; French 1985b: 21–3. He is known also for the doctrine that medical speculation does not transcend sense impressions.

[79] Joutsivuo 1999: 16, 22–3, 33–4, 41 (this quotation): 'et quoniam in hac dictione nostra non solum mentem Galeni proposuimus commentari, sed saepe digredientes aliqua incipimus, medicis non inutilia scitu, ideo plusquam commentum expositionem hanc appellavimus'; French 1985a: 50,

Siraisi suggests that the growth in the number and scope of medical commentaries in the Renaissance can be accounted for by a number of factors: the philological interests of humanists; the new translations of Greek works; the new religious and educational institutions; and emulation of biblical and patristic scholarship.[80] The guarantee of a good commentary is that it is written 'ex mente auctoris'; but this is acknowledged to be a construction.[81] As Cardano cynically observes, commentaries can be more informative about the commentator than about the author.[82] Notwithstanding this opinion, he himself not only wrote a number of commentaries but also expatiated over a number of years on the aims of exegesis. Argenterio, the acerbic critic of philological approaches to medicine and of Galen himself, also produces guidance for textual analysis, but this is largely negative and implicit, and is directed against authors and their authority where this is based on inconsistency, error, logical contradiction, incompleteness, negligence, long-windedness or false methodology. He neither produces Cardano's explicit order of operations on a text, nor does he elaborate a syllogistic justification for interpretation as a science in Aristotelian terms, as Dannhauer was to do later in his *Idea boni interpretis* of 1630, which was written to offer guidance to all branches of learning.[83]

From the outset, Cardano argues that commentary should be looked upon as a noble pursuit, partly because great scholars have engaged in it, and partly for a more ethical reason.[84] Certain kinds of knowledge – those associated with the arts such as medicine, which have an empirical component, with religion and its ceremonies, and with the history of nations and their leaders – can only be conserved in textual form;[85] for

citing Taddeo Alderotti's reference to *expositio* as a light to bring out the colours of a text. See Mugnai Carrara 1999: 257–8 (Manardo's attack on the 'plusquam commentator').

80 Siraisi 1987a: 176.

81 E.g. Bartolettus 1619: 255–9, who constructs an argument 'ex mente Galeni' (in the absence of texts he can cite). Argenterio 1606–7: 10 accuses some of his colleagues of putting forward explanatory opinions about other people's books and constructing a new sense never thought of by the author; see Siraisi 1990a: 168.

82 Maclean 1998a: 163; Siraisi 1997: 147, both citing Cardano 1663: 8.251.

83 Siraisi 1990a: 171. Whereas Cardano concerns himself with the interpretation of portents (albeit without the same constraints as he set himself as a commentator), Argenterio seems to want to have no dealings with them. The attribution of a theological, social or moral significance to monstrous or rare events precisely requires the suppression of rational procedures of interpretation which marks also the correspondence theory of signatures (below 8.8.6); this theory elides in a similar way the mediating function of mental or linguistic discourse, as critics of Paracelsianism point out: Bartolettus 1619: 259ff.

84 Cardano 1663: 1.58.

85 The 'empirical component' of medicine is the discovery by trial and error of remedies, which needs to be preserved in written form for future generations: Cardano 1663: 1.149: 'tria enim sunt

this reason, commentators and interpreters have to 'strain every muscle' to explain their texts correctly and fully according to a proper theory of transmission.[86] He believed that a professor of medicine should provide sound expositions of the set texts of the medical course, and began by elaborating his own theory of commentary in contradistinction to that of Galen. He accuses his illustrious predecessor of being indifferent to the truth value of a text, and of seeing the commentator's role as being nothing more than a grammarian, an expositor of the meaning of words.[87] Cardano insists that one needs to explain the 'mens' of an author, give a general account of his subject matter, and then unite these two. This entailed a commitment to the view that texts can be reduced to univocal meanings and that authors only write that which is worthy of note and not generally known, and do so without redundancy of expression or repetition.[88] This doctrine is combined with a rather strange version of the psychology of reading for which he was attacked by contemporaries:

The intellect is the thing itself which is understood, such that when I understand a horse, my mind is the form of a horse . . . For the intellect is of itself entirely separated from the body. For while I am at present writing these things, my mind is those things which you are understanding by my writing: when I write about medical matters, it is medicine; when I wrote about numbers, it was then number, and it follows necessarily that this happens to all others who write on diverse topics, so that while I am re-reading my writings, I seem to myself to be different from what I now am.[89]

quae vecordiae mortalium, perire sinentium bonas artes ac scripta, obstant: Rerum ipsarum inventio, velut Medicinae, quam necesse est constare scriptis, quod ars sit necessaria: ideo culta, et longa, ob id ut sensim augeatur, et Religio, quae caeremonias scriptis mandari vult, ut conserventur; Et principum studia, qui famam, gesta, vitam historiis consecrari cupiunt: his tribus tanquam principiis, res literaria constat.' See also Siraisi 1999.

86 Cardano 1663: 1.81, 122–3.

87 Siraisi 1997: 123 (citing Cardano 1663: 5.110, 257); Grafton and Siraisi forthcoming, citing Cardano 1663: 5.93–4. See also Cardano 1663: 8.513, quoted by Siraisi 1997: 295–6: 'adeo ut ausus sit dicere primo de Fracturis commentatoris officium non esse demonstrare quae dicuntur ab auctore esse vera, aut illum a calumniatoribus tueri, posse tamen nos id facere. Et alibi: "Officium boni expositoris non esse demonstrationes dictorum afferre sed solum quae ab illo dicta sunt verba explicare." Interrogo te, o Galene, in quo opus est medico ad interpretationem librorum medicinae si solum verba auctoris sunt explicanda? Nam si de dictionibus agendum est ac sensibus grammatici hoc opus est.'

88 Siraisi 1997: 135; also Siraisi 2000: 12 (on similar commitments by Girolamo Mercuriale). This contrasts with the view expressed by Pomponazzi about alternative readings or interpretations: see Perfetti 1999a: 459.

89 Cardano 1663: 3.583–4: 'intellectus res est ipsa, quae intelligitur. Veluti cum equum intelligo: intellectus meus est forma equus . . . ipse enim intellectus omnino a corpore per se separatus est. Nunc enim dum haec scribo, meus intellectus est ea quae per scripta tu intelligis: dumque medica pertracto, medicina; dum de numeris scriberem, tunc numerus erat, adeo quod aliis omnibus qui diversa scripserunt evenire necesse est, ut dum mea relego scripta, alius mihi

This sounds more neoplatonist than Aristotelian, and is difficult to reconcile with his claim that whereas in writing books one must obey nothing other than the imperative of truth, as an expositor one is held to reproduce the meaning of an author.[90] Yet what if the host text is wrong? I do not know of a place in which Cardano confronts this problem, although he is not above using the distinction between writing (the truth) and exposition (of the views of others) to get himself out of apparent contradiction.[91] One solution to his problem would be only to write commentaries on the texts of authors who got everything right; but this runs counter to his view (recorded above) that scholarship can be revised as well as being added to.

In his *De libris propriis* of 1562, he puts forward four guiding principles for practising commentary: one must first declare the sense of the author; then demonstrate in what way things are as he says they are; next amplify this; and finally defend him against unfair criticism (while accepting that he can make the occasional slip, for 'quandoque bonus dormitat Homerus').[92] He amplifies these principles in various ways. A commentator must communicate the style, words and senses of an author in a 'familiar' way; he must mediate his argument (i.e. demonstrate its structure); he must show how his logic works, and show that his thought is unified, for, just as Pascal would say a century later, an author must have a sense to which all the parts of his argument relate, or he makes no sense at all.[93] But he must also have knowledge of the 'continuitas textus seu sermonis' (that is to say, he must know what goes before and comes after the passage in question) which reveals the intention of the

---

fuisse videat ab illo qui nunc sum.' This passage, possibly inspired by the claim in the *De anima* that the mind can become all things (iii.5, 430 a 15), is mercilessly satirised by Scaliger who sets down a more conventional exegesis of the passage from the *De anima* (which concerns the self-consciousness of the mind of its own activity) and makes a rather predictable joke about it: 'intellectus Cardani est equi forma: ergo Cardanus equus est'; Scaliger 1592: 929–33 (xxxvii.6–7). According to Scaliger, Cardano is mistaken because the intellect only becomes the object of its scrutiny 'modo similitudinis et receptionis', and 'sola accidentia speciem efficiunt in intellectu'. On this see Maclean 1999b.

90 Cardano 1663: 1.139: 'in conscribendo libros scopus est, rei veritas; in explicandis autem libros aliorum, auctoris sententia'.

91 *Ibid.*, 3.390, quoted by Maclean 1984: 237.

92 Cardano 1663: 1.139: 'quatuor igitur sunt munia boni expositoris: auctoris mentem declarare, demonstrare quod ita sit quod dicitur, amplificare illius doctrinam, et tueri ipsum a calumniatoribus'; see also Siraisi 1997: 135, who quotes Cardano making a lesser claim; and Cardano 1663: 1.81, 122. The quotation about Homer is from Horace, *Epistula ad Pisones* (*Ars poetica*), 359.

93 Pascal 1963: 533 (*Pensées*, L257): 'tout auteur a un sens auquel tous les passages contraires s'accordent, ou il n'a point de sens du tout'; cf. Cardano 1663: 1.139: 'Sed si uni illi non omnia conveniant, scias te nondum mentem auctoris assecutum.'

author.[94] The context in which the author's thought must be placed is first that of the part of the work being discussed, then that of the whole work, finally in that of the whole oeuvre of the author.[95] A yet different (possibly later) exposition of his method finds him stressing first the relationship of the author's words to *empirical* confirmation of them as well as the general theory of the author, next, the need to spell out the implications of the text (to complete what is incomplete ('imperfectum')); then the need to clarify obscurities, to resolve any possible contradictions, and to supplement the author's arguments wherever possible. Here, even if he goes further than Galen in revealing the potential of the text, Cardano does not principally confront the author with the truth, but with consistency with himself.[96]

His most elaborate attempt to set down the rules of commentary and exegesis is to be found in his highly original *Dialectica* which appeared in 1566, which Johannes Albertus (Wimpinaeus) faithfully reproduces and uses in his own work *De concordia Hippocraticorum et Paracelsistarum libri Magni excursiones defensivae*, of 1615.[97] Cardano associates these rules with the name of Ptolemy, and describes the practice which they regulate as 'naturalis conjectura'.[98] We may note here a strange omission; there is no reference to the popular metaphor that nature was to be read like a book.[99] He uses Hippocrates 'who especially is worthy of being read first because of the clarity and profundity of his meaning'[100] to illustrate his method, which proceeds as follows: first expound the 'simplicem et universalem sensum'; then determine the meanings of obscure words to avoid nonsense. Thereafter seek the 'ratio' which we can easily find because the author would have proffered nothing without reason, redundantly or flippantly, knowing it to be absurd (the rule of economy)

---

[94] Cardano 1568: 462 (ii.74): 'cognitio continuitatis sermonis intellectu eorum, quae scribuntur, maxime pendet. Neque ego explanatori fidem adhibebo, qui rationem continuitatis textus non docuerit: nam neque illum intellexisse verisimile est authoris sententiam neque sine illa intellegi posse sperabimus: aut si non est in sensibus continuitas, quid est, quod teramus tempus in authore legendo, aut interpretando, qui a natura operibus alienissimus sit, cum illa nulli magis rei, quam continuationi operum suorum studuisse videatur.' Cf. the comments of Pascal on the 'économie de l'ouvrage' cited above (ch. 5, note 177). A possible source for Cardano is Cicero, *Disputationes tusculanae*, v.10.31: 'non igitur singulis vocibus philosophi spectandi sunt, sed ex perpetuitate atque constantia'; this is cited by Piccartus 1595: BIV.
[95] Cardano 1663: 1.139; also *ibid.*, 147 on 'genera scribendi'.
[96] *Ibid.*, 70.
[97] Albertus 1615: 3–5.
[98] Cardano 1663: 1.307.
[99] See Bono 1995.
[100] Cardano 1663: 1.303: 'qui praecipue ob claritatem et profunditatem sensuum dignus est legi primum'.

nor without it being consistent with experience and with the rest of his text (the rule of charity with respect to autopsy; the rule of internal coherence). We may obtain this 'ratio' from the mode of reasoning used by the author. Once this has been found, a number of operations follow:

> To submit to division, to reassemble, to amplify, to take excerpts, occasionally to call into question, to examine by means of the four causes, to apply it those things which pertain to it or which can be deduced from it, to compare with its opposites or to set out other things which are similar; thereafter one may refute the opinions which are contrary to the text. Then to teach its application, and finally to summarise everything in an epilogue.[101]

Cardano claims (through his commentaries written in this mode) to have stood out from the common run of exegetes, to have attracted admiration, and to have achieved a rich discussion of the text not so much through the authority of the great man who wrote it as by internalising and reproducing his deep and complex reasoning. We may especially note here the stress on the correctness of the text with respect to experience, and the importance of analysing the work according to correct mental norms of reasoning; and it is finally worthy of note that he refers not only to amplifying the text with illustrations but also excerpting or perhaps deleting passages from it and even disagreeing with it on occasions. A critical space has been opened up for the commentator. One can again point to the fundamental irreconcilability in his writing between a Platonic notion of thought and mental activity, a belief in human progress, and a highly developed awareness of the uncertain deductive bases (or fallible inferences) and the semiological procedures of certain arts such as diagnosis and dream interpretation;[102] these tensions are perceptible in the following passage from the 1562 version of his *De libris propriis*, written a decade after the passage on the same subject from the *De subtilitate* quoted above:[103]

> It is a very great pleasure for men to look at themselves as in a mirror, for the mirror which sends back to us our bodily image fills us with delight; yet the body is not part of us, but just the vehicle of ourselves. For man is altogether a spiritual

---

[101] *Ibid.*, 304: 'dividere, componere, amplificare, excipere, raro dubitare, per quatuor genera causarum examinare, applicare quae ad id pertinent vel quae ex illo deduci possunt, contraria contrariis comparare aut eadem aliorum exponere, tum etiam opiniones quae sententiae illi adversantur confutare licebit; demum tradere etiam ad opus, ac ultimo per viam epilogi colligere'.

[102] See Siraisi 1997: 174–91, and Le Brun 1994.

[103] See above, note 83; see also Cardano 1663: 1.76–7, 101 on how we know that we know, and the time delay implied in knowing that we know, and on 'reflexa proportio' in mathematics.

being ('anima'). Thus, when we read our writings, we contemplate ourselves as in a mirror. Moreover, the image of a body when absent dies away; but the image of our souls remains in the books, as though the author were still there; which is why you can perhaps compare books to pictures . . . but writings are different from pictures and statues, which are able to be seen by everyone, as immortal is different from mortal; for writings are renewed, and when translated [from one context to another] increase their authority; images die.[104]

A neoplatonist psychology of this kind seems on the one hand to leave no role for a history of meanings or for their mediation; yet on the other it specifically refers to the translation of meanings from one historical context to another, and their 'increase in authority'. This interest in psychology marks a clear difference from the doctrine on commentary recommended by Arnau de Vilanova two and half centuries before, as does the avoidance of specifically syllogistic analysis, and the requirements that the author be placed in the context of his own works and that his dicta be supported with empirical evidence.

6.4.2 Anthologisation: loci

The new critical space opened up for the commentator is especially noticeable in the matter of anthologisation, or fragmentation into loci; this has been studied as a humanist practice by Ann Moss and Francis Goyet, and described as a distinctive component of Renaissance philosophy by Eckhard Kessler, who sees in it a liberation from 'auctoritas' in the older sense and a discovery of the possibility of new configurations of argument.[105] In this he has the support of Vives, who warns that the process of citing authorities (including medical authorities) from florilegia removed their dicta from their original context and hence their true sense: 'How can the meanings of authors be understood if they are deprived and destitute of what can be said to be their basis in what went before and what comes after?'[106] But the extraction of loci is also looked

---

[104] *Ibid.*, 130: 'maxima voluptas est hominibus cum seipsos velut in speculo contemplantur: nam speculum cum corporis tantum effigie[m] referat, magna tamen cum voluptate nos afficit: tametsi corpus pars nulla est nostri, sed tanquam vehiculum solum. Etenim homo totus vere anima est. Scripta igitur nostra cum legimus, nos ipsos intuemur velut in speculo ipso. Adde quod effigies corporis ipso absente decedit: imago autem animae manet in libros, etiamsi homo ipse non adsit: quare forsan melius libros picturis et statuis comparaveris . . . distant praeterea scripta a picturis et statuis, quod in omnium conspectu sint: et ut immortale a mortali: nam scripta renovantur, augentque autoritatem translata: imagines amittunt.' Also Le Brun 1994.

[105] Moss 1996; Goyet 1996; Kessler 1999.

[106] Noreña 1970: 161, quoting *De disciplinis*, i.i.8. The full passage reads: 'Ita nunc Hieronymus, August[inus] Chrysost[omus] et prisci illi ac primi religionis nostrae scriptores, non ex suis

upon as a much admired ability: 'it is a sign of uncommon skill to perceive the mind and genius of authors from their scattered writings', as Sulcer writes.[107] In medicine, it is not a practice which generates unanimity. Whereas in law, anthologies of lemmata are nearly all consistent with one another, Galen's vast output and Brasavola's index giving piecemeal access to it meant that new Galens could be constructed by doctors. When, in the 1530s, Sylvius and Fuchs independently created dichotomous accounts of Galen's semiology by bringing together his various texts on the topic and excerpting from them, they come up with very different constructions; much later, in 1619, Bartolettus claims to have produced a quite different synthetic account from that of Argenterio who deliberately reconfigured the same texts in the 1550s in a way different from his predecessors of the 1530s.[108] Lacuna's epitome of all of Galen's work of 1571 is in itself an ingenious and original anthology; Valleriola's *Loci medicinae communes* of 1562 performs the same operation on the text in a different (more systematic) way, with different results. These variations undermine the claims of commentary to be determined exclusively by the parent text. The tendency to reconfigure the text and to alter its logical structures can be further exacerbated by the incipient Renaissance practice of including examples drawn from the commentator's own experience or reading of the consilia of others. This is especially true of commentaries in the practica tradition on such texts as the *Aphorisms* and *Epidemics* where the functions served by the commentary are not only pedagogical but also connected with the needs of practising physicians.[109] In all these ways, medical commentators may be said to become not the servants but the masters of the texts on which they write.

ipsorum monimentis cognoscuntur, sed ex collectaneis sententiarum Petri Lombardi, ex *Catena aurea* Divi Thomae, et aliis rhapsodiis eius notae: nacti sunt et medici suos decerptores flosculorum ex libris Galeni, Hippocratis, Avicennae: consuit centones jurisconsultorum Tribonianus; detruncatus est Lutetiae Aristoteles et traditus vix dimidiatus. Ne sic quidem breviaria haec lectores inveniunt, longum existimatur ea percurrere, sit satis indices aut rubricas inspexisse . . . qui possunt auctorum sensus percipi, deserti et destituti suis velut fulcimentis, nempe iis quae antecedunt, quaeque subsequuntur?'

[107] Manlius 1563: a8v: 'non autem vulgaris est artificis, ex lectione varia animadvertere spiritum et genium authorum'.

[108] See above 1.5.1. Bartolettus 1619: 259 claims that Argenterio confused necessary and contingent, soluble and insoluble and demonstrative and probable: i.e. that he was logically in error; Wear 1973: 249–50 quotes Argenterio 1606–7: 6 as being aware of the *hermeneutic* risk of what he was doing: 'spectamus enim in rebus probandis non quid ratio, et sensus nostri, quos natura nobis ad rerum cognitionem dedit, docere possint: sed quid Aristoteles, Galenus et quod deleterius est quilibet alius de ea re scripserit, illorum sententias colligimus, et libros nostros consarcimus, et detestanda temeritate edimus, laboramus praeter modum in authoribus conciliandis, quod nullus unquam ex praestantissimis authoribus fecit'.

[109] Siraisi 1997: 121ff.; 206–7.

6.5 CONCLUSIONS

6.5.1 Comparison with law

It may be helpful at this point to draw some comparisons with legal interpretation; some of these are noted by sixteenth-century writers. It is widely acknowledged that 'argumentum ab auctoritate est fortissimum in lege' and more frequently encountered there and in theology than in medicine.[110] Medicine, being an art relying on probabilities, facts and inference (or, more specifically, reasoning from effect to cause: see above 4.3.6), is determined not by dogmas, but by contingent 'res'. Thus historical meaning does not really apply, any more than historical intention; the construction of argument and the determination of reference is more important. Authorial meaning is only of value if it is consistent with logic and empirical fact. An indication of this is found in Sanctorius, whose *Methodi vitandorum errorum* is a set of precepts which, it is claimed, are scientific and not contingent and which at the same time are resolutely applied to contingent situations. Sanctorius's title may remind us of the legal maxim that 'negative commands bind without reference to time and place, but positive commands with respect to time and place';[111] but in fact there is no strong parallel to be drawn with such works as Herculanus's *De negativa probanda* because in medicine the positive context, which in law is verbal in character, is not dependent in any sense on words and intentions. So while there is self-evidence in medicine (7.1), it is not what is meant by 'plain meaning' in law but rather Aristotelian experientia.[112] Even though authority is cited in medicine, it is not anything more than the value of experience and reason combined; and even though there is signification through which medicine shares a linguistic structure with juristical inference from words to meaning, and thereby a hermeneutic character (in the sense of reading the world-book as a surface and its sense as a depth), this is not stipulative (see below 8.9.1); even though there are questions of verbal propriety, ambiguity and obscurity, these are all subordinate to the primary rule of reality, as Rodericus a Castro points out: lawyers depend only on other writings and on words, but doctors must be consistent with things themselves.[113] Lawyers can construct their reality with their 'verba', their 'mens legislatoris' and

---

[110] The quotation is from Coke, *1 Inst.*, 254a; see also Herberger 1981: 215–17; Maclean 1992: 91–5. See also Maclean forthcoming c.
[111] *Discourse* 1942: 35–6.
[112] Maclean 1992: 31; Dear 1995; above, 5.3.
[113] Castro 1614: 44–53.

their 'ratio legis'; the nearest doctors get to this power is in their selection and anthologisation of loci from classical authors, but even these have to be confronted with 'res'; 'interpretatio extensiva' and 'interpretatio restrictiva' do not apply, because although the meaning of words has to be fixed by the interpreter, it does not need to be tailored historically to a context; finally, there are few if any parallels with linguistic performatives found in the law. Incantation would be one example of such a performative, but it is rarely acknowledged to be a successful therapy by learned doctors (see above 4.2.4). This bias against incantations and prayer (or its reduction to an autogenic or occult cause) is symptomatic not only of learned medicine's rejection of folk practices but also of its rejection of words as anything more than instruments.

6.5.2 *Medical interpretation and modern hermeneutics*

We may finally gauge medical approaches to textual interpretation by comparing them with some of the major issues of modern hermeneutics. Five of these are pertinent here: (1) Do we create anew or rediscover the sense to a text? (2) Should we apply the same criteria to all forms of interpretation? (3) Are these criteria eternal or historically specific? (4) What sorts of meaning are to be discovered in texts? (5) Can we understand an author better than he understands himself? In relation to the first, doctors are committed to the view I rehearsed above that thoughts are expressed in texts and are unchangeable, which would seem to commit them also to the view that we recreate the sense of a text; but as we saw, Cardano also espouses a complex psychology of reading which seems to leave open the possibility of a revision of sense, as well as making the wry observation, when looking for an example of a true but generally not believed statement, that in commentaries one learns more about the commentator than the author.[114] On the second question, Renaissance doctors acknowledge that different sorts of writing have to be interpreted in different ways: thus Plato needs to be understood as writing in fables 'ironically' (the distinction is here between a literal and figurative meaning), and Vitruvius's text, because of its special nature, needs to be supplied with an assessment of architectural measurements

---

[114] See above notes 82 and 87. Cardano takes the view that we can understand any author *as well as* he has at one time understood himself, by realising through the active intellect the thought which he committed to paper in the form of its elements of ratio and experientia; but he does not comment on the risk of the active intellect misunderstanding the author.

as well as semantic explanation.[115] Cardano spends several pages in his *De libris propriis* of 1562 setting out the various 'modi scribendi' which all require a different form of analysis or exposition according to their disposition and other rhetorical features;[116] and the need to pay special attention to the exposition of aphoristic writing, a direct concern of doctors, is also recognised (above 4.2.5).

The issue of criteria does not arise, as doctors assume that human nature, although infinitely variable in its individual manifestations, is a constant, as are the natural objects which impinge on the medical art (even if their names can change over time). The question of meaning is therefore in the end reduced to a question of reference; the intention of the historical utterer or writer of a term or proposition is only of interest insofar as it designates an objective thing or mind-independent theory.[117] But on the last question, whether we can understand an author better than he understood himself, it is agreed that an interpreter has the right (even the duty, according to Cardano) to select and reconstruct the sense of a text by eliminating error from it, selecting loci, expanding on these, and configuring them anew. The claim made by doctors that to quote an authority is to quote its arguments and empirical data has the effect of generating a healthily critical attitude towards the classic texts of medicine; it also makes the commentators who practise this form of quotation potentially the masters of the texts they quote by their acts of excision (of spuria), dismemberment (by anthologisation) and paraphrase (by translation), and the creators thereby of 'authentic authors' having a coherent doctrine of their own devising.[118]

---

[115] Cardano 1663: 1.57, 69.

[116] *Ibid.*, 122–6, 134. On changes of style in the same author caused by subject matter and his evolution as a writer, see Siraisi 1997: 126.

[117] Cardano 1663: 1.123: 'verba propter res ipsas facta esse, non res propter verba'.

[118] I have not here dealt with the question of interpreting illustrations; some comments on this are to be found in 5.2.1.

CHAPTER 7

The content of medical thought

Medicine is the knowledge (scientia) of what is healthy, what is
morbid, and what is neither.

(Galen)[1]

7.1 INTRODUCTION

In this chapter I shall investigate medical discourse not, as in chapters 4
and 5, from the point of view of rational structures and argument but
from the point of view of content. This will involve me in examining in
turn what cannot be doubted; what is presupposed about natural principles; what nature is taken to be in general and in particular (humours,
spirits, causes); nature's relationship with art and custom; its unicity. Thus
far, the subject matter of this chapter is shared with natural philosophy,
and forms part of the debate discussed above about their relationship
(see 3.4); thereafter I shall turn to the terms of art and specific concerns
of medicine in respect of external and internal nature, health, illness,
monstrosity and mirabilia.

In medicine the same issue of self-evidence arises as in law, where it
is specifically enjoined on jurists not to attempt to prove or interpret the
self-evident;[2] in the case of medicine, the self-evident is nature itself in
the form of external reality which is 'maxime nota et evidens'(see above
4.3).[3] The 'evidentia' of nature are in the first instance accessible to sense:
we know that fire is hot, that heavy objects fall, that rhubarb purges bile,
and that someone wounded in the heart will die.[4] These and other such

---

[1] *Ars Parva*, K 1.307.
[2] Maclean 1992: 89–90.
[3] Vicomercatus 1596: 102r; but this is followed (104v) by a justification for defining 'self-evident'
   nature, using the same arguments as do the lawyers. See also Argenterio 1610: †1r; Cardano
   1663: 3.357; Porzio 1598: 138 (ii.3: 'quare definierit naturam philosophus, cum sit nota per se');
   Herberger 1981: 86, 92–6.
[4] Ingolstetterus 1597: 153: 'ignem esse calidum; gravia ferri deorsum; bis duo esse quatuor; omnis contradictionis unam partem veram, alteram falsam; rhabarbarum purgare bilem; unum

234

insights must be accepted as commanding belief;[5] no science can prove the existence of its subject matter; according to Porzio, 'things which are "nota per se" only need the support of weak induction'.[6] Problems immediately arise however (as they do for law): all knowledge, to be truly knowledge, has to be translated out of the order of sense into the order of the intellect, and it is not at all clear what should be done about intelligibilia which are not part of the perceivable natural realm (such as privation, or infinity, or the vacuum) or counter-sensory information (such as antiperistasis, by which a sense impression is intensified by an opposite quality: e.g., cold water intensifies the feeling of heat: above 5.3.4).[7] One route out of this problem is to acknowledge that part of those things 'nota per se' belongs to the order of sense, and part to prior knowledge ('praecognitio') (above 4.3); another is to recognise that there are limits to enquiry into nature of which one extreme is the utterly obscure and the other the self-evident, as was pointed out in the *Problemata* attributed to Alexander:

One must ask questions about things of a middling variety: that is, not those that are totally obvious of themselves, nor those that are so hidden and obscure that man cannot understand them; but those that, albeit difficult and obscure, can be explained by the erudition and understanding of men.[8]

This brings us back to Nicholas of Cusa's famous phrase, 'mens est mensura rerum'; things in themselves are beyond mankind's grasp; the mind of humans has to reduce everything to its own limitations. But natural philosophers and doctors are committed realists; as we have seen,

---

non nisi unum indicare; vulnerato corde mortem secuturam'; this list resembles that given by Melanchthon 1834–60: 13.150–1. See also Galen, *Methodus medendi*, i.4, K 10.38; *De elementis*, i, K 1.413–4 (elements are only known through reason: on this see Moraux 1981: 96); Biesius 1573: 158r: 'sunt autem omnibus nota principia demonstrationum omnium, quae axiomata vocant: ut totum esse quavis sua parte, de rebus omnibus affirmationem vel negationem esse veram. Sunt etiam certa, quae sensu bene constituto ab omnibus percipiuntur'; Goclenius 1625: 199: 'omne iudicium sumi ex aliquo praecognito, sive id sit sensibile, sive intelligibile'; L'Alemant 1549: 29v ('principia' are either theses ('praecepta') or 'axiomata' born of nature). Also Schmitt 1969: 109.

5 Aristotle, *Topics*, i.1, 100 a 30: 'things are true and primary which command belief through themselves and not through anything else; for regarding the first principles of science it is unnecessary to ask any further question as to 'why' but each principle should of itself command belief' (as against endoxa): cf. *Physics*, ii.1, 193 a 3: 'any attempt to prove that nature ... is a reality would be childish'; Blair 1997: 42 (citing Averroes); Dear 1987: 141 (citing Clavius); see also above, 4.3.

6 Porzio 1598: 138: 'quae sunt veluti proloquia solum opus habent tenui inductione'.

7 Galen, *De placitis Hippocratis et Platonis*, K 5.431 cited by Herberger 1981: 92. See also *ibid.*, 95–6; Horst 1621: 205 on antiperistasis: 'aqua frigida per antiperistatin auget calorem'.

8 Pseudo-Alexander, *Problemata*, Paris, 1541, 4–5, quoted by Blair 1997: 64. See also *Topica*, i.2, 104 b 2ff.

Sennert claims that things are the measure of our knowledge, not our knowledge of things; and things are not as they are because of how we know them, but because they are as they are, we must know them thus, if we want to know them correctly (above, 4.2.1). Nature in the form of external reality is thus paradoxically both self-evident and hidden; its reality is not questioned, but the ability of man's mind to capture it either fully or accurately either through the senses or through the intellect can be doubted.

7.2 UNIVERSAL AND PARTICULAR NATURE

Agricola Ammonius draws a well-known distinction between the principles of natural philosophy and those of medicine, the latter being derived from the former:

For philosophers contemplate things and their nature in themselves ('per se') and not in relation to the task in hand, and are content with contemplation of this sort and simple speculation. For the rest, doctors consider the dispositions of the human body as they do other natural objects in relation and application to the task in hand, nor do they forever stick fast to the roots [of the tree], which is more or less what the philosophers do, but through aspiration and effort they reach its branches and fruits.[9]

The sense of the phrase 'where the philosopher leaves off, the physician begins' ('ubi desinit philosophus, incipit medicus': see above 3.4.1) is taken here to be that natural philosophy provides the 'principia', and hence the 'praecognita', for medicine.[10] But the 'praecognita' of natural philosophy (basic metaphysical principles such as matter, form and privation, as well as substantial form, specific form, primary matter, substance and accident, potency and act, essence and existence, entelechy, elements, and qualities) are used directly in certain medical doctrines

---

[9] *Commentarii in librum artis medicinalis*, Basle, 1541, 45–6, quoted by Joutsivuo 1999: 75: 'contemplantur enim philosophi res et naturas rerum per se et absque relatione ad opus, contemplatione eiusmodi et speculatione ipsa sunt contenti. Caeterum medici humani corporis dispositiones, sicuti et alias res naturales considerant in relatione et applicatione ad opus: neque vero perpetuo in radicibus velut in salebra haerent, quod faciunt fere philosophi, sed adspirant eluctantur et pertingunt ad ramos et fructus ipsos'. Taddeo Alderotti had divided philosophy and medicine in this respect by distinguishing between 'iudicium intellectuale' and 'iudicium sensibile': *ibid.*, 42.

[10] Ingolstetterus 1596: A3 determines nature to have three separate meanings for the common man, for the philosopher, and for the doctor. The physical theories of the Stoics were known to medicine through Galen's *De placitis Hippocratis et Platonis*. The Paracelsian external and internal natural principles (salt, sulphur, mercury; 'constituentia', 'virtualia', 'hypostatica') are set out in various treatises: e.g. du Chesne 1609: 90. For the distinction between universal and particular nature see Goclenius 1609: 323–4.

such as that of the temperaments and humours.[11] It is possible for some of these terms to be modified without the general context being abandoned: Cardano (citing the authority of Hippocrates) talks of three (rather than four) elements and two (rather than four) qualities.[12] Other grounding principles which are alleged are the division of the sublunary and superlunary worlds, and the resultant doctrines of necessity, fortune and chance, space and time;[13] these last, together with motion and change, are the aspects of the sublunary world studied in the context of Aristotle's *Physics*.[14] The source of these principles and distinctions is both reasoning and the senses; it can also be given an origin in the 'lumen naturae', which is for Paracelsians and to some degree Philippo-Lutherans a specifically Christian doctrine (5.3.5), for others a neoplatonist one.[15]

The most important of all the concepts derived from these principles is that of nature, to which is attributed a bewildering range of meanings and functions. Perhaps the least typical of these is to be found embedded in John Cotta's *A short discoverie of the unobserved dangers of severall sorts of ignorant and unconsiderate practisers of physicke in England* of 1612:

The order of nature in all her works is constant, full of wonder, and unchanged truth in the continuall cohesion, sequence and fatal necessitie of all things, their causes and effects: wherein therefore how the Almightie Dietie hath commanded all things by an unchangeable law to be ordered, is both true and necessarie wisdom to understand, and the true patterne, rule and square of everie discrete, sober and wise designe and consultation. Hence upon the principles of nature stand everlastingly founded all arts and sciences ... And all true arts thus founded upon the undeceiving grounds of nature, in themselves are ever certain and infallible, whose rules although discretion according to circumstance continually diversly vary, yet can no time nor circumstance ever or at any time abrogate.[16]

---

[11] Doctors such as Biesius 1573 and Suterus 1584 set out in a pedagogical dialogue the meaning of these terms; see also Zabarella 1590; Vicomercatus 1596; Porzio 1598. See also Ottosson 1984: 202 on Giacomo da Forlì's three medical definitions of substance: that which subsists independently (as opposed to accident); that which is the essence (as heat is of fever); that which maintains the essence (as complexion maintains the essence of the human being).

[12] Cardano 1663: 3.381–2; Siraisi 1997: 64 (citing Hippocrates as a possible source).

[13] Peucer 1553: 79.

[14] See Des Chene 1996 for an exhaustive account of this in late Renaissance Catholic scholarship. The principia of nature are discussed in ways which do not necessarily exclude consideration of the forbidden propositions of 1270 and 1277, on which see above 3.6.1.

[15] On this see Lohr 1988; Copenhaver and Schmitt 1992: 309ff. (on Telesio, his cosmic vitalism, and his claim that the structure of the world and nature is to be derived not from reason but from the senses).

[16] Cotta 1612: 118, quoted by Wear 1995a: 171–2; see also Blair 1997: 20 (on Bodin's claim that nothing is uncertain in nature). Cf. Goldammer 1991: 19, who offers these meanings of 'natürlich' for modern readers: 'rational erklärbar', 'sinnlich-gegenständlich wahrnehmbar', 'empirisch verständlich', 'die Tatsachen entsprechend', 'kausalmechanisch die belebte und unbelebte Umwelt erfassend'.

We may note in this passage the coming together of the epistemological virtues (certainty, coherence, universality, truth) which Hollerius
carefully distinguishes (above 4.4); the principle of an undeceiving God
made famous later by Descartes; the derivation of arts and sciences from
natural principles; and the initial reference to the order of nature which
grounds logic and necessity itself. One may contrast this description with
the more cautious comment of da Monte in his commentary on Galen's
Ars parva: 'nature is not always understood in the same sense, and when
we say nature we do not always understand it in the way Aristotle defined
it . . . but more broadly'.[17] Here we are back to the familiar looser categories of medicine (see above 4.4); Montecatini even has a wider sense in
mind: 'some take all nature to be in the broadest sense everything which
subsists of itself'.[18] Such a portemanteau designation of sense is not very
helpful: but if all the available narrower definitions of the various ancient schools of thought are put together, incoherence can aggravate the
situation further, as Montaigne pointed out in his exercise in scepticism,
the 'Apologie de Raimond Sebond'; there he takes all the fundamental
theories about nature to be no more than plausible opinions.[19] If he is
right, then Renaissance scholars can aspire to no more than a weak description of nature, and not a scientific definition. To underpin medicine
with natural principles of this loose kind is to threaten the status of that
part of it which was claimed to be scientific (see above 3.1).

7.2.1 Universal nature: God

The very diversity of the following designations of universal nature
(which are listed variously by Pietro d'Abano, Valleriola, Piccolomini,
Goclenius and others) would seem to bear out his view: nature is God
(an identification found in Seneca) or is 'natura naturans' in the scholastic

---

[17] Da Monte 1587: 355: 'natura non semper eadem modo intellig[i]tur, ut cum dicimus naturam
non semper intellig[i]mus eo modo quo definivit Aristoteles . . . sed largiori quoque modo'.

[18] Montecatini 1576: 221: 'nonnulli latissime accipiunt naturam omnem pro omni re quae per se
subsistit'; cf. Biesius 1573: 1–4; Porzio 1598: 127–51.

[19] Montaigne 1965: 539–40 (ii.12): 'je ne sçay pas pourquoy je n'acceptasse autant volontiers ou les
idées de Platon, ou les atomes d'Epicurus, ou le plain et le vuide de Leucippus et Democritus,
ou l'eau de Thales, ou l'infinité de nature d'Anaximander, ou l'air de Diogenes, ou les nombres
et symmetrie de Pythagoras, ou l'infiny de Parmenides, ou l'un de Musaeus, ou l'eau et le feu
d'Apollodorus, ou les parties similaires d'Anaxagoras, ou la discorde et l'amitié d'Empedocles,
ou le feu de Heraclitus, ou toute autre opinion de cette confusion infinie d'advis et de sentences
que produit cette belle raison humaine par sa certitude et clairvoyance en tout ce dequoy elle
se mesle, que je ne feroy l'opinion d'Aristote, sur ce subject des principes des choses naturelles,
lesquels principes il bastit de trois pieces, matiere, forme et privation'. Not listed here are the
ideas of Hippocrates and the Stoics.

context given to this idea by Aquinas:[20] nature is the cosmos and all its contents, also known as the 'natura naturata' or 'God's art', a concept which is marked by a disagreement between Platonists, for whom the universe is a great living organism, and Aristotelians, who accept that the natural order of the sublunary world is distinct from that of the superlunary world, the latter not being subject to change in the same way as the former.[21] For the peripatetics, an account has to be given of how the two orders interact (above 3.6.4). This group of ideas is consistent with the view that nature is a gift of God, 'the essence and force given to each thing from its origin';[22] the grace of the act of creation can be identified with divine occasionalism, sometimes expressed as a world spirit diffused through all living entities; or it can simply act as the guarantee of the 'ordinary power of God in all things created', as Cotta puts it. Alsted's phrase 'organica ordinaria vis a Deo indita rebus creatis' expresses the same idea.[23] Some ancient authorities restrict the action of providence to the production of genera and species, but not individuals: a view which clashes with that of Aristotle, as the Conciliator points out.[24] There is also a related concept of nature as a life-giving force ('generatio viventium') not necessarily associated with a divine origin at all: a view implicit in the Plinian reference to a 'lusus naturae', and which was considered and rejected by Aquinas.[25]

7.2.2 Particular nature: the 'principium motus et quietis'

Thus far, we have considered the idea of universal nature; its dominant sense for medicine relates however to the individual. This is nature as the essential internal principle or cause of physical operations (movement and rest) in hylomorphic beings: the 'principle and cause of movement

---

[20] *Summa theologiae*, 1a 2ae 10.1 ('natura naturans id est Deus ordinans naturas omnium, sive auctor naturae, vel qui creavit omnes naturas'; other definitions given in 1a 2ae 2.1 and 2a 2ae 6.1.3); Pietro d'Abano 1548: 15 (ix); Biesius 1573:1–2, disputed by Vicomercatus 1596: 116–19.

[21] These ideas are drawn from the *Timaeus* and Plotinus, *Enneades*, iv.32. They raise the question of how the two worlds interact, on which issue see e.g. Melanchthon 1834–60: 13.179–80; Biesius 1573: 1–2; Porzio 1598: 127. Galileo's mathematical view is opposed to this: see Schmitt 1969: 124. On the sublunary world (and hence the human body) ageing and declining (a Lucretian idea) see Siraisi 1994b: 87.

[22] Blair 1997: 91 (citing Bodin).

[23] Alsted, cited by Camerarius 1626–30: 142 (ii.4).

[24] Moraux 1981: 99 (citing Alexander of Aphrodiseas); Pietro d'Abano 1548: 24v (xv). On the Stoic sources of this see Siraisi 1987a: 240 and Nutton 1988.

[25] See Findlen 1990: 293: nature's voluntary mutations of art or jokes are 'means of explaining something that would otherwise be without explanation, such as diversification'; Pliny, *Natural history*, xiv.42; Aquinas as cited in note 20.

and rest of an entity in which it is inherent primarily and of itself, and not accidentally', a definition adapted from Aristotle's *Physics*, ii.1 (193 a 28–30).[26] This definition is modified and expanded after the recovery of the commentaries of the Greek commentators Philoponus and Simplicius, without being radically transformed.[27] Other definitions related to this are derived from the same book of the *Physics* and recorded by the Conciliator: nature is matter, or form, or form-and-matter; it is the 'essentia cuiusque rei'; it is productive cause, propensity, rational principle.[28] Resembling definitions still less are the specifically medical designations found in Valleriola: 'the maker of all, whose minister is the physician'; 'the whole faculty which governs any animal'; 'the faculty which is the governor and ruler of the mind'; 'the faculty of lesser potency which we call vegetative or natural'; 'the origin of all movement in us'; 'innate heat'; 'complexion'.[29] What are here referred to are functions and dispositions; we have passed from the metaphysical or scientific question of what nature is to the question of what it does, and what its agencies are, a question which belongs to the sphere of art.[30]

---

[26] The Latin formulation is usually 'principium et causa motus et quietis entis in quo inest primo et per se et non secundum accidens'. The exclusion of 'accidens' gives rise to a problem for Renaissance taxonomists such as Fuchs and Rondelet who include accidents in their descriptions of plants and animals (see above 4.4.3); it also has implications for the relationship between illnesses and their symptoms, which were known in the Middle Ages as 'accidentia' (see below 7.5.3), but are said not to be so by Argenterio 1606–7: 76 (writing against Corti).

[27] Piccolomini 1600: 55 quoting Philoponus ('virtus quae per corpora effunditur, ea formantem et gubernantem: ac Principium, quo res, in qua est, moveatur et quiescat primo secundum se et non ex accidentia'); and a consensus of Aristotelians (*ibid.*, 54: 'forma rerum, natura constantium, ex materia pendens, finisque generationis et secundario materiae in qua significatione quaeritur eius definitio'). Porzio 1598: 138 offers a new version of the definition: 'ea quae est principium motus et essendi, essendi quidem, ut est actus et ἐντελέχεια: motus vero, ut notat propensionem ad transmutationem atque ad motum: atque iccirco Latini asseverunt, nomen naturae significare habitudinem'. See also da Monte 1587: 355; Weinrichius 1595: 24v ('id quod causa est, ut moveatur et quiescat, in quo est primo et per se motus ac quies non per accidens'). The degree of rephrasing is reminiscent of other late Renaissance fine tuning of definitions: for another example see Meier-Oeser 1997: 175–84 (definitions of sign).

[28] Pietro d'Abano 1548: 15 (xv). In the interests of completeness, the Conciliator also records the use of the word 'natura' to designate the female genitalia (as does Piccolomini 1600: 54).

[29] Valleriola 1577: 259: 'omnium opifex [cuius] minister [est] medicus'; 'omnis qua regitur animal facultas'; 'ea facultas animi imperium et ductum'; 'inferioris potentiae quae vegetrix dicimus facultas et naturalis'; 'principium in nobis motionum omnium'; 'nativus calor'; 'temperies'. Valleriola also gives sets of definitions from Aristotle and Plato. On specific form and idiosyncrasy ('temperies'), see Siraisi 1990c: 102–4, 136–52. Cf. Lommius 1558: 67–8, offering the following definitions for doctors: all elemental substances; human nature; 'calor naturalis' (relating either to the whole body or the heart); to these he adds a fourth: 'sub cuius nomenclatura passim occulta seu arcana proprietate significatur, quemque extra omnem mentis humanae captum posita, sola nosci experientia potest'.

[30] Cf. Piccolomini 1600: 56: '[Plotinus] non explicat quod natura sit sed quae sunt eius opera'.

7.2.3 Human nature: members, organs, humours

Nature also denotes human nature; or more generally the internal principle of life in individual human beings. Human nature is determined by the sanguine, phlegmatic, melancholic and choleric humours, related to the four qualities (wet, dry, cold, and hot), which are in turn related to the four elements (water, earth, air, and fire) and the four constituents of the human body (humours, homogeneous parts, spiritus, and innate heat respectively).[31] The humours are normally, but not always, said to combine into eight combinations which produce specific temperaments and distempers.[32] 'Complexio' or 'temperies' is a combination of humours which in theory could produce the perfect balance, although this seems to have been looked upon as an asymptote.[33] What the theory of 'complexio' makes possible (explicitly in Avicenna) is a thorough-going relativism; the substantial form of the individual is necessarily related to his or her 'complexio';[34] and in each individual, humours are dominantly, not absolutely, sanguine, phlegmatic, melancholic, or choleric.[35] They can even be redundant at certain times of the year. This means that humoral theory encompasses at once an argument from

---

[31] Horst 1609: 268. In some medical accounts of human nature, innate heat, organs and members are given also as its components. The organs are the dissimilar parts of the body, the similiar parts being muscles, membranes, tissues. In his account of the theoretical part of medicine, Stupanus 1614 includes a survey of parts of the human body, and relates this to the functionalism implicit and sometimes explicit in Galen's *De usu partium corporis*.

[32] Vega 1571: 637; Vallesius 1606: 18–23 (i.7). There are eight possible varieties of (intemperate) 'temperies', four simple (hot, cold, humid, moist) and four composite (hot and dry, hot and moist, cold and dry, cold and moist): Galen, *De temperamentis*, i, K 1.509ff. quoted by Sanctorius 1630: 14 and many others. Siraisi 1997: 64 records Cardano as speculating (on the authority of Torrigiano's commentary on the *Ars parva*) whether there are only three humours. García Ballester 1995: 132–3 says that for some purposes humours are reduced to two: radical moisture ('humiditas substantialis') and innate heat ('calidum innatum').

[33] This is the 'canon' represented by the statue of Polykleitos: see Galen, *De placitis Hippocratis et Platonis*, v, K 5.449; *De tuenda sanitate*, K 6.126; *De temperamentis*, i.5–9, K 1.534–51; *De optima corporis constitutione*, K 4.737–49; Cardano 1663: 6. 411–13 (i.6.9); Siraisi 1997: 48–9. The inverse problem is the 'fallacy of perpetual illness': Galen, *Ars parva*, K 1.317; see also the 'point of perfect health' in the 'latitudo sanitatis' (below 7.4.3), which is linked by Iulianus Martianus Rota in Torrigiano 1557: 26r to the statue of Polykleitos: 'per istud rotundum [a point in the diagram] intelligitur corpus optime sanum punctuale ac indivisibile, quod non est in latitudine, nec a medico consideratur, nisi ut aliorum mensura, ut statua Polycleti respectu aliarum et p[otes]t dici terminus latitudinis'.

[34] Siraisi 1987a: 82 quotes Vallesius accusing him of vapidity by thinking up 'supervacaneas quasdam et fictitias qualitates'.

[35] According to the *Ars parva*, K 1.331, humours are relative to parts of the body, not the whole body; see also Valleriola 1562: 94: 'humores alii in alia corporis parte magis dominantur'; 'humor quisque calidus, frigidus, humidus, aut siccus dicitur, a qualitate in eo superante'. Humoral theory can be made consistent with the Fall and with the individual sinner's original sin: Wallis 1995: 119.

dominance (its determination of 'complexio' in a given individual is a qualitative judgement) and a claim that humours are quantifiable in a given individual at a given time (see above 5.2.1).

7.2.4 Occult qualities

The humours are perceptible to the senses: there are components of human nature which are not. These include both occult powers and qualities (including qualities of the first degree), and the three spirits of Galenic medicine (animal, vital, natural).[36] Like formal and final causes, spirits are insensible but not necessarily immaterial and unintelligible, for there are effects in the real world which can be derived from their operation.[37] Where spirit is explicitly determined to be material, there is even a hint of an atomistic account of it as the subtlest component of matter.[38] An 'occult quality' is defined as that whose effects alone are known through the senses, and whose causes are not known to human reason through the 'praecognita'.[39] The principal examples of these are the symptoms of the 'morbus totius substantiae', sympathy and antipathy (including the magnet), and those functions of the body involving the connection between matter and spirit.[40] There are also qualities which lie beyond both the four primary qualities and the secondary qualities,

---

[36] According to Helm 1998, there are both two- and three-term divisions in Galen drawn respectively from *De placitis Hippocratis et Platonis* and *De usu partium corporis*, and reference is made to the Holy Spirit in relation to these powers. Temkin 1973: 142–3 and Joutsivuo 1999: 31 cite Argenterio's critical reading of Galen on this topic.

[37] Cf. Fernel 1610b: 1.75–6: 'Plato quidem rarius eam materiam calore perfusam spiritum appellavit, ignem frequentius, ut interdum calorem . . . est igitur spiritus corpus aethereum, caloris facultatumque sedes et vinculum, primumque obeundae facultatis instrumentum.' Henry 1997: 48–55 has a clear account of this doctrine.

[38] Richardson 1985: 178. There can be no doubt but that this doctrine was understood; a version of it is found in Fracastoro's theory of contagion through 'seeds' or 'animalia minuta' or 'bestiolae' which have the same explanatory force as atoms and secondary qualities: see Nutton 1990b: 232 (quoting Mercuriale, *Variae lectiones*, iv.6, Venice, 1598, 64r). There are contemporaries who accuse Fracastoro of Epicureanism: Nutton 1990b: 229. See also Siraisi 1987a: 248–66 (on 'minima naturalia' in Aristotle, Galen, Avicenna and the Conciliator). The implications of atomism for the teleology of nature and divine providence were clearly seen: see Melanchthon 1581: 281ff.; see also Copenhaver and Schmitt 1992: 303–9 and Wallace 1988: 214–15 on the debate about 'minima naturalia'.

[39] Nutton 1990b: 198–9; Pagel 1935; Copenhaver 1988: 283; Camerarius 1626–30: 20 (xiii.21); Blum 1992: 48ff. (citing *inter alia* Scaliger 1952: 1080 (344.8); Siraisi 1997: 51 (on Arnau de Vilanova); Keil 1992 (on occult qualities in the Middle Ages); Pittion 1987: 121 (citing Vallesius); Scribonius 1583: 10–11: 'occultae qualitates sunt quae diuturna tantum experientia cognoscuntur'; Thorndike 1923–58: 5.433–7, 550–62; Walker 1958: 75–84; Copenhaver 1978. Not all knowledge beyond immediate sense-perception is classified as occult: anatomy also falls under this category; see Galen, *Ars parva*, K 1.355.

[40] Sennert 1650: 1.139–67; Lloyd 1988; García Ballester 1988: 129 (on there being no statement in Galen of the precise relationship of 'krasis' to soul); Nutton 1988.

of which fifteen are listed by Galen;[41] being beyond sense, these may be ascribed to superlunary influence, or they may relate to the substantial or specific form of the organism, as was recognised in Padua even before the writings of neoplatonists such as Ficino appeared; the newly diffused neo-Aristotelian writings of the sixteenth century (notably Alexander) confirm this range of options.[42] By the end of the Renaissance, the discussion had broadened to include the 'causa continens' (see below 7.5.4), and occult qualities had been divided into five classes by Sennert (special, individual, inanimate, postanimate, 'secundum' or 'praeter naturam').[43] Recourse to such explanantia is open to the accusation of what has come to be known as recuperation, as late-seventeenth-century thinkers did not tire of pointing out.[44]

7.2.5 Spiritus

Another insensible is spirit, which is seen by neoplatonists as the instrument of vivification of a body or the medium of its descent into matter; as such, it can be viewed as diffused throughout nature, or as a sign of divine occasionalism; it prevents an identification of matter with life, as matter is inanimate unless implanted with the seed which inspirits it.[45] Fernel associates it with substantial form, which he derives not from matter as in a Thomist schema but directly from God who mediates it through celestial substances.[46] In a hylomorphic account on the other hand, nature is the 'substantia seipsam movens' through 'vires', 'virtutes' 'facultates'. Galen's account limits its effect to the natural faculties, the canonical three being animal (the source of rational thought and its lesser equivalent, the 'vis aestimativa', in animals), natural ('vis appetitrix', 'alteratrix', 'generatrix') and vital (which animates the

---

[41] *De usu partium corporis*, i.9, K 3.26–7; *De facultatibus naturalibus*, i.6, K 2.11f.; Sanctorius 1630: 642 (viii.1).

[42] Blum 1992: 48 (citing pseudo-Alexander, *Problemata*, i.2 a 2); Meinel 1992: 22ff. Substantial form determines the essential characteristics of the activity of any natural phenomenon; Brockliss 1993: 71 defines it as 'the principle that makes the object what it is: a member of its species'.

[43] Sennert 1650: 1.139–67.

[44] Culler 1972: 137: 'Recuperation stresses the notion of recovery, of putting to use. It may be defined as the desire to leave no chaff, to make everything wheat, to let nothing escape the process of assimilation ... to recuperate is to assimilate or interpret something ... to bring it within the modes of order which culture makes available.' For another example see Copenhaver 1988: 284 (citing Ficino on fascination). See also Hutchinson 1982. For Renaissance awareness of the problem, see for example Lodovicus 1540: aa3v: 'proprietatem non esse futile et inane nomen, sed substantiam'.

[45] Ingegno 1988: 238; Pagel 1935: 100 (on Augustine and Ficino); Blair 1997: 91.

[46] Brockliss 1993: 71 sees the consequence of this to be that a divine origin is attributed to transmittable disease.

heart).[47] There is a tradition of Christian thought which relates these faculties to the soul, to consciousness, and to the working of the Holy Ghost in the world.[48] The interaction of soul and body, which has profound theological consequences, arises as an issue both in the determination of mental dispositions and illness (as in Galen's *Quod animi mores corporis temperamenta sequuntur*) and in physiognomy.[49] Sympathy and antipathy constitute another pair of insensible effects; they are most discussed through the magnet and the doctrine of sympathetic cures (of which the most notorious is the weapon-salve). Sympathy is defined as an occult quality, a 'consensus between things without an obvious cause'; like spirit and occult qualities, it is subject to a taxonomy.[50]

7.2.6 Sense data

There is opposition to the recourse to spirits and occult causes. In a broader context, the name of Telesio springs here to mind, but I do not know of any doctor who explicitly cites his radical theories.[51] In a medical context, da Monte had modestly suggested that spirits and occult causes were not always needed to achieve a sufficient medical explanation;[52] later in the period, Sanctorius opposes both Fernel and Argenterio who rely on them, and claims on the authority of several Galenic loci that states of the body which cannot be given a full causal explanation through manifest qualities (because the four elements can be configured in infinite ways and are subject to infinite changes) can none the less in principle if not in practice be described as 'accidents

---

47 *De facultatibus naturalibus*, i, K 2.1–73; Temkin 1973: 147; Scaliger 1592: 1072–3 (343) adds also 'attractrix', 'concoctrix', 'retentrix', 'expultrix'.

48 On the Augustinian and Christian neoplatonist sources of this, see Pagel 1935; Walker 1958; Melanchthon's syncretism is discussed in Helm 1998; see also Blair 1997: 91 (on Bodin).

49 On these issues, which include the ability of human beings to correct predispositions to certain mental and affective states by the exercise of the will, see above 3.6 and below 8.8.1.

50 Mizauld 1554; Jessenius 1599; Bono 1995: 85–122; Pagel 1958: 52–3; Cardano 1663: 3.638 ('sympathiam voco consensum rerum absque manifesta ratione: velut antipathiam dissidium': a definition whose second part is contested by Scaliger 1592: 1074–6 (344.2): 'aliud est dissentire, aliud contrasentire'); Chiaramonte 1625: 3; the locus cited in Galen is his *In epidemica*, vi.6.5, K 17b.325–37; Goclenius 1625:)(3 (distinguishing between primary, secondary and tertiary qualities, and identifying five 'gradus' of sympathy or antipathy: natural things which have congruence with certain humours and bodily members (e.g. rhubarb and bile); antipathy between plants (e.g. brassica and vines); sympathetic action between animals (e.g. swallows curing blindness in chickens by applying grasses); antipathy between animate species (e.g. that between wolves and lambs); sympathy between metals and stones on the one hand and organs or illnesses on the other (e.g. that between emerald and epilepsy)). *Ibid.*, 171ff. also discusses the weapon-salve, on which see also Foster 1631 and Fludd 1631. Goclenius's views on the weapon-salve are attacked by Forerus 1624: 249–80.

51 See Copenhaver and Schmitt 1992: 309–14.

52 Nutton 1990b: 211.

pertaining to the predicament of quality'; since they are curable by the application of contraria, they must belong to the category of quality, and hence be potentially knowable.[53] The continuation of this debate can be found in the writings of Harvey, who argues that one should stick to 'spirit' as a 'mode of being' not, as in a dualistic system, as the partner of matter, and warns against using occult quality as a recuperative device through which God acts continually on nature, which in his view should be looked upon as 'self-operating'.[54] This view is consistent with a utilitarian attitude appropriate to the medical art: a remedy may only be explicable through a non-manifest cause or process, which can be acknowledged without being fully grasped.[55]

7.2.7 Nature and custom

Nature and human nature are constituted by humours, causes, spirits, faculties, members, organs; these can be contrasted to things such as contingencies which do not bear on the given nature of an object;[56] they are related to custom and art in a different way. The topos 'custom is second nature' ('consuetudo altera natura'), derived from various Aristotelian and post-Aristotelian loci[57] is found in natural-philosophical and medical writing; in the former it is related to nature in the form of the 'habitudo' of our matter and form, and its propensity to transmutation, both of which seem to allow for the development of acquired characteristics.[58] Even a force external to the body can become in some

---

53 Sanctorius 1630: 659–61 (viii.6, referring *inter alia* to Galen, *Methodus medendi*, xii, for the argument that 'qualitates reconditae habent contrarium, ergo qualitates reconditae non erunt substantiae'; *De constitutione artis medicae*, viii, K 1.251–4 and *De locis affectis*, ii (for the argument that the 'infinitae alterationes elementorum' prevent manifest qualities being seen as such). See also Pagel 1935: 115 (quoting Valleriola, who, unlike Roger Bacon, accepts that occult properties can rise from the mixture of elements) and Bates 1998 (on Harvey's claim that spirits are recuperative causes, and that God acts on inert matter by instrumentalising it). Wolf 1620: A4 (on poor analogy, tautology and the petition of principles in the writings of those who defend the existence of occult qualities).

54 Bono 1995: 107–22.

55 Ingolstetterus 1597: 38 (quoting Mercuriale and Fernel on the doctor's interest in the occult being limited to the effectiveness of remedies). A remedy is defined by Liddel 1628: 605 as a '[contrarium] [quod] non solum quae manifestis facultatibus inter se pugnant sed etiam quae occulta facultate et specifica forma: praeterea privantia, et tam ea, quae ex accidenti et potentia talia sunt, quam per se et actu'. See also Sennert 1650: 1.522–5 (on sympathy of physical constitution, function and contiguity).

56 This is the category of 'neither natural nor contrary to natural'; a negation of the sort described in *Prior analytics*, i.46, 51 b 6ff.

57 *Rhetoric*, i.11, 1370 a; *De memoria*, 452 a 28; Peucer 1553: 537 gives Hippocrates as the source.

58 Piccolomini 1600: 54–5; Porzio 1598: 130, 135 ('habitudo materiae et formae nostrae': 'propensio…ad transmutationem atque ad motum'); even physiognomy allows for the effects of upbringing (Porta 1593: 50–2 (xv): 'quod a nutricibus etiam in morum cognitionem devenire possumus').

way natural; in other words the non-naturals, which belong to the sphere
of nature in spite of their name (see below 7.4), can be internalised.[59] Yet
it is also asserted that 'custum cannot be converted into nature'; it can
only become second nature; as Vallesius puts it, referring to Galen's *De
motu musculorum*, ii.7, K 4.452, custom is 'an alien form of nature' ('natura
adventitia').[60] The problem arises that it is very difficult to tell the difference between nature and this sort of second nature, as Sanctorius's
Aristotelian definition of 'consuetudo' using the four causes makes plain:
'the disposition of a natural constitution introduced through the senses by
the assiduous exercise of agent and reagent, such that agent and reagent
are made similar to each other'.[61] This definition exposes a general difficulty with the definition of nature itself, which is characterised as both
passive and active.[62]

7.2.8 Nature and art

The relationship of nature to art is crucial to such practices as alchemy,
which is associated with medicine in our period and for some time
before.[63] In the *Physics*, nature is defined as the internal principle of motion in individual natures, as we have seen; it is also said (ii.8, 199 a 19–21)
that art 'completes what nature cannot bring to a finish, and apes her';[64]
yet this does not imply that it is anything other than 'weaker than nature'
(*Meteorologica*, iv.3, 381 b 4–6). What is at stake for experimental science
here is the justification for undertaking experiments and drawing conclusions from their results; this entails the rejection of the received doctrine
that it is impossible for composite matter to revert to its elements, and

---

59 Campilongo 1601: 5v (on external things becoming 'quamvis secundam naturam', leading to
    the conclusion that non-naturals should be treated as though they were inherent to the body);
    cf. Siraisi 1994b: 83 (on the deformity of some skulls explained by custom).
60 Vallesius 1606: 364ff. (viii.5): his long discussion of the topic is not settled decisively.
61 Sanctorius 1630: 378–83 (iv.7) : 'ostenditur consuetudinem non posse converti in naturam'; *ibid.*,
    384: 'consuetudo est dispositio constitutionis naturalis sensim introducta ab assiduo exercitio
    agentis, et reagentis ut agentia et reagentia reddantur inter se similia'. In this definition, the
    formal cause is 'sensim introducta'; the material is 'constitutio naturalis'; the efficient is 'assiduum
    exercitium'; the final is 'ut agentia et patientia reddantur similia'. Sanctorius, who does not
    believe that custom can be converted into nature, also argues, citing Aristotle, *Metaphysics*,
    ii.3, 995 a 1ff., both that custom is an impediment to truth (1630: 365), and that 'a longa
    consuetudine et usu externarum causarum corpus in varias et aliquando contrarias naturas
    mutari posse' (361–72 (iv. 5)).
62 Porzio 1598: 140: 'natura habet impetum ad illa, ut perficiatur vel motu vel quiete, ab intrinseco';
    ibid., 149: 'naturae vero impetus et inclinatio non est, nisi ad recipiendum motum: et propter
    hoc potius appellatur principium passivum ab Aristotele, quam activum'; also Sennert 1650:
    1.13–14.
63 Crisciani 1996a.
64 See also *Politics*, vii. 15, 1336 b 37–1337 a 3. Cf. Derrida 1967: 207–9 (on supplement).

be reconstituted out of those elements. As William Newman has shown, this has in turn implications for the theory of forms.[65] It is also pertinent to note that the positive attitude to experimentation has as its corollary a progressivist view of science: to discover the hidden forces of nature will, according to Pereira and others, lead to greater human accomplishments in the sublunary world.[66] The issue for medicine here arises from the general claim that the art is 'ministrix naturae' and the particular claim which we have already met (3.2.3) that doctors themselves correct nature in her errors.[67]

7.3 NATURE AS PRODUCER AND PRODUCT

In these descriptions and designations of nature, a number of difficult issues arise which it is pertinent to mention before turning to the specific natural issues concerning doctors. Nature emerges as a producer (in the forms of 'vires', 'virtutes', 'facultates', and a generative internal principle); a product (the hylomorphic being, with its internal principle of movement and rest), and a process (also in the form of cause, 'vis' or function).[68] Another way of expressing this combination is through the distinction between act and potency; nature is both an active 'forma informans' and passive in respect of the necessity which governs it, and which can thwart its purposes: 'many things happen by necessity which are not brought about by the intention of nature'.[69] It is therefore both sufficient to itself, and incomplete; both autonomous and subordinate.

7.3.1 Intention and teleology in nature

Insofar as nature is a process and a producer, it is pertinent to ask whether it has an intention which it expresses through the functionality of its

---

[65] Newman 1997. This doctrine is derived from *Metaphysics*, viii.5, 1044 b 30f.: 'a return from privation to habitus in generations of natural things is not conceded'. Agriculture and medicine are associated with alchemy through the view that art can exceed nature.

[66] Blum 1992: 59 citing Pereira, *De magia*, Cologne 1612, 24–5.

[67] E.g. Cardano 1565: 83 (i.3.21: 'medicus an debeat imitari naturam recte operantem?'): 'respondeo, operantem naturam recte debemus imitari: non tamen quiescente natura semper medicus debet quiescere'.

[68] Galen, *Methodus medendi*, i.9, K 10.70.

[69] Henning Arnisaeus, *De iure connubiorum*, Frankfurt, 1613, 150, attributed to *Physics*, ii.9, 200 a 10ff.: 'multa fiunt ex necessitate quae non fiunt ex eius intentione'. Lenoble 1969; Daston and Park 1998: 209; Sennert 1650: 1.14; Porzio 1598: 150–1 (on Deus, 'electio', 'casus' and art as principles of action in nature). See also *Physics*, ii.9, 200 a 32ff.; *De generatione animalium*, iv.4, 769 b 32ff.; ii.5, 197 b 33ff.; ii.6, 199 a 11–15.

creatures, and whether this is a regular feature of nature. From *Physics*, ii
(198 b 25–199 a 1), it is argued that if nature is a cause, it must embody
at least a tendency if not an intention. This is deduced from the requirement of a final cause, and from the evidence of design.[70] But this does not
necessarily mean that nature has a mind, or that its personification as a
mother, 'opifex', and so on refers to anything more than a potency in it
which incorporates a purpose when in act.[71] Its teleology can be reduced
to mere material causality, as it was to be by Bacon;[72] others, however,
cling to it as a bulwark against atomism.[73] Hence the rehearsal of the
argument from design, and the claims that 'nature makes nothing in
vain', and that 'in its works, nature is neither lacking in what is necessary,
nor does it abound in what is superfluous', claims which characterise it
by its activity, purpose, economy, self-regulation and consistency.[74] This
can of course be represented paradoxically: as Montaigne puts it, 'il n'y
rien d'inutile en nature, pas mesmes l'inutilité'.[75] For doctors, function is
at issue here; the *De usu partium corporis* suggests that all parts of the body
are there for a purpose, 'ruled by that nature which rules, manages and
governs all things with supreme reason and supreme foresight'.[76] Physiological functions are supported by arguments from design derived from
anatomical structure.[77] From these comments it would seem therefore
that nature is a self-contained, self-causing, self-existing, and self-effecting
machine or organism.

---

[70] Cardano 1663: 3.545; Porzio 1598: 155–7; *Physics*, ii.8, 198 b 25–199 a 1.

[71] Vicomercatus 1596: 123–8; Vallesius 1606: 383–4 (viii.8): 'natura cum non ratiocinetur, nihil
tentat nisi quod per se fertur in bonum finem'.

[72] Against Aristotle, *De partibus animalium*, ii.15, 650 b 15, Bacon 2000: 87 argues that eyelashes
should not be looked upon as protection for the eyes but as pilosity in the vicinity of a moist
orifice. Ironically, this 'modern' insistence on the material cause is exactly what Molière satirises
in the following exchange from *Le Médecin malgré lui*:

> GÉRONTE: La cause, s'il vous plaît, qui fait que [ma fille] a perdu la parole?
> SGANARELLE: Tous nos meilleurs auteurs vous diront que c'est l'empêchement de l'action
> de la langue.

[73] Melanchthon 1581: 281ff.

[74] Aristotle, *De generatione animalium*, ii.4, 739 b 19–20; cf. *Mechanics*, 847 a 15–16: 'nature always
acts consistently and simply'; Porzio 1598: 131; Piccolomini 1600: 54–5; Silvaticus 1601: 430:
'naturam ipsam in suis operibus non deficere in necessariis, neque abundasse in superfluis';
Blair 1997: 24; Parisanus 1621: BIV: 'nihil in natura sive natura sive causa naturali fieri; propterea
perbelle post hosce Aristoteles, Eorum omnium, inquit, quae Naturae lege fiunt certas esse . . .'

[75] Montaigne 1965: 790–1 (iii.1); Maclean 1996: 118.

[76] Wear 1973: 95 (quoting Piccolomini on the spleen); *ibid.*, 142 (citing Bauhin on multifunctionalism
in nature, based on book ii of Aristotle's *De generatione animalium*).

[77] Bylebyl 1985a: 224–5 (on Vesalius); cf. Capivaccius 1596: 143 contains a logical approach
to function as a combination of 'agens' (e.g. 'anima'), 'instrumentum' (e.g. 'cerebrum') and
'objectum' (e.g. 'in quo agit facultas, et a quo facultatis organum afficitur').

7.3.2 Beyond nature

This is reminiscent of the characterisation of nature in the *Timaeus* as an infinitely changeable enclosed seething mass of energy and action, 'un immense vivant aussi rebelle aux formes fixes de la pensée que la vie elle-même aux équations mathématiques et aux lois rigoureuses', as Lenoble puts it.[78] Yet there are other forces outside nature in the sublunary world: not only chance, human inventiveness in the form of art, and the capacity of natural objects to act on themselves, but also the influence on these objects of 'necessity' (which may include all or some of these forces) and the superlunary world.[79] Whether a deterministic account of nature is possible is a vexed question with strong ideological overtones, as the Pomponazzi affair revealed (see above 3.6.1).[80] The issue comes to the fore in natural philosophy and medicine through the question of infinity. This is usually denied as a possibility: 'infinity is repugnant to nature and to its principles; for the infinite cannot exist in [informed] matter, still less in its principles'.[81] Aristotle however concedes that one possible form of the infinite which can be found in nature is that which to all intents and purposes is immeasurable or uncomputable.[82] It is a universally acknowledged fact that nature's productions constitute an infinite variety of mixtures and temperatures.

7.3.3 Underdeterminations: residues and redundancy

The same issue of determinacy is also perceptible in the question of re-dundancy, residues and errors of nature.[83] This question is detectable in

---

[78] Lenoble 1968: 279–90.

[79] Vicomercatus 1596: 123–8.

[80] Copenhaver and Schmitt 1992: 107–10; Ingegno 1988: 242–5 (on Pomponazzi and Cardano).

[81] Vicomercatus 1596: 17v: 'infinitudo et naturae et principiis repugnat. Infinitum namque in materia [sc. informata] nullum esse potest, multo minus in principiis.' But infinity can be a property of primary matter; see Maclean forthcoming d.

[82] *Physics*, iii.3–8, 202 b 30ff.; *Metaphysics*, xi.10, 1006 a 35ff.; *De caelo*, i.5–7, 217 b 1ff.; iii.4, 302 b 10ff. Five definitions of infinity are derived from these loci: what cannot be divided or 'traversed'; the limitless; the too large to measure; the indefinite; what can always be added to or further divided. The formal definition given in *Physics*, iii.6, 207 a 1f. is 'that which after subtraction always leaves a residue'. Galen refers also to the sense of 'too large to measure', e.g. in his reference to an 'infinite number of diseases': *Methodus medendi*, ii.6, K 10.115: see also Camerarius 1626–30: 21 (i.33). It is in this sense that the individual lies beyond the grasp of art: Campilongo 1601: 7r (referring to Galen, *Methodus medendi*, iii.7, K 10.309–13 and *Ars parva*, ii, K 1.309–13).

[83] See Herberger 1981: 67ff., 178–81 on regula and rule, and Daston and Park 1998; Maclean 2000b; Rossi 1970: 67; Siraisi 1994b: 62, who claims that sixteenth-century life sciences have a 'conception of nature that no longer exhibited the feature of uniformity'; see *ibid.*, 68–71, 87 on variation in the no longer canonical human body.

the organisation of textbooks, in which one finds such catch-all categories to accommodate these residues as 'res diversae', 'praeterea', 'classis extra ordinem', 'variorum'.[84] The art of medicine moreover excludes a category of evidence from its doctrines: these are the 'rarissima' ('things which occur very infrequently do not fall within the scope of the art'),[85] the 'supervacanea' ('inutilia', 'subtilia'), and the radically individual case. This means that the art can both recognise that 'the external sources of signs are numberless', and then proceed to a finite division whose claims to adequacy are undermined by the inclusion of unclassifiable residues.[86] Such underdetermination of nature by art can be matched by its overdetermination, through which it is possible to do what is not possible in the natural world.[87]

Excess also exists in nature itself. Even though Aristotle claims in *De generatione animalium* that nature does nothing superfluous (ii.24, 739 b 19–20), his pupil Theophrastus provides a locus for the contradictory claim, pointing out that nipples in males, hairs in the nose and antlers on the heads of stags all constitute examples of redundancy.[88] Individual natures can have plethoras or superfluous humours.[89] The whole issue of exceptions in nature, which operates only 'for the most part' in respect to its own rules, is linked to the excess and defect of the moment of generation of natural beings.[90] Yet natural defect, referred to both inside and outside the terms of art of medicine as 'praeter naturam' and 'contra naturam' is, as we have seen, also a contradiction.[91] These schemata lead to the problem of recuperative argument which we have already met:

---

[84] Maclean 1999a: 18; García Ballester 1993b: 44 (citing Arnau de Vilanova).

[85] Silvaticus 1601: 27 (citing Hippocrates): 'res eventu rarissimae sub arte non cadunt'.

[86] Oddi 1564: IV; Argenterio 1610: 1691–1701. Capivaccius 1603: 10 ('fontes signorum externi sunt innumeri') sets out the rules for division, including the division of signs, (*ibid.*, 1036ff.), without making reference to the difficulty noted earlier.

[87] Bennett 1998: 214, quoting Gemma Frisius, *De astrolabo catholico liber*, Antwerp, 1556, 4v: 'nam per geometriae inventa faciemus, quod naturam rerum non permittit'.

[88] Theophrastus, *Metaphysics,* vi, 10 b 5ff. (the *editio princeps* is in the fourth volume of the Aldine Aristotle of 1497), cited by Valleriola 1577: 45. On this passage see Lennox 1985. There is an entry in Brasavola 1556: 312v which reads 'natura aliquid fecit frustra' (referring to *De anatomicis administrationibus*, ix), but ten other loci are cited which refute this. Galen opposed the view that there is redundancy in nature, which he associates with Erasistratus: see Galen 1991: 95 (Hankinson, citing *De naturalibus facultatibus*, ii). On Aristotle's support for the view that there is nothing superfluous in nature, see *De generatione animalium*, ii.4, 739 b 19f. and iv.4, 770 b 28ff.

[89] Campilongo 1601: 51r: 'qui laeduntur a similibus et iuvantur a contrariis habent superfluos humores, v.g. quos calida et sicca iuvant, pituitam superfluam habent; quos frigida et humida, bilem, et sic de caeteris'; see also Chapman 1979: 290 (on plethora).

[90] Cf. *De generatione animalium* iv.4, 770 b 35ff.

[91] Siraisi 1997: 218–19.

something which is not 'for the most part' in nature has to be provided with an explanatory framework which threatens the whole system on which the exception is based. In other words, a mode of explanation is adopted in which some catch-all principle is adduced to account for those things which otherwise lack explanation; this can appear however to be no more than a verbal trick. An early example of this is Nicolas Oresme's use of God as a universal explanans;[92] a famous Renaissance example of awareness of the problem is Scaliger's phrase 'asylum inscitiae' (later referred to as 'asylum ignorantiae').[93]

7.3.4 *Variability*

It is also pertinent to point out that note is increasingly taken of the variability of nature. This is not only through the recovery and edition of such texts as Hippocrates's *Airs, waters, places*, but also through the empirical work of anatomists, botanists and zoologists. Even though theories such as that of idiosyncrasy and the use of extended lists of circumstantiae *qua* variables in diagnosis and therapy are in themselves admissions of the diversity of forms in the physical world, the abandonment of strict taxonomy (above 4.4.3) and a post-canonical approach to the constituents of the human body greatly accentuate the loosening of the conceptual bonds of what is taken to be natural.[94]

7.4 MEDICINE'S TERMS OF ART: NATURALS AND NON-NATURALS

I come now to the 'praecognita' and terms of art of medicine proper relating to nature: these are bound to show some of the effects of the incoherence, inconsistencies, even paradoxes inherent in the meanings of nature given above. Medicine is an art dedicated to the end of health, which sets it aside from other arts;[95] it is therefore to be expected that the

---

[92] Blair 1997: 93 (quoting Oresme); see also Ottosson 1984: 237–8 (on Giacomo da Forlì's invention of a fourth humour in blood which is indistinguishable from the other three).

[93] Scaliger 1592: 1080 (334.8); Blum 1992: 58.

[94] Siraisi 1994b.

[95] Haly Ridwan, quoted by Ottosson 1984: 71: 'nam scientia harum rerum est genus omnium artium factarum a principiis sumptis ex scientia naturali, sicut agricultura et curatio bestiarum, et pastoralis scientia animalium, et medicina. Et differentia eius est sermo eius cum sanitate et aegritudine, et cum dispositione in qua non evadit homini sanitas neque aegritudo. Haec enim differentia discernit essentialiter medicinae ab omnibus artibus factis a principiis sumptis ex scientia naturali.' The question arises whether perfect health, like perfect temperament

terms relating to nature will relate to this useful end: namely, external nature in relation to individual nature, health and sickness and the various
states between them, monstrosity and mirabilia. This division is also that
between 'res naturales', 'res non naturales', and 'res contra (or praeter)
naturam' which is adopted with little change from medieval sources.[96]
The most important of these terms is 'praeter naturam', which covers
a very large field including illness, abnormality and rarity, as we shall
see. The natural things are elements, complexions (or temperaments),
compositions (or humours), members, virtues, and spiritus (or 'vires', or
'facultates'); we have met many of these as part of individual human nature above. The non-naturals are those things in the realm of nature 'not
to do with the constitution of the body': some resemble circumstantiae
as external factors, some relate (in a way somewhat alien to a modern
outlook) to the human will, and are ordered by human nature.[97] The following constitute the traditional list: air, food and drink, sleep and vigil,
motion and rest, evacuation and repletion, and the 'passiones animi', in
which sexual activity is included (it also is in part evacuation, and in part
motion).[98] Fabio Paulino even argues that sex is a seventh non-natural,
on the authority of both Galen and 'alii recentiores'.[99] Basing himself

(see above, 7.2.3) is a natural state, and whether, if it is, the conservation of health is a part of
medicine or not: Mikkeli 1999: 10. This arises also because the neutral state is both analeptic in
the case of convalescence and prophylactic in the case of those declining into illness: *ibid.*, 52–3
(citing Sennert and Cardano); cf. Celsus *De medicina*, i.l: 'sanus homo qui et bene valet et suae
spontis est nullis obligare se legibus debet, ac neque medico neque iatralepta egere'; Lommius
1558: 1. On listening to the voice of your own body and being your own physician, see Mikkeli
1999: 16–18.

[96] Ottosson 1984: 253ff. Capivaccius uses 'praeter naturam' and 'contra naturam' interchangeably
in some contexts: 1603: 12, 15.

[97] Mikkeli 1999: 20: patient–doctor relations are also defined through this distinction, there being four factors involved ('res naturales'; 'res non naturales'; 'res contra naturam'; 'externa
accidentia': see García Ballaster 1993b: 44–8). On the distinction between necessary changes
in body caused by the res naturales as opposed to non-necessary changes (sword wounds, maul-
ings by wild beasts), see Galen, *Ars parva*, K 1.367.

[98] Mikkeli 1999: 54–8, giving the Galenic source of the six as *Ars parva*, K 1.367 and Arnau de
Vilanova's list of six principal and seven subsidiary non-naturals (seasons, locale, sex, occupation,
play, bathing, and habits). On passions of the soul in respect of moral vices (the matter of
philosophy and law) as opposed to effect on body (the matter of medicine) see Ottosson 1984:
260; on environmental factors Mikkeli 1999: 15 (referring to Hippocrates, *Airs, waters, places*).
Ibid., 59–60 on food as a non-natural regulated by circumstantiae or variables in respect of size,
complexion, age, gender, season, region, exercise, sexual activity, emotion and the nature of the
food. Mikkeli also makes the point (*ibid.*, 51) that through the inclusion of food the non-naturals
clearly have a place in regimen. See also Starobinski 1982. Frölich 1612: A3v uses 'non-naturalis'
eccentrically to mean 'neutralis'.

[99] See Galen, *Ars parva*, K 1.371; Paulino in Avicenna 1608: A2v: '[Venus] quam collocamus non
solum auctoritate Galeni, qui seorsum eam collocavit in arte medicinae, sed etiam aliorum
recentiorum, licet vulgus medicorum partim motui partim excrementis subjiciant'.

on Galen's *De tuenda sanitate*, v.10, K 6.358, Sanctorius reduces the list of six to four.[100]

7.4.1 Secundum naturam: health

The epithets 'secundum naturam', 'praeter naturam' and 'contra naturam' are used in a wide diversity of ways. In respect of the first, Vicomercatus repeats Simplicius's distinction between 'kata phusin' ('secundum naturam': which is to do with health) and 'phusei' (rendered as the ablative 'natura': that which arises from the conditions of generation, such as being thin or fat, or having a hooked or squat nose).[101] In respect of the second and third epithets, the Latin language can provide a distinction which is not present in the Greek: 'para phusin' embraces both 'praeter naturam' and 'contra naturam', as Argenterio points out.[102] 'Praeter naturam' is distinguished in various ways from 'secundum naturam', 'super naturam', and 'contra naturam'. Fernel uses 'contra naturam' for disease, and 'praeter naturam' for minor blemishes such as freckles, warts and calluses; his usage is eccentric.[103] A more widespread example of 'contra naturam' in the sphere of nature is the kidney stone, which is a body of a foreign material composition inside the human being.[104] Tumours are almost universally described as 'affectus praeter naturam', as in the Latin title of the Galenic treatise on them. Beyond nature lies the supernatural (either superlunary or celestial), otherwise known as the extranatural and innatural; Vicomercatus eccentrically locates this as a middle term between 'praeter naturam' and 'contra naturam'; but he also refers to a category of the supernatural which is 'truly beyond nature' and thus not constrained by contingency (time, place and movement). He points out moreover that 'supra naturam' has a meaning in theology ('those things which could never be brought about by any natural power') which he as a natural philosopher would wish to render as 'praeter et contra naturam'; and he adds a category 'post

---

[100] Sanctorius 1630: 421 (v.2); the four are 'ea quae assumuntur', 'ea quae fiunt animo vel corpore', 'ea quae excernuntur et retinentur' and 'ea quae foris adhibentur'.

[101] Vicomercatus 1596: 141v; Simplicius 1882: 269; *Physics*, ii.1, 192 b 32.

[102] Argenterio 1610: 230.

[103] Fernel 1610b: 1.180–1 (*Pathologia*, i.2: a chapter on 'quid contra naturam' and 'quid praeter naturam'); cf. Brasavola 1556: 314r cites a locus in *Methodus medendi*, viii distinguishing between 'non naturaliter' and 'praeter naturam'.

[104] Argenterio 1610: 230–1: 'sit ergo illud contra naturam quod nullo modo fieri potest ob naturae repugnantiam, differens ab eo, quod est praeter naturam: quippe hoc fieri possit, et si non a propria sua natura, vel non utraque'. Vicomercatus 1596: 144r reserves the term 'contra naturam' for fictional (i.e. artificial) objects.

naturam' which he designates as referring to 'supercaelestia et mentes divinae, et ens item'.[105] 'Praeter naturam' also impinges on the supernatural in Thomist theology, where it refers to the state of souls after death deprived of a body.[106] A non-theological context is given to these terms by Pomponazzi, who refers to occult properties and unknown superlunary influences in the category of 'praeter naturam' or 'contra naturam';[107] they are later excluded by Bacon from his triadic nature 'in her course', 'erring' and 'altered'.[108] Others (of neoplatonist persuasion) describe the influence of the stars as 'secundum naturam'.[109] These distinctions have other identifying features: 'praeter naturam' has a life cycle ('principium', 'augmentum', 'statum', 'declinationem') where the 'res naturales' have no life cycle;[110] and 'secundum naturam' has symmetry and is 'unum veluti regula et mensura', whereas 'praeter naturam' is 'varium et multiplex'; Vicomercatus is thereby drawn to comparing the former with the truth and the latter with lies.[111] An extensive Renaissance debate on these terms was occasioned in Germany by the affair of the Golden Tooth.[112] Such fluctuating terminology is a sign of the flexibility of doctors in their use of words (see above 4.2.1).

7.4.2 Praeter naturam: death and putrefaction

Argenterio's discussion of 'praeter naturam' (which he links to a discussion of monsters: see below 7.6.1) is one of the fullest of its time. He examines critically Simplicius's and Fernel's ideas on this matter. For the former, 'secundum naturam' applies to 'what occurs through the course ("ratio") of nature, and those things which have their own perfection';[113] so to be born blind is 'praeter naturam' (although not all blindness is so),

---

[105] *Ibid.*, 144v: 'illa vero supra naturam dici possunt, quae extra coelum sunt posita, nec locum, nec tempus, nec motum participantia, vitamque beatam perpetuo degentia, cuiusmodi sunt Aristotele etiam docente mentes divinae. Supra naturam rursus, quae religio nostra asserit, quae nulla vi naturae effici unquam potuerunt, quae et eadem physicis praeter et contra naturam dicerentur. Sunt et aliqua post naturam, de quibus opus est Aristotelis Metaphysica, id est, de his, quae post res naturales sunt posita. In quibus et ea sunt, quae supra naturam diximus, supercoelestia videlicet, et mentes divinae . . .'

[106] *Contra gentiles*, 4.79.

[107] Clark 1997: 263.

[108] Bacon 2000: 63.

[109] Ingegno 1988: 238.

[110] Campilongo 1601: 11v.

[111] Vicomercatus 1596: 143v.

[112] See 2.3.2.

[113] Argenterio 1610: 228: 'quod fit secundum rationem naturae, et quae habent propriam perfectionem'.

but illnesses are not 'praeter naturam', because their effect on the patient is their perfection and 'per actionem naturae'. Simplicius also agrees with Aristotle that putrefaction is 'secundum naturam', 'ex naturae principiis, et a natura ipsa', as is death; the very monsters described in *De generatione animalium*, iv.4 (see below 7.6.1) are 'secundum naturam' in a certain way, even if not perfect in their nature. Argenterio's own view is elucidated in the context of these claims. For him, the natural is to do with both form and matter (more the former than the latter); and so those in whom both form and matter are in a state of perfection are certainly 'secundum naturam', those in whom neither form nor matter has been brought to perfection cannot be described as 'secundum naturam': and those who have the perfection of either form or matter but not both are partly 'secundum naturam' and partly 'praeter naturam'. A number of *cas-limites* are examined (the 'mola mulierum', which depends for its classification on its degree of deformation; death, which if it arises from internal principles, and is accompanied neither by illness nor pain, is natural;[114] and 'putredo', which is natural in respect of its coming about through the action of the four elements, but praeternatural in respect of its effect on the body in which it inheres).[115] Argenterio's conclusion is that 'health and illness differ not in species and form, not by true contrariety, as white and black, but only by degree of more and less'.[116] Argenterio concludes his discussion with a refutation of Fernel's use of 'praeter naturam' to designate 'those things which exert no force on nature, and all light affects which because of their slightness cannot be noticed by our senses or those of the patient'; Argenterio argues that it should only be used for 'that which not only exceeds nature's limits, but also exerts a force on it, and interferes with its powers and functions'.[117] He accuses both Fuchs and Fernel of being Galenists who 'assign arbitrarily

---

[114] Cf. Ottosson 1984: 251; Liddel 1628: 596–600; Vallesius 1606: 280 (vi.1); the conflict between Galen and Aristotle over the question 'an per tuendae valetudinis artem possit mortis devitari in aeternum?'

[115] Aristotle, *Meteorologica*, iv.1, 379 a 11–b 9; Vicomercatus 1596: 140v; Ottosson 1984: 251; Sanctorius 1630: 691–5 (viii.13): on Zabarella's failure to distinguish 'putrescibile', 'putredo' and 'putrefactum' (potency, process, and object): Erastus 1590; Baldutius 1608: 3–20. Putrefaction was to play an important role in iatrochemistry, as it betokened the fermentation and effervescence of humours to which iatrochemists appealed as a means of explaining the nature of diseases.

[116] Argenterio 1610: 230: 'differunt ergo sanitas et morbus non specie et forma, non vera contrarietate, ut album et nigrum, sed solum gradu per magis et minus'. On the logical implications of this see above 5.2.3 (Kepler).

[117] *Ibid.*, 230–1: 'illa quae naturae nullam vim inferunt . . . et omnis levior affectus, qui ob parvitatem, nec nostris, nec laborantium sensibus animadverti potest . . . quod non solum naturae limites excedit, sed etiam illi vim infert, eiusque vires et functiones manifeste interturbat'.

senses to Galen's words', informing them that they have the sanction only to reproduce them, and repeats his conclusion that Galen describes those things as 'praeter et contra naturam' which 'exceed the appropriate ('conveniens') and functional ('utile') condition of the healthy body.[118] Argenterio has produced a touchstone of functionality here, as well as a somewhat uncharacteristic procrustean attitude to words which contrasts with the general laxity of terminology noted above. He has also produced the notion of a force beyond nature, which interferes with its operation; this can only be a general nature interfering with individual natures, or a supernature interfering with general nature.

7.4.3 The neutrum and the latitude of forms

One feature of Argenterio's debate of these issues – the use of the phrase 'gradus plus et minus' – is worthy here of further elucidation: we have met already this phrase in the debate about the latitude of forms (4.4.2). This debate involves not only qualities, which may or may not be said to permit of degrees,[119] but the whole discipline of medicine: 'medicine is knowledge ('scientia') of all things in their latitude, from the first to the last degree', as da Monte puts it.[120] The best example of latitude is that which exists between health and sickness.[121] Discussion of it is marked not only by the disagreement between the texts of Aristotle and Galen, but also by internal inconsistency in the texts of Galen himself, who among other things had debated whether there was such a thing as perfect health.[122] Da Monte argues that as healthiness is not an unchanging state, perfect health could only be a fleeting moment, a 'sanitas punctualis' in terms of Victorius's diagram (fig. 5.4 above); for him, it is nothing more

[118] *Ibid.*: 'cum ipsi medici sint et Galeni sectatores, debebant non ex suo arbitrio vocabulorum significationes effingere: sed ex solo Galeno eas transcribere. Atque, ut antea ostendimus, Galenus ea praeter et contra naturam vocat esse, quae excedunt convenientem et utilem sani corporis conditionem.' There is a problem here with the notion of incurable disease: see Cardano 1583: 243 (on whether everything can in principle be cured, as Hippocrates claimed), and Seidelius 1593.

[119] Vallesius 1606: 8–11 (i.4): Is quality a mediate or immediate contrary? Can there be degrees of cold? Can hot and cold overlap? Can one be both hot and cold? This is an example of the logical alternatives of mediate and immediate contrary being shown to be inadequate: Vallesius ends up by describing 'warm' as follows: 'fit illud medium participatione extremorum, calore et frigore coniunctis, non amborum defectu'. On qualities as state or condition, natural capacity, affections and shape or form see *Categories*, viii, 8 b 25f.

[120] Joutsivuo 1999: 117, quoting da Monte, *In artem parvam Galeni explanationes*, Lyon, 1556, 151: 'est enim medicina scientia omnium in latitudine, et a primo gradu ad ultimum'; cf. Joutsivuo 1999: 157 (citing Fernel, *Opera medica*, Venice, 1565, 223–4 on gradual differences between bodies).

[121] Others are the latitude of monstrous forms (see below 7.6.1) and the opposition of sex, on which see Maclean 1980: 37–45.

[122] Joutsivuo 1999: 45–61; Mikkeli 1999: 41 (on *De sanitate tuenda* vs. *Ad Thrasybulum*).

than a useful concept. Matteo Corti (1475–1564) claims that perfect health is possible if considered with some latitude (again, as in Victorius's diagram); Cardano, and later Salvo Sclano, suggest that like the 'canon of Polykleitos' (the statue with a perfect physique), it is a norm against which all 'more or less' perfect bodies can be measured; a comparison used by Galen and later the Conciliator in their discussion of the possible existence of a perfect temperament.[123] We are brought back to the form of contrariety associated with dialectics, which does not have to have fixed termini (4.3.1).

Galen declares in his *Ars parva* that medicine is the science of 'salubria', 'insalubria' and 'neutra'.[124] According to him, and the majority of doctors who follow him in this respect, the opposition health/illness can be accorded a middle term, or even degrees ('gradus') of a middle term:[125] namely the 'neutrum', set between the natural state of health and the praeternatural state of illness. Health is 'secundum naturam', complete, 'aequalis' (balanced or symmetrical); it is characterised by the right admixture of homogeneous parts and the right balance of heterogeneous parts.[126] Sickness is the contrary of this; neutrality, the middle term, is partly 'secundum naturam', partly 'praeter naturam', or a degree between the state of health and the state of illness.[127] The existence of such a middle term, whether it is assumed to partake of the properties of both extremes, or of one, or of neither, means that to expel illness is not synonymous with introducing health.[128] Some argue from sensory data alone that there can be no 'neutrum'; abdominal pain, headache or a bitter taste in the mouth are neither states of health, nor illnesses, nor degrees between the two.[129] Others claim that they are examples of the middle term of a complex mediate contrary. In Jakob Jokissus's account, 'neutrum' has three possible meanings: a middle term which is disjunctive in respect of the extremes of health and sickness; a middle

---

[123] See above 7.2.3; 7.4.2.

[124] K 1.307.

[125] Argenterio 1610: 228: his (Aristotelian) example of a 'gradus inter illa quae sunt praeter naturam' is a black grape which appears in a bunch of white grapes; the grape vine is 'between' a black and white nature: see *De generatione animalium*, iv.4, 770 b 20f.

[126] Ottosson 1984: 155; Galen, *Ars parva*, K 1.309–10.

[127] Argenterio 1610: 230, citing Galen, *Methodus medendi*, xiv.14, K 10.990–2; Gavassetius 1586: 2–3. It can be associated more with health or more with sickness: Joutsivuo 1999 argues that it is more associated with the latter in our period.

[128] Liddel 1628: 601–2. Health also relates differently to the homogeneous parts (where it is the right mixture) and the heterogeneous parts (where it is the right symmetry): Ottosson 1984: 155, and Galen, *Ars parva*, K 1.309–10.

[129] Joutsivuo 1999: 77 (citing Antonio Cittadini); Galen, *Ars parva*, K 1.358–63.

term which is conjunctive 'per confusionem'; and a conjunctive middle term 'per complicationem'.[130] Others distribute the medial status of 'neutrum' according to the different categories or predicaments to which it can be assigned:[131]

not altogether healthy or sick	relating to quantity
not more healthy than sick	relating to degree (quantity)
between healthy and sick	relating to location
partly healthy, partly sick	relating to quantity (or quality)
sometimes healthy, sometimes sick	relating to time

This schema is derived remotely from Galen's *Introductio seu medicus*, and is the product of sustained discussion by the Arabs and by medieval doctors. Timo Joutsivuo has shown how complex the reception of this issue is in the Renaissance, and has elucidated its connection with debates not only about the nature of health[132] but also about the nature of form, temporal and logical modes (ut nunc/ut multum/semper/simpliciter), and modes of opposition.[133] The 'latitudines' of theoretical medicine may indeed be, according to Giovanni Filippo Ingrassia (1510–80), things

[130] Jokissus 1562: ix. 'Per confusionem is glossed as 'κρᾶσιν'; 'per complicationem' is glossed as 'ἐπιπλοκήν'. Unfortunately, Jokissus's diagram does not survive.

[131] Sylvius 1539a: 25; Vega 1571: 324 (referring to categories); Ottosson 1984: 167, 169 (referring to the Galenic *Isagoge* on 'qualitate, quantitate aut tempore').

[132] Joutsivuo 1999: 106ff. gives a full account of the Renaissance discussion of the question whether absolute health exists, which arises from Galen's *De tuenda sanitate*, i, K 6.14 (where it is alleged *inter alia* that there are shades of health as there are shades of white). The issues of the fallacy of perpetual pathology (Galen, *Ars parva*, K 1.317) and the status of health as habitus and disease as a disposition arise here. Da Monte argues that perfect health is only a concept; Sclano (after Victorius and Altomare) argues that it is a latitude. Joutsivuo (106–7) argues that there is a difference between scholastic and humanist commentaries on the neutrum: the quaestiones technique of the former leads to an acceptance of all individual authoritative statements as equally true, where the latter tend to highlight conflicting alternatives. For an exposure of the logical problems in da Monte's ninefold model of the neutrum, see *ibid.*, 204–6. See also *De sophisticis elenchis*, 166 b 20–7 (on the distinction between 'simpliciter' and 'secundum quid' as qualified in respect, place, time or relation).

[133] Galen, *Ars parva*, K 1.308: 'the "generally" healthy … has two senses: that of "always" and that of "for the most part" … the "neither", as cause, sign and body, both generally and with application to the present, has three subdivisions in each case. The first is the sense of having no part in either of the opposites; the second that of participating in both; the third that of participating sometimes in one, sometimes in the other. And of these, too, the second admits of a distinction; for it may participate in both equally, or in one more than the other.' See also Galen, *Ad Thrasybulum*, K 5.816 (referring to two neutral states); Oddi 1564: 62–3; Argenterio 1610: 100–1 (against the views of Manardo); Mikkeli 1999: 15, 53, 43 ('in general, during the sixteenth century, the neutral state of the body became increasingly a kind of subspecies of the healthy body, while in the previous centuries it had still been a middle state between healthy and sick bodies, or even a subspecies of the sick body instead of the healthy one'); Joutsivuo 1999: 76–7 (on Manardo's views), 127–53, esp. 148–9 (on Argenterio's argument in favour of an overlap between perfect/imperfect and permanent/temporary).

about which philosophers speculate idly with more or less rigour; but the issues, whether there is a continuous series of forms, or successive forms, whether the 'neutrum' is a 'medium transitus', or a 'medium formae', expose some of the fundamental problems of Aristotelian physics.[134] Health and sickness are also the subject of a major disagreement between authorities: Aristotle cites the opposition variously as an immediate or a privative contrary, and Galen claims that it is a mediate contrary permitting of degrees.[135] By the end of the sixteenth century, the most widely accepted view seems to be Galen's; the 'neutrum' is accepted as a 'latitudo', a 'gradus imperfectae sanitatis'.[136] Between eight and fifteen 'differentiae corporum' are identified, and made visible in diagrammatic form.[137] It was seen as important for doctors to identify these states, which play a part in progressive or degenerative conditions such as convalescence, falling ill, and ageing, and even determine the division of patients between different sorts of hospital in this period.[138]

7.5 PRAETER NATURAM: DISEASES

I come now to the concept of disease ('morbus'; 'affectus praeter naturam'), which even Galen recognised as being as manifold, complicated and varied as any element of the discipline.[139] Of all parts of medicine, pathology is probably the most debated in the sixteenth century, both because of the occurrence of hitherto unknown diseases and

---

[134] Ingrassia, quoted by Joutsivuo 1999: 74: 'haec philosophis speculanda dimittantur. Vel tamquam logicae ac vanae ipsis Dialecticis'; also 64 (the relationship of latitude *qua* continuous succession of forms to the problem of Eucharist in the medieval period); 70 (Averroes and the 'medium transitus' as 'a medium which differed from extremes only by degree' (i.e. quantitatively) as opposed to the 'medium formae', which differed in species from both extremes) and 74 (the connection of this debate to that which concerned the intension and remission of forms).

[135] *Categories*, 12 a 10–12; a full list of loci in Joutsivuo 1999: 58ff.

[136] Ottosson 1984: 176–7; Liddel 1628: 13; Thriverus 1592: 4; Campilongo 1601: 8v; Fernel 1610b: 1.182–3 (*Pathologia*, i.5).

[137] Thriverus 1592: 8 (eightfold division); Cardano 1663: 5.107–8 (ninefold division of health and illness from perfect to wholly ill); Mikkeli 1999: 52–3. Jokissus 1562 has ten stages by having 'insalubris' not coincide with 'aeger'; Joutsivuo 1999: 113 (citing da Monte's fifteen degrees (nine of neutral); *ibid.*, 134, 156 (Oddo degli Oddi's and Salvo Sclano's diagrams: Joutsivuo argues that Oddi's diagram is better at representing the latitude than Victorius's medieval one: see above fig. 5. 4 and 5.2.1).

[138] Argenterio 1610: 501–2; Liddel 1628: 12–13; Rondelet 1586: 582–3; Brockliss 1993: 78 (citing Le Paulmier's view that mankind as a whole is growing more unhealthy as the world gets older); Joutsivuo 1999: 163 (on different hospitals for those infected, those suspected of being infected, and for convalescents).

[139] Galen, *De experientia medica*, iii–iv, quoted by Hankinson 1995: 69.

the plethora of books of practica which reflect on them. Are diseases infinite in number? Do the Galenic genera and differentiae account for all diseases, or can there be new species? Do diseases occur as constant and stable 'affectus', or can they change in the body? Can they arise as composites? Are they local to given regions? How should they be analysed? These questions arise because it is perceived that one disease can impede the functioning of another; that some occur in most cases in the company of others; that some diseases cause other diseases; that some diseases are transformed into other diseases; and that all diseases are subject to circumstantiae and vary in their manifestations. In the account of these questions which follows, I shall be relying in large part on the excellent article of Nancy Siraisi which has elucidated the complexities of Renaissance thought on this matter.[140]

7.5.1 Taxonomy

All disease corresponds to asymmetric or unbalanced states of the body (as opposed to the symmetry of health); it is a predisposition of the body unable to function as usual; Galen's division into three genera is almost universally cited, although it does not go unchallenged.[141] The three kinds are 'intemperies' (imbalance of humours affecting the homogeneous parts), 'mala compositio' (the malfunction of an organ; an 'actio laesa' of a heterogeneous part) and 'solutio continuitatis' (or 'unitatis': a trauma to the body caused by an external agent).[142] Disease is said to have a life cycle, and to possess five significant features: appearance, magnitude, character, movement, and outcome.[143]

---

[140] Siraisi forthcoming (the source of some of the references below): for some instances of these issues, see Vallesius 1606: 256 (v.17): 'species [morborum] perpetuae sunt, secundum speciem, carentes principio et fine'; Camerarius 1626–30: 21 (i.33): 'morborum . . . infinitus numerus et species'; Nutton 1983: 15 (on Lange's disagreement with Fracastoro both on the number of diseases and the possibility of new diseases); Bertotius 1588: 7–16; Fuchs in Galen, Aliquot opera, Paris, 1549, 57v–58r quoted by Siraisi forthcoming (on 'morbi fientes', discussed in relation to views of Valleriola); Fernel 1610b: 1.186–8 (Pathologia, i.10); Siraisi 1997: 218 (on Cardano's distinction between 'morbus', 'vitium' and 'symptoma'); see also Rondelet 1586: 582ff. (on distinguishing between diseases).

[141] Vega 1571: 689; Argenterio 1606–7, vol. 2 passim (a radical critique of Galen); Cardano 1583: 3 (four, not three, genera of disease). As well as this division, another is found, drawn from a wide range of Galenic loci, which comprises 'idiopathia', 'sympathia', 'antipathia', 'protopathia' and 'consensus'; see Vallesius 1606: 209–15 (iv.6) and Sanctorius 1630: 117–33 (ii.1–4).

[142] On this standard part of Galenic doctrine, see Ars parva, K 1.380ff.; Vallesius 1606: 256 (v.17); Bartolettus 1619: 218ff. (a very coherent account); Sanctorius 1630: xx (i.4); Siraisi 1997: 218, 324.

[143] Liddel 1628: 560. No loci are given, but this is clearly a composite part of Galenic doctrine.

7.5.2 *Disease, symptom and cause*

A difficulty is encountered in the distinguishing between cause, symptom and disease. In Siraisi's words:

> According to Galen, every condition of a body declining from its natural state was one of three things: cause of disease; disease; and symptom. Disease was a constitution different from the natural that damaged function; cause of disease was an antecedent effect producing the disease that damaged function, and symptom was something different from the natural in the body accompanying or following disease. These three things were thus separate and distinct: diseases were not the same as causes or symptoms of disease; causes of disease were not the same as diseases or symptoms; symptoms of disease were not the same as either causes of disease or diseases. But in both the *De morborum differentiis* and the *De symptomatum differentiis* Galen surrounded these and other apparently clear distinctions with qualifications that made them a good deal murkier. For example, he reported with disapproval the view that some conditions could be either diseases or symptoms, depending on the situation in which they arose (so that convulsions associated with 'phlegmone' would be symptoms, but convulsions directly caused by imbalance of temperament alone would be diseases); but he also asserted that it was 'only a controversy about names' when some people called symptoms diseases. Nevertheless, symptoms were not diseases because they did not necessarily involve either an *affectus* (as most of the translators latinized diathesis) of the body or damage to function – yet his own triple classification of symptoms categorized them as either *affectus*, or functional damage, or both.[144] Moreover, he also asserted that damage to function in and of itself constituted a symptom. Furthermore, he claimed that since the broadest definition of symptom was anything other than natural that happened to the body, disease itself – or even a cause of disease – was also 'in a certain way a symptom'. And although he asserted that the narrower definition was more correct, Galen allowed that under the broadest definition even diseases and causes of disease imperceptible to sense could be described as symptoms.[145]

This confusion was clearly perceived in the Renaissance: Capivaccius points out that 'things are mutually conjoined, such as the praeternatural states of disease with another disease, disease with cause, disease with symptom, cause with another cause, cause with symptom, and symptom with another symptom'.[146] It is principally Paduan or Paduan-inspired manuals of *practica* which dwell on these definitional confusions.

---

[144] See Bylebyl 1991: 166 (on Joubert's distinction of 'affectus' and affected part). On affection not being identical to the disease see Galen, *Methodus medendi*, i.9.1, K 10.67, ii.3, K 10.86–91, where disease is not identified with disposition, but known through place, quality and activity.

[145] Siraisi forthcoming: the Galenic references are to *De symptomatum differentiis*, i–ii, K 7.42–55; *De morborum differentiis*, v, K 6.848–55.

[146] Capivaccius 1603: 5 'coniunguntur res invicem, ut praeternaturales (morbus cum morbo, morbus cum caussa, morbus cum symptomate, caussa cum caussa, caussa cum symptomate,

7.5.3 Symptom

It is convenient to intercalate here a discussion of symptom and cause, both of which are complex terms, before returning to the topic of disease. Symptoms are often said to be easier to recognise than illnesses, even though they may vary in quantity and quality. They were known to the Middle Ages as events and accidents, and taught through the medium of a verse mnemonic.[147] They are subjected to various classifications (see below, 8.2.2). Liddel gives their 'latissima significatio' as 'what is praeternaturally present in any animate body', and records Galen's division of symptoms into 'common' and 'proper and special'.[148] It is possible to distribute symptoms logically and chronologically: by their association with prior causes of disease or subsequent effects; by their manifestation through impaired function or changes in excreta; by their occurrence after the onset of disease, or after the coction of matter; by their indication of crisis, or prognostic force.[149] Argenterio disagrees with Corti as to whether a chance event ('casus') can be a symptom.[150]

7.5.4 Cause

The doctrine of causes is yet more convoluted, and subject to competing distributions. Some, like Peucer, seek to distribute causes across the whole field of creation; his four classes of cause are God; secondary causes (the Aristotelian quartet of final, material, formal and efficient) in the operation of which God alone can intervene; the will of man (a final cause); and chance.[151] Avicenna stresses the four Aristotelian causes, with the final cause being seen as the dominant of these; one Galenic locus adds a fifth, the instrumental cause, to these, which provokes a debate in the

---

symptoma cum symptomate), naturales et praeternaturales, naturales et non naturales, non naturales et praeternaturales'. The example given for the last combination is 'febris cum aere (regione, tempestate) calida'.

[147] Ottosson 1984: 189; Siraisi 1987a: 50.

[148] Liddel 1598: A4r: 'quod animato corpori praeter naturam inest': the categories are 'communiter' and 'proprie et speciatim': 'ut [symptoma] a morbis et morborumque causis distinguitur, pro ipsis omnibus tantum, quae morbis consequuntur aut a morbis proveniunt', referring to De differentiis symptomatum, i–ii, K 7.42–55.

[149] Campilongo 1601: 13r: 'a natura rei signatae; ab effectu; a causis; a simili et dissimili; a natura optimae constitutionis causarum et effectuum eiusdem'; Bartolettus 1619: 221–2: 'ex antecedente'; 'ex consequente'; 'ex supposito [i.e. actio laesa, excrementa mutata]'; Cardano 1568: 602 (iii.39): 'quae sequuntur morbum', 'quae sequuntur materiam', 'quae sequuntur coctionem materiae', 'quae crisim significant', which are subdivided into 'quae praedicunt et praecedunt [crisim]'; 'quae fiunt cum ipsa [crisi] et pendent ab illa'; 'quae sequuntur ab illa'.

[150] Argenterio 1610: 174.

[151] Peucer 1553: 79.

Renaissance.[152] The Conciliator stresses material and efficient causes, as does Clementinus.[153] Torrigiano, the 'plusquam commentator', distributes causes by the two variables of frequency and power.[154] Valleriola argues that the investigation of the nature of the four causes belongs more to metaphysics, with its primary concern for truth, than to medicine: for doctors, who are principally concerned with the utility of their art, the more significant duo are proximate and remote, both implicitly belonging to the category efficient.[155] Other Renaissance debates concern the questions whether illnesses can have infinite causes,[156] and whether rules about causes are no more than rules of thumb;[157] but the most persistent discussion concerns the causes of diseases as these are described in Hippocrates and Galen. Hippocratic loci suggest that there are two (primary and predisposing) or three (including the triggering cause);[158] Galen declares variously that there are two (preceding and antecedent) or three causes, made up of two material (the first called variously cohesive, 'contentiva' or 'continens', affecting the state of the organs prior to their malfunctioning; the second antecedent, denoting the predisposition of the body) and one efficient (called variously initial, 'praeincipiens', procatarctic or external, involving the non-naturals and the broader range of circumstances governing the disease).[159]

---

[152] Aristotle, *Physics*, ii.3, 194 b 24ff.; Avicenna, *Canon*, i.1.1.1; Galen, *De symptomatum differentiis*, i, K 7.42–53; *De usu partium corporis*, vi.12, K 3.464–5 (citing the instrumental or organic cause); Brunus 1623: EIV; Argenterio 1610: 501–2; Cesalpino 1593: 170–2; Harvey 1653: 262–4 (I) (on the relationship of instrumental to efficient). See also Bates 1995: 139–41; Moraux 1981:86ff.

[153] Cadden 1998 (on Pietro d'Abano); Clementinus 1535: 4–5.

[154] Torrigiano 1557: 26v: 'debiles frequenter occurrentes'; 'mediocres communiter occurrentes'; potentissimae raro occurrentes'.

[155] Avicenna, *Canon*, i.1.1.1 (on causes for utility rather than truth); Valleriola 1562: 378: 'propter quid, a quo, ex quo, per quod', but he adds: 'de his in universum tractare ad metaphysicum magis quam ad medicum pertinet'; also Bylebyl 1991: 188 (citing da Monte); Pittion 1987: 117ff.; Campilongo 1601: 2v ('medicina est prius scientia corporum et signorum quam causarum'); *ibid.*, 49–50 (on efficient, material, proximate and remote causes); *ibid.*, 93r (on doctors having better knowledge of proximate than remote causes).

[156] Vallesius 1606: 256 (v.17).

[157] Campilongo 1601: 51v (citing a material cause giving rise to a rule which is not 'perpetuae veritatis'); Pittion 1987: 120 (on Burton's critique of Fernel).

[158] The loci listed by Valleriola 1562: 384–9.

[159] *De usu partium corporis*, vi.12, K 3.464–5; *Methodus medendi*, i.8, K 10.65–6 (for primary as opposed to proximate cause); *De morborum causis*, ii, K 7.2–10; *De causis procatarcticis*. According to Siraisi 1990a: 172, Argenterio was among the first to make use of this last treatise. See also Nutton 1983: 27; Pittion 1987: 118–19 (citing Gorris); Clementinus 1535: 5 (who translates Galen's causes into material and efficient). The persistence of the doctrine can be seen in Cunningham and Williams 1992: 4 (citing R. Hooper's *Lexicon medicum* of 1831 on predisposing external (procatarctic), antecedent and immediate causes). Sanctorius 1630: 67 (i.27) argues on the authority of *De differentiis febrium*, i.4, K 7.282–7 that procatarctic causes are not truly causes but merely occasions of illness.

There is a fierce debate in the Renaissance about this Galenic doctrine. Avicenna had resolved these causes into three classes: external, internal, and a combination of the two. Leoniceno, and Fuchs after him, argue against him on philological grounds that only two causes come into question for diagnosis: the 'externa' or 'primitiva', and the 'interna' or 'antecedens'.[160] Fuchs is widely attacked for this view, both by traditionalists and Paracelsians.[161] Most of these want to keep the third cause, which is the conjunction of the first two.[162] There are more radical positions, such as that of Schegk, who seems to define the 'causa continens' as 'Deus per omnia penetrans', aligning it with neoplatonic spiritus, that of Sanctorius, who claims that procatarctic causes are in fact not more than occasions, and Argenterio, who attacks the three-cause model on yet other grounds, and produces, as we have seen, an eightfold model (above 4.4.4).[163] Of these eight, the instrumental cause is attacked in turn as a heretical addition by later Aristotelians.[164] What is happening here is a loosening of the physical rules by which a cause is identified; this is very apparent in both Peucer's account, and those of Valleriola and Campilongo. Peucer has a number of logically generated causes (from the five predicables and the distinctions 'per se'/'accidentaliter' and 'separabile'/'inseparabile');[165] Valleriola refers to 'causa manifesta' and 'causa obscura', of which the second is of occult but not necessarily celestial origin; 'causa per accidens'; 'causa conservatrix', 'causa preservatrix', 'causa instrumentaria', 'causa sine qua non', 'causa adiutrix qua rem assequatur facilius'.[166] Campilongo has a similarly loose list ('interna', 'externa', 'juvans', 'laedens', 'efficiens', 'conservans', 'per se', 'ex accidenti').[167] At the end of our period, Bartolettus tries to re-establish order by producing a list reduced to four classes ('per se'/'per accidens'; 'extra corpus'/'intra corpus'; 'antecedens'/'coniuncta'; 'sine qua non',

---

[160] Fuchs 1530: 44; Fuchs 1546: 103v (against Avicenna, *Canon*, ii.1).

[161] Horst 1629 (a full account of the debate); also Valleriola 1562: 378 (quoting Sylvius and Fernel, among others); Valleriola 1577: 350–67(against Fuchs); Albertus 1615: C3r (citing Schegk, Fuchs, Valleriola, Johannes Baptista Peregrinus 'et multi alii').

[162] Ferdinandus 1611: 217–21(a nuanced position).

[163] Schegk 1540: 6r–9r; Sanctorius 1630: 67 (i.21): 'procatarcticas [causas] non operari, et ipsis non esse morborum culpam attribuendam . . . ipsas demum procatarcticas esse occasiones, et non causas' (citing Galen, *De differentiis febrium*, i.4, K 7.2–10 as authority); Argenterio 1610: 499–501 (attacking da Monte).

[164] Brunus 1623: E1r.

[165] Peucer 1553: 67–9.

[166] Valleriola 1562: 378–80; see also Copenhaver 1992.

[167] Campilongo 1601: 13v, 49–50.

also called 'adiuvans').[168] As is apparent from all these attempts, the categories 'accidens' and 'adiuvans' permit of an impossibly broad etiology, and the nature of humoral theory and empirical therapy makes the category 'instrumental' very imprecise.

Causes are not the same as qualities although sometimes difficult to distinguish from them, as in the case of contagion.[169] According to many, they are neither the beginnings of diseases nor their occasion, yet they can affect the action of the body.[170] If the 'causa continens' in question is material, it can actually be an illness, according to Fernel (though not Vallesius or Valleriola); if efficient, it can be either an illness or a symptom. Causes must be known to the rational doctor through methodical examination before an illness can be known because 'scire est rem per causas cognoscere' (4.4.4), but as contrary causes can give rise to the same 'compositi morbi', this is not easy to achieve, especially as it is conceded that the 'fontes causarum' are not identical to the 'fontes essentialiter inhaerentium'.[171] The relationship of cause to sign, like that of symptom to sign, is also fraught with difficulties (see below 8.2).

7.5.5 Diseases as entities

I am now able to return to the concept of disease in itself. As is well known, the idea of disease as an ontological entity having independent existence in the body is subsequent to the period under discussion here; only foreshadowings of it are to be discovered in Renaissance writings, notably by Paracelsus, Fracastoro and Joubert.[172] Doctors did however

---

[168] Bartolettus 1619: 215–16 (on reducing all causes to these four categories): 'etenim causa continens, seu elicitiva per actionem imminentem dicta in morbis non datur. Nulla enim causa morbifica intra se formaliter morbum tanquam effectum producit, quia morbus in partem viventem, tanquam in subiectum dimittitur. Causa, quam appellant propriam, est ipsa causa morbifica coniuncta. Causa, quam appellant impropriam, cum sit, vel urgens, vel principalis, ambae ad antecedentem reducuntur: urgens quidem, sive ratione suae entitatis, ut materia venenata; seu ratione loci, ut pituita in cerebro, ad causam antecedentem reducitur: similiter causa principalis, quae simpliciter dicitur antecedens causae coniunctae.'

[169] Nutton 1990b: 205 (on da Monte's attempt to distinguish air, putrefaction and poison as primary, secondary and tertiary qualities respectively).

[170] Oddi 1589: 2: 'vestigium leporis, quod leporis principium non est, sed duntaxat investigationis et notitiae eius' (citing *Methodus medendi*, i.5, K 10.39–45; *De optima secta*, i, K 1.106–8); Valleriola 1562: 377.

[171] Campilongo 1601: 93v (citing Galen, *Ars parva*, K 1.366–8); Horst 1621: 114–16 (iv.3: 'an detur causa continens a morbo distincta?').

[172] Siraisi 1987a: 236 argues that Sanctorius changes much by concentrating not on the individual and the rebalancing of his or her humours (as does Galen) but on the identification of disease and its treatment in different people; cf. above 5.2.1, on Hasler. See also Nutton 1983; 1990b

ask to which of the Aristotelian predicaments 'morbus' belonged. Was it, as Averroes had suggested, and Argenterio agreed, a 'qualitas'? or a 'quantitas' of a 'qualitas', about which Oddi speculates? or a 'substantia', for which Vega opts? or an accident, as Fuchs believes? or a relation, which Vega also considers a possibility? or a passion, as Aristotle himself had suggested (*De sensu et sensato*, 436 a 17–21)? or a constitution or disposition (not strictly a predicament, unless in the mode 'habitus' or possession), a view taken by Fuchs from Galen? or a privation (an 'absentia sanitatis': also not strictly a predicament, unless taken as the negative state of possession), as Horst thinks? or a combination of two or more of these (a possibility considered by Fuchs and Fernel, who think in terms of a combination of relation and passion, but denied by Bartolettus, who argues that nothing can belong to more than one predicament)?[173]

7.5.6 'Morbi occulti'

These alternatives suggest the subtle, even abstruse nature of the distinctions and argumentation which doctors employ; it would perhaps be enlightening to see these in action in the case of two concrete examples. The first concerns the question whether there are such things as 'occulti morbi', and how (if they exist) they should be cured: an issue made famous by Fernel's aside concerning diseases of the whole substance in his *Pathologia*,[174] which provoked early responses from Cardano and Argenterio.[175] A summary of the debate is to be found in a 1619 disputation by Paulus Müncerus, a Silesian student at Basle, which consists of 'forty contradictions'. Among other things, he makes the case for dividing the class of disease known as intemperies into two classes, one 'manifest', the other 'occult', citing Paracelsians, anti-Paraclesians (among them Riolan), Italians (Vidi, Falloppio, Cesalpino, Argenterio), his Basle teachers (Stupanus, Bauhin), and doctors teaching in Germany (Horst, Sennert, Liddel). Given the complexity of the subject, we should not be surprised to find natural philosophers also cited, including Zabarella and

(on Fracastoro); Paracelsus 1567 (attributing to disease a 'physiognomy'); Bylebyl 1991: 166 (on Joubert); Aubéry 1585:15 (on the physiognomonic syllogism, correlating disease with remedy).

[173] Oddi 1589: *passim* (for rehearsal and refutation of the views of Argenterius and Vega); Horst 1629: 114; Fernel 1610b: 1.179–89; Galen, *De morborum differentiis*, K 6.836–80; Siraisi 1990a; Siraisi forthcoming; Bartolettus 1619: 218–19 ('non enim potest dari una ratio abstrahibilis duobus praedicamentis universa'). See also Ferdinandus 1611: 217.

[174] Siraisi forthcoming points out that the discussion of this topic occupies only a part of one chapter: Fernel 1610b: 1.184 (i.7). See also Blum 1992: 60–1.

[175] Siraisi 1997: 168 (Cardano); Siraisi 1990a: 170 (Argenterio); see also Richardson 1985: 175ff.

Julius Caesar Scaliger, the 'subtilitatum magister', and author of the jibe that occult qualities are the 'asylum inscitiae' (above, 7.3.3). His references to contemporary sources reveal not only the diversity of opinions about occult qualities, but also in a certain way their agreement, in spite of the polemical stances adopted in the literature, about the importance of the issue.[176]

7.5.7 *'Morbi totius substantiae'*

Müncerus cites Horst's *Pathologia* of 1612; but a more complete examination of the question whether there are occult diseases which are called diseases of the total substance ('an dentur morbi occulti quos vocant totius substantiae') is to be found in Horst's *De morbis, eorumque causis ac symptomatibus liber* of 1629. He first lists the reasons of those who deny the existence of occult illness: health and illness occur to the body in respect of its accidental, not its substantial form; the illness cannot come about separate from the body in which it inheres; the operation of the substance of parts of the body is not direct, but is effected through mediate qualities; the whole substance of the body is constituted as an indivisible entity, and cannot be stretched or reduced, yet it is host to diseases in a greater or lesser degree. Against these reasons, he continues, a number of 'recentiores', including Fernel, Falloppia, Colombo, and Stegghius, have argued that occult disease exists on the following grounds: the impaired function of homogeneous parts of the body cannot always be attributed to dyscrasic qualities or to an external vitiating factor; it is (on Scaliger's authority!) impertinent to deduce everything from manifest qualities, or a singular cause; Hippocrates posits a sacred (θεῖον) element in certain diseases which cannot be derived from manifest qualities; the substance of a part of the body can be lost through putrefaction and corruption, such as gangrene, which are not corruptions of qualities alone. He goes on to examine closely Fernel's account of the 'morbus totius substantiae', which he finds in various respects wanting; and ends by giving his approval to Falloppia's argument that all 'res naturales' consist of the four elements and a number of 'nobiliores formae' which are the locus of occult disease and the place through which also they are cured: 'there are in the parts of our body both a manifest and a formal complexion: in respect of the former there are manifest diseases; but diseases of the whole substance have their origin in the latter: in respect of the former

---

[176] Müncerus 1616.

rhubarb acts as a hot and dry agent; it attracts bile through the body's formal complexion'.[177] Horst's preferred explanation does not relate occult qualities to the 'vitale principium' of the various parts of the body, nor to the subject's 'forma coelestis',[178] nor to the operation of salt, sulphur and mercury as spagyric explanatory principles; he remains within Aristotelian natural philosophy and broadly within Galenism, accounting for Galen's silence on the subject by claiming that we can only know and cure these diseases by experience alone, whereas Galen explicitly calls for an etiological approach to diagnosis, as we shall see, which rules out purely empirical knowledge of illness (8.6.1).[179]

7.5.8 Plague and contagion

A second revealing discussion concerning the status of disease (as either ontological or physiological) is that inspired by Fracastoro's work on plague, contagion and fever. The unvarying clinical pattern of plague and certain fevers, and their regional character, raised the possibility that they were to be explained as entities, and not dispositions of the body.[180] Paracelsus had moved in the direction of an ontological explanation in the *Opus paramirum*, and had later spoken of disease as having a 'physiognomy';[181] inside the camp of learned medicine, Fracastoro elaborated an approach in the terms of the university debates of his day. In comparison to Pietro d'Abano's scholastic treatment of the transmission of disease, and the widespread attribution of plague to divine intervention in nature,[182] his explanation is altogether more empirically apt; so much so that it was very quickly adopted by even the most traditional of his contemporaries.[183] Plague is attributed to either bad air or contagion or both: Fracastoro defined contagion as 'a similar corruption of the substance of a particular combination which passes from one thing to another'. Airborne 'semina' have direct contact with the victim, leaving behind tinder ('fomites') which are not occult causes; according to this explanation, different seeds become responsible for different contagions,

---

[177] Horst 1629: 25: 'dari in partibus nostris temperaturam manifestam et formalem, unde respectu illius morbi manifesti: at huius rationis morbi totius substantiae nascuntur: illius respectu Rhabarbarum calefacit et siccat; at per formalem temperaturam bilam trahit'.
[178] Valleriola 1577: 422–3 makes this neoplatonist suggestion explicit.
[179] Horst 1629: 25.
[180] Temkin 1977: 442–3 cited by Nutton 1983: 21ff.; Lonie 1981: 30.
[181] Pagel 1935: 105–6 (citing *Opus paramirum*, iii.1); referred to by Bartolettus 1619: 259.
[182] Nutton 1983: 21 (citing Pietro d'Abano's commentary on the *Problemata*, vii.7); Nutton 1990b: 210; Horst 1629: 88–9 (iii.8–9).
[183] *Ibid.*; Crusius 1615: 106; Pagel 1935: 278 (on Fludd on 'seminaria' carried by the wind).

in a way which foreshadows a naturalistic and ontological account of plague.[184]

7.6 PRAETER NATURAM: MONSTERS AND MIRABILIA

7.6.1 Monsters

The issue of monstrous births and abnormality relates also to the category of the praeternatural. The locus classicus on this topic is in Aristotle's *De generatione animalium*, iv.4 (770 b 10ff.):

> A monstrosity... belongs to the class of things contrary to nature although it is contrary not to Nature in her entirety, but only to nature in the generality of cases. So far as concerns Nature which is always, and by necessity, nothing occurs contrary to that... Unnatural occurrences are found only among those things which occur as they do in the generality of cases, but which may occur otherwise.

The monstrous or the abnormal (which is distinguished from the pathological) is the product of defect or excess in animals, but does not occur in stones or metals:[185] most often this excess or defect is attributed to the intervention of a higher power, or to the moment of generation, which is subject to unquantifiable circumstances, or to primary matter, which is beyond predication.[186] Cardano follows the usual division in separating monsters into those which degenerate into an alien form, those which have features of more than one species, those which are lacking in some respect, and those which have hypertrophic members.[187] In his discussion of the Aristotelian locus, Argenterio stresses the inclusion of the monstrous in universal nature, examines various degrees of 'praeter naturam' (possession of a sixth finger is less monstrous than someone with a reversed spleen and liver), and ends up by confessing that the matter is obscure and uncertain, because the principles and definitions of the topic have not been established; the commentators on and translators of

---

[184] Nutton 1983; 1990b: 201 (on meaning of 'fomites'); and Pittion 1987: 116.

[185] Argenterio 1610: 500: 'morbi non ea ratione dicuntur esse praeter naturam, ut monstra, quae agentia naturalia non sibi proponunt, tanquam finem sui operis, sed ex errore aliquo contingunt'; Weinrichius 1595: 54–5; Waldungus 1611 (on *cas-limites*); Céard 1996; Roger 1997: 68ff.

[186] Toletus 1615: 75–6: the causes given are 'defectum materiae'; 'materiae abundantia'; 'qualitas activa quae in semine est potissimum calor'; 'malitia continentis foetum'; 'imaginatio matris'; 'caelum', either through the work of demons or through divine punishment. Cf. Piccolomini 1600: 224: 'conspicuus egressus ex ordine lege communi recessus ab instituto Naturae ob materiae impedimenta'. See also Liceti 1634.

[187] Cardano 1568: 662: 'quae in alienam formam degenerant', 'quae multiplicia sunt', '[quibus] aliquid deficit', '[quod] membrorum magnitudinem habet ultra mensuram'.

the second book of Aristotle's *Physics* could, he avers, make it clearer, but they merely confuse matters.[188] It seems that in arguing this he implicitly reduces all physics to an endoxical status.

As is well known, monsters ('ostenta', 'prodigia', 'portenta') were frequently taken to be portents; but for this to occur, they had, according to Peucer, to be very remarkable indeed.[189] The interpretation of such portents fell to theologians rather than doctors, just as the distinction between monstrous and non-monstrous had a theological dimension in the question of the preservation in life of abnormal births (see above 3.6). From the early Middle Ages, it was believed that monsters of this prodigious kind must have been intended in the divine mind; lesser versions could however be treated naturalistically as though the product of the 'voluntas naturae'.[190] The Paracelsian account of monstrosity stresses the fact that monsters are destined for this state *ab ovo*.[191] In traditional medicine, the explanation depends on the distinction between particular and universal nature: they are included in the latter, in spite of being 'praeter naturam' according to the former.[192] For this

---

[188] Argenterio 1610: 227–8: 'praeterea est locus in *lib 4 de gener anim 4* ubi Aristoteles scribit, aliquid esse monstrosum, esse rem praeter naturam, sed praeter eam, inquit, quae magna ex parte fit; nam praeter eam, quae semper et necessario est, nihil est. Verum in rebus his, quae magna quidem ex parte ita fiunt, sed aliter etiam possunt fieri, evenit, quod praeter naturam consistit: nam et inter eas ipsas, quibus accidit quidem praeter hunc ordinem, sed numquam quolibet modo, minus monstruosum esse videtur: quoniam quod praeter naturam fit, idem secundum naturam quodammodo est, cum natura materiae, naturae formae non superat'; but these things are 'obscura et incerta, quia definitiones et principia eorum non sunt posita'. On a sixth finger not being a morbus, see Galen, *De morborum differentiis*, K 6.862 and Fernel 1610b: 185 (*Pathologia*, i.8); on degrees of the praeternatural, *ibid.*, 1.180 (*Pathologia*, i.2); and Siraisi 1994b: 82 (quoting da Monte's commentary on *Avicenna*, *Canon*, ii.1). See also Vicomercatus 1596: 142; Daston and Park 1998: 116 (citing Albertus Magnus).

[189] Peucer 1553: 321ff.; cf. Zeisoldus 1638: D2v: 'an prodigia semper et ex necessitate aliquid significent?'; answered affirmatively, with the rider 'quod significent necessario necessitate non consequentis sed consequentiae'. See also Daston and Park 1998: 180. Cf Melanchthon 1581: 289ff. (he is forced to construe monsters as portents because he is so deeply committed to the argument from design).

[190] Daston and Park 1998: 50 (citing Isidore of Seville, *Etymologiae*, xi.3.1–4); Gemma 1575: 81: 'quanquam si magis cum Christo sit philosophandum quam cum gentilibus hisce philosophis [i.e. Aristotle], nihil penitus fortuitum Deo, nullum etiam naturae formatricis erratum apto sermone dicemus. Utrumque enim nostri comparatione quid tale videtur, ipsa tamen divina mens, et certo fine, et instrumentis ceu mediis, in illum convenientibus, agit maximeque ordinata incedit via, secundum intelligibiles mundi abditissimas rationes. Natura enim autem mutabilis illi obtemperans, etsi iuxta inferioris mundi seriem a solita lege deflectat, rapitur tamen divini spiritus vi, iam seipsa prope divinior facta: quippe quae legi antiquiori porrigens manum, toti se subjiciat totam, atque conspicuo, divinae illius providentiae fatum augustius multo, atque sublimius esse demonstret.' See also Liceti 1634: 28–9.

[191] Dorn 1584: 67.

[192] Barbarus 1579: 12 (i.16) (citing Philoponus's commentary on *Physics*, ii): 'ut autem causae quaedam improprie sunt efficientes ita quoque effectu reperiuntur, quae dici monstrifica consueverunt. Et illa quidem tametsi non ex sententia particularium causarum eveniunt: ab universali tamen natura fine quadam et ratione donantur.'

reason 'natural defect' can be said to be a contradiction in terms, or to disguise an ambiguous use of 'natural'.[193] It is thus not surprising that monsters can only be defined by the logic of 'magna ex parte' as Argenterio points out after Aristotle: 'a monstrosity is beside the course of nature ("praeter naturam"), but only in the sense of besides the ordinary course of nature ("praeter ea quam magna ex parte fit"); for there is nothing besides nature itself, which is what it is always and by necessity'.[194]

7.6.2 Mirabilia

The final category to be considered in this chapter is that of 'mirabilia' ('mira', 'miranda', 'admiranda'); this is related to the very extensive literature discussing remarkable events and phenomena and the secrets of nature.[195] Medical mirabilia constitute a category of remarkable and causally not fully explicable cases or cures, often collected from the experience of one or more doctors. Antonio Benivieni's *Libellus de abditis nonnullis ac mirandis morborum et sanationum causis* of 1507 sets a trend for similar books in the sixteenth century;[196] the cases described were all witnessed by the writer, who recognised that the explanatory force of medicine was inadequate to account for them, but none the less showed unwillingness to attribute their unusual features to astrological or other supernatural factors.[197] For doctors writing after Benivieni, these cases include 'rara' (for the guidance of general practitioners: 'nova' (such as syphilis, or the sweating sickness), 'monstrosa' and 'admiranda' (not conforming to accepted laws of nature: 'contra naturam').[198] This last category is the most problematic, because it impinges on two other discourses: theology and law.[199] The element of astonishment and sometimes horror implied in the encounter with the extraordinary case can be an occasion

---

[193] Siraisi 1997: 218–19.

[194] Argenterio 1610: 227–8, cited above, note 188. See also Monti 2000 (on the thirteen causes of monsters (including God and the devil) cited by Ambroise Paré).

[195] On these see Maclean 1984: 234–6; Eamon 1994; Findlen 1994; Céard 1996; Clark 1997; Daston and Park 1998; Siraisi 1997: 150–2; Grafton and Siraisi 1999.

[196] Benivieni 1529; Cardano 1663: 1.82–95; Valleriola 1573; Dodoens 1581: A6v–7v, who recognises that Benivieni initiated the genre, names Fernel, Hollerius and Valleriola, and includes excerpts from the writings of Benivieni, Tarantano, Benedetti, Matthias Cornax, Aegidius Hertogius and Achilles Gassarus; Libavius 1599b; Schenck 1609a; Smetius 1611; Donatus 1613.

[197] Siraisi 1997: 153–8.

[198] Schenck's title is *Observationum medicarum rararum, novarum, admirabilium et monstrosarum volumen*.

[199] The Roman Catholic Church had a clear doctrine of miracles; they are treated with great caution by the various protestant churches at the end of the sixteenth century. Calvin denied that there were any miracles after Christ's death; and Luther only recognised miracles occurring up to the end of the primitive church. But both Calvin and Luther recognise God's

for religious awe; but in Aristotelian terms, it is the stimulus to philosophical enquiry and the sign of ignorance.[200] Thus the more that can
be discovered about nature by diligent investigation, the greater the number of events which will not require classification as 'supra naturam' or
miraculous: a procedure which is in harmony with the view enunciated
by Peucer that it is possible to distinguish miracles from rule-governed
events.[201] Before him, Pomponazzi had declared in a more aggressively
naturalistic way about such events that 'things are not miracles because
they are totally against nature and besides the order of celestial beings;
they are only called miracles because they are unusual and rarely occur
and are not in the common course of nature except if this is seen over
long periods of time'.[202]

Some Renaissance doctors thus stress the urgent need to investigate the
fact ('to hoti') first before having recourse to supernatural explanations;
in other words, to assume that the 'latent causes' of miracles of nature
are not only to be found 'in the immense power of God' but also 'in

direct intervention into His world through the overriding of the operation of secondary causes
(i.e. those causes governing the working of nature which man is permitted to know). The Roman
Catholic categorisation of miracles (as opposed to the doctrine), derived from Aquinas, *Summa
theologiae* 1a 105.7–8 and 1a 110.4, seems to have been widely accepted, and was enshrined in
civil law by Bartolus (ad D 22.5.§57); and set out in a logical form by Zacchia 1630: 4.1–13, who
divides effects with unknown causes into non-miraculous and miraculous, and the miraculous
into wholly supernatural (e.g. the sun standing still in the sky), partially supernatural, which
is subdivided into 'contra naturam' (e.g. levitation, or moving mountains) and relative (events
which are miraculous because of the subject in which they occur), 'supra naturam' (e.g. the dead
coming to life again, or the blind seeing) and 'praeter naturam' (e.g. a sudden cure or the sudden withering of fig tree). What the tacit adoption, even by protestants, of this categorisation of
miracles permits is the examination of a 'remarkable' occurrence by investigators from outside
the Church without there being any infringement of the authority of the Church (or reference
to it); that is to say, they can investigate all phenomena as if the unknown causes were natural.
The eventual authority by which an event is described as miraculous of course lies only with the
Church, but secular authorities, whether legal or medical, are not prevented from describing
events as diabolical, or explaining how events can be accounted for within the realm of nature (a realm which includes nature's aberrations and the operation of secondary causes). The
problems which then arise are the question of God's direct intervention in the world, and the
role that this might play as an explanatory device in medical matters, the extent of the powers
to be attributed to the devil, and whether recourse has to be had to causes above secondary
causes to provide an adequate explanation of given events. See Clark 1997; Daston and Park
1998.

[200] *Metaphysics*, i.2, 982 b 12–13; Ingolstetterus 1597: 13: 'admiratio certissimum indicium ignorantiae
est'.

[201] Peucer 1553: 13–19, 291, 321–8 (eclipses are rule-governed events, but monstrous births are
not).

[202] Kessler 1994b: 41, quoting Pomponazzi 1567: 294: 'non sunt autem miracula quia sint totaliter
contra naturam et praeter ordinem corporum coelestium, sed pro tanto dicuntur miracula,
quia insueta et rarissime facta et non secundum communem naturae cursum sed in longissimis
periodis'.

the intimate secrets of nature'.[203] Even Paracelsians recognise that the powers which inhere in the living body and in the corpses of saints are all in the sphere of nature.[204] These arguments can generate speculation which goes in the opposite direction, and points to the amazing things in nature which surround us and which we take for granted: Vega cites an infant suckling and the movement of muscles as two of these.[205]

7.7 CONCLUSIONS

The philosophical context and content of medical thought thus supplies doctors with a concept of nature which is predominantly that of individual natures; universal nature is in part a determinant of these individual natures, but is capable of erring in respect of its goals, although never of the necessity which governs it in turn. The doctrine states that it can be overridden by this necessity and of course by its creator God, but recourse to explanations based on this tenet became less frequent in medical discourse as the century progressed. The specific premisses of medicine relate to the humours, spirits and members which make up the human being, and to the opposition health/sickness, of which the 'neutrum' is a complex middle term. It is, as we have noted, conceded at this time that medicine is only a science in an improper or loose sense of that term, whereas it is certainly a conjectural art, and an art is, according to the popular definition taken from Porphyry, 'the finite doctrine of infinite things' (see above 4.4). An art must deal with singular events, which are infinitely variable and are known through the senses: our intellect only grasps things at the level of species and genera. For this reason it is commonly claimed that 'rarely occurring events do not fall under the art [of medicine]', whose role it is to explain and make accessible the commonplace (the specific or generic) to the intellect.[206] Yet at the same time, it was acknowledged that doctors needed to be

---

[203] Siraisi 1997: 164 (referring to Cardano 1663: 6.480); Liceti 1612: 1.152 (ii.172–3): 'certe hoc sensu non reclamabo, ieiunium huiusmodi tam diuturnum quoddam esse naturae miraculum, cuius latentes caussas non ex immenso Dei virtute solum, sed ex intimis naturae penetralibus hauriri debet physiologus'. See also Daston and Park 1998: 122 (citing Aquinas, *Contra gentiles*, 3.102.2; see also *ibid.*, 3.99.9 and *Summa theologiae*, 3a 77.1 ad 1, on recognising that grace can none the less override the 'communis lex naturae').

[204] Webster 1995: 416 ; for another view, see Siraisi 1999a.

[205] Vega 1571: 893 (vii.54); 'sunt sane multa non tantum in humano corpore, sed extra ipsum quae nobis frequenti usu sunt, et eadem quotidie inspicimus, portenta maxima, quae ea ratione in miraculorum censu non habentur, quod eadem quotidie videamus'.

[206] Silvaticus 1601: 27: 'res eventu rarissimae sub arte non cadunt'; see also Argenterio 1610: 1694–1701.

apprised of the rare, the novel, the monstrous which others encounter, to supplement the direct experience they might have of disease. Just as the praeternatural is the other of nature within nature, the monstrous, novel and rare is the other of art within the art. There are therefore two orders of knowledge in medicine: that which falls under the 'certa praecepta', and which justify the doctrine's status as a 'science': and the record of mirabilia and monsters, about which there is knowledge, but of a less organised kind. This division is rather different from the more commonly encountered one, according to which the science of medicine is its theoria, and the art the operative knowledge by which cures are effected in the individual case.[207]

Nature also harbours other potential inconsistencies. As well as being economical and purposeful, it is redundant and excessive; as well as being a producer, it is a process and the product of that process; as well as being finite and finitely located in the sublunary sphere, it is infinite and subject to celestial and astral influences. All of these features of nature – the governing concept of natural philosophy, and one of the governing concepts of medicine – are known to Renaissance scholars: they are not the blind victims of their thinking, although they are obliged often to set aside its incoherence. In Cardano's *Contradicentia*, Siraisi has found not only the clash of Aristotelianism with Galenism, Aristotelianism with the new science, and Galen with Galen, but also both the competing claims of experientia and the rational critique of natural philosophy, both scholastic method and self-expression, both an interest in universals and an interest in particulars, and both rationalism and occultism.[208] These conflicts reveal the mental juggling acts required of those doctors who at this time try to set down the rational bases of their discipline.

The specific medical concept of health, with its opposite sickness and its mediate term neutrum, is also fissured; it is impossible to reconcile the latitude of forms, which a scale from healthy to sick presupposes, with the requirements of logic; there is need to establish classes of things and to develop a concept of disease which reveals the limitations of Aristotelian physics. The confusions of medical theory in this area no doubt brought awareness of the indeterminacy of some aspects of Galenic thought, as well as a realisation of the multiplicity and complexity of the material phenomena which were the subject matter of medical diagnosis, as Siraisi

---

[207] Cf. Cardano 1565: 83 (i.3.20), on the division of arts into 'certa per se' (e.g. arithmetic), 'certa per se', 'coniecturalis in exercitatione' (e.g. medicine and agriculture), 'coniecturalis per se et in exercitatione' (e.g. divination).

[208] Siraisi 1997: 69.

has suggested.[209] For all this, there is no sign that most doctors despaired of their art, or were so dismayed as to wish to abandon the edifice of Galenic medicine and the underpinning of Aristotelian logic altogether. This might be attributed to the fact of their intellectual passivity; but it seems to me more plausible to see the logic and the premisses with which they were working as a viable and living conceptual if shambolic system, with enough flexibility to allow for progressive changes in doctrine and even the reconciliation of Galenism with both Paracelsianism and a version of atomism in the work of Sennert at the very end of the period which we are considering.

[209] Siraisi forthcoming.

CHAPTER 8

The doctrine of signs

Il faut que le medecin sçache en les maladies les causes, les signes, les affections, les jours critique . . . car pour exemple, comment trouvera il le signe propre de la maladie, chacune estant capable d'un infiny nombre de signes? Combien ont-ils de debats entr'eux et de doubtes sur l'interpretation des urines?

(Montaigne)[1]

8.1 SEMIOLOGY AND MEDICINE

We are used to reading in Renaissance texts claims about the dignity, nobility, excellence and difficulty of subjects: in the case of semiology we may for once believe them. Vega claims that it lies at the origin of the whole art of medicine; Capivaccius declares that nothing is more useful or more difficult than the doctrine of signs, a point which Argenterio develops as follows:

For what, I ask, is more difficult than to distinguish between all those present, past and future things which befall our bodies, which is the task of this part of medicine? Because they are often so hidden that they seem not to be able to be grasped by any certain indication, and because their very discussion covers so many and so diverse heads, that even when the matter has been investigated, it is extremely difficult to explain them through a secure method of teaching.[2]

As one of the five divisions of medicine, semiotic or semiology sits in both theory and practice: the theory covers the relationship of physiology to

---

[1] *Essais*, ii.37, 773A.
[2] Vega 1571: 159: 'a signis inchoanda est ars tota'; Capivaccius 1603: 9: 'nihil utilius difficiliusque doctrina de signis'; Argenterio 1610: 1676: 'quid enim quaeso difficilius, quam praesentia, praeterita, futuraque omnia, quae corpori nostro accidunt, quod haec medicina pars promittit dignoscere? Cum saepe ita lateant illa, ut nullo certo indicio deprehendi posse videantur, et tam multa, tamque varia capita ipsa tractatio obtineat, ut etiam re ipsa perspecta, omnia certa docendi ratione explicare sit difficillimum.'

276

signs, the practice that of pathology to signs.[3] The theoretical textbooks
are usually presented 'to dioti': there is a definition followed by divisions.
The practical manual, although going from cause to sign in textual layout, is usually governed by a presentation 'to hoti' of illnesses in sequence,
from head to toe; it is much closer in appearance to modern textbooks
of pathology.[4] It has a very long and relatively stable history, stretching
from Avicenna's *Canon* and Bernard de Gordon's *Lilium medicinae* in a
more popular mode at the beginning of the fourteenth century to Ercole
Sassonia (Saxonia) in the seventeenth.[5] Its generic layout (cause-sign or
symptom; or cause-sign or symptom-remedy) is ubiquitous, and is even
found in Renaissance popular or layman's handbooks of therapy.[6]

8.1.1 Ancient and medieval sources

The ancient and medieval sources of semiology help explain why there
are so many versions of sign theory in Renaissance medical texts. As
late as Diderot's *Encyclopédie*, Hippocrates is celebrated as the founding
father of semiology: he is praised there for his observational skills, un-
systematic presentation of material and terse delivery of judgements.[7]

---

[3] Campilongo 1601: 1–4, who seems to be reflecting the demands of Paduan students for practica
rather than theoria (see above 1.5.1) ('omnes medicinae partes vel sunt actu, vel potestate
factivae'); see also Sennert 1650: 1.447, and Frölich 1612: A2r, who point out that the final cause
of semiology is not 'cognitio curationis' but 'curatio'.

[4] Peucer 1553: 207v: 'signorum in tota arte medica, ea est ratio ad res significatas, quae vel
causarum ad effectus, vel effectuum ad causas, vel eorum quae causis et effectibus adiuncta
cohaerent, ad eorumdem correlativa'; Campilongo 1601: 2 (referring to Galen, *Ars parva*) says
that the 'cognitio causarum' precedes the 'cognitio corporum et signorum' in teaching the art
of medicine, but in its practice the order is reversed. 'To hoti' here has both senses: the question
of fact and the passage from effect to cause. *Ibid.*, 15r makes the point that the 'demonstratio
quia ab effectu' is the most suitable for semiology. Also Jokissus 1562: viii (on Galen's *Ars parva*):
'ratione scientiae et naturae sic sese consequuntur: causa, corpus, signum, ratione vero artis et
sensus hoc modo collocantur; signum, corpus, causa. Sed ratione scientiae et artis simul isto
ordine recensentur: corpus, signa, causae, quem ordinem Galenus in arte medica sequitur.'

[5] Saxonia 1603; Cardano 1583; Betrutius in Heyll 1534: 47 affords the following example of the
first category on the condition 'defectus odoratus': 'causa est virtutis odoratae laesio. Ablatione,
cum ex odoribus bonis nil percipi potest. Diminuta, qui nisi fortia et acuta odoramenta, nullum percipitur. Corrupta, cum odores percipiuntur, a re praesenti odorabili alieni. Quod sit
a cerebri calida vel frigida ultimate in temperie, potissimum in poro eius. Ab oppilatione
narum aut colatorii. Casu vel percussione, inducente tortusitatem in ossibus et chartilagine
nasi. Signa caliditatis: siccitas narum cum odore. Non sentiuntur odores calidi, sed frigidi.
[Signa] Frigiditatis. Frigiditas nasi. Foetidos vel calidos odores tantum odoratur. [Signa] op-
pilationis. Gravitas capitis. Ex naribus vel palatu nihil egreditur. Difficulter attrahitur aer per
nares.'

[6] E.g. Duport 1584 (many editions in the following century).

[7] *Encyclopédie*, Neuchâtel, 1765, 14.938: 'de tous les auteurs qui ont écrit sur la *sémeiotique* Hippocrate
est presque le seul dont les ouvrages méritent d'être consultés, et surtout celle qui regarde les
maladies; tous les autres n'ont fait que le transcrire ou le défigurer'.

The Hippocratic *Prognosis* and *Aphorisms* (especially i.12, together with Galen's commentary on this aphorism) form part of the central canon of medieval pedagogical texts. Their importance was recognised by Galen, who wrote widely read commentaries on both. Galen himself composed a number of tracts on pathology with a strong semiological content: *De symptomatum differentiis*; *De pulsuum differentiis*; *De morborum causis et differentiis*; *De locis affectis*; *De crisibus*; *De diebus decretoriis*. His dispersed remarks were known in the compilation *De accidenti et morbo* in the medieval period, and had been already recast into systematic form by the Arabs, notably Avicenna (*Canon*, i.2.3), whose version of the doctrine appeared in editions of the *Articella*, together with the *Isagoge* of Joannitius, and also contains a brief much-quoted account of semiology.[8] In the medieval period, these texts were subject to a series of influential commentaries by Gentile da Foligno, Jacques Despars, Dino del Garbo, Taddeo Alderotti and Ugo Benzi, among others.[9] Galen also wrote about the theory of semiology (*Ad Glauconem*; *Methodus medendi*; *Ars parva*; *De simplicibus medicinae facultatibus*, ii.1–4, K 11.459–71). Altogether his writings form a vast body of disparate knowledge requiring ordering and anthologisation. With the republication in the 1520s of a number of relevant Galenic texts in Greek[10] came the first series of these reworkings: a certain Stephanus Dutemplaeus or Dutemple published a visual dichotomy in Lyon in about 1530, distributing the material in an anacephaleotic or dialectical way (see above 4.4.3) which as a pedagogical innovation would later be attributed to Ramus.[11] He was followed in this initiative by two much more famous doctors, Leonhart Fuchs of Tübingen and the Parisian Jacques Sylvius (Dubois), who brought out similar distributions of material in 1537 and 1539 respectively. Thereafter an impressive number of new orderings of the material are elaborated in Italy: by da Monte, Argenterio, Cardano,

---

[8] Avicenna 1608: 131–9; Paolino in Avicenna 1608 (a dichotomised version of Joannitius); Arrizabalaga 1998.

[9] Torrigiano 1557; Siraisi 1987a.

[10] Durling 1961: 252f. gives the full bibliography; there were near-simultaneous translations of the most relevant texts by Guillaume Cop and Thomas Linacre which appeared in 1523 and 1524 respectively, in Paris and London. The trigger of expository activity seems to have been the publication in Paris in 1528–9 of the *De crisibus* (by Chrétien Wechel), the *De differentiis morborum* and the *De causis morborum* together, the *De differentiis symptomatum* and the *De causis symptomatum*, also together, and the *De diebus decretoriis* with other texts (all by Simon de Colines).

[11] Maclean 2001. As well as Dutemplaeus, Fuchs and Sylvius, Huggelius 1560, Zwinger 1561, Weckerus 1576, Capivaccius 1603, Paolino in Avicenna 1608 and Fabricius 1626 produce dichotomised distributions of semiology. The first textbook to appear at Tübingen after the university's rejection of Arabic manuals was on semiology: see Fuchs 1537a.

Capivaccius, Campilongo, Bartolettus. Many of these (not least the last) insist that they are the first to have attempted to sort out this field of medicine.[12]

8.1.2 Renaissance semiologies

There seem to be two reasons why the field was seen to be so susceptible to reorganisation by sixteenth-century doctors, and was so worked over. The first is the extent of the textual material to be reworked; over 400 entries in Brasavola refer to sign, symptom and indication, and his brief descriptions of these loci is suggestive of how many ways they can be arranged into patterns. The second reason is the mismatch between the logic of signs which most doctors learned from Aristotle, the debate about epilogism and analogism, and the nature of signs themselves (5.1, above). We have seen that doctors try to save the certainty of their art by claiming that its 'praecognita' are necessary and only its 'exercitatio' conjectural, but in so doing allege a 'praecognitum' (nature) which cannot of itself be necessary as it is under certain circumstances contingent and imperfect (see above, chapter 7); in a similar way, medical semiologists construct systems which cannot be more than endoxical divisions or distributions, as we shall see. As emerged from the discussion of the logic of signs (5.1), there cannot be an adequate sequence of differentiae of signs for a number of reasons: because of their ambivalent status, which may be either intelligible or sensible or both;[13] because signs may have their own entity, or may be identical with their signata, or may be no more than signs of something else; because they relate to various states of health, and to temporal moments in the past, present and future; because as species they are subject to differentiae which cannot logically be combined (e.g. common/proper, early/late, substantial/accidental); because they may be mediate or immediate, certain or uncertain, permanent or labile, and more besides. My own ordering of material in this chapter is beset with the same organisational problems as those which sixteenth-century doctors faced when confronted with this bewilderingly diverse doctrine,

---

[12] Bartolettus 1619: 246. On the republication of the Galenic texts, see Durling 1961. Da Monte follows the sequence of *Canon*, i.2 but develops it by reference to Galen's semiological texts: Siraisi 1987a: 54–6. A new lectureship on this text was established in 1551 in Padua; its first occupant was Antonio Negri: Facciolatus 1757: 2.383.

[13] In Joannitius and Avicenna, signs and symptoms are treated together; but the former (in Avicenna 1608: A6r) makes the point that signs are what are perceived by the doctor (through his intellect), and symptoms ('accidentia') by the patient through his or her senses. See also Arnau de Vilanova 2000: 110ff. and Rondelet 1586: 592–7.

elements of which are to found scattered throughout the Hippocratic and Galenic corpus. These can be anthologized in different ways, and drawn upon to support a variety of theoretical constructions. The majority of writers follow a fairly similar sequence, based more on Joannitius than Avicenna, but there is considerable variation of content.[14] I shall not be able to claim, any more than the writers on this topic to which I shall refer, that what follows is a necessary or neat progression. All that follows should be read in the context of the logical and methodological discussion of signs, which has been examined in detail above (5.1), all or part of which is to be found in Renaissance discussions of the medical sign.

Semiology can be looked upon as a general discipline of which medical semiotic is only one branch. From the medieval period onwards, physicians were active as writers and commentators on the broad range of conjectural arts, which include astrology, physiognomy, chiromancy, metoposcopy, dream interpretation and weather forecasting; in the Renaissance, the Paracelsian doctrine of signatures can be added to this list. The inclusion of all of these arts in this chapter is justified by their

---

[14] Both Fuchs 1537a and Sylvius 1539a distribute Galen's books on the causes and differentiae of illnesses and symptoms, and introduce other material (Sylvius's is a fully fledged practical manual). Avicenna's distribution begins with time, then passes to degrees of health, substantial signs, proper signs, 'assidentia' and 'emergentia', primary and secondary illnesses, complexions, temperamental balance and imbalance, 'repletiones', dominant humours, 'oppilationes', 'ventositates', apostemata, pulse and urine; Paolino in Avicenna 1608 distributes Joannitius as follows: '1 significationum seu signorum genera sunt tria et alia sumuntur a 1.1 significatis quae sunt alia 1.1.1 sanitatis 1.1.2 aegritudinis 1.1.3 neutralitatis; a 1.2 tempore quod triplex 1.2.1 praeteritum 1.2.2 praesens 1.2.3 futurum; a 1.3 specie signorum quae in aegro dicuntur accidentia, in medico signa et sumitur horum divisio vel 1.3.1 absolute 1.3.1.1 virtus 1.3.1.2 qualitas 1.3.1.3 exiens a corpore [vel] 1.3.2 respective 1.3.2.1 intrinsecus cuius modi sunt sex 1.3.2.2 extrinsecus cuius modi sunt tres (my numbering). This is a very clear account of the text in *Articella* 1515: 8v (cf. Liddel 1598). Sylvius 1539a (*De signis*) begins with the distinction sēmeion–tekmērion (above, 5.1); combines time and health (below 8.6), and then passes to signs of (healthy) temperament; organs and parts; illnesses; critical signs; and finally neutral signs. Fuchs 1604: 1.215–16 (in the *Institutiones medicae*, iv.1) is a simpler version of this; da Monte 1587, Argenterio 1610, Capivaccius 1603, Campilongo 1601, Liddel 1628, Sennert 1650 all follow approximately the order of Galen's *Ars parva* (a definition, followed by a division of health (salubria, neutra, insalubria), a division of signs according to time (diagnostic, prognostic, anamnestic), a discussion of their 'vis'; thereafter an account of the 'fontes signorum', followed in some cases by discussion of pulse and urine, and critical and decretorial signs). But inside this broad distribution, there are many local differences. Huggelius 1560 begins with critical signs; Weckerus 1576: 272–92 begins with the distinction between essential and accidental, the former being subdivided into formal (under which primary (humoral) and secondary (sensory) fall), and material (composition, conformation, figure, size, etc.). Under accidental, there is a distribution by action (of the principal organs) and passion (non-natural extrinsic factors). Frölich 1612 offers yet another distribution into the three 'fontes' (signs drawn from 'res naturales', 'neutrales' (which he eccentrically calls 'non naturales'), and 'praeter naturales'; the last considered in respect of the differentiae external/internal, supernatural/natural, diagnostic/prognostic, cause/effect/similarity; he ends with a short passage on critical signs.

commonly accepted affinity to medicine in this period. Some doctors, notably Gemma and Peucer, approach medical semiology through the general field of conjectural practices; the former, concentrating principally on astrology, makes use of a neoplatonist hierarchical distribution (divine, metaphysical, paraphysical, natural) as well as a traditional sublunary one (weather, health/sickness, peace/war, politics). The latter, whose theme is divination, surveys in turn signs of oracles, theomancy, magic, incantations, sacrifices, auguries, spells, dreams, medicine, weather, astrology and teratology.[15] In the more specialised area of medical semiology in the late Renaissance, Italian names dominate: Jessenius a Jessen's bibliography in his edition of Campilongo of 1601 shows the strength of the Paduan tradition (da Monte, Capivaccius, Campilongo); Jacchinus and Argenterio are also mentioned, as is Rondelet of Montpellier. A chronological survey of books reveals the richness of the field, as well as the development of tendencies if not schools. In the first generation, Sylvius, Fuchs, da Monte, Vega of the Complutense and Thriverus of Louvain are prominent; the 1550s see the emergence of Argenterio, Cardano, Fernel, Jacchinus, and Rondelet; by 1590, a new influential figure – Capivaccius – has appeared, who opposes Argenterio's doctrine. Thereafter a number of lesser writers declare themselves the disciples of either Argenterio (Le Thielleux and Aubert) or Capivaccius (Campilongo, but with reservations).[16] At the very end of the period we are discussing, an eclectic approach can be detected in the writings of Liddel and Horst, and there is the consolidation of the Paracelsian theory of signatures, in defence of which du Chesne and later Croll write (see below 8.8.6).

8.2 MEDICAL SIGNS

8.2.1 Sign and cause

Semiology is the 'knowledge of all indications of a therapeutic method, discovered by rational doctors through their own mental resources (instrumenta), for the sake of effecting a cure'.[17] The medical sign has,

---

[15] Peucer 1593; Gemma 1575.
[16] See also Alonso 1598: 21, who discusses Argenterio's sign doctrine, and Liddel 1628: 520, who accepts his use of arguments from proportion and analogism (where Sanctorius 1630: 501–3 (vi.1) rejects them). Varanda 1620: 15–19 discusses aspects of both Altomare's and Argenterio's semiology.
[17] Campilongo 1610: 16r: 'cognitio omnium indicantium methodi curatricis, a dogmaticis per propria instrumenta inventa, gratia curationis'.

as we have seen, its own definition: either as a substitutive term, in which no ratiocinative process is involved, of which smoke as a sign of fire is the standard example; or, in Capivaccius's words, as 'a proposition, produced by the intellect from objects perceptible to the senses, demonstrating a posteriori something unknown in the medical art'; or a middle term in a syllogism (above 5.1). It is agreed by all that signs always precede an illness, and are always accompanied by a cause: da Monte claims that signs cannot exist without causes, nor causes without signs; one is attached to the other as the shadow is to a body.[18] They pose a peculiar difficulty because they can simultaneously be a symptom, or a cause, or even an illness, or even both of these latter; this problem had long been recognised.[19] As Cardano points out, there are 'pure signs' (such as bad colour), signs which are simultaneously causes (he cites pain and wakefulness as two of these), signs that are identical to illnesses (epilepsy and jaundice are cited here) and signs which are in different respects both causes and illnesses.[20] We have already encountered the difficulties which arise when attempts are made to clarify the Galenic doctrine of the distinction between sign, cause, illness and symptom, which Argenterio persuasively claims to be confused;[21] this is compounded by the complexity and untidiness of the doctrine of etiology, which has already been examined (above 7.5.2–4). Valleriola's brief excursion into this doctrine offers an example of this: he distinguishes *inter alia* between manifest causes, which are evident to sense: obscure and hidden causes which have various non-sensory signs not discoverable by rational activity, including causes known only *qua* causes to God; and the causes of rare and unusual events.[22]

8.2.2 Sign and symptom

Causes, being of the same order of non-material entities as other 'entia rationis', are intelligible through necessary signs; symptoms on the other hand are sensory, accidental and variable. Cardano declares

---

[18] Diocles of Carystus 1572: 2v: 'nullus praeter naturam affectus homines corripit nisi certis praecurrentibus signis ille indicatus fuerit'; da Monte 1554: 67v: 'unde sumuntur signa est locus affectus, et causa faciens affectum, ideo dicitur signum, quia accidens est sequens locum affectum, et causas, sicut umbra corpus, quia signa sine causis esse non possunt, neque causae sine signis'.

[19] Argenterio 1610: 933; Peucer 1553: 204v; Ottosson 1984: 198 (on Averroes).

[20] Cardano 1582: 444–5.

[21] Siraisi 1990a: 171, quoting Argenterio 1592: 91.

[22] Valleriola 1562: 381–2 (citing Hippocrates, *De flatibus* as the source of this distinction, although it is not explicit there).

that signs (*qua* intelligible species), unlike symptoms, never change.[23] For Argenterio, these latter are signs insofar as they are 'effects of an illness'.[24] According to Sanctorius, there are first- and second-order symptoms; the second order (a symptom of a symptom) can be translated into the first, and thus for him (though not for all) be rightly described as a sign.[25] Two prominent sources of symptoms are pulse and urine; the former is intimately connected with the vital and animal faculties;[26] the latter, together with faeces, sweat, spit, vomit, and so on, is an excretion.[27] According to Galen's *De constitutione artis medicae*, they are privileged means of determining the condition of the patient;[28] the procedures of inspecting and assessing both were revised in the Renaissance. Struthius's book on the pulse, which claimed to have recovered the full scope of the Galenic lore which had been lost for 1,250 years (a claim whose chronology at least is remarkably accurate), sold 800 copies on the day it appeared in Padua; it led to a number of subsequent studies, of which the most elaborate is the *Monochordon symbolico-biomanticum abstrusissimam pulsuum doctrinam, ex harmoniis musicis dilucide, figurisque oculariter demonstrans* (1640) of Samuel Hafenrefferus.[29] Uroscopy was also revised both by da Monte (his teachings are reproduced by his pupils Bassiano Landi and Franciscus Emericus) and later by Capivaccius, and was subjected to new tests by Paracelsians.[30] According to Vivian Nutton, it lost credit in certain quarters in the course of the sixteenth century, and became in the end, when not accompanied by other diagnostic tests, the mark

---

[23] Cardano 1568: 616 (on Hippocrates, *Prognosis*, iii.41). Silvaticus 1601: 27 seems to contradict this by dividing symptoms into 'antecedentia', 'post apparentia', and 'semper existentia', unless 'semper' is taken here to have a loose sense.

[24] Argenterio 1610: 168.

[25] Sanctorius 1630: 19–25 (i.6) (it should be noted that this view is consistent with Sanctorius's argument that all information relevant to diagnosis can be derived from the senses); García Ballester 1995: 143; cf. Sylvius 1539a: 8–12 (here symptoms are said to follow illnesses as shadows follow the body); Donatius 1591: 31 says that both signs and symptoms which generate indicia are derived from the senses, but Heyll 1534: A2r has signs derived from symptoms ('signa sunt symptomatum notae'). Willichus 1582:11 takes the two terms to be synonymous.

[26] A standard definition is taken from Galen, *De differentiis pulsuum*, iv as cited by Valleriola 1562: 456: 'actio peculiaris cordis, deinde arteriarum, quae distentione, ac contractione moventur a facultate vitali, quo caloris nativi mediocritas retineatur, generetur autem in cerebro spiritus animalis'.

[27] Valleriola 1562: 456ff.; Liddel 1628: 532–42.

[28] Albertus 1615: B5v points to the inspection of pulse and urine as sources of the doctor's authority over his patients.

[29] Durling 1961; Hafenrefferus 1640; Bylebyl 1985a.

[30] Landi 1543: 31ff.; Emericus 1552 (R2v has a cautionary tale about the wrong way to diagnose from urine); Daca 1577; Capivaccius 1595; Rhenanus 1614; Argenterio 1610: 1831–70 is a treatise on urine written against da Monte.

of a quack.[31] A debate arose as to whether the pulse or the urine yields better information, in which it is possible to find proponents of either and neither side.[32] Both pulse and urine are conjectural as symptoms (or signs derived from symptoms).[33] Like all symptoms, all they can do is yield better information through the application of a correct method: signs derived from symptoms 'do not have the status of eternal truths'.[34] The objections expressed here by Sanctorius are straightforwardly derived from the Aristotelian doctrine of sensible and intelligible, individual and general data (above, 4.3).

8.2.3 Sources of signs

There are three sites or sources of signs: the patient, his or her attendants (the 'astantes'), and the doctor himself.[35] The signs given by attendants at the bedside concern the history of the patient's disease, and a non-subjective view of its progress; the doctor is the site of knowledge, in which the sensory signs from the patient and his environment are translated into intelligible 'indicantia'. There are at least three Galenic loci discussing the signs derived from the patient. The most commonly cited is taken from *De locis affectis*, i.5 (K 8.44), and identifies the following five sources of signs in the patient: impaired function; excreta; the site or position of bodily parts; the nature of the pain; finally, 'propria accidentia', which sound like a logical oxymoron (property and accidence being two different predicables), and refer to inseparable but variable accidents of the kind discussed at length by Boethius in his commentary on Porphyry.[36] From the account given of morbid signs in the *Ars parva*, Peucer deduces the following five headings: changes perceptible to the senses such as size, colour or shape, in number and site of bodily parts, in qualities such as hardness, softness, heat or coldness; impaired function; pain; excreta; abnormal tumours.[37] A third set of differentiae is taken from Galen's *De symptomatum differentiis*,

---

[31] Forestus 1589; Nutton 1996.
[32] Vallesius 1606: 117–19; Emericus 1552: 51r; Nutton 1985a: 94.
[33] Sanctorius 1630: 487–8 (v.13).
[34] *Ibid.*, 499 (vi.1): 'non sunt aeternae veritatis'.
[35] Argenterio 1610: 169.
[36] Fernel 1610b: 1.209; Wolf 1620: A2v; Bartolettus 1619: 248; Horst 1609: 132: 'actio laesa'; 'excreta'; 'partium situs atque positus'; 'doloris proprietas'; 'propria accidentia'; he adds tumours to this list. Frölich 1612: A4v claims that 'propria accidentia' can be subsumed under the four other classes. See also Boethius, *In Porphyrium*, PL 64.55–70.
[37] Peucer 1553: 212r: 'In arte parva hos fontes in quinque contrahit [Galenus] capita, Alterationes praeter naturam accidentium subjectorum sensibus, ut magnitudinis, coloris, figurae, numeri, partium, sitis, duriciei, molliciei, caloris, frigoris; Laesas actiones; Exeuntia; Dolores; Tumores praeter naturam.'

ii (K 7.53) and *Methodus medendi*, xii.1 (K 10.311): the altered state ('affectus', 'diathesis') of the body; functional damage; or both, principally in the form of abnormal excreta and retenta.[38] These together are conflated in various ways.[39] Inspired no doubt by the Fernelian 'morbus totius substantiae', Liddel adds 'interconnected phenomena or the consensus of bodily parts'.[40] Sanctorius's six 'fontes', which claim to guarantee a certain diagnosis, are derived from external (procatarctic) causes, the disposition of the patient, the symptoms, the affected places, and the signs which, by showing what alleviates or aggravates the condition, can reveal to the doctor the illness which is affecting the hidden parts of the body.[41] These signs have to be read in sequence; they are not straightforward, as the pain may not be situated in the affected part, and the impaired function not relate to the affected organ. In these classifications, we may again note the confusion of categories (objective/subjective, sensible/intelligible, cause/symptom/disease) which both reveals the fragility of the doctrine, and the need to inculcate a flexible mental approach in doctors who, in grappling with symptomatology, need to be aware that the evidence they derive from the patient and his attendants is potentially both ambiguous and obscure.

8.3 THE SIGN DISTRIBUTED

We come now to the distribution of signs. The medieval tradition divided substantial from accidental: the former relating to the homogeneous parts in respect of primary and secondary qualities (hot/dry; cold/moist; hard/soft and colour) and to the heterogeneous parts in respect of form, quantity and position; the latter governed by the distinctions good/bad

---

[38] 'qualitates mutatae', 'laesae operationes', 'exeuntia', 'detenta': Cardano 1583: 1–3; Campilongo 1601: 13v; also Valleriola 1562: 389–92; Liddel 1628: 228 identifies three 'principal' kinds of symptom: 'quod facultatem, facultatis functionem respicit' ('actio laesa'); 'quod in contentis consistit' ('excrementorum et humorum vitia'); 'quod in solidis partibus [invenitur]'('qualitas mutata'); Ferdinandus 1611: 211 (iii.4) produces a threefold division, the first consisting in the four listed here, the second arising from the three faculties of the body, and the third being those things detected by the senses; see also Lonie 1981: 32 (the three classes of diathesis) and Hankinson 1995: 69–70 (citing Galen, *De experientia medica*, ii–iv). Argenterio 1606–7: 76 writes to refute Corti's fourfold division of the sources of symptoms ('a propria substantia membri'; 'ex necessario consequentibus'; 'a necessario accidentibus'; 'ab operationibus').

[39] E.g. by Peucer 1553 ('accidentia; actiones laesae; excrementorum qualitates; tumores praeter naturam; dolores; colores partium aut corporis universi'). These can be reduced to three: 'ex constitutione et habitudine; ex essentia partium; ex annexa forinsecus'.

[40] Liddel 1628: 515.

[41] Sanctorius 1630: 34–6 (i.9).

and perfect/imperfect, indicating changes in operative ability (such as indigestion), changes in quality (such as jaundice) and changes in excretion (such as black urine). There is a complication here, as the word 'accidens' can also in medical parlance refer to any symptom.[42] A logical accident is said not to yield any 'scientia'; but some symptoms ('propria accidentia') can do this, presumably because a link is taken to exist between the symptom and the cause of the illness. The same sign can relate to either the substantial or the accidental; it can be mediate (as function) or immediate (as urine); it can be ephemeral or permanent; it can be true, mostly true, or not true.[43]

8.3.1 The differentiae of the sign: time and health

It is not possible to create a Porphyrian tree out of the differentiae of the sign, but there are some forms of exhaustive distribution. Sylvius derives one of these in his De symptomatibus from Galen's Isagoge (see above 5.2.1 and fig. 5.1);[44] by this diagram, signs are distributed in relation to time (past, present, future) and to the mediate opposition of health and sickness, with neutrum as a middle term. The same distribution is found in non-schematic form in many other writers.[45] It requires that health be defined in respect of the individual patient's temperament, which needs first to be determined:[46] and as we have seen, the 'neutrum' is not a straightforward mediate term, being a place of passage of health to sickness or sickness to health in which quantity is not always physically specifiable.[47] There are other problems with this model which are made explicit by doctors. Vega points out that only corpora, and not signs themselves, are healthy, sick or neutral; Campilongo, following Galen, shows that all three temporal classes of signs can be used in prognosis ('praenuntiativa'); Crusius, following Fernel, reduces the right-hand column of Sylvius's schema to two (relating to diagnosis and prognosis); Argenterio thinks that a fourth category ('lethalia') should be added to the left-hand column.[48]

---

[42] Pietro d'Abano 1548: 123v (lxxviii). This ordering is broadly followed by Weckerus 1576: 264ff.

[43] Ottosson 1984: 203–4; cf. Alonso 1598: 21–5; Fonseca in Jacchinus 1615: 277 (on ephemeral common signs in fever).

[44] Sylvius 1539a: 25f.

[45] Capivaccius 1603: 15 has an exhaustive combinatory of disease, cause and symptom; Liddel 1628, Thriverus in Laurembergius 1621, Horst 1609 are writers who use degrees of health and time to distribute signs.

[46] Nance 1993.

[47] On neutrum and latitude of forms, see 4.4.2, 7.4.3.

[48] Vega 1571: 159; Campilongo 1601: 10v; Argenterio 1610: 1698; Galen, Ars parva, K 1.364.

8.3.2 The differentiae of the sign: common and proper

A bewildering set of differentiae and categories of signs are referred to, some logically grounded, some not. Perhaps most important is the differentia common/proper, which in one Galenic locus (*De febrium differentiis*, iii) is expressed as separable/inseparable; we have encountered the discussion of these before (above 5.1). Various senses are given to these distinctions when they are taken together. All are agreed that the proper and inseparable sign is the pathognomonic sign, to which I shall return; but Vega thinks that there are also common and inseparable signs (e.g. pain); Liddel and Sennert understand common and separable ('assidentia' or 'synedreuonta') to refer not to signs of the essence of an illness, but to its duration, strength or development; Campilongo associates proper signs with greater, and common signs with lesser degrees of certainty; and only Cardano mentions the fourth possible category (proper and separable), but he gives no example of it.[49] Pathognomonic signs are agreed to be unambiguous and unique indicators of given diseases, and are very rarely encountered singly; they are most often met in the form of syndromes or 'concursus' of common signs.[50] Common signs have to be disambiguated (because common); they rely on the 'praenotio' of the professionally trained doctor.[51] Another distinction, borrowed, as we shall see, from physiognomy (as is much of this doctrine) is that between perpetual and contingent or labile signs, such as those which are linked to states of fever.[52] The distinction between 'epiphenomena' ('mox apparentia') and 'supervenientia' is also found; it raises the problem of time and etiology again (since supervenience may not imply a causal link), as does the category 'epigenomena' ('comitantia').[53] These last show the mutation of the illness by coction or crudity.[54] There are also signs of recovery or death, which are linked to critical or decretorial signs.[55] 'Gnorismata' are indications encountered at the beginnings of illness.[56] The distinction between mediate and immediate signs is also found.[57]

[49] Vega 1571: 368–9; Liddel 1628: 511–12; Sennert 1650: 1.124; Campilongo 1601: 15–16; Cardano 1582: 47–8.

[50] Rondelet 1586: 591 (citing *Aphorisms*, ii.30); da Monte, cited by Siraisi 1987a: 346.

[51] Peucer 1553: 85.

[52] Crusius 1615: 175; see also below, 8.8.1, and *Physiognomica*, ii, 806 a 8ff.

[53] Sennert 1650: 1.323; Vega 1571: 1073 derives the distinction 'propria/mox apparentia/assidentia' from Galen, *De crisibus*, i.5, K 9.562–3.

[54] Sennert 1650: 1.527: 'coctionis signa nunquam mala sunt'.

[55] *Ibid.*, 323; Vallesius 1606: 119; Valleriola 1562: 423–5; Valleriola 1577: 422; Fracastoro 1574: 140ff.; Peucer 1553: 210–11; Pagel 1935: 107; also Siraisi 1997: 140 (on Luca Gaurico).

[56] Fabricius 1626: A4v–B1r.

[57] Argenterio 1610: 168; Ingolstetterus 1597: 146 (on natural signs).

8.4 PATHOGNOMONIC SIGNS: SYNDROMES OF SIGNS

Pathognomonic signs pose a particular problem. There can be such a
sign, which is the proper of one illness; but such signs are acknowledged
to be 'very rare', if at all found; and even if they were found they would
not yield a secure method, because it is held that there can be no
method or knowledge of such things.[58] Proper signs are here said not
to be present in the subject *simpliciter*, but rather *ut nunc*; but they also
are of no demonstrative force any more than are proper names (see
above 4.2.3), and possess no significatory function.[59] A single sign is
not to be trusted; this doctrine is cited by Alonso in a discussion about
prognosis on the authority of the *Physiognomica*.[60] So signs have to come
in syndromes, and be common.[61] But even syndromes of signs can fail
to yield scientific information if they include, like those of the empirics,
signs which are derived from analogy or proportion ('ex similitudine
et ex proportione'), which Sanctorius in refuting Argenterio denounces
as 'mere analogisms'.[62] Sanctorius's method ensures both that only
appropriate common signs are taken into consideration and that their
contingency and 'ut multum' probability (a necessary feature of common signs which can indicate more than one illness) are purged by
submitting each syndrome to the six 'fontes' method (see below 8.6.1).
Sennert makes a similar statement in his own study of medical signs:

> For although nothing certain about an illness can be legitimately deduced from
> [common signs] if they are considered singly, if, however, they are taken together,
> and are determined in [the way I have shown], they will necessarily lead the
> doctor to knowledge of the underlying humour.[63]

This is a very strong claim; syndromes can be 'infallible, eternally true,
and scientific'; Sanctorius declares to have supplied enough elements

---

[58] Sanctorius 1630: 30 (i.8): 'methodum certam de signis propriis tradere non possumus, cum de
illis quae non sunt semper nulla methodus vel scientia detur'.

[59] Platter 1625: 105: 'quare non uni alicui signo credendum, sed pluribus simul collatis morbi
sedem, speciem causasque indagare, et de morbis statuere oportet. Horum enim incertitudo,
nobis Medicam artem coniecturalem facit, et morbo non plene cognito, curatio erit vel nulla,
vel plane perversa, aut fortuita'; Sennert 1650: 1.448: 'plerumque signa pathognomonica
constituitur ex pluribus coniunctis, quae si seorsim sumantur, pathognomonica non sunt'.

[60] Alonso 1598: 24: 'signo uni credere fatuum est neque signum unum ita fidele est, ut exquisite
ostendat singula ex futuris temporibus' (cf. *Physignomica*, ii, 806 b 38).

[61] These points are made in various places in Galen's works, including *De methodo medendi*, ii.4,
K 10.100–1 and *De sectis*, iv, K 1.79–83, where the use of the syndrome is attributed to the
empirics.

[62] Sanctorius 1630: 501–3 (vi.1).

[63] Sennert 1650: 1.516: 'Licet enim si singula [signa communia] separatim considerantur nihil
certi ex iis de morbo concludere liceat, tamen si coniunctim sumantur, atque ita [viz. seriatim]
determinantur, necessario medicum in latentis humoris cognitionem deducunt.'

in his method to eliminate all possibility of ambiguity.[64] The totality of signs in a given case is described elsewhere by Galen as 'the harmony of a choir', much in the same way that François Hotman describes a legal rule as producing a polyphonic harmony.[65] But there are also sometimes very unchoirlike dissonances: signs sometimes contradict one another; and sometimes they point to different inferences, depending on whether the greater number of consistent signs or those with the greater strength are given precedence. Then only a 'medicus expertissimus' can discern their meaning.[66]

8.4.1 Pleurisy and the critique of syndromes

The locus classicus for the harmony of a syndrome is the illness known as pleurisy as described in Galen's *De constitutione artis medicae* and elsewhere, the traditional four signs being coughing, fever, difficulty in breathing, and a stabbing pain in the right side.[67] There are two problems in taking these four signs together to be a pathognomonic sign. One is logical, as Sanctorius points out:

A logical error is committed, because these four pathognomonic signs taken as a group (*universaliter*) constitute an argument from the consequent to the antecedent, as in the example: A is a man, A is an animal, but A is an animal, therefore A is a man, which is invalid... The following argument errs in many ways, as we have shown elsewhere: there is a pain in the side, a cough, difficulty in breathing and acute fever, therefore there is pleuritis; it is invalid unless the [individual] terms become convertible, as in the example: there is a stabbing pain in the side, therefore there is pleuritis, and so on; if we want to draw certain conclusions from proper signs, they must be limited and constrained as they are [in my method] below.[68]

Sanctorius's chapter (i.24) points to the consequences both of taking each sign in turn and not considering other signs, and to the fallacy of

---

[64] Sanctorius 1630: 30 (i.8): 'syndromen infallibilem, aeternae veritatis et scientificam'; *ibid.*, 536 (vi.7): 'idcirco tot locos proposuimus ad tollendam omnem ambiguitatem'.

[65] Galen, *Ad Glauconem*, i.2, K 11.9; Hotman 1569: 324: 'leges esse tanquam voces, et sonos singulos: regulam vero esse tanquam harmoniam et concentum'.

[66] Liddel 1628: 523–5 (on signs being mutually contradictory, and on the need for an expert doctor: see also *Physiognomica*, i, 805 b 1); Argenterio 1610: 1723–4 (on how to interpret signs which vary according to difference in humours); Jacchinus 1615: 187: 'oportet coniecturam facere considerando non solum numerum signorum sed vim et magnitudinem'; and above 5.2.2.

[67] Galen, *In aphorismos*, i.12, K 17b.380–400; da Monte 1554: 302r; Peucer 1553: 207; L'Alemant 1549: 29–30; Lemosius 1598: 39–40; Liddel 1628: 511–13; Aubéry 1585: 16; Campilongo 1601: 15v; Melanchthon 1547: R7v; Alonso 1598: 22. Sanctorius 1630: 85 (i.24) points out that Galen adds a fifth symptom (fast and shallow breathing) in *De locis affectis*, v.3, K 8.306f.

[68] Sanctorius 1630: 84 (i.24), quoted above, ch. 5, note 53.

the consequent (above 5.1.1). He cites also the critique found in Galen (*De locis affectis*, iii, K 8.136–47), where the sorites argument is used to show that the simple enumeration of signs will never yield a definition of disease. Both of these arguments are in defence of rational medicine against unguided intuition or the formulaic application of empirical rules.

8.5 SIGNS AS EVIDENCE: CERTAINTY AND UNCERTAINTY

The word 'conjectural', which doctors use to describe their practice of inference from signs (see above, 5.1.1), raises the more important issues of certainty and uncertainty, ambiguity and redundancy: as Silvaticus puts it, 'the art of medicine, which in those things which pertain to signs is almost wholly conjectural and hardly logically necessary or scientific at all, can be said to be defective'.[69] Long before him, Celsus had pointed to the possible elements of redundancy in medical diagnosis.[70] That signs are ambiguous is pointed out by the medieval commentator Giacomo da Forlì; and it is also evident from the Aristotelian locus in *Physiognomica*, i (805 b 1), which points to the problem of opposite characters producing the same facial features.[71] We have already met the problems of certain ('tekmēria') and uncertain ('sēmeia') signs (above 5.1.1); the former having the characteristic of necessity, the latter of probability in one of its guises.[72] Division of signs into certain and uncertain or ambiguous is commonly found; it is sometimes associated with the vexed problem of psychological certainty (above 4.3).[73] In the sphere of *practica*, the

---

[69] Silvaticus 1601: 83: 'defectuosa dici ars potest medica, quae in his quae ad signa attinent tota fere est coniecturalis et minime necessaria, sive demonstrativa'.

[70] *De medicina*, ii.2–6.

[71] Ottosson 1984: 275 (quoting Giacomo da Forlì); Fontanus 1611: 31.

[72] Campilongo 1601: 92v (citing Averroes's commentaries on *Prior analytics*, ii): cf. the use of tekmēria by Hippocrates cited in García Ballester 1981: 29; and Emericus 1552: P3v (on Galen, *In prorrhetica*).

[73] Donatius 1591: 32–6: 'certae notae appellantur, quae rem, cuius notae esse dicuntur, minime dubitanter aperiunt. Incerta vocamus, quae ambigua sunt, ex quibus certam coniecturam efficere non possumus. Haec a Graecis simpliciter σημεῖα, illa τεκμήρια appellantur. Quemadmodum enim duplices sunt rerum naturae ex quibus medici futura praenunciant; oratores vero non necessariae. Item veluti quaedam observatione empirica, quaedam ratione consecutione, quae plane demonstratio est, comprobantur; ita et nomina diversa rebus inter se maxime discrepantibus imponere antiqui voluerunt. Certa signa sumuntur ab iis morborum signis, quae quasi mores aegritudinis ostendere solent, non ab iis, quae iudicia praenuntiant; multo minus ab iis symptomatibus quae a caussa extrinseca non a corporis aegritudine excitantur; haec enim nullam certam habent praesagitionem . . . Signa quaedam dubia quaedam certa. Aperta et dilucida signa sunt, quae admistione dubiorum quasi liberata, pura, integra et sola sunt . . . dubia, quae difficiles explicatus habent, aut propterea quod minima sunt, aut quod pauca, aut quod ambigua, incerta et fallacia sunt.' Liddel 1628: 511 begins his chapter on signs with the sentence 'scopus autem doctrinae signorum est ex infallibilibus notis

only certain signs are 'signa coctionis'.[74] At the other end of the scale lie 'signa decretoria' which are 'altogether untrustworthy, and have no certainty in them; because the same signs which reveal a good crisis are those which show a bad one'.[75] Some writers accept that all signs have degrees of certainty ('gradus certitudinis') implicitly suggesting thereby that there are no absolutely certain signs, rather in the way that there is no absolutely perfect state of health or balance of temperament (above, 7.4.3).[76] There are two sorts of semiological certainty in question here: the first refers to the sign that is certainly right some of the time;[77] the second to the sign which of its nature is not sufficient to be used in a scientific demonstration.[78] In this latter case, the only route towards certain knowledge is afforded by the aggregation of more or less certain signs which leads nearer and nearer to the truth.[79] The conjectural nature of the art of medicine arises from the element of uncertainty in the sign, as is frequently repeated in the Renaissance.[80]

8.5.1 Redundancy, ambiguity, obscurity

This sentiment finds its way in the Middle Ages into the commentary on the law of evidence by Baldus.[81] As in the case of law, the problem

et evidentibus signis, omnem corporis constitutionem, omnesque affectus, affectuum sedes et causas patefacere et manifestare': but as has been noted above (5.1.2), he abandons this claim to completeness and certainty in his subsequent account of signs.

74 Vega 1571: 1195 (citing Galen, *De crisibus*, i.14); Emericus 1552: 02r: 'Galenus ait signa coctionis omnium esse firmissima, certissima, ac semper fida, et quae ultimo veritatem declarant.' Sennert 1650: 1.527: 'coctionis signa nunquam mala'.

75 Vega 1571: 1195: 'omnino infida; ex se nullam habent certitudinem; quoniam eademet signa, quae ostendunt bonam crisim, ostendunt etiam malam'.

76 This was already known to the Middle Ages; see Ottosson 1984: 204, quoting the passage from Haly's commentary on the *Tegni*, ii.1.7, cited above in ch. 5, note 61. Similar divisions of substantial signs into true (immediate or accidental), almost true (mediate and accidental), or not very reliable are found in Emericus 1552: 02r; Liddel 1628: 511ff.; Fonseca in Jacchinus 1615: 187 derives 'tres gradus signorum' from Hippocrates, *Aphorisms*, ii.19.

77 E.g. Campilongo 1601: 13r referring to 'symptomata [quae] non necessario consequantur, saepiusque vel raro vel aequaliter morbo superveniant'.

78 Liddel 1628: 514: 'licet *plerumque* communia quaedam signa sunt, quibus semel affectum aut partem affectam et causam deprehendimus: imo *pauca sunt* signa affectuum, quae non simul locum et causam demonstrant, ut Galenus 1 de locis [affectis] admonet' (my italics); Argenterio 1610: 1723: 'quaenam signa [humorum] ex tanta multitudine certa omnino existant, et numquam fallere valeant, quae vero incertiora et duntaxat coniecturalia, quidque in singulis observandum, ne hallucinemur. Itaque notae, quae a natura humoris sumuntur, perpetuo verae esse non possunt.'

79 Sanctorius 1630: 94–116 (i.28–33), on diagnosing pregnancy from aggregating signs (amenorrhoea, vomiting, appetites for strange foods), which separately could indicate something else.

80 Platter 1625: 97: 'signorum tractatio maxime [est] apud medicos necessaria et operosa simul, eorumque incertitudine conjecturalis et dubia fiat nostra ars'.

81 See Baldus 1615: 35r (ad C 4.19.rubr.12–15), quoted below, note 189.

facing doctors is how to translate the conjectural sign into an evidential sign,[82] or to put it differently, because 'not everything signifies everything', a rule needs to be found to validate or warrant an inference from a sign.[83] Argenterio sees the 'via divisiva' as the route to maximising certainty; Sanctorius (as we shall see) looks to the six 'fontes' method of mutually negating or confirming orders of signs, and that of aggregation; Martinengius proposes the conditional proposition (if x then y) as the way forward; Rondelet tries exclusion as a method of differential diagnosis.[84] These methods can lead to 'artificial certainty', that is to say, to the intellectual product of the mental procedure; but it cannot yield knowledge of the individual case; it leaves unjudged the issue of which signs in a group are more or less to be trusted, and provides no rule of thumb for the elimination from all assessment of superfluous or meaningless signs.[85] Aristotle's *Liber de divinatione per somnum*, i refers to certain signs which do not represent an effect of the things they signify if a subsequent cause intervenes; according to Alonso, this means that signs indicating future events are uncertain, because among their latent causes they have ones which could potentially impede the as yet not

---

[82] García Ballester 1981: 34 (quoting Galen's commentary on Hippocrates, *Prognosis*, iii.44).

[83] Argenterio 1610: 1688: 'non omnia significant omnia'; the phrase is cited from the *Rhetoric to Alexander*, xii, 1430 b 30ff., quoted above, 5.1.1.

[84] Martinengius 1584: 38–67; his 'method' also stresses that prognosis is more important than correct diagnosis, and he approaches the exposition of it through a commentary on selected cases from the *Epidemics* (68–95); Porta 1593: 38–9 (on *a contrario* determination of meaning; i.e. the absence of a sign indicates the opposite meaning to that which its presence would indicate). A mystical approach to negative knowledge of this kind (connected with physiognomics) is found in Skalich de Lika 1556: 15: 'habes leonem aut cervum, utique et nomen ex hoc sensibili signo, impositionem significativam continens, quae signa sequuntur occulta occultorum. Quid igitur est agendum in eliciendo, ab obiecto sensibili, occulta occultorum praeter occulti considerationem? . . . cum in nominis significatione affirmationem senseris, ad mentem negationem contendas, tum habebis verissimum modum a sensibili obiecto eliciendo occulta occultorum.'

[85] Varanda 1620: 3 (citing Hippocrates, *De glandulis*): 'medicus parum delinquat; cum exactum certitudinem in arte medica, ut in aliis coniecturaliter, raro reperire liceat. Nos igitur ad eiusmodi artificiosam certitudinem, quae methodo comparatur, properantes, quaedam remorantur, quorum cognitio ad non necessaria existit, nimirum: quae sint in universum medici munera et actiones; quae conditiones in eiusmodi actionibus exercendis requirantur; quibus instrumentis perficiantur; quot rationes seu modi, quibus uti possit medicus ad eiusmodi instrumentorum inventionem'; Campilongo 1601: 7v (referring to Galen, *Ad Thrasybulum*, viii, K 5.817–19): 'medici munus est distinguere symptomata utilia ab inutilibus' (no rule is given); Vega 1571: 1154 (citing Hippocrates, *Prognosis*, iii.15): 'signum, ex quo nihil certi praesagiri praecipit, nisi aliis adiunctis signis, illud non esse de fortibus et dignioribus in significando' (again, no rule is supplied). On the presence of redundant signs, see also Agrippa 1992: 66: 'fateor praeterea magiam ipsam multa supervacua et ad ostentationem curiosa docere prodigia', on which see also Maclean 1984: 236; Argenterio 1610: 1780. On redundant willed signs ('nulls' used in Renaissance cryptology), see Bacon 2000: 121–2, and his sources (Joannes Trithemius, Giambattista della Porta and Blaise de Vigenère) as identified by the editor (318).

realised effects.[86] The conjectural art relies on the 'peritia' of excluding irrelevant information, for which, it appears, no rational rules can be laid down.

8.6 SIGNS AND TIME: ANAMNESIS, DIAGNOSIS, PROGNOSIS

We come now to the issue of signs and time; diagnosis and prognosis.[87] The *degré zéro* of both is the position of an empiric, who prescribes a remedy without engaging in either mode of judgement; but rational doctors are obliged to engage in both as linked activities on the authority of a number of Galenic texts.[88] The first aspect of both is the gleaning of information from the sickroom, the attendants, and the patient. This involves taking a history; Capivaccius's schema 'de modo interrogandi aegrotos' recorded by Campilongo is the most sophisticated account of how to do this.[89] Noteworthy here is the use of the nurses and attendants as sources of information, and the sequence of questions, which reveals not so much a sensitivity to the issue of unfolding narrative and of progressive revelation of the patient's condition as a rigorously directed series of enquiries structured by medical theory.[90] Among the signs to be discovered are anamnestic signs, which are not only signs of what has happened in the past to the patient, but also those which are relevant to the present in a complex temporal mode, and those which can be gleaned by autopsy after death to prove the internal and hitherto invisible symptoms which reveal the cause of death.[91] Cardano makes a strong claim in respect of these signs that he is the first in his age, and perhaps of

---

[86] Alonso 1598: 25: 'signa aliqua sunt quae null[o]s effectus eorum quos signabant consequuntur, adveniente superiori causa, quasi diceret propter hanc rationem signa significantia futura fiunt incerta, quia habent causas potentes impedire effectus nondum ad extra productos, sed solum in suis causis latitantes' (citing Aristotle, *De divinatione per somnum*, 463 b 20ff.).

[87] There is a connection between the preference for prognosis over diagnosis, which is uncertain, and therapy, which is even more so, and the literature abour cautelae: see Siraisi 1990c: 153, and above 3.7.

[88] Cf. García Ballester 1981: 16: 'Galen, like the Hippocratics, was not distinguishing between a diagnostic judgement (the scientific knowledge of what a patient has) and the prognostic judgement (the conjecture about what will happen to him). For him to understand a clinical case technically, to "diagnose" was, among other things, to know with greater or lesser certainty the outcome for the patient, to "prognosticate". Prognosis, then, is one of the essential problems and most important objectives of Galenic diagnosis.'

[89] See also Argenterio 1606–7: 253–81 ('De consultandi ratione').

[90] The past history of the patient's illness is investigated by questions about the three vital faculties and excretions which have the effect, among others, of increasing the patient's confidence in the doctor and his authority over them: Campilongo 1601:)(8r; Liddel 1628: 511–12.

[91] Siraisi 1997: 116.

all ages, to have made proper use of them.[92] A feature of time in respect of diagnosis which is rarely dwelt on, but which is none the less significant, is the fact that diagnosis itself extends over a given period, and may result from a sequence of visits, hypotheses about the patient's condition, and suggested treatments; southern French doctors from Arnau de Vilanova onwards allude to this, as does Argenterio, and it is implicit in the practice of clinical precepting.[93] This feature of decision-making (or determining the truth) contrasts with the law's procedure on this point, which although the relevant information was possibly gleaned over a period of time, none the less settles the facts in a stipulative way by the decision of the judge;[94] it also contrasts, according to J. J. R. Christie, with Paracelsus's 'semiotic', which has, similar to the law, a peremptory look about it: 'Diagnostic art was then identification of the *entia* [responsible for disease] and with reference to which particular internal star of the body which was being caused to act abnormally. The human body in Paracelsian discourse . . . was, as a patient, first of all semiotic.'[95]

8.6.1 Diagnosis

The method and order of diagnosis are variously set out. Hippocrates does not explicitly prescribe these, although it might be said that the case histories of the *Epidemics* and the terse clues given in the *Aphorisms* constitute a method. As described by Sextus Empiricus, the Hippocratic approach is to observe individual cases ('aisthēsis'), document the experience of the patient, those attending him or her, and other doctors ('logos'), and draw inferences from one set of circumstances to another

---

92 Cardano 1663: 8.705–6: 'unde emersit tertium genus signorum nobilissimum [the first two being diagnostic and prognostic signs], in quo ego fortunatissimus fui, qui id aetate mea, et forsan primum omnium etiam ante nos, qui id introduxerim, aususque fuerim in medium praeponere, atque tentare'.

93 Arnau de Vilanova is explicit about this (on trying in sequence remedies such as clyster, calefactorium, and bath): 1585: 1702; Rondelet 1586: 592: 'neque erit statim inclamandum heureka heureka'; a doctor should check his diagnosis three times as a merchant checks his receipts and outgoings three times. Rondelet also stresses the importance of the 'initium investigationis' (presumably taking a history). Ferrier 1592: 107–17 (a chapter entitled 'de complicatione, contrarietate, et concursu indicantium'); Argenterio 1610: 1780–1: 'nam quae ab initio obscura incertaque fuerant tempore patefaciunt'. See also the comments of the annalist of the German nation at Padua quoted by Bylebyl 1979: 351. Sydenham 1848–50: 1.11–24 is sometimes credited with the first practice of progressive diagnosis, but even in the ancient Greek literature, the reference to gnorismata (signs associated with the onset of disease) makes this claim dubious.

94 Maclean 1992: 130.

95 Christie 1998: 278.

('logismos').[96] Galen, as one would expect, readily yields up a number of rules which are not necessarily consistent with each other. One of these suggests that one should begin by distinguishing redundant from necessary elements in diagnosis (that is, incidentals from causes);[97] another suggests that one should begin with an investigation of the 'res praeter naturales' and then pass to the 'res naturales';[98] a third rule, implicit in the *De locis affectis*, recommends localisation as the first step.[99] Other accounts record Galen's method as the following three steps: divide illnesses into species and subspecies; typify the disease; determine its strength.[100] Against Argenterio's accusation that Galen betrays himself as confused, Bartolettus defends him on the grounds that these rules answer different diagnostic needs.[101]

Renaissance methods are more directive. Vega's universally applicable way ('via omnis') of getting to the illnesses and affected parts investigates in turn the essence, causes, effects, similarities and differences, and things bringing relief or aggravating the condition. His order seeks to identify in turn the 'morbi genus', the 'species', the 'locus affectus', its 'magnitudo', 'affectus et mos', finally the 'tempora et fines'.[102] Argenterio's (according to Bartolettus) is very similar: passing from the essence of the part of the body, to the efficient causes of the part, the effects which overtake the affected part, and finally to the similarities and proportionality of the rest.[103] Sanctorius, to whose method I shall return presently, rejects the last part of this method as logically invalid, and offers a sequence of investigation through the six 'fontes', which he sees as an answer to the empirics, whom he condemns for relying on common signs, moving from particulars to universals, and looking to the patient's symptoms without

---

[96] García Ballester 1981: 24.

[97] *Methodus medendi*, ii.3.11.

[98] García Ballester 1981: 24, on Galen's prescribed sequence – first pulse then other signs, then the non-naturals – set out in *De prisca medicina*, i, *Ad Glauconem*, i.9, K 11.25–42 and *In prorrhetica*, i.4, K 16.511–24; Campilongo 1601: 18r.

[99] Temkin 1977: 446; García Ballester 1981: 21–3; *De locis affectis*, i.1, K 8.1–20.

[100] Bylebyl 1991: 181–2; García Ballester 1981: 18–19 (giving the Galenic loci from *De constitutione artis medicae*, K 1.293–5, *De crisibus*, i.5, K 9.563–4 and *Ad Glauconem*, i.11, K 11.36–7).

[101] Bartolettus 1619: 254.

[102] Vega 1571: 369.

[103] Bartolettus 1619: 255–9, cf. Argenterio 1610: 929. Argenterio's work resembles a combination of the practical emphasis of Parisian doctors such as Sylvius (with whom, or under whom, he studied), and the 'via divisiva' recommended by da Monte (see above, 4.4.3). Sanctorius's critique of his use of proportion runs as follows: 1630: 501 (vi.1): 'fons igitur a proportione positus ab Argenterio est, verbi causa, si aliqua saeviret endimia in populum, et medici nescirent, quibus humoribus danda esset endimiae culpa, et propterea cadavera aperirent, viderent esse atrum succum: dicit ex hoc experimento oriri fontem a proportione dicendo sicut in cadavere erat ater succus; similiter in alio homine eadem aegritudine vexatio est similis ater succus'.

determining the relationship of symptoms to signs. Rational doctors, according to him, begin with convertible signs (thus avoiding the fallacy of the consequent), move from the universal to the particular, and proceed by way of the symptoms of causes, to the symptoms of the affected parts and the affected virtues or faculties.[104]

What is actually practised may be different from these recommendations. The disposition of manuals of practica (cause–symptom–disease–remedy) may not be a guide either to teaching or to practice.[105] Prominence is sometimes given to taking a patient's history.[106] In his De locis affectis, Galen shows both the need for this to be taken in the most thorough way and for flexibility of thought, to the extent of making counterintuitional deductions (that is, ones where the site of the pain or lesion is misleading, or particular conditions of the medical event alter the significance of the evidence).[107] Were Sanctorius's twenty-two circumstantial categories (see 5.1.3) to be exhaustive and to constitute the basis of the interrogation of patients, it would be impressive enough, but it is in fact open: Sanctorius ends by referring to 'other specific natures and conditions of which some are found in many causes, rarely, however, in all', stressing thereby the need for an art to master the infinitely bewildering complexity of the individual case;[108] this recommendation is also remarkable in that it is a clear statement of a polythetic approach in the work of a committed Aristotelian.[109] A variety of techniques are recommended to help in this process. Altomare draws attention in turn to cause, locus, cure, and sequence of treatment if several diseases are in question; da Monte starts from proper signs, complexion, symptoms, causes, essence of disease, and part, to end with proximate cause; Campilongo follows this order rather than the recommendation of Rhazes espoused by Jacchinus, which is to move from impaired function, to quality, to the

---

[104] Sanctorius 1630: 782–8 (xii.4).

[105] An equivalent modern problem is referred to by Beck, Francis and Souhami 1974: ix: 'while most patients present with symptoms, most textbooks are written in the form of descriptions of diseases'.

[106] Bylebyl 1991: 187 (on da Monte); Campilongo 1601:)(8r.

[107] García Ballester 1981: 32–3 (relating the story in De locis affectis, i.6 K, 8.56–8 where Galen, on discovering that a patient's fingers were lacking sensation, discovered by interrogation that he had suffered trauma to the back, and proceeded to treat the back); Campilongo 1601: 41r (relating the story in In Hippocratis de officina medici, i where Galen correctly diagnosed a dislocation by taking a history); ibid., on the need for social contextualisation (a nobleman breaking wind in another's company is a sign of madness or uncontrollable pain, but if he is alone it indicates nothing). On the individuality of cases, see 3.7.3 (Sennert's example of a patient in good health who idiosyncratically has the facial signs of imminent death).

[108] Sanctorius 1630: 742 (xi.5): 'et aliae specificae naturae et conditiones, quarum aliquae in multis invenientur, raro tamen omnes'.

[109] On polythesis, see Needham 1975.

affect of the part, to the causes, and to end with the remedy; Sanctorius and Argenterio have yet other sequences to offer.[110] Among signs, says Liddel, begin with the most common, then consider the less common, and finally the proximate and 'maxime speciales'.[111] Ferdinandus, on the other hand, starts with 'essentia generica', then passes to 'differentiae rei praeternaturalis'.[112] The Paracelsian Albertus starts with location, passes to the nature of the illness, then considers treatments and finally the viscid excrements.[113] The last component in the sequence of practical medicine – remedy – is not always applicable; there is a debate as to whether all diseases are curable.[114] One may perceive a great deal of similarity in all these approaches in respect of the elements they take to be significant, as well as some degree of disagreement as to the sequence of signs to interrogate. As the method betokens order of enquiry, we may take these disagreements to be significant to the actors, even if to the modern eye they may not appear so.

The most impressive descriptions of diagnostic method I have found are those of Fernel, Rondelet and Sanctorius. Fernel suggests a system based on Galen's *De constitutione artis medicae*, which begins with the symptom, next moves to the affected part, to the other supporting symptoms, to the discordant symptoms, then to other parts in a sort of heuristic sequence involving revisions of views at every stage:

Every investigation leads from that which is perceptible to sense to abstruse and hidden causes . . . But some symptom – whether it was damaged function, or abnormal excrement, or pain . . . – first leads us to the suspicion of the affected part; then one should think over whether there are other symptoms in the suspected part that support this belief. For almost no symptom exists alone, but in one and the same disease many always go together. Therefore when one has heard everything related and thought over everything, if the symptoms agree in signifying one and the same affected part, the affected site should be investigated. But if the symptoms do not agree with one another, the investigation should be diverted to another part . . . For example, suppose we are asked to decide something about difficulty of breathing. Because when that function is impaired, it is established that one of the organs that serve breathing is affected, [first] see if there is any defect peculiar either to the throat or trachea. If nothing appears

---

[110] Bylebyl 1991: 171, 176–88 (on Altomare and da Monte); Campilongo 1601: 49v; Jacchinus 1563: 5; Argenterio 1610: 1694–1706; Sanctorius 1630: 3–9 (i.2).

[111] Liddel 1628: 605.

[112] Ferdinandus 1621: 2

[113] Albertus 1615: D4. Paracelsus argues that there is a precondition to diagnosis which is the determination by providence that the patient and the physician will meet at a certain time: Christie 1998: 281.

[114] For Cardano 1568: 15, this raises the question of common illness (epidemic) and divine providence. On incurable diseases, see ch. 7, note 118.

to be wrong with these, the cause must be in the lungs or thorax or abdomen. If the patient's breathing is stertorous and he or she has a painless cough, the lungs are defective. If pain presses in the chest, on the false ribs of the right side, the condition should be observed and diagnosed from other signs. For if there is sharp pain and continuous fever, it is a sign of pleurisy . . . That should be the method of investigation.[115]

Rondelet's explicit method is set out in his *De dignoscendis morbis liber*, published posthumously in 1586 with his *Methodus curandorum omnium morborum*.[116] He begins with circumstantiae, the history of the patient, and information from those present ('astantes'); thereafter he proceeds by a negative route similar to modern differential diagnosis. He illustrates it by an example to show how he sorts out symptoms which are relevant to a given affection (especially if the patient is suffering from more than one illness).[117] He describes this process through the metaphor of sorting out a pile of grain into its component elements of millet, pepper seeds, beans, chickpeas, vetch and wheat. The diagnostician begins by removing the biggest seeds, and then engages in a 'substratio aliorum generum',

---

[115] Fernel 1610b: 1.210–11(ii.9), quoted in the translation given by Siraisi forthcoming: 'omnis investigatio ab eo quod sensuum perspicuum est in abstrusas occultasque causas deducit: quodque ortu et causarum ordine potissimum est, investigatione primum occurrit: nempe aut morbus aliquis manifestus, aut certe symptomata. Hoc autem sive laesa functio, sive excrementum, sive dolor fuerit, tum ex situ tum ex specie nos in aliquam partis affectae suspicionem primam adducet: deinde percontandum num etiam alia existant suspectae partis symptomata quae primae coniecturae consentiunt. Etenim nullum fere symptoma solitarium existit, sed unius eiusdemque morbi multa semper occurrunt. Quum igitur omnia quae tum narrando tum percontando audita sunt, in unius eiusdemque affectae partis significationem congruunt explorata compertaque est affecta sedes. Sin vero illa inter se dissidunt atque discordant, in alterius partis investigatione divertendum, dum quaedam deprehendatur, quae certorum signorum testimoniis affecta confirmetur. Si omnium symptomatum significationes eodem pertinent, neque ullum alio quoquam deflectat, pars unica laborat. De hac praeterea disquirendum, proprione affectu an alterius partis consensu laboret, et quaenam ea fuerit. Si proprius est affectus, isne etiam primarius sit, an ex alio antecedente profectus, omnium quippe eiusmodi distinctio in primis est ad medendi rationem necessaria. Quendam (exempli gratia) statuamus de spirandi difficultate queri. Quum ex ea actione laesa constet instrumentum aliquod eorum quae respirationi inserviunt affici, perscrutandum quidem fauces an aspera arteria peculiari vitio tenetur. Si nihil in his apparet, causa aut in pulmones, aut in thoracem, aut in septum transversum, aut in vicinas partes conferenda. Quum stercor respirando obauditur, et tussis molesta est sine sensu doloris, pulmones in vitio sunt. Quum dolor in thorace premit, idque circa nothas costas dextri lateris, ex aliis signis dispiciendus est. Si enim pungenti similis fuerit cum febre assidua, cum tussi qua maxime cruentum expuitur, pleuritidis est index . . . ea sit igitur investigandi ratio.'

[116] Dr R. G. Lewis has pointed out to me that he, together with his Montpellier colleagues, eschew long logical introductions to their works, and even deduce the qualities of illnesses from the (contrary) qualities of the remedies that are known empiricially to alleviate them; in this, they could possibly be the targets of Sanctorius's attacks on empirici in the twelfth book of the *Methodi vitandorum errorum*. Rondelet 1565 does not explicitly make this point about deduction, but the text is consistent with such an approach.

[117] Liddel 1628: 513ff. considers the same problem.

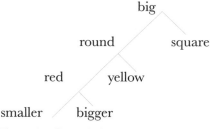

Figure 8.1. Rondelet's method of diagnosis
(to be compared with Porphyry's tree, above,
fig. 4.3)

separating them out by shape, size and colour until there is only one left:
see fig. 8.1.[118] This constitutes a passage from 'genus generalissimum'
through the 'genera subalterna' to 'species', which in medical terms
begins with 'affectus manifestior', passes to 'species doloris', 'partem
affectam' and so on until an unambiguous result is reached:

> Let there be a 'genus generalissimum' of disease in which not only causes, but
> also illnesses and symptoms are included, in which whatever befalls the body –
> whether 'intemperies', 'mala compositio', or 'solutio continuitatis' [all versions
> of illness: see above 7.5.1], whether a changed quality, something retained or
> evacuated by the body, pain, a tumour, an impaired function, an adnate or a
> skin blemish [all symptoms: see 7.5.3] – has to be represented as it were in a
> table.[119]

We may note here that Rondelet relies on elements of dogmatic medicine
(classification of disease, symptom and so on) which we have seen to be
riven with conceptual difficulties. This is one reason why his method
is not reducible to a tree diagram (suggested here by 'veluti in tabella
quadam picta'); it is rather a dialectical or endoxical division, because
its quarry, the illness(es), is not necessarily singular, nor is it definable by
its own tree (see above 4.4.3).

Rondelet's approach, although unusually explicit and comprehensive,
is not unique in its constituents: Cardano also uses elimination as a means

---

[118] Rondelet 1586: 597–8. Mixed seeds in a jar are an example of composition, not mixture, in
Aristotle, *De generatione et corruptione*, i.10, 328 a 2ff.

[119] Rondelet 1586: 598: 'Sit igitur genus generalissimum affectus praeter naturam in quo genere et
causae et morbi et symptomata compraehenduntur, et veluti in tabella quadam picta habere
oportet, quod quicquid praeter naturam accidit in corpore, vel est intemperies, mala con-
formatio aut solutio continuitatis. Qualitas mutata, retentum aliquid, reiectum, dolor, tumor,
functio laesa, adnatum, et vitium cutis'. On 'repraesentare veluti in tabella' see Maclean
1992: 96.

of diagnosis,[120] and Capivaccius employs a dichotomous approach which does not specify the order of operations but specifies the elements.[121]

Sanctorius's method is more explicitly logical, and involves the progressive analysis of a syndrome of signs. Because, in the theory of the humours, every patient is completely idiosyncratic, physicians cannot, as they can today, identify an illness from its objective signs alone: and there are illnesses mentioned which have contrary symptoms but the same cause, or which at an early stage have almost indistinguishable symptoms.[122] Sanctorius's method is designed to overcome these problems. There are six sources ('fontes') of diagnostic signs: procatarctic causes; the disposition of the patient; internal efficient causes; symptoms; affected parts; finally, those things which aggravate or alleviate the condition. Sanctorius gives a number of examples of this: the one which sets out the diagnosis of a stomach ulcer is found in the seventeenth chapter of the first book of his *Methodi*. The procatarctic causes are given there as bitter foods and medicaments; the anatomical and digestive dispositions predisposing a patient to stomach ulcers are next described; the third source consists in bitter humours; the fourth source (the consequent signs, or symptoms) involves the rehearsal of the range of symptoms, including stabbing pain, loss of appetite, thirst, bad breath and belching; the fifth sign is bloody vomit, which reveals the location of the ulcer by the time delay after ingestion and the nature and exact site of the pain suffered by the patient; the final confirmation is found in the treatment (bitter and sharp preparations aggravating the condition, emollient ones relieving it).[123] Sanctorius's first and sixth books are devoted to examples of this kind; for the most part, Sanctorius makes strong claims about

---

[120] Siraisi 1997: 210 gives an example taken from Cardano 1663: 10.501.

[121] Capivaccius 1603: 5–8.

[122] Liddel 1628: 523–5 (looking at factors such as age, region, and season which can disguise the true nature of symptoms); Rondelet 1586: 586ff. points to the opposite problem (distinguishing between illnesses whose symptoms are very similar, especially at an early stage): 'morbi cum inchoantur, herbis nascentibus similes sunt, quae non nisi exercitatissimis discernuntur. Pauci enim Lactucas a Betis primo distinguunt, si certi morbi aliqui adeo inter se sunt similes, ut sit difficilimum illos ab invicem distinguere. Pauci febrem spuriam duplicem a quotidiana distinguunt: inflammationem lateris a Peripneumonia, et iis maxime qui pulmones costis alligatos habent: aut hepatis inflammationem a pleuride partis dextrae: item febres continuas vix a se invicem distinguunt. Huius rei causa est materiae similitudo, affectiones eaedem vel similia accidentia, partim vicinitas, aut continuitas, vel situs vel consensus vel morborum multorum concursus et symptomatum vehementia, quae morbos occultat.' Galen, *In prognostica*, iii.39, K 18b.309, makes the claim however that signs never wholly change in their nature, even if they indicate different things: 'namque symptomata et ex malis quodammodo fiunt bona, et ex bonis mala. Signa vero nunquam in contrariam naturam vertuntur, sed maioris minorisve mali aut boni testimonia sunt.'

[123] Sanctorius 1630: 57–8.

having removed all ambiguity and uncertainty from his conclusions by considering a sufficient number of 'fontes'; the examination of the symptoms occupies the greatest space, and involves in many cases differential diagnosis through the comparative study of similar complaints. In one case alone, the example is listed in the index under the less ambitious phrase 'when there are several [competing] signs, which is the more to be believed' ('signa dum plura sint, quibus magis sit credendum').[124] This is a very long way from Ramus's 'via una et simplex' and even from Galen's claim (repeated by Vega) that 'there is common method for all issues'.[125] If we take into account that chance is given a role by some in the discovery of remedies[126] and that different parts of medical practice determine method both for teaching and for application,[127] we have moved a very long way from demonstrative 'science'.

8.6.2 Prognosis

Prognosis (alias 'praecognitio', 'praenotio', 'providentia'; not however strictly the same as 'praedictio', which relates only to the communication of future events to the patient or his or her attendants) is said to be the main task of the doctor:[128] medicine and prophecy are related, since Apollo is the author and father of both arts.[129] According to Donatius, medical signs are mainly in the service of prognosis; this is the first aim of medicine, which has the advantage also of avoiding the problems of

---

[124] Sanctorius 1630: 19–25 (i.6) (for method); *ibid.*, 522 (vi.4): '[ut] virtute signorum aliorum fontium contingentiam et probabilitatem expurgemus'; 532 (vi.6): 'hic non per unicum signum in re difficili est incedendum, sed per signorum syndromen, quae sola vehere potest nos ad veritatis apicem'; 535 (vi.7): 'si [fontes] invicem non viderimus dissentire, certum et exploratum iudicium faciemus . . . ab hac concordia locorum colligemus, quae scientiae demonstrativae aequiparari potest'; 536 (vi.7): 'tot locos proposuimus, quot sufficerent ad tollendam omnem ambiguitatem'. In spite of these claims, I would argue that these 'fontes' in sequence can only be transcribed into an endoxical, not a Porphyrian tree.

[125] Vega 1571: 369 (on the 'via omnis'); *De symptomatum causis*, iii (Galen 1550: 3.30): 'methodus est communis in omni re'.

[126] Ferdinandus 1621: 266 (on the role of chance in the discovery of remedies: he cites a number of Renaissance doctors on this topic, including Antonio Benivieni, Franciscus Valleriola, and Johann Lange).

[127] Argenterio 1610: 15–16.

[128] Liddel 1604: ddiv ('praesagitio' is 'praenotio in mente'; 'praedictio praecognita per vocem efficitur'); Linden 1999 (on Zerbi); see also Ficino 1576: 2.1616 on 'praedicandi modi' ('arte, casu, natura, daemone, deo'), where he points out the relative superiority of doctors and farmers in the very uncertain practice of prediction ('si agricolae et medici in re certiore saepius falluntur, caeteri praedictores saepissime falluntur').

[129] Siraisi 1997: 183; García Ballester 1981: 16; *De locis affectis*, iii.7, K.8.168 and *De constitutione artis medicae*, K 1.292 are loci which oppose diagnosis to prophecy to divination.

identifying and assessing cause and cure.[130] The major ancient sources of the art of prognosis are in Hippocrates, whose *Prognosis* is to be found in many medieval compilations of texts, and in the *Articella*, where it is accompanied by Galen's commentary; his *Prorrhetica* is also known in the Renaissance.[131] Galen's *De praecognitione* was edited in the sixteenth century by Jacchinus; his *De differentiis symptomatibus*, *De crisibus* and *De diebus decretoriis*, which were frequently reprinted in our period, also contain relevant material.[132] The intention behind this literature is to instruct doctors in an 'artificiosa cognitio' of the future outcome of the illnesses of the human body, whether good or bad, whether leading to recovery or death, based on the clues ['indicia', 'symptomata', 'signa'] contingent on the illnesses of the affected body.[133]

These symptoms or clues fall, according to the Galenic tradition, into five temporal classes: 'past clues of the past'; 'past clues of the present'; 'present clues of the present'; 'present clues of the past'; and 'present clues of the future'.[134] All these come from proximate causes: it is logically impossible for information to be obtained from future effects.[135] Cardano sees four purposes in prediction: to apprise hidden things from manifest signs and external causes; to recognise manifest things from those which

---

[130] Donatius 1591: 32–3; García Ballester 1981: 16; Wallis 1995: 120; Cocus 1601: xvi: 'indicare et praecognoscere sunt idem'.

[131] Durling 1961; *Prognosis*, iii.15 is particularly important. On the distinction in sense between prognosis and prorrhetica, see Martín Ferreira 1995: 118 (citing Vega).

[132] *Ibid.*, for a full list; Jacchinus in Galen 1540; Valleriola 1540; Vega 1571: 900ff.; Victorius 1551.

[133] Victorius 1551: 8: 'edocere medicum prognosticari de futuro termino morborum corporis humani aegroti ad bonum, vel malum ad salutem vel mortem, per indicia assumpta a symptomatibus contingentibus morbis eiusdem aegroti'; cf. Liddel 1628: 579; Martinengius 1584: 7; Alpini 1601: 6 (on predicting the outcome of the 'battle' between the illness and nature, an image taken from Galen's *De constitutione artis medicae*); Varanda 1620: 15: 'prognosis igitur medica nihil est aliud, quam artificiosa cognitio futurorum eventuum et mutationum in morbis, constans signis habentibus connexionem naturalem cum re significata'. See also 3.7.2 (on cautela and prognosis).

[134] This division is that given in Galen, *Definitiones medicae*, K 19.396–8 (Galen 1556a: 1.46r): 'Indicativum signum est, quod primas sibi vendicat in minus manifesti alicuius deprehensione idem bonum consequentis. Suggerens memoriae signum est, ut aiunt empirici, res, quae apparet, atque ex antegressa observatione innotescit, utilis rei, quae cognoscitur, ad memoriam revocandae: praesentium praesentia signa sunt pathognomonica omnia affectuum indicativa; haec cum fiunt atque adsunt, adsunt perinde et affectus; cum cessant, morbi quoque solvuntur. Praesentia praeteritorum sunt signa, ut facti prius ulceris cicatrix. Praesentia futurorum, ut cadaverosa facies, mortis. Praeterita autem sunt praeteritorum signa, ut cum remissio a declinatione, deferbuisse morbum significat. Praeterita praesentium, ut esse ab aspi ad demorsum inter exitalia censeri. Sunt, qui hoc modo dicant: praeterita praesentium, ut tenue intestinum vulneratum esse, pernitiosis admunerari. Praeterita futurorum, ut confracto contritaque osse tofum contrahendum: ei nanque oportet tofum abduci, dum ad pristinum statum redit. Non nulli vero sic. Praeterita futurorum, ut de capite dempto osse cicatricem sequituram.'

[135] Liddel 1628: 558ff.

are hidden (here 'genus', 'species', 'modi' and 'qualitates' come into question); to learn future things from those present and past; and 'living things from the dead' (that is, information from post-mortem autopsy relating to the lethal illness).[136] The progress, duration and eventual outcome of the illness are to be foreseen with the help of past history and a knowledge of symptoms.[137] Attention is to be paid to the signs of recovery or death, the signs of digestion or failure to digest ('signa coctionis et cruditatis'), the decretorial information and the possible outcomes ('modi eventus').[138] The prognosticating doctor should ask himself the following questions: Will there be death or recovery? Will the recovery be complete or incomplete? Will it be easy or difficult? certain ('fida') or uncertain?[139] Prediction is acknowledged to be not always right; it is an 'ut plurimum' procedure based on conjecture.[140] Sometimes it is not discursive at all: Cardano records seeing patients and pronouncing imminent death or recovery without knowing why.[141] This is analogous to the process of forming or reaching indications (below 8.7) and is reminiscent of the debates about the empirical practice of epilogism (see above 5.1.2).

8.6.3 Astrology

In determining the future course of illnesses, the stars can be said to have a role; astrology therefore comes into question. Pietro d'Abano accords three tools from other disciplines to doctors: logic, which is its 'salt'; natural philosophy, which supplies the 'scientific' principles for medicine; and astrology, which gives direction to the doctor's judgement.[142] This last was associated with the name of Hippocrates in the Middle Ages;[143]

---

[136] Cardano 1568: 2 ('ex manifestis obscura cognoscere'; 'ex obscuris manifesta'; 'ex praesentibus futura'; 'ex mortuis viventia').

[137] Galen, *De crisibus*, i.3, K 9.705–10; Alpini 1601: 1–2 (his 'praevidenda' are 'ex morbis praevidendis, ex praeteritis, ex symptomatum cognitione, ex longitudine et brevitate morborum, ex praesagienda morte et vita').

[138] Liddel 1628: 558ff.; Taurellus 1581:):( ):(3r.

[139] Capivaccius 1603: 17–18.

[140] See Galen, *In prorrhetica*, i.2.37, K 16.594; *In epidemica*, vi.1.16, K 17a.861–3; cf. Aquinas, *Summa theologiae*, 1a 86.4; Campilongo 1601: 71–87 (the more or less certain ends, procedures and results of prognosis). Liddel 1604: dd1r–v (referring to Hippocrates, *Aphorisms*, ii.19) mentions three factors which make prognosis uncertain: error in the prescription of a remedy by the doctor; the patient not following the prescription of the doctor; chance. For this reason all predictions should be made conditionally.

[141] Siraisi forthcoming; Cardano 1663: 7.262.

[142] Siraisi 1990c: 14–16 (on Pietro d'Abano). This section is heavily indebted to the forthcoming article by Grafton and Siraisi; I am very grateful to them for allowing me to see it.

[143] Siraisi 2000: 11.

in the Renaissance, Ptolemy comes to be seen as its principal authority. His version of the art is said by Cardano to be more noble than other forms of prediction, including medical prognosis, because it dealt with causes; stars are for astrologers 'causae, non signa'.[144] Part of the computations concerning stars is numerological: another part concerns location, which may not be quantitative, but it is intricate; a third part concerns variables connected with human beings and geography. In the *Tetrabiblos* (i.2), Ptolemy discusses the conjectural nature of the art of astrology, and compares it specifically to the practice of medicine, which also is made up of certain precepts combined with variables; from this passage, Cardano derives a particular sort of dialectical reasoning (the Ptolemaic).[145] The stars provide one of the most easily observed examples of natural regularities; it is therefore not surprising that correlations between their movements and sublunary medical events should be attempted. Influence was attributed to them over conception, crises in life and health, medication and parts of the body, through a system of correspondences; phlebotomy and surgical interventions were also governed by their position, which it was incumbent on the learned doctor to know.[146] Siraisi avers that astrology grew in importance in the fourteenth and fifteenth centuries; this growth can be charted through the concomitant rise of the genre of medical prognostication.[147]

Ptolemy admits (*Tetrabiblos*, ii.8) that astrological predictions are necessarily approximate, and that it is a hopeless and impossible task, given the number of possible combinations of planetary influences, to mention the proper outcome of all of them, and to enumerate absolutely all their aspects.[148] Pietro d'Abano had furthermore shown that the medical month of twenty-six days and twenty-two hours is not a secure basis for

---

[144] Cardano 1663: 5.93: 'artes autem quae futura hoc modo, cognoscere docent, sunt Agricultura, Nautica, Medicina, Physiognomia et illius partes, Somniorum interpretatio, et Magia naturalis, ac Astrologia. Harum nobilissima astrologia est, quia de omnibus est, alia autem sunt certi generis. Est etiam per causas semper atque eas nobilissimas, reliquarum nulla semper, sed etiam per signa docet futura praedicere.' Cardano looked upon himself as the scholar who made the *Tetrabiblos* available for his contemporaries in the same way that Galen's Hippocratic commentaries had made Hippocrates accessible for his: Cardano 1663: 5.105. Also *ibid.*, 5.556 on 'astra esse causas non signa'.

[145] 1663: 1.307.

[146] The chapter 'Medico necessariam esse astrorum scientiam, adversus quorundam assertionem' in Valleriola 1577: 368–70, makes the general point that doctors need to know as much about causes as possible, which must include knowledge about stars, which manifestly affect human beings.

[147] Siraisi 1990c: 133–6; Macdonald 1981: 24–30.

[148] Cf. Cardano 1663: 5.204: 'impossibile [est] describere hanc mistionem vel remissionem qualitatum', associating the difficulty with the problem of the latitude of forms (see above 7.4.3). See also *Tetrabiblos*, i.2, where Ptolemy admits that predictions fail sometimes, but claims that individual errors do not detract from the truth and beauty of the art as a whole. Also Cardano

calculation; but this did not deter thinkers such as Pomponazzi and his medieval predecessors from considering the question of astral determinism at the moment of generation, with its implications for divine freedom of action and human free will.[149] For him and for his contemporaries, astrology is seen as dual: judicial astrology attempts to predict specific future events; natural or medical astrology studies the influence of the stars on climate, environment and health, and the causation of epidemic disease and its transmission; it investigates alterations in the four humours of the body and mind as these are affected by the moon, sun and stars (the moon governing the course of acute diseases, the sun of chronic diseases). Some Renaissance opponents of astrology attack it on a broad front (this is the case of the most famous of the attacks on the art, the *Disputationes adversus astrologiam divinatricem* of Pico della Mirandola, which appeared in 1496, and of the critiques of doctors such as Manardo and Fracastoro); some attack only the judicial version.[150] It is not necessarily the case that an attack on astrology coincides with progressive cosmological views; it is perfectly possible to be a student of Copernicus and an astrologer, as is the case of Giovanni Antonio Magini of Bologna.[151]

8.6.4 Decretorial and critical days

Medical astrology involved the use of the stars to predict the course of a disease by constructing a celestial figure from the outset;[152] it was associated with the alleged sympathy or affinity between plants, herbs, talismans, colours, sounds, odours and stars; and it was employed in the determination of critical and decretorial days.[153] Renaissance thinkers

---

1663: 5.93: 'est autem ars haec philosophiae pars prognostica et praecognoscere dicens, unde non vere scientia, sed ut ad medicinam se habet liber praedictionum Hippocratis et Galeni, ita hic ad totam philosophiam'; see also Trinkaus 1985 (citing the cautious view of Pontano).

[149] Cassirer 1963: 73–122; Canziani 1988: 211–12.

[150] Grafton and Siraisi forthcoming.

[151] I am grateful to Nancy Siraisi for this point, and this example.

[152] This could even give rise to an experimental testing of the success of such prediction, as seems to have been undertaken by Boderius 1555, although his preface and opening passage seem to suggest that what he calls 'philosophia iudicaria' is not only necessary for medical prognosis, but even can claim the status of scientia through its involvement with astral causality.

[153] On critical and decretorial days, see Hippocrates, *Aphorisms*, ii.24: 'the fourth of the set of seven is indicative. The eighth is the beginning of another set of seven. But the eleventh is also worthy of consideration, for it is the fourth of the second set of seven. Again the seventeenth will be considered: it is indeed the fourth from the fourteenth, but the seventh from the eleventh'; Galen, *De diebus decretoriis*, iii.2, K 9.902–3 (linking decretorial days to the moon); Huggelius 1560: 7 (the above in tabular form); Ferrier 1549a (offering a variety of arithmetical versions). This, together with the notion of sympathy, gives some credence to the claims of Foucault 1966: 32–59 concerning Renaissance semiology, although his claims do not fit with other parts of Renaissance learned discourse; see Maclean 1998a.

were aware that the alignment of parts of the body with heavenly bodies could be looked upon as arbitrary:[154] a more telling critique of critical days was delivered by Liddel on the authority of Averroes:

> Averroes thinks that the whole rationale of critical days depends on the proportion of nature acting to illness resisting; indeed, since this proportion is variable, it is impossible for a calculable ratio ('enumerandi ratio') to be obtained from it; nor will one be able to know why a crisis on the seventh day is better and safer than one on the sixth or eighth.[155]

In spite of the evidence of such quotations, Chapman alleges that 'by 1600 astrology had come to incorporate so much of the explanatory apparatus of classical medicine...that any thoroughgoing scepticism about astrological system was likely to shake confidence in orthodox medicine'.[156] This may be true of the English texts to which he refers; it is true of Paracelsian medicine;[157] but it is not true of the learned profession as a whole. Astrology has of course its proponents; but one only has to consult the long and sustained polemic against astrology in the sixteenth century to see that it was controverted with considerable vigour.[158] It has been argued that its authority and influence were upheld in part because astrological predictions can always be adjusted to appear right in retrospect; they furthermore enjoy what others have called a 'confirmation bias', that is to say their proponents suffer from the psychological condition of being able only to remember the successes of their art.[159] The signs on which the art is based are not necessarily ambivalent in themselves; the construction placed upon them is however necessarily contentious, depending on the perceived relationship of the superlunary and sublunary worlds and the significance accorded to the coincidence of celestial movements and changes in the human body.

8.7 INDICATIONS

I come now to the signs most closely connected to therapeutics: indications, contraindications, coindications, 'correpugnantia'. These,

---

[154] Chapman 1979: 275ff. (quoting Perkins); Aristotle, *Metaphysics*, xiv.6, 1093 a 1ff.

[155] Liddel 1628: 584–5: 'Averrhoes arbitratur, totam hanc dierum criticorum rationem dependere a proportione naturae agentis et morbi resistentis: verum, cum proportio illa varia sit, unde certa enumerandi ratio sumi nequit; nec scire poterit cur crisis septimo die melior et tutior sit quam sexto aut octavo.'

[156] Chapman 1979: 300n.

[157] Goldammer 1991: 122–7; Christie 1998; Fabricius 1626.

[158] For a bibliography, see Lipenius 1679: 58f.

[159] Grafton 1999: 328; Siraisi 1990c: 133–6.

according to Argenterio, constitute the true semiotic of medicine.[160]
One ancient source which deals with this is to be found in Galen's
De constitutione artis medicae, where it is described as a method.[161] It is
an 'insinuatio' ('endeixis'), involving persuasive powers and the non-
ratiocinative application of hypotheses on the basis of incomplete correlations, whose enthymematic form is various called a 'practical syllogism'
and a 'physiognomonic syllogism' as we have seen (above 5.1).[162] In
Valleriola's version, Galen's definition runs thus:

A prompting to follow a certain course or to act ['sequentis sive agendi insinuatio']; by it only what to do is suggested and urged; it will not prescribe how,
at what time, in what order, in what quantity, and with what help to undertake
the required action; these the doctor determines himself, having reviewed the
possibilities of remedial action, by reference to the nature of the illness, the
strength, age, habit, mental state, and so on, of the patient.[163]

In a more explicitly logical way, Gemma calls 'indicatio' a 'kind of demonstration of the similar or opposite things necessary to the action of the
doctor', referring to the two unstated premisses 'contraria contraria curantur' and 'similia similibus conservantur', here expressed as 'finding
similar things in conserving [conditions of the body]' and 'finding opposite things in destroying and conquering'. These species 'are only for
the determination of the categorial class; for similarity and contrariety,
in these broad terms, are different according to substance, and different when applied to quantity, quality, place and time'.[164] Liddel follows Galen in distinguishing between 'primary indications' (of illnesses,
causes and faculties) which anyone can see; and 'secondary indications'
('coindicantia', 'contraindicantia', 'correpugnantia'), such as feebleness
('vires debiles') or the non-naturals (indicating 'vires fractas') which 'show'

---

[160] Argenterio 1606–7: 2.175–96.

[161] Valleriola 1577: 133; Kudlien 1991: 103ff. *Methodus medendi*, ii, iii, ix, x contain a great deal on indication.

[162] Liddel 1628: 606–7; Justus 1618; Valleriola 1577: 560; Varanda 1620: 16–17; Schegk 1579a; Aubéry 1585: 15.

[163] Valleriola 1577: 560: 'sequentis sive agendi insinuatio, ab ipsa tantum suggeritur et insinuatur, quid agendum est: sed quomodo, quo tempore, ordine, mensura, quibus praesidiis id agere oportet, non praescribit, quod medicus ipse facit: propositis sibi medendi scopis, a morbi natura, aegrotantis viribus, aetatis, consuetudine, animi, constitutione, et caeteris huiusmodi' (cf. the definition given in *Subfiguratio empirica*, quoted below, 8.7.2). Many doctors use the phrase 'agendi insinuatio'; see Liddel 1628: 606; Rosenbachius 1620; Capivaccius 1603: 12.

[164] Gemma 1575: 218–19: 'demonstratio quaedam similis aut contrarii ad actionem artificis nec-essaria . . . species tantum pro categoriae classis discrimine tribuuntur; nam similitudo, contra-rietas, latius accepto vocabulo alia est secundum substant[iae] alia quantitatis, qualitatis, loci, temporis'; Schegk 1579a: A2r compares discovering indications to following Ariadne's thread.

through something other than themselves.[165] Other accounts speak not
of demonstration, but of demonstrative inference ('illatio demonstrativa')
or an inferential process leading from the 'indicans' perceived by the intellect to the unknown 'indicatum' or illness.[166] Da Monte calls indication
a 'relatio' or 'quoddam relativum'[167] at one point, but elsewhere shows
himself to be less concerned with its logical status:

An indication reveals the intention which of itself is indistinct and confused,
and the more that these indications are distinct, the more also that the intention
to act will be clear. For an indication comes after an intention. So intention
is principally to be considered by the doctor. But what is it that distinguishes
indications? The 'methodus divisiva' [above, 4.4.3]. Let us look at the argument
for this. I intend to cure an illness; it is therefore necessary for it to be indicated
to me what the illness is. What distinguishes an illness? Nothing other than the
divisive method, which distinguishes the indication, and thereafter the intention.
Because the intention is to cure the illness, and illnesses are many in number,
they must therefore be submitted to division.[168]

Da Monte's account, which is inspired by that of Rhazes, conflates indication with diagnosis, and applies the same method (progressive division)
to both. He refers to purpose, but does not link this to the practical syllogism; he refers also to correlation, but does not reduce this to Aubéry's
minimalist 'physiognomonic' reasoning.[169]

8.7.1 Indicans and indicatum

The 'indicatio' is distinguished from both the 'indicatum' and the
'indicans', which here designates not a sign ('which signifies something')

---

[165] Liddel 1628: 607–8, referring to *De methodo medendi*, ii.7, K 10.126ff.

[166] Bartolettus 1619: 3: 'processus illativus ab indicante noto secundum intellectum ad ipsum
indicatum ignotum ceu ad affectum'.

[167] Da Monte 1554: 67–8: 'indicatio est quoddam relativum . . . talis est natura relationis, ut secundum varietatem rei indicatae ac habitudinem varietur relatio, quot ergo erunt fundamenta, ad
quae indicationes referuntur, tot erunt indicationes, et quot modis variabuntur fundamenta,
tot etiam indicationes variabuntur, quia semper erunt sub relatione fundamenti sui'.

[168] Da Monte 1587: 849: 'Indicatio ostendit intentionem quae ex se est indistincta et confusa,
et quanto istae indicationes sunt magis distinctae, tanto intentio agendi quoque magis erit
distincta. Indicatio est enim posterior intentione. Intentio autem principaliter est consideranda
a medico. Si quid est, quod distinguitur indicationes? Methodus divisiva. Videmus hoc in
discursu. Intendo curare morbum, oportet ergo indicari mihi, quis sit iste morbus. At quid
distinguit morbum? Nihil aliud quam methodus divisiva, quae distinguit indicationem, et
postea intentionem. Cum igitur propositum sit curare morbum, morbi autem sint multiplices,
ideo et ipsi dividendi sunt.'

[169] Bylebyl 1991: 178–9; Liddel 1628: 606–7; Aubéry 1585: 15. Argenterio 1606–7: 176–7 refers
to a combination of 'observatio', 'analogismus', 'ratiocinatio', 'agendo insinuatio' and 'cognitio
iuvantis ac nocentis'.

but a motivation to apply a cure ('which indicates something which must be done in the use of materia medica').[170] Some designations, such as that of Liddel, may make the relationship of 'indicans' to 'indicatum' sound less logical than semantic (see below 8.9.1):

[An 'indicans'] is something observed and identified in a healthy or sick body, by virtue of which something is said to occur which must be done to it; or again, it is anything healthy or sick which is not revealed to the intellect, leading to an understanding of the appropriate treatment. The 'indicatum' is that very treatment, or is that which is consistent with the 'indicans', or follows from it in the interests of restoring health.[171]

His indication is a prompting to action, but is separate from experience, and drawn from the nature of the object being treated or a consideration of its scope without observation or rational deliberation; there is no reasoning process involved, although it can be represented as a practical syllogism (see above, 5.1).[172] According to the more orthodox Aristotelian Sanctorius, the 'indicans' is the Minor of a such a syllogism, whose force ('essentia specifica') is jussive or purposive; the Major is the remedy and the third term is an 'individuum aliquot'. Those who say that there are more than three 'indicantia' (including Galen, *Methodus medendi*, x.2) are in error; there can only be three because there are only three terms in syllogistic logic.[173] The 'indicans' can be 'genericum', 'subalternum', 'specificum', even 'proprium' (of a logical particular, not an individual); it is better known than its referent (the 'indicatum') being manifest to sense; it is not external to the body, but is that which itself is cured. Neither symptoms, nor the site of the disease ('locus affectus'), have the power to indicate; the 'indicans' is distinct from antecedents and consequents: that is to say, that it is neither sign, symptom nor

---

[170] Argenterio 1610: 1677.

[171] Liddel 1628: 607: 'quoddam in corpore secundum aut praeter naturam observatum et designatum cuius gratia aliquid fieri dicitur, quod ei conferre debet: sive omne quod secundum aut praeter naturam intellectu manifestum non est, ducens ad rei iuvantis comprehensionem. Indicatum vero est illud ipsum iuvans, sive id quod indicante congruit aut consequens agendum gratia sanitatis restaurandae'.

[172] Liddel 1624: 606–8: 'agendi insinuatio, sive ratio dirigendi actionem, seiuncta ab experientia, et sumpta a natura rei sive contemplatione scopi citra observationem aut expressam ratiocinationem ... modus procedendi indicationibus ad indicatum sine expressa ratiocinatione fit et tamen ad expressam reduci poterit ... ea ratiocinatio syllogismus factivus est, cuius tota vis ex duobus principiis dependit: contraria contrariis curantur; similia similibus conservantur'. The example is 'Plato febricitat; ergo est refrigerandus', used also by Campilongo 1601: 4r, and is probably Galenic in origin.

[173] Sanctorius 1630: 729–30 (xi.2). The three terms are described as 'causa quae efficit', 'res affecta' and 'subiectum', which are analogous to 'aedificator', 'aedificium' and 'materia aedificii'.

cause in any straightforward way.[174] It can show quality better than quantity.[175]

Sanctorius's negative description of 'indicantia' makes them sound mysterious and elusive; others list their sources less enigmatically, and in ways reminiscent of lists of naturals and non-naturals, circumstantiae, symptoms and external observations. Auger Ferrier of Toulouse in fact finds that there are sixteen ways of proceeding to an indication, which relate to external bodily clues of one kind or another ('ab effectu'; 'a temperamento totius corporis'; 'a parte affecta'; 'a viribus aegrotantis'), environment ('ab aere ambiente'), the state and nature of the patient ('a consuetudine'; 'ab aetate'; 'a naturarum proprietate'; 'a sexu'; 'a vitae munere et arte'), the progress of the illness itself ('a longitudine et brevitate morbi'; 'a quatuor morborum temporibus'; 'a particularibus morborum accessionibus'; 'a quotidianis, ordinatisque aliis naturae functionibus'), the effect of the treatment ('a medicamentorum facultatibus') and finally the stars and planets ('a lumine et influxu corporum caelestium'). His sophisticated discussion, which expands on these categories, includes a moderate defence of astrology, a denunciation of those who attack it out of ignorance and contrariness, and a method for resolving the problem of choosing between indications of equal weight ('indicationes aequaliter pollentes').[176]

8.7.2 Mental processes

The central problem concerning indication is whether it is a matter of the (trained) intellect alone, or of the intellect and the senses, or intuition (of a nature not clearly specified) without explicit ratiocinative procedures. In his polemical tract *Subfiguratio empirica*, Galen defines an indication as a

logical transition based on the nature of things . . . [which] lays hold of knowledge. But the empirical variety relies on what is discovered by experience, not because it is persuasive or plausible, that the similar should be productive of something similar, or require similar things, or undergo similar things . . . but on

---

[174] Campilongo 1601: 5–7.

[175] Sanctorius 1630: 763–6 (xi.13); Argenterio 1606–7: 176–7.

[176] Ferrier 1592: 107: 'pari modo mihi cavendum est ne insensos mihi reddam eos qui contradictione, ignorantiae pedisequa, non ratione feruntur in caelestis disciplinae calumniam' (on unjust criticism of astrology); *ibid.*, 107–17 ('de complicatione, contrarietate et consensu indicantium') gives a method for disambiguation of competing indications, which is to look first at non-naturals, next distinguish 'signa communia' from 'signa propria', then distinguish by magnitude and dignity of indication.

the basis of the fact that [empirics] have discovered by experience that similar things behave in this way.[177]

He is arguing here that it is necessary to have a theory of pathology to obtain therapeutic information from indicative signs: in the *Methodus medendi*, ii.7 (K 10.126–7) he declares that therapeutic method is independent of experience and that everything distinct from experience is called indication.[178] Sanctorius makes explicit this anti-analogistic and anti-empirical approach by setting out to demonstrate on the basis of the same text and Aristotelian syllogistic logic that indication is the only way to approach the choice of remedy.[179] Silvaticus says that indication arises from 'praecepta medica' and can work even better than the resolutive method.[180] This is not a claim which Sanctorius finds persuasive. He prefers to translate the indication into a syllogistic form.

Campilongo points to another possibility: that indication can lead us to counter-intuition, what he calls non-consenting knowledge: 'anamnestic signs lead to knowledge of effects to which the intellect assents . . . signs of healthy and sick things lead us to a kind of knowledge in which the intellect does not assent'.[181] This seems close in various ways to the intuition or 'nous' of *Posterior analytics*, ii.19 (100 b 8), and recalls the reference in the *De interpretatione* to the meaning of words or phrases intended by the speaker.[182] The reference to counter-intuition is difficult

---

[177] Galen 1556a: 1.33: 'porro rationalis transitus . . . ab indicantis rei natura innotescat. Empiricus vero ea potius imitatur, quae sensu praecognita fuerint, non quidem quia probabile videtur simile a simili generari, aut agere, aut pati . . . sed quod experimento cognoverint ita se invicem habere, quae sunt similia'.

[178] Capivaccius 1603: 12 uses this topos, but derives from it the following definition of indication: 'agendi insinuatio, haec est eius virtute manu ducimur in artem administrandorum auxiliorum. Ut autem sciamus, non solum in genere, quid sit agendum; sed etiam distincte. Indicatio sumetur ex indicante: ergo qu[ot]uplex est indicans, tot etiam erunt indicationes. Indicantia autem sunt triplicia, sc[ilicet] res naturales, non naturales, contra naturam. Ergo ut indicationes ex his sumantur, haec tria accurate consideranda erunt. Consideramus autem haec vel singula vel mixta, praesertim sibi invicem nonnunquam opposita, ubi sane cum indicantia opponantur, non ita facile indicationes inveniuntur.'

[179] Sanctorius 1630: 726–32 (xi.2).

[180] Silvaticus 1601: 374 (on the question of purging pregnant women): 'est sine dubitatione verum, et a Galeno pluries determinatum, quod in resolutiva methodo ultimum obtinet locum, illud idem ex executione, sive in curatione primum sibi vendicare: tamen et interim posse ac debere ordinem huiusmodi variare, et immutare, decrevit ille idem in lib 7 meth. medend. cap. 2. Porro id quod magis urget, et a quo maxime discrimen aegro impendere cognoscitur, illud est, quod dictum ordinem potissimum evariat. At id observans medicus tantum abest, ut irregulariter incedat, ut potius praecepta medica, artis nixa principiis recte et congruo ordine dicatur observare; omnis vera indicatio ipsius artis est, huicque satisfaciens, medicus regulariter prorsus incedere dicendus est.' See also above 4.3.

[181] Campilongo 1601: 10v, 19v; *De interpretatione*, iii, 16 b 19.

[182] Hankinson 1995: 74.

to reconcile with the role accorded to experience (here it is the habitus developed from past practice of the doctor) which leads to 'artificiosa coniectura' and the affirmation of the importance of the precepts of the art.[183] Others correlate indication with circumstantiae (as do Ferrier and Argenterio) and make each indication a unique act.[184] The Montpellier doctor Rondelet, in a way perhaps characteristic of the practical, even anti-theoretical bias of that school, gives more place to 'observatio et experientia' in the assessment of dosage than in the identification of the correct materia medica.[185]

Two late accounts stand out, which point up this problem of indication being either intelligible or sensible or both, and leading either to objective or psychological (non-objective) certitude. That of the Montpellier doctor Jean de Varanda describes indication in terms now familiar to us of something which is persuasive or dissuasive of a course of action; it is not the same as empirical evidence, which does not have the power to suggest a remedy; it does not operate by analogy; it is not even the same as reasoning, because there is no discursive process involved. This raises for him the question whether any layman or even plebeian ('idiota aut vulgaris homo') could be as effective in prescribing cures as a doctor, if indications are persuasive in themselves and need no rational processing. The reply given is characteristic of a doctor writing in defence of his profession: for indications to persuade, they need to be heard in the context of a knowledge of available treatments, of an ability to distinguish causes from symptoms, of a grasp of the norms of health, and an ability to judge the degree of strength of a disease: in other words, in the context of professional medical training.[186] For all the ingenuity of this argument, there is not a clear determination of the relationship of brute evidence (in this case the circumstances of the case) and the rational procedures by which it is evaluated; as in the case of the law, there is a smudging of the line between fact and non-discursive interpretation, and a penetration of hermeneutics into logical analysis.[187]

---

[183] Valleriola 1577: 558; Frölich 1612: A2r describes 'mens medici' as the efficient cause of semiology.
[184] Argenterio 1610: 928.
[185] Rondelet 1586: 291–2: 'quis enim ratiocinando tantum intelligeret medicamenta quaedam proprio peculiarique humori exigendo idonea esse? Horum etiam cognitionem experientia primum veteribus tradidit et usu comprobat; ut et medicamenta... quantitas asservatione dehinc artificiosa coniectura cognita'. See also Schegk 1579a: B4r–v who refers to the need for specialist knowledge, sensory information and skill.
[186] Varanda 1620: 16–18.
[187] Maclean 1992: 142–58.

Varanda's contemporary Joannes Justus, a Basle disputant whose theses on indication were defended in October 1618, draws on both da Monte and Valleriola, and produces a definition including a reference to semantics ('significatio'), and involving demonstration, observation, comprehension, experience and 'insinuatio', all dependent on 'praeexistens cognitio' (see above 4.3):

Indication is a prompting, representation, or signification of action or following a certain course. Indication is also the perception without observation or reasoning of the appropriate treatment together with the understanding of the inappropriate . . . Indication can also be defined as a perception or comprehension of the 'indicatum' together with a grasping of the 'indicans' without empirical or rational activity . . . Indication falls under the rule of relation ('pros ti'), and has a relation to the things to which it relates. Therefore the prompting or understanding through which indication occurs cannot be caused in our intellect unless by preexisting knowledge.[188]

These accounts, and especially the last, show the relationship which has to be made with (active or passive) modes of cognition; and the connection with the modes of cognition in the law known as 'praesumptio', 'suspicio' and 'coniectura'.[189]

A number of other points emerge from these discussions which are pertinent here. First, 'indicantia' possess the force to co-indicate or

---

[188] Justus 1618: N3r: 'Indicatio [est] quod sit sequentis sive agendi insinuatio, repraesentatio vel significatio. Est quoque indicatio perceptio iuvantis adveniens cum comprehensione nocentis adveniens sine observatione et ratiocinatione . . . Potest quoque definiri, quod indicatio sit perceptio seu comprehensio indicati cum comprehensione indicantis citra experientiam et ratiocinationem . . . Est enim indicatio ex numero τῷ πρός τι et relationem ad sua relata habet. Insinuatio igitur sive comprehensio, per quam indicatio fit, non potest causari in nostri intellectu, nisi a praecedente cognitione.'

[189] On active and passive modes of cognition, see Maclean 1999a; on sign, conjecture and judge's intuition, see Farinacci 1606: 300–12 and Maclean 2000b; Farinacci is quoted by at least one doctor (Horst 1606: 67, in respect of the 'indicium magnum, verum, verisimile, credibile, proximum' as opposed to the 'certa, extrinseca et cognita praesumptio'; cf. C 4.19.25 on 'indicia indubitabilia'). A complication in law is the issue of witnesses, which is not at issue in 'indicationes' but which is very important to natural philosophy in the following century and can be sensed in the issue of syndromes of signs: below 8.8.1 and 8.9.1. On 'suspicio', see Baldus 1615: 35r (ad C 4.19. rubr. 12–15): 'suspicio vero est passio animi non eligentis firmiter aliquam conclusionem . . . et est modicae virtutis in indicando. Scias quod Iudex est sicut Medicus. Medicus enim cognoscit aegritudinem tripliciter; uno modo figuraliter, et improprie per urinam . . . videt enim infirmitatem sicut homo videt aliquid in speculo per quandam umbram, sic se habet Iudex q[uoniam] videt speculando, et intra se conferendo, per verisimilia et proxima ad veritatem cognoscendam. Secundo m[odo] videt Medicus per tactum pulsi, sic Iudex se habet q[uoniam] tangit veritatem per aperta testimonia. Tertio m[odo] videt Medicus a remotis, prognosticando; ita Iudex cum annexa suspicatur, q[uod] non pertinet ad condemnationem in genere. Dubitatio vero est animi passio cum praecisa ignorantia extremorum unde dicit Arist[oteles] dubitatio est aequalitas priorum ratiocinatorum . . . omne probatio reducitur ad quinque modos . . . q[ui] not[antur] hoc versu: *vox, scriptura, nomen sacrum, confessio, visus.*'

contraindicate very much in the way words have illocutionary force.[190] Second, they come in forms which are auxiliary to each other negatively or positively;[191] indications are secondary in these oblique forms, having the power to 'show' not directly but through the medium of something else; in this they resemble certain classes of signs, such as tavern signs (see above, 5.1).[192] Third, the absence of explicit reasoning creates problems when contradictory indications occur: if a doctor is forced to choose between these, he may become 'like a directionless sailor who sets the sail to the winds and tides'.[193] Galenic rules of thumb are however given for such circumstances by Liddel, drawing on the tenth book of Galen's *Methodus medendi* (K 10.661–733), which discusses the persuasive power of the competing indications, and Ferrier, referring to the following book of the same work (K 10.734–809) and *De febrium differentiis*, ii.8–10 (K 7.363–771), from which he sketches out a method based on a hierarchy of 'indicantia'.[194] Fourth, the learned doctor becomes the embodiment of indication, which is necessarily a performative and contingent act even if performed on the basis of past training in the art of medicine, in the same way that he becomes the embodiment of the art of medicine and its precepts at the bedside of his patients.

8.7.3 *Fictional cases*

A final point may be made, which has its parallel in law, where the jurist, in order the better to understand or teach the law on a given topic, may choose to make up an imaginary case ('fingere casum').[195] Doctors also can consider whether to draw pedagogical examples of cases from real experience or from their own imagination ('utrum medicus exempla ex se fingat an extrinsecus petat'):

[For it is evident that] a doctor makes up in his own head various examples of preserving or restoring health which are like conceptions, the reasons of which suitably guide his consultations, and through which he cures illnesses and protects health. For what is suggested to the mind of the doctor by an indication

---

[190] Capivaccius 1603: 15. The parallel with illocutionary force is made explicit by the use of 'vis permittendi, limitandi, repugnandi, removendi'.

[191] Varanda 1620: 15 points out that the term 'correpugnantia' had been coined by the 'recentiores'.

[192] Liddel 1628: 609–10.

[193] Gemma 1575: 194f.: 'tanquam otiosa nauta [qui] ventis et fluctibus vela committit'.

[194] Liddel 1628: 610: 'semper eam [indicationem] praeferre quae violentior est et magis urget'; Ferrier 1574: 21–106 (see note 176 above).

[195] Uldaricus Zazius, quoted in Maclean 1999c: 8.

drawn from something's essence can be derived from his own reflections and be pressed into use as a conclusion of a sort. Indeed, nature suggests indications to the doctor, from which he logically derives the connected procedures of the cure . . .[196]

This passage from Valleriola again shows the complex interaction of past experience, present case, ratiocination and decision theory. The importance of this fictional approach is seen also in the matter of counter-intuition: all indication can be undone by counter-intuition, as Maiolus points out in respect of dosage: a correct decision can be reached which 'can appear astonishing and almost incredible'.[197] Galen's self-glorifying narratives of his counter-intuitional diagnoses in the *De locis affectis* are pertinent here too (see above, 8.6.1).

8.8 CONJECTURAL ARTS OR SCIENCES

8.8.1 Physiognomy

I come now to the sign-based conjectural arts or sciences which were often looked upon as inferior to medicine but often practised and written about by doctors: physiognomy, metoposcopy, chiromancy, oneirocritics, divination.[198] All of these have ancient roots; and all are much written about in the course of the Middle Ages and Renaissance. Physiognomy is an art devoted to the distinguishing of sensory signs;[199] it is defined as 'a method (ratio) of investigating natural characteristics (mores) from fixed signs which are in the body and accidents which change the signs';[200] it is derived from 'the movements, shapes and colours, and from habits appearing in the face, from the growth of hair, from the smoothness of the skin, from the voice, from the condition of the flesh, from the parts

---

[196] Valleriola 1577: 559: 'nam in comperto est medicum varia sibi in mente sanitatis vel tuendae vel resarciendae exempla ac veluti ideas quasdam effingere, ad quarum rationem consilia sua commode dirigens et morbos curat et sanitatem tuetur. Quid enim medico ab indicatione a rei essentia sumpta in mente suggeritur, id ex se effingit ut consecutione quadam in usum ducit. Natura quidem indicationes medico suggerit, quibus innexas ratiocinatione curandi rationes sumit' (citing *De constitutione artis medicae* and *De methodo medendi*, iii). Michael McVaugh has informed me that Arnau de Vilanova makes up cases. Cf. the remarks of Porzio 1598: 92 on 'corpus mathematicum'.

[197] Maiolus 1497: 7v: 'mirabile videtur et propemodum incredibile'.

[198] Cf. above, 4.4 (the classification of divination as conjectural both in doctrine and practice in Cardano 1565: 83r).

[199] Fontanus 1611: 34: 'physiognomia tota sita [est] in signis sensibilibus dignoscendis'.

[200] Porta 1593: 55: 'morum inspiciendorum Naturae ratio, ex iis quae corpori insunt fixis signis, et accidentibus quae signa mutant'.

of the body and the general character of the body' (*Physiognomica*, i, 806 a 35f.).[201] For some, it is a 'disciplina practica' with a 'methodus analytica seu resolutiva'; for others a 'scientia speculativa'.[202] Guglielmo Gratarolo (1516–68) suggests that it is a necessary science in respect of animals (who have no means of regulating their natural inclinations and aptitudes by reason), but a 'scientia ut in pluribus' in rational man, who has some power of self-determination.[203] Physiognomy's privileged ancient source is the work of that name attributed to Aristotle, which enjoyed several new editions and commentaries in our period; indeed, it is rewritten in a new order of propositions by one scholar (Jacques Fontaine (Fontanus) (d.1621)) to expose more clearly its logic.[204] There is also an important passage in *Prior analytics*, ii.27 which uses physiognomy in a logical example (see above 4.3.3). Its premisses are recorded by the most famous Renaissance writer on the question, Giambattista della Porta: that each class of creatures must have a passion common to all of them; that in other classes, this passion is to be found in some individuals, but not in all of them; and that a sign is in all who have this passion, and is not present in those who do not have it.[205] Other ancient writers on the topic are Adamantius (whose tract appeared in Paris in Greek in 1540, and was published in Latin in Janus Cornarius's translation in 1544)

---

[201] Fontanus 1611: 49.

[202] Moldenarius 1616 links physiognomy, chiromancy, metoposcopy and oneirocritics as practical disciplines; Schmitt and Skinner 1988: 271–2 (on Achillinus); Porta 1593: 8, who describes physiognomy as a 'scientia'. See also Aubéry 1585: 15, quoted above, ch. 4 note 122, who gives the name 'physiognomonic syllogism' to reasoning of this kind: 'coltsfoot is associated with pulmonary congestion; [therefore] pulmonary congestion is associated with coltsfoot'.

[203] Gratarolo in Indagine 1603: 216: 'omnibus animalibus commune est agere vel pati ab inclinatione naturali, quae in brutis impetus, ita in hominibus propensio dicitur (ut in cholerico est ad iram inclinatio) . . . Inclinationes ergo istae in hominibus morum atque affectuum semina dicuntur, quoniam ratione regulari possunt; in brutis vero mores et affectus, quoniam sensibus et appetitu vivunt. Ex hoc quidem patet Physiognomiam scientiam esse necessarium, quo per ipsam praedicimus aptitudines naturales et affectus vel mores: quo vero per ipsam praedicimus affectus vel mores actuales, nec est scientia necessaria, nec firma: verum quia homines plerunque vivunt sensu, et non nisi sapientes vivunt ratione, ideo physiognomia est scientia praedicandi mores actuales et effectus ut in pluribus, quoniam plures appetitu et sensu vivunt, quam ratione, quam etiam ob causam Bias Prienaeus dicebat plures esse malos quam bonos.'

[204] Porta 1593 seems to accept the doctrine of both Aristotle and Polemo, and has chapters on the errors of Philo (who sees physiognomy as concerning facial appearance only), Plato (who considers the whole animal), Trogos (who relies on the dispositions of the heavens and of place: against which Porta argues that there are clever Scythians and stupid Athenians); see also *Infinita nature secreta* 1515; Willichius 1538; Lacuna in Aristotle 1541; Fontanus 1611, Baldus 1621.

[205] Porta 1593: 57–8: 'considerandum est animalium genus unum, cui in universum insit ea passio; alia genera invenienda quae non universale, sed particulariter eiusdem passionis sit capacia; quae nota omnibus insit, quibus inest illa passio et similiter removeatur ab illis, quae eiusdem expertia sunt'.

and Polemo (whose treatise was first printed in Greek in 1545 and translated seven years later by Nicolaus Petreius).

The theory of signs given in these works is both workable and sophisticated (indeed, some of its precepts are taken over into diagnostic medicine); it rests on a number of distinctions. We have already met that between common and proper signs (above 5.1, 8.3.2);[206] there are also permanent and evanescent signs, of which only the first properly belongs to the science of physiognomy.[207] Signs can be plural (even contrary) in signification, and can relate either to accidentia or substantial features;[208] although Aristotle's *Physiognomica* claims that 'no animal has existed such that it has the form of one animal and the disposition of another' (805 a 10) at least one commentator questions this, pointing out that it is not consistent with metempsychosis, lycanthropy and the theory of the microcosm.[209] There are signs of masculinity and femininity, which Giambattista della Porta systematises from the scattered remarks of the *Physiognomica*.[210] Signs are different in their relative force: Baldus explicitly introduces a dominance argument in considering 'in which signs more or less trust is to be placed', and arguing that it is rational to ask 'whether all sources of signs have the same degree of

---

[206] Gratarolo in Indagine 1603: 216–17 makes a distinction between 'duo signorum genera': 'aliqua quae a qualitate elementaria sumpta animi affectiones significant, ut thoracis pilositas, quae iracundiae est indicium, ex corde calido. Quaedam a proprietate, ut capitis in dextrum inclinatio, quae signum est c[i]naedi, nec ex causa calida aut frigida, sed proprietate colligitur. Peripatetici vero (ut Aristoteles secundo priorum) supponunt nulli homini inesse aliquam affectionem, aut aliquem morem a natura, quin illum in corpore comitetur signum per quod illa passio aut mos possit significari.'

[207] Fontanus 1611: 41; a 'signum permanens' would be redness of face: a 'signum fugax' would be blushing. Cureau de la Chambre 1662: 324 seems however to take the reading of labile signs to be part of the detective function of the physiognomist: 'rien de considérable se forme dans l'esprit qui ne se puisse découvrir par le visage, par la parole, par les effets et par les circonstances dont on tire des coniectures asseurées, ou du moins fort probables'. He also has interesting things to say about the detection of simulated passions (*ibid.*, 325f.).

[208] Porta 1593: 28–9; Fontanus 1611: 31, 43 pointing out that the same accidental features of the face can be shared by those of opposite character ('aliqui tametsi dissimiles moribus eadem habe[nt] vultus accidentia'), and recording the disagreement between the view of Aristotle that facial accidents cannot signify character (the pallor of the mathematician arises from his lifestyle, not his accidental profession), and that of Rhazes, who in his own *De physiognomia* claims that accidents like the profession of philosophy can generate physiognomic signs. The difference of opinion is reconciled by Fontanus: 'illa signa esse eius qui aptitudinem ad Philosophiae capescendam habet, non eius qui sibi habitum Philosophiae labore comparavi'. Porta 1593: 36–9 points out also (against Philo) that our faces change over time by 'formae mutatio'.

[209] Fontanus 1611: 25–6; but Porta 1593: 15, 50–2, supports the Aristotelian line: 'necessarium est tale corpus talem animam ipsius speciei convenientem sequi'.

[210] *Ibid.*, 30.

certainty, or whether some are more certain than others'.[211] Syndromes
of signs partake of this dominance argument, which is also probabilistic
in implication, since syndromes are said to be more trustworthy than
single signs: Fontanus points out that the truth of physiognomy cannot
be established by one or two signs, but by a greater number all of which
are consistent with each other.[212] This view is expressed in Aristotle and
Adamantius, who not only points to the issue of confirmatory signs but
also that of a hierarchy ('signa potentiora') to settle cases of doubt; indeed, this is one of the rare points at which a negative approach to the
construction of knowledge through doubt is employed in anything but a
destructive way, as by sceptics. A further implication of sign syndromes
is the use which can be made of negative or contrary evidence and absent signs as means of confirmation.[213] They arise also in the topic of
natural kinds (best known through Theophrastus's *Characters*) in which
the danger of interpreting proper signs without subsidiary confirmation
is stressed (as it is also in Aristotle).[214]

For all this sophistication in its approach to evidence, physiognomy
was part of secrets literature in the Middle Ages, and became associated in the early Renaissance with neoplatonism and occult explanantia,

---

[211] Baldus 1621: 41: 'quibus signis maior quibus minor fides sit adhibenda'; 'numquid omnes
[fontes] aequaliter ostendant, an aliqui certiores sint aliis'; according to him, Aristotle's answer
runs as follows: 'signa quae sumuntur ab apparentia, quam vocant morem, et a motibus, et
a figura corporis, omnino aliis sunt efficaciora, vel quoniam minus ab voluntate pendent, vel
quoniam magis ab ea animae parte, quae virtus est in corpore, et immediatius nascuntur,
faciei enim apparentiam pro libito non mutabis, neque corporis formam, aut saltem maxima
cum difficultate, quare non immerito Terentius Chremes admirabatur, quod vultum pro libito
fingeret Syrus servus . . .' Porta 1593: 52 gives a hierarchy of common signs (whether by
presence or absence), of which the more certain are in the face, and the least certain the lower
body. Fuchs 1615:):(8v quotes 'Loelius' on the problem of our failing to hear what signs have
to say for us: 'multis signis natura declarat quid velit, ac quaeret, ac desiderat: absurdescimus
tamen nescio quo modo, nec ea quae ab ea monemur, audimus' (cf. also Adamantius, ii.1).

[212] Fuchs 1615:):(7v: 'id nosse expedit, quo ex uno signo per se, et ex duobus constans pronuntiatio
[of the truth of physiognomy] fieri non potest, sed ex pluribus et maioribus, quae omnia inter
se mutuo consentiunt'; it might seem that this point, which is made in Aristotle's *Physiognomica*,
ii, 806 b 38 ('generally speaking, it is foolish to put one's faith in any one of the signs: but
where one finds several of the signs in agreement in one individual, one would *probably* have
more justification for believing the inference true [my italics]'), is not consistent with the passage
in *Prior analytics*, ii.27, 70 b 12ff. which claims that a physiognomonic sign is only valid if one
sign corresponds to one affection. Burnyeat 1982 says that such a sign is an inference yielding
generalisations: the example given in *Physiognomica*, iii, 807 b 5–12 is: 'he is a coward because
his eyes are weak and blinking and his movements constrained'. Interestingly, Fontanus leaves
out the dominance argument in respect of the syndrome in his reordering of the text of the
Physiognomica.

[213] Baldus 1621: 41, quoted below 8.9.

[214] Gratarolo interestingly develops a political dimension of physiognomy by stressing not only
national differences but intranational differences: Canziani 1988: 217.

imagination, spirits and powers.[215] Its growing popularity (which may be gauged by the number of new works published on the subject) can be accounted for by the apparent power it affords to those versed in it over the secret thoughts and inclinations of others The titlepage of Giambattista della Porta's treatise announces that it is for 'all categories of those seeking knowledge, so that they may be seen to penetrate the secret recesses of the mind' ('omnium ordinum studiosi, ut intimos animi recessus penetrare videantur'); this appeal can be felt as late as 1662, in Cureau de la Chambre's *L'Art de connoistre les hommes*, which again promises to impart such insights to the reader. In the sixteenth century, its influence can be felt in the writings of Paracelsus;[216] somewhat later, it attracts the attention of a range of authors. These include Cardano, who said of it that 'physiognomics without doubt contains great truth', and that, like chiromancy and oneirocritics, it can 'make as certain predictions as can medicine'; Lemnius; Gratarolo, who produces a typology of physiognomic signs; Peucer, who derives his account from Galen's *Animi mores sequuntur temperamenta corporum*, and is realistic about the variability of these signs:[217] and finally Chiaramonte, whose *Semeiotike* of 1625 is a sophisticated account of the subject in a quasi-probabilistic way, and whose method for reaching inferences from physiognomonic signs has already been examined in detail (above 5.2.2).

8.8.2 Chiromancy and metoposcopy

Practices associated with physiognomy are chiromancy, in which Paracelsus took an interest;[218] metoposcopy; ophthalmoscopy; and oneirocritics. Joannes ab Indagine's work on several of these conjectural arts begins with a section on chiromancy; after 1586, when Sixtus V issued a bull condemning the practice (although not physiognomy), the announcement of the subject was omitted from at least one titlepage,

---

[215] *Ibid.*, 220; see also Porter 1997. But it was prescribed to be read in the University of Freiburg in the mid-fifteenth-century statutes 'si lecti per magistros fuerint': Ott and Fletcher 1964: 46.

[216] See also Schmitt and Skinner 1988: 271–2, citing Cocles, Scot and Achillini; Paracelsus 1567 extends the concept to disease itself.

[217] Cardano 1568: 8 (i): ' physiognomia haud dubie magnam continet veritatem . . . facere praecognitionem adeo certam ut medicina'; Lemnius 1582: IV, 150v (on the body betraying the passions of the mind); Gratarolo in Indagine 1603: 216–17, quoted above, note 206 (on the two 'signorum genera' in physiognomy, 'a qualitate elementaria' and 'a proprietate'; an example of the former is a hairy throat, which indicates anger; of the latter, a head leaning to the left which indicates homosexuality). See also Peucer 1553: 258–69.

[218] Webster 1998: 69.

although not from the text.[219] Cardano's late-published account of
metoposcopy (its first edition was in 1658) contains a bibliography;
Hagecius ab Hagek, Goclenius, Moldenarius, and Fuchs also give references to Renaissance contributions to the subject.[220] Cardano avers that
all metoposcopic signs are ambiguous or plurivalent; but that does not
deter him from describing the subject in positive terms, claiming in his
De libris propriis of 1562 that it is a 'highly rational consideration, based on
semiotic postulation, and employing the dialectical rules of Ptolemy'.[221]
Fuchs links metoposcopy to ophthalmoscopy and quotes Epictetus as
an authority on the inefficacy of both practices: 'every sign shows only
what something is; it does not truly bring about what it designates'.[222] It
is linked by Hagecius to astrology and physiology;[223] he points out that
it is a branch of knowledge which had died out and needed to be redis-
covered. He classes it as a form of signature (see below 8.8.6), but one
which is imperfect, yielding only probable ('plaerumque') knowledge;
like physiognomy, its signs have only a limited predictive force in men:

As far as the certainty of this art is concerned, people should reflect on the fact
that it is, like medicine and astrology, an art which although it is more polished
than either of those, and is built on a certain method, is, however, linked to things
which occur not always but only for the most part ('plaerumque'), because
it deals with such things. Indeed, natural disposition ('ingenium'), character,
fortune and chance can be known in a clear way, and we have several signs of
most certain [future] events, and time will reveal many things. This art cannot
be so internally consistent and unchanging in human nature as in the natures
of beasts, because the latter are placed under the instruction of nature alone,
whereas the former, even if they have a [natural] propensity, are modifed to
some degree ('plaerumque') by upbringing and education.[224]

---

[219] Canziani 1988: 220; Indagine 1603 (cf. Taisnierus 1583); Cardano 1663: 3.385–8 (lxxix).
The eighteenth-century owner of the copy of Indagine's book in the Herzog-August-
Bibliothek, Wolfenbüttel wrote on the flyleaf 'Chyromantia habet fundamentum in Psalmo 39';
the reference is not clear to me.

[220] Hagecius ab Hagek 1562; Goclenius 1625; Moldenarius 1616; Fuchs 1615.

[221] Cardano 1663: 1.104.

[222] Fuchs 1615:):(7r (referring to Arrianus, *Epicteti Enchiridion*, i.14): 'omne signum, tantum quid
sit, ostendit: non vero efficit, quod designat'.

[223] Hagecius ab Hagek 1562: B4r.

[224] *Ibid.*, B1v: 'Quod ad certitudinem huius artis attinet, id cogitare singuli debent, artem esse
qualis Medicina et Astrologia, quae quanquam utraque cultior sit hac nostra, et certa Methodo
constituta: tamen quia versatur circa ea, quae plaerumque accidunt, in eo cum eis communicat.
Ingenium, mores, fortuna, et casus quidam non obscure cognosci possunt, et plaeraque signa
habemus certissimorum eventuum, et plura profert dies in lucem. Non potest etiam haec ita
sibi constans et perpetua esse in hominum naturis, ac in brutorum animantibus, propterea
quod haec solo naturae instructu feruntur, illae vero etsi ad quaedam sunt propensae; tamen
institutione et educatione plaerumque mutantur.'

8.8.3 Oneirocritics

Perhaps the richest part of the field of conjectural arts is oneirocritics, which has an ancient medical connection through the work of Hippocrates on dreams and Galen's *De dignotione ex insomniis*, which enjoyed six editions between 1531 and 1562.[225] Other ancient texts to emerge on this subject include those of Artemidorus (published in the Greek in 1518, and in the Latin translation of Cornarius in 1539) and Synesius, which Ferrier edited in 1549, and Cardano thirteen years later. The standard typology of dreams, however, is that to be found in the medieval encyclopaedia of Isidore of Seville, in which the 'somnum' (which is obscure, and needs interpreting) is distinguished from the 'visio', an image of a future event, the 'oraculum', which is the intervention of a (dead) parent to deliver a warning to his or her offspring or reveal the location of lost objects, and finally the 'insomnium' or 'visum' which is biological or digestive in origin, and reveals bodily failings through a set of mainly self-evident and univocal images (such as cisterns betokening bladders, or bladder trouble).[226] Ferrier, who links dream interpretation directly to medical semiotic, divides dreams into 'vana', 'naturalia' and 'vatidica'; this last category being subdivided into dreams of divine origin and those demonically inspired.[227] Another typology divides dreams into divine, supernatural and natural:[228] Cardano is cautious about this division. He would also wish to include categories of dreams which warn of future danger and impart medical advice, dreams in which the dreamer's spiritus is influenced by celestial forces, and dreams which are directly caused by evil demons, about which he says little.[229] These latter categories are imperfect dreams, being mixed, deformed, or transposed in some way.[230] All writers are agreed that dream signs with very rare exceptions are not univocal, and that their meaning is established by a mode of aggregation or conjunction of plausible readings of the signs. Signs are therefore only significant 'magna ex parte'; they can be uncertain, wholly individual and plurivalent. Their individual,

[225] Durling 1961: 286.
[226] Siraisi 1997: 181; Boriaud 1999. Among writers on medical semiology, Frölich 1612: B4v–C1r is one of the few to offer a typology of dreams.
[227] Ferrier 1549b: 13: 'hanc philosophiae partem non minus esse certam, quam ea sit medicinae portio, quae a graecis σημείωτική vocatur'. 'Divine dreams' are subdivided into allegorical and speculative: *ibid.*, 17–36, 50 (where Ferrier admits to the difficulty of distinguishing between the 'susurrum diaboli' and the 'vox Dei').
[228] Camerarius 1626–30: 2.83–5 (citing du Chesne and others); Ingolstetterus 1597: 157.
[229] Siraisi 1997: 186, 178–9; Grafton 1999: 165ff.; Isidore of Seville, *Etymologiae*, iii.6, iv.13.9.
[230] Boriaud 1999; Siraisi 1997: 180 (citing Ferrier 1549b: 29–33).

contingent nature also has as a consequence that each dreamer (in the Greek, if not the Old Testament tradition) is his own best interpreter, in stark contrast to learned medical diagnosis, for example, where professional training is taken to be a prerequisite.[231] The popularity of the genre of books on dream-interpretation no doubt arises from the hermeneutic autonomy of the dreamer. Dream signs also can be redundant or include redundant information, as Agrippa points out: 'there is as it were no dream which does not have something insignificant in it, just as there is no grain without straw'.[232] It might be claimed that this view should be seen in the context of Agrippa's polemic against all sign-based arts;[233] but even proponents of these conjectural arts are prepared to admit that their basic units of information are untrustworthy and weak.[234]

8.8.4 Divination

Weakest of all these practices, by common consent, is divination, on which Peucer and Gemma write at length, and which involves prognostication, judicial astrology, oneirocritics (witness Sanches's *De divinatione per somnum*), and, insofar as it concerns the prediction of future events, prognosis.[235] Much divination involves the interpretation of natural signs as though they were pregnant with meaning. It is their association with this dubious practice which creates the need in learned doctors to distinguish the precept-based and scientific nature of their discipline (a discipline which requires them to know about astral conjunctions, as we have seen, for purposes of phlebotomy and other treatments) from acts of foretelling which are manifestly exposed to charlatanry at every level. It is also why learned doctors engage in prognostications; not only as a way of earning money, and of establishing their authority, but also as a warning against unauthorised and potentially harmful interpretations of the future. It is therefore commonplace to find denunciations of judicial astrology in these little tracts.

[231] Siraisi 1997: 184 cites Synesius as explicitly making this point.
[232] Hallyn 1995: 93 (quoting Agrippa).
[233] Zambelli 1992: 85–6 (referring to *De vanitate*, xxxii–xxxvi).
[234] Peucer 1553: 183v–203r; Gemma 1575: 1.126–8; 2.6, 145–56.
[235] Siraisi 1997: 190. There are many other kinds of 'ars aretifii' (characters of planets, images, significance of motion of birds, animal song, virtues of herbs), according to Cardano 1663: 3.312.

8.8.5 Natural signs: weather

I come now to natural signs not used in divination, which according to Luke 21:25–33 were given to man for him to interpret: of this class of signs, those relating to the weather form a coherent body of doctrine. The most sustained treatment of the subject in ancient texts is to be found in Theophrastus's *On winds*, which deals with the rising and setting of stars, the configuration of terrain, animals and their habitat, and the sun and moon.[236] It is explicitly probabilistic in its approach to signs, accepting both dominance and degrees of certainty: its information is derived from *experientia*; according to Gratarolo, who wrote a short alphabetical list of signs of weather which can be read in the natural world, this is something which all creatures share, and which is attested by the Bible.[237] He takes weather and those things which reveal its future course to be influenced by the lunary and superlunary spheres; but that does not mean that there are occult sources in this art, which is compared to medicine by being conjectural in application and precept-based in doctrine.[238] It can inspire contemplation of the deity, but this should not lead to the expectation that natural events are divine signs, these being set apart by being pronouncedly counter-natural (i.e. against the fundamental laws of nature).[239]

8.8.6 Natural signs: signatures

The most contentious of natural signs are signatures, which we have met already in a metoposcopic context: Hagecius claims that lines on the forehead are 'signatures of the highest architect'.[240] Signatures are related to the single pathognomonic sign and to locality; they are also connected to the 'lumen naturae' in one of its two guises: either the

---

[236] Bonaventura 1593 (an edition and commentary of Theophrastus *inter alios*); Burnett 1999 (on Al Kindi); also Bos and Burnett 1998. They point out (27) that Cardano 1663. 3.663–6 is among those with a positive view of weather forecasting in the Renaissance.

[237] Gratarolo in Indagine 1603: 281: 'animantes omnes natura mutationes temporum sentiunt, quoniam naturali quodam instinctu ex impressione corporum caelestium producto, movuntur pro ratione dispositionis aeris ad temporum cognitionem, ut necessarium est suis naturis, super illud Hieremiae capite octavo [Jeremiah 8:7]: milvus in coelo cognovit tempus suum . . . animalia enim minus occupata, et corpore imbecilliora, mutationes temporum praesentiunt'. Nifo 1540 is a treatise on weather signs which surveys all the available sources, but does not speculate on competing signs or degrees of certainty in signs.

[238] Bonventura 1593: 228; Gratarolo 1554: 195 (on peacocks predicting rain by screeching).

[239] Cardano 1663: 1.105, 144, 147; Peucer 1553: 235v–278r; Ingolstetterus 1597: 147; Zacchia 1630: 4.1–13 (on miracles and natural events; see ch. 7, note 199).

[240] Hagecius ab Hagek 1562: a2r; Bianchi 1987.

divine light given through faith, or the 'naturalis ratio' which is the privileged instrument for the interpretation of nature (see above 5.3.5). The
doctrine of signatures is most commonly associated with the name of
Paracelsus, whose 'ars signata' rests not only on the ability of the believing doctor to see the significance of visual correspondences, but also on
the premiss that the cures for human ailments are to be found in the
localities in which they occur: a view which is not at odds with traditional learned medicine.[241] What is less in tune with such doctrine is the
quasi-cratylic presupposition that the connection between the sign and
what is signified is not conventional or arbitrary but rather essential.[242]
Thus Giambattista della Porta's natural magic and even du Chesne's
relatively sober account of signatures are in this respect in conflict with
traditional learned medicine (although not with country lore and empirical wisdom).[243] Not all aspects of this are necessarily mystical and
unscientific: the fact that illnesses are said by Paracelsus to have a physiognomy prepares the way for seeing them as ontological entities; the fact
that urine has a signature predisposes later doctors to look at its composition analytically; the same might be said to be true of the investigation
of balsam.[244]

Having said this, the correspondence theory of signatures in plants
is what is best known of this doctrine, and is its most contentious manifestation. It is worth quoting in full the rejection of this theory by a
contemporary botanist, Rembert Dodoens, as it reveals how resistant
the learned world was to a theory which Foucault (quite wrongly, in
my view) made the cornerstone of the Renaissance episteme:[245] on the
proposition 'signatures are found either in the form or shape of a plant
or any of its parts, or are derived from its colours or juices, or are taken
from other properties', he writes:

That the faculties of plants can be known from the characters or signs which are
in them or are sometimes to be observed in their parts, is a doctrine not found
in the most trustworthy authors among the ancients; this has been discovered,
or rather made up by several authors of later date and some of our own time.

---

[241] Cardano 1568 (on Hippocrates, *Airs, waters, places*); Sanctorius 1630: 791 (xii.5) (on region). Cf.
also Aubéry 1585: 15 (on the 'physiognomonic syllogism'), which although it does not specify an
essential relation between the plant and the illness it cures, none the less offers a loose means
of associating them.
[242] Pozzo forthcoming.
[243] Porta 1589; du Chesne 1609: 88 (a reading list).
[244] Paracelsus 1567; Kühlmann 1992: 118–19; Severinus 1571: 17–27.
[245] Foucault 1966; Maclean 1998a.

These last think that nature has marked very clearly whatever it has pleased her to create with its peculiar signature, and they teach that, through these, mainly hidden powers and faculties can be known with certainty: in the same way (so they say) that by the inspection of the face and other parts of the body the art of physiognomy perceives the characters and affections of men. But physiognomy is attested by Aristotle and other ancient philosophers; whereas the doctrine of the signature of plants has been attested by no one ancient writer who is held in any esteem; furthermore, it is so changeable and uncertain that it seems absolutely unworthy to be held to be either science or doctrine.[246]

Dodoens argues that all similarities of this type are 'fortuito casu'; and that the theory of signatures fails to distinguish between significant and insignificant similarities. He links signatures with occult properties (which are undemonstrable), and tries to untie the theory from Aristotelian physiognomy which its proponents quoted as a supporting doctrine. In his attack on Paracelsianism, Bartolettus goes one step further, and reduces the doctrine to categories within the Galenic system.[247]

A long, cogent and somewhat oratorical defence of signatures is to be found in du Chesne. He argues that nature makes nothing in vain, and that the correspondences which can be perceived in nature must be there for a purpose;[248] and that man as the microcosm is in this sense a mirror of all nature (or rather nature is a mirror of man), and as such the correspondence has to do with the management of man's health. He concedes what signatures reveal is uncertain, but claims also that they can yield infallible information: this leads du Chesne to conclude that the occult properties of plants are to be deduced 'ex similitudine formae atque figurae, cum animantium tum inanimantium'.[249] Even

---

[246] Dodoens 1583: 16: 'signaturae autem vel in forma figurave stirpis aut alicuius eius partis, reperiuntur, vel ex coloribus aut succis deprehenduntur, aut ex aliis proprietatibus accipiuntur...ex characteribus sive signis quae in stirpibus, aut earum partibus observari contingit, ipsarum cognosci facultates posse, a probatis inter veteres auctoribus traditum non reperitur: nonnullorum posterioris aetatis et nostri saeculi recentiorum haec inventa, aut verius commenta sunt. Qui naturam quodlibet a se procreatum suis peculiaribus signaturis manifestissime notasse existimant ac docent per quas vires et facultates praesertim occultae et latentes, certo cognoscantur: haud aliter (ut aiunt) quam ex inspectione vultus et nonnullarum corporis partium φυσιογνωμία mores et affectus hominum percipi: sed physiognomia ab Aristotele ac aliis veteribus philosophis probatur: doctrinae vero de signaturis stirpium, a nullo alicuius aestimationis veterum testimonium accepit: deinde tam fluxa et incerta est ut pro scientia aut doctrina nullatenus habenda videatur.'

[247] Bartolettus 1619: 262.

[248] This is a heuristic principle used by the investigators of zoology at this time: see Rondelet 1554–5: 1.78.

[249] Du Chesne 1609: 70–4: 'haud vane a Platone, eiusque sectatoribus mirabile illud, et prima fronte παράδοξον visum pronunciatum: Plantam esse hominem inversum. Hae si quidem,

among the proponents of the theory of signatures, therefore, the system of correpondences is not taken up in the sterile and Procrustean form described by Foucault, but is translated into a functional system which its proponents can defend rationally.[250] It must be conceded that when represented in tabular form, as it is later in the seventeenth century by Kircher and as earlier by Fabricius in his schematic presentation of all Paracelsian doctrine, the theory has altogether the appearance of constative mystical thought which was once thought to characterise primitive societies: in the latter's dichotomous presentation, for example, physical types ('encrasiae') are associated with the seven planets and the four humours through 'signaturas magicas' in an apparently inflexible way.[251] The juxtaposition in Fabricius's work of this with a tabular account of Galenic semiotic is stark. Whether this is tantamount to saying that there is a paradigm difference between occult and scientific mentalities, a position which Brian Vickers espouses, is not altogether clear however, as this would require the historian to argue either that Fabricius was intellectually schizophrenic in treating these incommensurable discourses serially, or unable to perceive the incoherence of his adoption of both.[252]

si rem ipsam exacte et oculo attento, sagaci, atque curioso, hoc est philosophico, intueamur, magnam, non tantum cum homine, sed caeteris quoque animantibus habent similitudinem. Quin imo ad naturae illam ἀναλογίαν rerum considerandarum ductricem oculos, et mentem attenderimus, ex iisdem, aut certe non usque adeo ab similibus plantas cum homine habere quandam proportionem animadvertemus... Haec et similia, mihi crede, non vane a natura in mundi hocce theatro sunt producta: Namque, ut verissime habet axioma, Deus et natura nihil faciunt frustra. Non itaque existimandum frustraneas atque fortuitas esse istas signaturas, sed in certum aliquem finem a natura productas. At in quem potius alium productas illas signaturas dicamus, quam in finem hominis? In bonum, inquam, imaginis divinae, cuius gratia cuncta creata, cunta producta sunt, cunctaque perenni successione propagantur atque conservantur? Et certe videtur nobis natura eo ipso, ceu speculo quodam ob oculos ponere, cui quaeque appropriata, propria atque utilia, et in quem finem singula ab ea producta sint. Nihil enim, uti dictum, facit frustra. Cui igitur simile potius comparabis, quam suo simili? A quo remedia desumes, quam ab eo, quod parti affectae, atque ipsi adeo naturae est simillimum? Non absurde itaque philosophati sunt, qui plantas resque omnes a natura signatas, animantibus brutis haecque rursus omnia, cum illis creaturarum perfectissimo nobilissimoque homini naturae, virium quadam similitudine statuerunt.' There is an inconsistency in du Chesne, in that at one point he relies on the presence of a strong teleology in nature, and at another (on seminal doctrine of illness, which is quasi-atomistic) he seems willing to see nature as unteleological.

[250]   Maclean 1998a; Kühlmann 1992: 117. It is of note that at least one traditional rational doctor includes signatures in his account of semiology: Frölich 1612: A2v: '*Signaturas externas rerum* accuratissimus Osvvaldus Crollius proponit.'

[251]   Fabricius 1626: BIV.

[252]   Vickers 1984b: 1–55; Vickers 1988b; Kühlmann 1992: 113 (on Croll) argues that hermetic philosophers of this time espouse a hermeneutics of nature which treats nature as a place of meaning, not a site for deductive reasoning.

8.9 CONCLUSIONS: PROBABILITY
AND THE CONJUNCTION OF SIGNS

It is pertinent to end this chapter by pointing out some common features of the theories of signs set out above, and by suggesting a few modern parallels. The first general point concerns probability: or to put it in the form in which it occurs in Renaissance texts, how to compute the likelihood of a sign or of several signs having a given signification. There is a class of signs which are certain (tekmēria) and unambiguous; they can be used for apodictic demonstration (see above, 4.3.5 and 5.1); but in medicine, they are 'rarissima', by common consent. So it is on syndromes of common signs that inference rests; and traditional syllogistic logic can do no more than reach conclusions from plural minor premisses which are 'magna ex parte' true only. The weakest of all inferences is derived from one 'ut plurimum' or polyvalent sign; the syndrome yields stronger but variable results. Some of these are conditional (which is the case where quantification can be employed: again a rare case); they can be interpreted seriatim, but no judgement about an increasing likelihood of outcome can be made. Negatively employed, syndromes can eliminate as in differential diagnosis. These points emerge from Baldus's careful assessment (after Aristotle) of evidence of both positive and negative (or present and absent) sorts:

I note however that two things are required if we want to affirm anything with certainty; one is that there be several signs which testify to the same thing, the other that there is no sign present which designates the opposite affection, or from which the opposite affection can be deduced; as when I say, this man is courageous, firstly because he has large extremities, a broad and hairy chest, a big mouth, and firm flesh; secondly because in the same man none of the signs appear which betoken fear, or mental weakness, or avarice, two of which are not inconsistent of themselves with courage, but usually accompany fear.[253]

What is not mentioned here, and indeed is very rarely treated, is the problem of conflicting evidence (one or more discordant signs in a concursus); Argenterio is one of the few to mention the issue, and he does

---

[253] Baldus 1621: 41: 'nota autem, ut aliquid certi dicere possumus duo requiris, unum est, ut plura signa sint, quae idem testentur, alterum est, ut nullum quod designat contrarium affectum, vel consequens ad contrarium, adsit, ut dico fortem hunc esse, primum quoniam habet magnas extremitates, latum pectus, pilosumque, os grande, carnem duram, deinde quoniam in eodem non apparet quid quam eorum signorum, quod vel timorem arguat, vel animi mollitiem, vel avaritiam, quae duo per se quidem non opponuntur fortitudini, at comitari soleat tamen timiditatem'. On a parallel discussion of negative evidence in law, see Herculanus 1584.

not elaborate on it.[254] Where the concursus of signs all indicate one conclusion, they can be treated either finitely (where the elimination of other conclusions can be definitively made); aggregatively (where the accumulation of evidence is allowed to induce persuasion);[255] or even infinitely, if the persuasion arises from an incomplete or incompletable set of signs. Many of these claims obey the logic of 'magna ex parte' premises set out in 4.4; this is unmathematical, as has been said, and leads to the treatment of two uncertainties together as yielding a higher degree of certainty.[256] In all this an important element of interpretation has crept in, because judgements are being made about dominant meanings, and about the elimination of obscurity and ambiguity. This hermeneutic element reinforces that which we noted as part of the dialectic of medical thought: namely the intrusion of interpretation into its theory, its evidence and its very notation. It is worth noting in passing that the source of the most sophisticated thought about signs in groups and about probable or dominant constructions to be placed upon them is the very 'science' – physiognomy – which is most decried in later ages for its lack of rigour and scientificity.[257]

8.9.1 The grammar of signs

Most striking however is the way in which the signs themselves and their treatment correspond to a grammar rather than a logic. One might well suspect such a claim of presentism and anachronism. Anthony Grafton points out that 'current intellectual fashion dictates the comparison of events to texts'; but he also concedes that some Renaissance figures noted this themselves, citing the example of Pontano, who in his *De rebus caelestibus* of 1512 avers that the language of the stars is the language of humans.[258] As I have argued elsewhere, the body of doctrine which we would call semantics is distributed across a number of classical texts, and has to be reconstituted by Renaissance jurists for their own purposes.[259] Medical doctors do not need to probe the relationship between 'verbum'

---

254 Argenterio 1610: 1688, 1780; also Liddel 1628: 524 notes that 'signa aliquando sibi mutuo contraria esse', and require a 'medicus expertissimus' to 'discernere' them.
255 Cf. Cohen 1980 (on the basis of decisions made by juries).
256 Hagecius ab Hagek 1562: B2v: 'qui Genethialogicam huic arti [metoposcopia] coniunxerit, certius de eventibus praedixerit'; Chiaramonte 1625: 1–6.
257 E.g. the judgement of Burnyeat unpublished: 'a low-level codification of unreflective prejudices, accepted ideas and supposed observations of men, women and animals'.
258 Grafton 1998; Trinkaus 1985: 458; Blumenberg 1989; Bono 1995.
259 Maclean 1992.

and 'voluntas', between speaker's sense and hearer's sense, nor even (except incidentally) that between 'verbum' and its historical sense. But they have to determine the relationship of word to referent, the meaning of signs in context, and sometimes treat signs as though they were articulated with each other in a sort of syntax. These relations were of course investigated with great subtlety in the domain of metaphysics, epistemology and language; it does not seem that these discussions left a very direct impression on those in medical writings.[260] But the link between 'signum' and 'significatio' is made explicit in less formal terms in the texts I have been investigating. First, there is the relationship between 'signum' and 'signatum', which is described as a 'connotans' by Campilongo;[261] Capivaccius explicitly links his sign theory to the linguistic conventionalism of the *De interpretatione* (above, 5.1.1); Horst talks of a sign as a 'quasi rei alicuius significatum', and a 'conceptus quidam mentalis';[262] Liddel says of the relationship between 'indicans' and 'indicatum' in quasi-linguistic terms that they refer to each other, the indicatum being known from the indicans.[263] Second, there is an echo of the grammar of the modistae in the references to 'significandi modi'.[264] Signs, like nouns, are proper and common; and if all were proper, it is agreed that there would be no rational discourse and no communication.[265] Signs have tenses (past, present and future, and even more complex tenses: past of the present etc.).[266] They can be constructed in such a way as to minimise or eliminate ambiguity and obscurity, as Sanctorius's six 'fontes' method demonstrates.[267] They have, in the shape of indication, an illocutionary force: a 'vis insinuandi'; Capivaccius even speaks a 'vis coindicandi, permittendi, imitandi, contraindicandi, repugnandi, removendi'.[268] In a certain sense, every act of indication is performative of the medical

---

[260] Meier-Oeser 1997: 171ff.; for a distribution of signs by efficient and final causes, by the differentiae natural/artificial and real/verbal, by signata and modi significandi, appropriate to a theological or metaphysical rather than medical discourse, see Freedman 1988: 412–36 (on the distribution of Clemens Timpler); Sdzui 1997: 84–92 makes extensive use of the Conimbricenses in his account.

[261] Campilongo 1601: 12r.

[262] Horst 1609: 131–2.

[263] Liddel 1628: 607: 'se mutuo referuntur, et ex indicante indicatum cognoscitur'.

[264] Argenterio 1606–7: 148; Heath 1971; Maclean 1992: 99.

[265] See above 4.2.1.

[266] Galen 1556: 1.46, cited above, 8.6.2.

[267] Sanctorius 1630: 533–6 (vi.6).

[268] Capivaccius 1606: 14. It might be possible to push this analogy further, and seek adjectival, adverbial and verbal properties in signs; but such a mapping would not be in the spirit of a Renaissance approach, which would be much more likely to attempt an analysis through the four Aristotelian causes: see for examples Frölich 1612; Jensen 1990.

competence of the doctor, which resembles his linguistic competence. Finally, just as we have to deal with new sentences which have never before been uttered, but which our linguistic competence makes comprehensible to us, so also does the learned doctor engage in a completely new act of diagnosis with every patient, who is ex hypothesi unique in his humoral composition; and his production of this diagnostic act is thanks to the 'coniecturalis ars' which, according to Cardano, is Ptolemy's peculiar dialectical method. These parallels to language analysis are rarely if ever made explicit, however, even if da Monte on one occasion compares elements of natural philosophy to elements of grammar.[269] When pressed to justify their modes of thought, doctors almost invariably turn to the syllogism and to reduction to the first figure (if at all possible). This has the effect of giving priority to the sign as a proposition or as a middle term, rather than as a linguistic token.

8.9.2 Modern parallels: diagnosis

I come in conclusion to some sketchy and incautious parallels with more recent diagnostic practices. The debate about the sensory or intelligible status of the sign persists, and may be found in much later texts: in the late nineteenth century, the sign is said by Hecht to be 'le résultat d'une opération intellectuelle' as opposed to a 'phénomène particulier organique et fonctionnel survenu dans l'économie sous l'influence de la maladie' and as late as 1986, Barondess's distinction between a sign as that which is a manifestation of a disease perceptible to the observer as opposed to a symptom which is observable by the patient (a distinction found in writings as early as those of Joannitius).[270] Professor Rosenberg's paper on the 'tyranny of diagnosis' highlights, it is true, some of the ways in which no parallels may be made:[271] there is no straightforward Renaissance equivalent for 'statistically meaningful prediction indications'; nor did sixteenth-century doctors rely on statistics as 'aggregated consensual truth', although they had a dominance rule to cover the former of these, and a rule of authority to cover the second. But I hope to have shown that the distinction he draws (with many others) between management and diagnosis, where the former makes no claim to providing a remedial pathway or even a complete account of the relevant pathology, has echoes in the past, not only in the distinction between

---

[269] Siraisi 1987a: 100.
[270] See above, note 13; Hecht 1864–86; Barondess 1986: 308–11.
[271] Rosenberg forthcoming.

empirical and rational medicine, but also in Jakob Horst's modest assessment of the powers of doctors,[272] and the care taken with evolving therapy by attendance on the patient and meticulous history-taking. Rondelet's cautious approach to the patient is exemplary in this: he advises doctors to listen carefully to the patient and his or her attendants, but to make no positive diagnosis on the first visit; to offer a very mild palliative, and not to rush to apply strong remedies; to try to treat the seat of the condition without necessarily alerting the patient to what he is attempting to do; to try treatments in succession, and to employ common sense at all times.[273]

There is a clear sense of Veyne's 'allongement du questionnaire' up to the present day in respect of diagnosis,[274] as it evolves from Hippocrates, *Aphorisms*, i.12 through objectified versions of uroscopy, pulse-taking, scrutiny of facial colour, percussion, galvanism and auscultation to modern sophisticated tests and procedures.[275] The usual terminus a quo of this development is taken to be Sydenham's *Observationes medicae* of 1666; but this seems to me to pay too little credit both to Sanctorius, and to the medieval quantificatory approaches which McVaugh and others have revealed. I have pointed above also to the parallel between the negative or elimination approach of Rondelet and modern differential diagnosis, a method including both tests for exclusion and for keeping options in play. Finally, Professor Rosenberg's plea for a return to the pragmatics of diagnostic negotiation between the patient, those around him or her, and the doctor, his caution against too markedly positivistic approaches, and his implicit call for an awareness on the part of doctors of their role not as 'scientists' dealing with objective knowledge but as 'artists' negotiating in a broad cultural as well as therapeutic sense with their milieu has its echoes not only negatively in the satire directed at pretentious doctors in the Renaissance but also positively in their own accounts of their professional caution ('cautela') and the limited efficacy of their art.[276]

8.9.3 Modern parallels: semiology

Parallels can also be drawn with modern theories of signs. I hope that I have shown that signs are indeed tokens of something else, and are

[272] Horst 1585.
[273] Rondelet 1586: 593–7: cf. Arnau de Vilanova 1585: 1704–20.
[274] Veyne 1978: 141–56.
[275] These are the diagnostic procedures listed in the nineteenth-century *Catalogue méthodique des sciences médicales* of the Bibliothèque Nationale in Paris.
[276] Rosenberg forthcoming.

independent of those who use them in arguments, and that there is
in this sense such a thing as evidence in the theory and practice of
Renaissance medicine.[277] The deployment of both Stoic and Aristotelian
theories of the sign creates a somewhat intricate (if not slightly incoherent)
doctrine which is informed by distinctions (such as sensible/intelligible,
act/potency, types of cause, etc.) which have no place in modern semiological discussions. If we take but one of these, that of C. S. Peirce's
triad of symbol (the conventional sign), index (as smoke of fire) and the
icon (the sign of similarity); and we try to map medical signs on to this
distinction, we quickly discover that because of the overriding realism of
the discipline, only the last two categories come explicitly into question
(the first, although known to doctors, being deemed irrelevant by them),
and that there is no clear distinction made between these categories
(smoke as a sign of fire, for example, is both a Stoic commemorative sign
and an Aristotelian natural sign).[278] What is more, Renaissance loose
logic as deployed by doctors allows *inter alia* for redundancy, plurivalence,
polythesis, 'magna ex parte' signification, all of which are abhorrent to
Peirce's system. It might be said that this loose logic is no more than
a *post hoc* justification for operative decision-making by doctors in their
acts of diagnosis, in the same way that topical argument is said to operate for lawyers, who deploy any argument *in utramque partem* which has a
contingent use, and for whom rhetorical force, professional standing and
the securing of the correct outcome are more important than 'truth'.[279]
But this does not necessarily make the medical art a failure as a system, for it allowed its theorists and practitioners to teach their pupils,
to communicate rationally with each other, to argue about individual
(or at least specific) cases, and to achieve a grasp on the reality around
them sufficient for their knowledge of it.[280]

---

[277] This against the already-mentioned claim made by Hacking 1975: 32 that in the Renaissance
there is 'no concept of evidence qua that by which one thing can indicate contingently the state
of something else'.

[278] Peirce 1931–58.

[279] Maclean 1992.

[280] Cf. *ibid.*, 6–7; 212–13 for parallel considerations about the discipline of law.

Postscript

> Who does not feel as I do that at this very time the causes and
> remedies of diseases can be so successfully investigated that we will
> hear no more the oft repeated axiom: *there is no certainty in Physick?*
>
> (Connor)[1]

It is not easy to draw together the threads of this study into a single,
harmonious conclusion. On the one hand, the story which has been
sketched out here is of a static discourse in which certain lines of thought
did not evolve, and intellectual change was slow to occur. On the other,
the discourse has been shown to engage successfully in acts of intellectual
bricolage, some elements of which prefigure the developments of later
centuries, some of which have subsequently disappeared from view. The
discourse itself has been characterised in its own terms with respect to its
logical procedures and its dogmas; and these have also been shown to be
embedded in institutional, professional, and sociocultural contexts which
inflect these same procedures and dogmas. In view of these differing
perspectives, I shall attempt by taking one exemplary text summarily
to distinguish the Renaissance both from the medieval discourse which
preceded it and from the 'new science' of the seventeenth century; I
shall next assess the effect of the various contexts I have chosen on the
discourse itself; point to the problems which arise seen both from inside
and outside the discourse; and finally speculate about the continuity and
discontinuity which this may be argued to reveal in medical discourse
over the *longue durée*.

It is pertinent to take as representative of the medieval outlook Arnau
de Vilanova's commentary on the first aphorism of Hippocrates ('ars
longa, vita brevis'), which touches on a broad range of topics relevant

---

[1] Connor 1697: 2.28–9: 'qui non mecum illico sentiet, posse nimirum morborum causas atque
remedia non incassum ad examen vocari; adeoque protinus evanescit decantatum isthoc Axioma,
Medicinae scilicet *nihil inesse Certitudinis*'.

333

to this study.[2] Arnau's 'expositio' is concerned to make explicit Hippocrates's intention in writing, to show the need for the written form of the aphorisms, and to defend the doctrine set out in them. This involves him (in the version of his text received in all Renaissance editions)[3] in borrowing a passage from Avicenna to locate the 'perfectio medicinae' in relation to the three speculative disciplines of metaphysics, physics and mathematics; to show the need for rational medicine, and to reveal the specific nature of medical rationality; and to exemplify the practical issues about diagnosis and prognosis, about the treatment and the relationship of the doctor to his patients, those nursing them and the circumstances in which they find themselves. These four elements – the doctor himself, the patients, their nurses, and the attendant circumstances of the illness – are the objective and subjective sources of all the information at the doctor's disposal. The trained (Galenic) doctor (or doctors) determines the questions to be asked by a 'premeditatio inquirendorum', proceeds to a 'collectio signorum', and comes to conclusions on the basis of the medical art by assembling the sensory signs from himself, patients and nurses and setting them out in a methodical order ('tabulare omnia'). This involves him in a succession of negotiations with patient and nurses, and an evolving series of judgements about the disease and its treatment. Many pieces of sound practical advice are offered, and are made concrete by the presentation of exemplary cases.[4] This is not to say that elements of scholastic analysis are absent: there is, for example, a long logical analysis of the part of the text opposing 'long' to 'short'; but the dominant mode of the passage is one of sturdy practical teaching offered for the benefit of the practitioner. As Arnau (or a later editor) points out at one point, he caters for the theorist separately, in a long excursus on the principles of the science of medicine which he advises his practitioner readers to skip.[5]

A comparable Renaissance commentary on the same text is that of Antonio Musa Brasavola, which appeared in 1541. This is based on a

---

[2] Arnau de Vilanova 1585: 1677–1722.

[3] See above ch. 3, note 23; Michael McVaugh is preparing an edition from a manuscript which contains not this excursus but a remarkable passage about the practical problems of consultation.

[4] *Ibid.*, 1706–22: Arnau advises the doctor to be cautious about telling the patient too much; to admit to ignorance; not to tell indiscreet nurses bad news; to be aware of the life cycle of all illnesses; how to deal with a colleague being present; how to deal with contingent and rare circumstances; what to take into consideration (e.g. the orientation of the bed with respect to the windows); how to deal with a sequence of attempted remedies (clyster, calefactoria, baths); to prefer 'ratio' to experientia, except where the latter manifestly is at odds with doctrine.

[5] *Ibid.*, 1679: 'haec autem prima lectio solum est necessarium volentibus doctorari: quia tota est speculativa, sed aliae duae sunt valde necessariae volentibus proficere in exercitio medicinae'.

different translation; it contains long quotations in Greek; it is followed by Leoniceno's commentary, and Brasavola's notes on the Galen commentary which was widely known through its inclusion in the *Articella*.[6] Brasavola begins with a historical account of previous commentators on the text. He considers, as does Arnau, the questions of intended readership, the choice of aphoristic form; and the sources of information (sense and intellect) to which it refers. His phrase by phrase commentary cites the Greek text, with passages quoted from ancient commentators (principally Galen, Oribasius, and Philotheus). Like Arnau, he reviews the whole of medicine as a combination of speculative and practical ('activa') art, and discusses the nature and range of information available to physicians about their patients. Brasavola's notes on Galen's commentary are designed to amplify his meaning, to disambiguate his text, and to supply a full philological analysis of the Greek.

If we set aside the humanist interest in the textual history of Greek and the omission of formal logical analysis, we may be struck by how similar the two commentaries of Arnau and Brasavola are. No significant advances had been made in therapeutic procedures; there is the same attention paid in both to the patient's history and to the *circumstantiae*; the same kind of asseverations is to be found about the nature of medical science. The return to the Greek *fontes* and the advances in anatomy, in botany, in surgery hardly touch the diagnostic and prognostic approach. If anything, as the sixteenth century draws to a close, there is a sort of convergence with the practical concerns of Arnau, which is detectable in later commentaries such as those of Oddo degli Oddi, Hollerius and Heurnius.[7]

Where changes can be perceived is in the argumentation which underpins the doctrine. As we have noted, dialectical argument is explicitly used to ground semiology in the Renaissance; an increasing desire to quantify data is to be detected; new taxonomies of signs, symptoms, causes and illnesses are being produced. Indeed, the great stress laid by many theorists on the importance of dialectical division and *differentiae* to medicine at various levels might lead one to think of it as a discipline characterised by the 'via divisiva'. This feature of medical theory is, it is true, new; but it was accompanied by a progressive and eclectic appropriation of the past, with increasing weight being accorded to setting

---

[6] Brasavola 1541: 5: 'vita brevis, ars vero longa, occasio autem praeceps, experimentum periculosum, iudicium difficile. Nec solum se ipsum praestare opportet opportuna facientem, sed et aegrum, et assidentes, et exteriora'.

[7] Oddo degli Oddi 1564; Hollerius 1582; Heurnius 1637.

out doctrine in modes other than the purely Aristotelian, although these are still employed by certain Italian thinkers such as Sanctorius. One writer exemplary of this eclecticism is Duncan Liddel; his own position is not as 'advanced' however as that of Daniel Sennert, who even tries to incorporate Paracelsian doctrine into a modified Galenism, a move which Liddel rejects.[8] It is tempting to suggest that we can distinguish at this time backward-looking doctors who argue the case for astrology, avoid quantification, and show hostility to new nosological theories from the heroes of a progressivist history of medicine, which would include da Monte, Paracelsus, Vesalius, Fracastoro, Cardano, Fernel, Argenterio and those who support them; but I think this underrates the similarity in outlook which is found in texts at the end of our period. From the evidence of even those who oppose new theories such as Paracelsianism (Zwinger and Bartolettus among them), it is possible to argue that there are not two distinct mentalities – the rational and the hermetic – but rather one, informed by the looser dialectical logical categories which were set out in chapter 5. This claim may be associated with the frequently encountered argument that trained physicians combine reason with experience, and hence can accommodate information from both; it may be related also to the fact that the lowly science of physiognomy is the source both of crude and arbitrary generalisations about human types and a sophisticated theory of signs. Only where the correspondence tables of hermetic medicine are given prominence (as they are by Fabricius, in his *Medicinae utriusque Galenicae et hermeticae anatome philosophica* of 1626) is it plausible to argue that a quite different mentality is in question. The totalitarian nature of these correspondence tables contrasts strongly with the aphoristic approach; there only those precepts and principles are alleged which are necessary for the context of the aphorism in question; systematisation is made secondary to satisfactory explanation of a small area of medical practice. This approach often focusses on the single case at the expense of general theory, in a way which may be thought to prefigure the accounts of experiments in the new science of the seventeenth century.

Where it is more plausible, in my view, to claim a paradigm shift is in the passage from a logical outlook on syndromes and on argument from propositions which involve the quantifier 'most'. Sanctorius is here an interesting transitional case; he insists on the only valid form of syllogism (camestres) permitting the reasoner to use syllogistic form to conclude

---

[8] Sennert 1650: 3.697–862.

about individual cases, but claims to be able to construct arguments from six sources of information ('no more, no less') which allow him to claim that he can eliminate all ambiguity and uncertainty from diagnosis. He distinguishes these procedures from those which use syndromes of signs as a single convertible minor proposition to reach conclusions (a procedure which he rejects). These is a mixture here of protomathematical reasoning (from a number of different sources) which one might expect to result in the degrees of probability which Chiaramonte enunciates in a different context: but Sanctorius does not proceed in that direction, remaining attached to an Aristotelian concept of proof. A similar transitional position seems to be reflected in the adapted logical diagrams illustrated in chapter 5, and in Kepler's move to quantify the predicate quoted in the same chapter.

What is the relationship of medicine's relaxed structure of thought to the new science of the seventeenth century? One way to measure this would be to look at Hooke's rules for the new experimental philosophy set out in the preface to his *Micrographia* of 1665. He alleges six; of these, some seem to me to be perfectly compatible with the practice of Renaissance doctors. The injunction to assess critically the evidence of others, and to collate it with one's own, is obeyed; it is even true that wherever possible, late Renaissance doctors use instruments to supplement the power of their senses, as Hooke recommends. His precept that one should abstain from any prior metaphysical notions (such as matter, or occult qualities) as this will prejudice the eye as it observes 'the subtlety of the composition of bodies, the structure of their parts, the various texture of their matter, the instruments and manner of their inward motions, and all the other possible appearances of things' relates to the degree of unconscious presupposition in scientific observation; it seems to me to be arguable that Renaissance doctors are capable of knowing what presuppositions subtend their arguments, even if they do not discard them, whereas Hooke's anti-metaphysical stance is in fact unrealistic, since it implies a state of freedom from presuppositions in the enquirer into nature which he himself arguably did not achieve in his own micrographical descriptions. His insistence that experiments should be repeated and subjected to as precise measurement as possible, and that their results should lead the enquirer to engage in a kind of hermeneutical circle, a 'continual passage round from one Faculty [of hands and eyes, memory and reason] to another' can be reconciled with Arnau de Vilanova's careful account of progressive diagnosis and treatment: and Pereira's stricture about the constraining force of observation and empirical fact over theory (cited above, 5.3.2) also suggests that some Renaissance doctors recognised the need for a sort of constant revision of theory through observation. The much-advertised combination of experientia and ratio which they embody also sounds something like the practice of the new science of the seventeenth century, although 'ratio' here is to be understood primarily as Galenic method and medical precepts. The most striking difference between Hooke's rules and the practice of Renaissance doctors and jurists lies in the rule that nothing should be omitted; we have seen that medicine is a finite and motivated ('propter utilitatem') art which recognises that some available knowledge is excluded on grounds of practicality. Thomas Sprat's accusation against Aristotelians of being 'over-hasty and praecipitant [in] concluding upon the <u>Causes</u> before the <u>Effects</u> have been enough search'd into'[9] seems here to be a telling critique which marks a watershed.

But there are also reasons for according to medicine the status of precursor of the new science: the empirical nature of sixteenth-century anatomical, zoological and botanical investigation; the strong concern for efficient and material causes; the use of protomathematical calculation rather than purely qualitative explanations; the development of diagrams; the stress on the need for accurate observation, which culminates at the end of our period in the measurement of temperature and the pulse through the thermometer and the pulsilogium.

The case against seeing medicine as protoscientific is also strong. Not only is it explicitly wedded to precepts which have no foundation in sensory experience (insensible qualities, occult causes), and to the treatment of effects without a knowledge of causes; it is also happy to embrace a highly complex form of explanation involving modes, function, forms and qualities, which contrasts with the demand for simplicity and elegance of the new science. Moreover, it does not seek to explain all the data at its disposal, and is willing to include recuperative devices such as faculties, powers and spirits in the explanations it offers. Most damningly, however, it locates the rational grasp of the doctor in him as a practitioner, rather than in the objective facts of the cases with which he deals, as we have seen; this is a point to which I shall presently return. For these reasons, it can only be said to prefigure the new science in a very tenuous way; it may have protoprobabilistic elements, its diagrams may be non-representational and abstract, and it may treat its evidence in a sophisticated manner, but its approach to the signs with which it

9 Sprat 1667: 103.

works does not disincorporate them altogether from the doctor who derives sense from them. Paula Findlen has suggested that sixteenth-century natural philosophers move between the various philosophical approaches to knowledge (of the time), combining intellectual categories and experiental data in ways that now seem inherently conflictual;[10] I believe the same to be true of doctors, who allow (in some cases knowingly, in others apparently not) their data to be inflected both by the theory through which they understand it and by the means by which they interpret it.

This brings me to the question of the real and the constructed: and to the effect which the social, technological and institutional contexts in which the discipline of medicine is embedded affect it. I have argued that its incorporation into universities and colleges of physicians reflects both guild interests and disciplinary rivalry. Both predispose doctors to make strong claims for the necessary rationality of their art, to distinguish themselves from empirics and unlicensed practitioners on the one hand and, on the other, from their rivals in other faculties. Medicine has to struggle to maintain its status and its authority over the human body which it claims the right to treat; both theological issues (among them astrology and determinism, the soul–body relation, the setting of priorities in the treatment of categories of patient) and legal issues (involving precedence, authority, and professional standing) help determine the strategies of protectionism and independence and the claims made for the scientificity of the discipline. Even in the ancient world, medicine was acknowledged to be a necessarily scriptural discipline; the advent of printing, the organisation of book fairs, and the exploitation of the market for medical books by entrepreneurs are among the factors which help to unify the discipline and pedagogy of medicine across Europe, and stimulate the polemics which both reflect its internal dissensions and at the same time help define it as a coherent and relatively independent discourse. One effect of this is the fostering of eclecticism through the accumulation of medical texts of all kinds in libraries; another effect, linked to the humanist concern for purified texts, is the confrontation of authorities both with each other (as had already happened in the medieval period) and with empirical observations which clashed with them. This leads doctors to acknowledge the primacy of the real in a way which often makes them seem forward-looking. The practices of translating, reading, interpreting and restating doctrine in a

---

[10] Findlen 1990: 296.

logical mode specific to medicine also reinforces the realism of the profession. The loose logic which it comes to adopt allows for the modification of doctrines, such as those concerning anatomy and nosology, within a general framework; a modification which is as much due to new empirical discoveries as new theorising. The same loose logic allows for the penetration of a degree of hermeneutics into logical procedures, which mirrors the involvement of the practising doctor in the real world of infinitely variable human natures. He incorporates performatively medical rationality, which becomes thereby a strange amalgam of the subjective and the objective, and is quite unlike the decision-making of the law, which is always presented in terms of non-contingent equity, even if the contingency of decisions is acknowledged.

These methods of enquiry and their physical site and mode of communication affect directly the doctrine in more troublesome ways. Andrew Cunningham has elegantly shown how the order of investigation into illness affects its classification:[11] some similar disciplinary effects were noted in the Renaissance, some were not. The distinctions between a finite art and an infinite sphere of investigation, and between operative and theoretical knowledge, were noted; as was the more complex issue of the uncertain frontier between the incorporated rationality of the doctor as he contingently intuits an indication and the necessary rules by which this is achieved; objectivity and subjectivity are not rigorously kept apart. A similar rift exists between the precepts of the art, which are characterised as certain and immutable, and the far less rigorous ways in which they are applied. Finally, the need almost universally felt to reduce signs to syllogistic notation is to be set alongside the actual articulation of these signs in something akin to a linguistic fashion. This last aporia is not noted in the Renaissance, but the preceding ones are. Increasing unease is detectable in certain writers (notably those of Montpellier such as Joubert, who were not as wedded as were the Paduans to Aristotelian logic) about the relationship of the precepts of the art described by some as true, certain, universal and internally coherent, to the experience of practitioners; and the division made between the science (the precepts) and the skill (the application of them in individual cases) turns out not to be in itself sufficient to calm this unease. Whether this can be described in terms of a collapse of Galenism is less clear; if one returns to Arnau's text, one finds the same modesty about the claims of the skill married to a confidence in the precepts which constitute its basis. I am rather

---

[11] Cunningham 1992.

more inclined to see it as a sort of coexistence of opposing features which medieval and Renaissance physicians alike were prepared to tolerate; and to argue, as Charles Schmitt has done for Renaissance Aristotelianism, that there are many Galenisms at the end of the sixteenth century, and that they betoken the vigour, not the demise, of the tradition. Equally, it seems to me that the *bricolage* which characterises their art constitutes a sophisticated and effective grasp of the reality with which they were faced, and the limited means through which they could act on it.

As I indicated in the introduction, there seems to me to be a clear discontinuity in medical discourse, which is manifest in the following recent categorisation of data in an evidence-based medical journal:[12]

1. Strong evidence from at least one systematic review of multiple well-designed randomised controlled trials;
2. Strong evidence from at least one properly designed randomised controlled trial of appropriate size;
3. Evidence from well-designed trials without randomisation, single group pre-post, cohort, time series or matched case controlled studies;
4. Evidence from well-designed non-experimental studies from more than one centre or research group;
5. Opinions of respected authorities based on clinical evidence, descriptive studies or reports of expert committees.

It is not necessary to spell out the mathematical procedures implicit in much of the technical vocabulary of this passage for it to be clear that the only form of evidence available even to the late seventeenth century is the endoxical sort referred to in the fifth point; and we are dealing here only with the issue of evidence, not that, for example, of nosology, or morbid anatomy, or bacteriology, or genetics. The phrase 'to think like a doctor' has therefore, so it seems to me, a quite different semantic content in 1600 and 2000, unlike the phrase 'to think like a lawyer'; even if several points can be cited which unite the two sorts of thinking. I shall not dwell here on medical ethics, which may have changed in its content but not (many would argue) in its fundamental tenets.[13] In conclusion, I should like to point to the perennial medical problem of the division between the objective and the subjective; between the physician and the patient, between the internal suffering of the latter and the external

---

[12] *Bandoleer*, 12 (Feb. 1995), 1.
[13] Schleiner 1995 and Rütten 1999 would suggest that ethics have changed in nature; Debus 1999 not.

investigation of the former, the individual nature of the latter and the genera or species to which the doctor is constrained to reduce it, between the objective data of tests and histories and the interpretation to which the doctor must subject it, which will contain inevitably some trace of his own processes of thought; and finally between the treatment as observed by the therapist as opposed to its direct experience by the sufferer. The privileged example of this in the Renaissance is indication, an intuition which relies on an incorporated non-discursive rationality. It is striking that the phrase 'x was indicated' implies even today the combination of a trained mind with a quantitative judgement which we found expressed in the semiological texts examined in this book. But for all this similarity, the other components of Renaissance medical discourse which predispose doctors to 'think like doctors' – a reasonable grasp of syllogistic logic, a view of nature and human nature which acknowledges both the imperfect character of these and the incomplete grasp of the human intellect of them, and a practical art which is founded on a physiology, a pathology, and a theory of humours, qualities and contraries – are so alien to a modern medical outlook as not to constitute in any way its forerunner.

Bibliography

References to Frankfurt are to Frankfurt am Main, unless otherwise stated.

ABBREVIATIONS

K   Galen, *Opera omnia*, ed. C. G. Kühn, 22 vols., Leipzig, 1821–33
PL   *Patrologiae cursus completus, series latina*, ed. J. P. Migne, 222 vols., Paris, 1844–1904

PRIMARY SOURCES

MANUSCRIPTS

Biblioteca Ambrosiana Milano B Ambr. N 26 Sup.: Selecta ex Aristotel. hist. de animalibus et partibus
Bodley Rawl. D 274: Day, John (1589) Liber Joannis Daij Londiniensis
Valladolid, Archivo Histórico Provincial, Protocolos 1629

PRINTED BOOKS: PRIMARY SOURCES

Achillinus, Alexander (1515), *De proportionibus motuum*, ed. Claudius Achillinus, Bologna, excudebat Hieronymus de Benedictis, fol.
Agricola, Rudolph (1967), *De inventione dialectica* (facsimile reprint, Cologne, 1523)
Agrippa, Cornelius (1992), *De occulta philosophia*, ed. V. Perrone Compagni, Leiden, New York and Cologne
Akakia, Martin (1549), *Claudii Galeni ars medica quae et ars parva*, trans. et comm. Martin Akakia, Venice, ex officina Erasmiana Vincentii Valgrisii, 8vo
Albanesius, Guidus Antonius (1649), *Aphorismorum Hippocratis expositio peripatetica*, Padua, typis Pauli Frambotti, 4to
Alberius, Claudius, *see* Aubéry, Claude
Albertus, Jacobus, *see* Aubert, Jacques
Albertus, Johannes Wimpinaeus (1615), *De concordia Hippocraticorum et Paracelsistarum libri*, Strasbourg, impensis Pauli Ledertz, 8vo

343

Albertus, Salomon (1585), *Tres orationes*, Nuremberg, in officina typographica Catharinae Gerlachiae, 8vo

Aldrovandi, Ulisse (1599), *Ornithologiae hoc est de avibus historiae libri xxi*, Bologna, apud Franciscum de Franciscis, fol.

Alexander of Aphrodiseas (1541), *Problemata*, trans. Joannes Davio, Paris [Edmée Tousan], 8vo

Alonso y de las Ruyres de Fontecha, Juan (1598), *Medicorum incipientium medicina, seu medicinae Christianae speculum*, Alcalá de Henares, ex officina Joannis Gratiani, apud viduam, 4to

Alpini, Prospero (1601), *De praesagienda vita et morte aegrotantium*, Frankfurt, apud Jonam Rhodium, 8vo

    (1611), *De medicina methodica libri tredecim in quibus medendi ars methodica . . . restituitur*, Padua, apud Franciscum Bolzettam ex typographia Laurentii Pasquati, fol.

Altomare, Donato Antonio (1559–60), *De medendis humani corporis malis*, Lyon, apud Joannem Frellonium [excudebat Symphorianus Barbierus], 8vo

    (1574), *Omnia, quae huiusque in lucem prodierunt opera*, ed. Giovanni Altomare, Venice, sumptibus Jacobi Anieli de Maria bibliopolae Neapolitani, fol.

Arentsehe, Henningus (1601), *Disputationum physicarum secunda. De natura et causis continens ea quae in 2. Libro Physicae Auscultationis ab Aristotele explicatur*, resp. Wolfgangus Piscator, Helmstedt, excudebat Jacobus Lucius, 4to

Aretaeus of Cappodocia (1554), *De acutorum et diuturnorum morborum causis et signis libri iiii*, Paris, apud Andraeum Turnebum, 8vo

Argenterio, Giovanni (1578), *In artem medicinalem Galeni commentarii tres*, 2 vols., Paris, 8vo

    (1592), *Opera*, Venice, apud Joannem Baptistam Ciottum et socios, fol.

    (1606–7), *Opera*, Venice, apud Iuntas, 2 vols., fol.

    (1610), *Opera ex exemplari Veneto revisa*, Hanau, apud haeredes Claudii Marnii, fol.

Aristotle (1541), *Liber de physiognomicis*, trans. Andreas a Lacuna, Paris, excudebat Petrus Calvarinus, 8vo

Arnau de Vilanova (1975), *Opera, vol. 2: Aphorismi de gradibus*, ed. Michael R. McVaugh, Barcelona

    (1585), *Opera omnia*, ed. Nicolaus Taurellus, Basle, ex officina Pernea per Conradum Waldkirch, fol.

    (2000), *Opera, vol. 1: Tractatus de intentione medicorum*, ed. Michael R. McVaugh, Barcelona

    (forthcoming), *Repetitio super canonem Vita brevis*, ed. Michael R. McVaugh

Articella (1515), Lyon, per Joannem de la Place impensis Bartholomei Troth, 4to

    (1529), ed. Hieronymus de Salijs, Venice, in aedibus haeredum Octaviani Scoti ac sociorum, fol.

    (1557), *see* Torrigiano 1557

Aubert, Jacques (1596), *Semeiotike sive ratio dignoscendarum sedium male affectarum*, [Lyon], apud Jacobum Chouet, 8vo

Aubéry, Claude (1578), περὶ ἑρμενείας *seu de enuntiationibus, quas propositiones vocant, in quibus verum et falsum primo diiudicantur*, Lausanne, excudebat Franciscus le Preux, 8vo

(1584), *Organon, id est, instrumentum doctrinarum omnium in duas partes divisum, Nempe, in analyticum eruditionis modum, et dialecticam, sive methodum disputandi in utramque partem*, Morges, excudebat Franciscus le Preux, 4to

(1585), *De concordia medicorum*, Lausanne, excudebat Joannes le Preux, 8vo

Avicenna (1608), *Libri Canonis*, ed. Joannes Costaeus and Joannes Paulus Mongius; *additis Librorum Canonis oeconomiis, necnon tabulis isagogicis in universam medicinam ex arte Humani id est Joannitii Arabis per Fabium Paulinum*, Venice, apud Iuntas, fol.

Ayrer, Christophorus Henricus (1592), *Apologia sive defensio medicinae rationalis contra empiricos, uromantes, circumforaneos, et alios*, Nuremberg, excudebat Nicolaus Knorr, 4to

Bacon, Francis (1878), *Novum organum*, ed. Thomas Fowler, Oxford

(2000), *The advancement of learning*, ed. Michael Kiernan, Oxford

Baldus, Camillus (1621), *In Physiognomica Aristotelis commentarii . . . opus Hieronymi Tamburini diligentia et sumptibus nunc primum in lucem editum*, Bologna, apud Sebastianum Bononium, fol.

Baldus de Ubaldis (1615), *Commentaria in IIII et V Codicis librum*, Venice, apud haeredes Georgii Varisci, fol.

Baldutius, Valerius (1608), *De putredine libri duo*, Urbino, apud Bartholomaeum et Simonem Ragusios fratres, 4to

Barbarus, Hermolaus (1579), *Compendium scientiae naturalis*, Lausanne, excudebat Franciscus le Preux, 8vo

Barlandus, Hubertus (1532), *Velitatio cum Arnoldo Nootz*, Antwerp, ex aedibus Henrici Petri Middelburg[ensis], 8vo

Bartholin, Thomas (1674), *De peregrinatione medica*, Copenhagen, sumptibus D. Paulli, 4to

Bartholinus, Casparus (1608), *Enchiridion metaphysicum ex philosophorum coryphaei Aristotelis optimorumque eius interpretum monumentis adornatum*, Basle, typis C[onradi] Waldkirchii, 12mo

Bartolettus, Fabritius (1619), *Encyclopaedia hermetico-dogmatica sive orbis doctrinarum medicarum physiologiae, hygiinae, pathologiae, simioticae et therapeuticae*, Bologna, typis Sebastinani Bononij, 4to

Bauhin, Caspar (1602), *Josephi Struthii Ars sphygmica seu pulsuum doctrina super MCC annos perdita . . . accessit Hieronymi Capivaccii De pulsibus elegans tractatus et Caspari Bauhini Introductio pulsuum synopsis continens*, Basle, impensis Ludovici Königs, 8vo

(1614), *De hermaphroditorum monstruosorum partuum natura ex theologorum, jureconsultorum, medicorum, philosophorum, et rabbinorum sententia libri duo*, Oppenheim, typis Hieronymi Galleri, aere Johan-Theodori de Bry, 8vo

Benivieni, Antonio (1529), *Libellus de abditis nonnullis ac mirandis morborum et sanationum causis*, Basle, per Andream Cratandrum, 8vo

(1588), *Therapeutica, sive methodus generalis medendi, ex Hippocratis, Galeni et Avicennae placitis scripta*, Lyon, apud Antonium Candidum, 8vo

Bertotus, Alphonsus, Alphonsus (1534), *see* Heyll 1534

Biesius, Nicolaus (1558), *Theoreticae medicinae libri sex*, Antwerp, apud Martinum Nutium, 8vo

(1573), *De natura libri v*, Antwerp, apud Philippum Nutium, 8vo

Boderius, Thomas (1555), *De ratione et usu dierum criticorum opus recens natum, in quo mens tum ipsius Ptolomei, tum aliorum astrologorum hac in parte dilicudatur*, Paris, excudebat Andreas Wechel, 4to

Bodier, Thomas, *see* Boderius, Thomas

Bodley, Thomas (1926), *Letters to Thomas James*, ed. George William Wheeler, Oxford

Boethius (1492), *Haec sunt opera . . . quae in hoc volumine continentur . . .* Venice, per J et G de gregoriis, fol.

Bonaventura, Federicus (1593), *Anemologiae pars prior, id est de affectionibus, signis, causisque ventorum ex Aristotele, Theophrasto, ac Ptolomaeo tractatus*, Urbino, apud Bartholomaeum et Simonem Ragusium fratres, 4to

Brasavola, Antonio Musa (1541), *In octo libros Aphorismorum Hippocratis, et Galeni, Commentaria et annotationes*, Basle, in officina Frobeniana, fol.

(1556), *Index refertissimus in omnes Galeni libros qui ex Iuntarum tertia editione extant*, Venice, apud Iuntas, fol.

Brisianus, Hieronymus (1596), *Nova medicina*, Venice, apud Damianum Zenarium, 4to

Brunfels, Otto (1534), *Ὀνομαστικόν medicinae*, Strasbourg, apud Joannem Schottum, fol.

Brunus, Jacobus [praeses] (1623), *Disputatio viii de infinito ex cap. iv–viii lib. iii Physic.*, resp. Johannes Alberti, in *Aphorismorum physicorum centuriae duae . . . quas ad normam Peripateticam in inclyta Norimbergensium Altdorphina privatae disquisitioni subjecit [M. Jacobus Brunus]*, Altdorf, typis exscripsit Balthasar Scherffius, 4to, sigs. E–H

Buteo, Joannes (1560), *Logistica, quae et Arithmetica vulgo dicitur in libris quinque digesta*, Lyon, apud Gulielmum Rouillium, 8vo

Cachetus, Christophorus (1612), *Controversiae theoricae, practicae in primam Aphorismorum Hippocratis sectionem*, Tulle, apud Sebastianum Phillippi, 8vo

Camerarius, Johannes Rudolphus (1626–30), *Sylloges memorabilium medicinae et mirabilium naturae arcanorum centuriae duodecim*, Strasbourg, sumptibus Eberhardi Zetzneri bibliopolae, 12mo

Campilongo, Emilio (1601), *ΣΗΜΕΙΩΤΙΚΗ seu nova cognoscendi morbos methodus, ad analyseos Capivaccianae normam expressa*, ed. Johannes Jessenius a Jessen, Wittenberg, typis Laurentii Seuberlichij, 8vo

Campolongus, Æmilius, *see* Campilongo, Emilio

Capivaccius, Hieronymus (1593), *Nova methodus medendi*, Frankfurt, apud Joannem Feyerabendium, impensis Henrici Osthausii Iunioris, 8vo

(1595), *De urinis plane recens ex bibliotheca D. Laurentii Scholzii in lucem prodiens*, Zerbst, excudebat Bonaventura Faber, 8vo

(1596), *Methodus practicae medicinae*, Lyon, apud Jacobum Roussin, 8vo

(1602), *Josephi Struthii Ars sphygmica seu pulsuum doctrina super MCC annos perdita . . . accessit Hieronymi Capivaccii De pulsibus elegans tractatus et Caspari Bauhini Introductio pulsuum synopsis continens*, Basle, impensis Ludovici Königs, 8vo

(1603), *Opera omnia*, ed. Johannes-Hartmannus Beyerus, Frankfurt, e Paltheniana curante Jona Rhodio, fol.

(1606), *Medendi methodus universalis tabulis comprehensa*, Frankfurt, e Collegio Paltheniano, fol.

Capo di Vacca, Girolamo, *see* Capivaccius, Hieronymus

Cardano, Girolamo (1565), *Contradicentium medicorum libri duo*, Paris, apud Jacobum Macaeum, 8vo

(1568), *In Hippocratis Coi prognostica . . . commentarii*, Basle, ex officina Henricpetrina, fol.

(1570), *Commentarii in Hippocratis de aere aquis et locis opus*, Basle, ex officina Henricpetrina, fol.

(1578), *In Cl. Ptolomaei de astrorum iudiciis . . . commentaria*, Basle, ex officina Henricpetrina, fol.

(1582), *Commentaria in librum Hippocratis de alimento*, Basle, apud Sebastianum Henricpetri, 8vo

(1583), *Liber de causis, signis ac locis morborum*, Basle, apud Sebastianum Henricpetri, 8vo

(1663), *Opera omnia*, ed. Charles Spon, 10 vols., Lyon, sumptibus Joannis Antonii Huguetan, et Marci Antonii Ravaud, fol.

Cardosus, Fernandus Rodericus (1620), *Tractatus absolutissimus de sex rebus non naturalibus*, ed. Petrus Uffenbachius, Frankfurt, typis Pauli Jacobi impensis Jacobi de Zetter, 8vo

Carrerus, Petrus Garcia (1628), *Disputationes medicae et commentaria in fen primam lib[ri] quarti Avicennae*, Bordeaux, apud Gullielmum Millanguium, fol.

Caselius, Johannes (1580), *Explanatio loci Rhetoricorum Aristotelis περὶ εἰκότων σημείων*, Rostock, typis Stephani Myliandri, 8vo

Castellanus, Honoratus (1555), *Oratio Lutetiae habita, qua futura medico necessaria explicantur*, Paris, apud Michaëlem Vascosanum, 4to

Castro, Rodericus a (1614), *Medicus-politicus: sive de officiis medico-politicis tractatus*, Hamburg, ex Bibliopolo Frobeniano, 4to

Catalogus (1637), *Catalogus librorum in diversis Italiae locis emptorum anno 1636 . . . qui Londini in Caemeterio Sancti Pauli ad Insigne Rosae prostant venales*, London, typis Johannis Legatt, 4to

Cellini, Benvenuto (1956), *The autobiography*, ed. George Bull, Harmondsworth

Cesalpino, Andrea (1588), *Tractationum philosophicarum tomus unus, in quo continentur I. Philippi Mocenici universalium institutionum ad hominum perfectionem contemplationes II. Andreae Caesalpini quaestionum peripateticarum libri v III. Bernardini Telesii de rerum natura iuxta propria principia libri xi*, [Geneva,] excudebat Eustathius Vignon, fol.

(1593), *Quaestionum peripateticorum libri v; Daemonum investigatio peripatetica; Quaestionum medicarum libri ii; De medicamentorum facultatibus libri ii*, Venice, apud Iuntas, 4to

Champier, Symphorien (1516a), *Symphonia Platonis cum Aristotele: et Galeni cum Hippocrate. Hippocratica philosophia. Platonica medicina de duplici mundo: cum eiusdem scholiis. Speculum medicinale platonicum et apologia literarum humaniorum*, [Paris], apud Badium, 1516, 8vo

(1516b), *In libros demonstrationum Galeni Cathegorie medicinales*, Lyon, per Johannem Marion, 8vo

Chiaramonte, Scipione (1625), *De coniectandis cuiusque moribus et latitantibus animi affectionibus σημειωτική moralis seu de signis*, Venice, ex officina Marci Ginammi, 4to

Claramontius, Scipio, *see* Chiaramonte, Scipione

Clementinus, Clementus (1535), *Lucubrationes*, Basle, excudebat Henricus Petri, fol.

Clessius, Joannes (1602), *Unius seculi: eiusque virorum literatorum monumentis tum florentissimi tum fertilissimi: ab anno . . . 1500 ad 1602 . . . elenchus . . . librorum*, Frankfurt, ex officina Typographica Joannis Saurii impensis Petri Kopffii, 4to

Cocus, Jacobus [praeses] (1601), *Theses medicae pro disputatione σημειωτικής prima eaque generale. De signorum discretione*, resp. Paulus Reinholdus, Wittenberg, typis Meisnerianis, 1601, 8vo

Collado, Theodorus (1615), *Adversaria seu commentarii medicinales critici, diacritici, epanorthotici, exegematici, ac didactici*, [Geneva,] ex typographia Jacobi Stoer, 8vo

Columbo, Gerardus (1601), *Disputationum medicarum de febris pestilentis cognitione et curatione libri duo*, Frankfurt, excudebat Beatus Bilschius, 8vo

Connor, Bernard (1697), *Evangelium medici: seu medicina mystica; de suspensione naturae legibus sive de miraculis*, London, sumptibus Richardi Wellinton, Henrici Nelme, Samuelis Briscoe, 8vo

Coras, Jean de (1591), *Tractatus de iuris arte*, in *Tractatus de iuris arte duorum clarissimorum iurisconsultorum Ioannis Corasii et Ioachimi Hopperi*, Lyon, excudebat Gabriel Carterius, 8vo

Cotta, John (1612), *A short discoverie of the unobserved dangers of severall sorts of ignorant and unconsiderate practisers of physicke in England*, London, [R. Field] for W. Jones and R. Boyle, 4to

Crato von Krafftheim, Johannes (1595), *Isagoge medicinae*, Hanau, apud Gulielmum Antonium, 8vo

Crellius, Fortunatus (1621), *Isagoge logica, cum notis Henningi Arnisaei*, Stettin, impensis Johannis Thymij exscripta a Samuele Kelnero, 8vo

Crusius, David (1615), *Theatrum morborum hermetico-hippocraticum, seu methodica morborum et curationis eorundem dispositio*, Erfurt, typis Nicolai Schmuckii impensis Johannis Episcop[i], 8vo

Cureau de la Chambre, Marin (1662), *L'Art de connoistre les hommes, premiere partie*, Paris, chez Jacques d'Allin, 4to

Daca, Alphonsus (1577), *Libri tres de ratione cognoscendi caussas et signa tam in prospera, quam adversa valetudine urinarum deque earum veris iudiciis et praenunciationibus opus praeclarum,* Seville, apud Alfonsum de la Barrera, 4to

Decas (1618–31), *Decas I [–VII] disputationum medicarum ... de novo recusarum per Johannem Jacobum Genathium Acad[emiae] Basil[iensis] Typographum,* Basle, 4to

Descartes, René (1996), *Œuvres,* 11 vols., ed. Charles Adam and Paul Tannery, Paris

Diocles of Carystus (1572), *Epistola de morborum praesagiis et eorundem extemporaneis remediis,* ed. Antoine Mizauld, Paris, apud Federicum Morellum, 8vo

Discourse (1942), *A discourse upon the exposicion and understandinge of statutes. With Sir Thomas Egerton's Additions,* ed. Samuel E. Thorne, San Marino

Dodoens, Rembert (1581), *Medicinalium observationum exempla rara,* Cologne, apud Maternum Cholinum, 8vo

    (1583), *Stirpium historiae pemplades vi sive libri xxx,* Antwerp, ex officina Christophori Plantini, fol.

Donatius, Joannes Baptista (1591), *Rei medicae studio stipendia sex,* Frankfurt, apud Joannem Wechelum et Petrum Viscerum consortes, 8vo

Donatus, Marcellus (1613), *De historia medica mirabili libri sex [liber septimus* by Gregor Horst], Frankfurt, impensis Johannis Jacobi Porsii, typis Erasmi Kempfferi, 8vo

Dorn, Gerhard (1584), *Dictionarium Theophrasti Paracelsi, continens obscuriorum vocabulorum quibus in suis scriptis passim utitur definitiones,* Frankfurt, [Christoff Rab], 8vo

Draut, Georg (1625a), *Bibliotheca classica,* Frankfurt, impensis Balthasaris Ostern, 4to

    (1625b), *Bibliotheca exotica,* Frankfurt, impensis Balthasaris Ostern, 4to

du Chesne, Joseph (1606), *Diaeteticon polyhistoricon,* Paris, apud Claudium Morellum, 8vo

    (1609), *Liber de priscorum philosophorum verae medicinae materia, praeparationis modo, atque in curandis morbis, praestantia,* Geneva, apud Johannem Vigum, 8vo

du Laurens, André (1595), *Opera anatomica,* Frankfurt, excudebat Gulielmus Antonius, fol.

    (1596), *De crisibus libri tres,* Frankfurt, ex officina Paltheniana sum[p]tibus haeredum Petri Fischeri, 8vo

Dubois, Jacques, *see* Sylvius, Jacobus

Duport, François (1584), *De signis morborum libri quatuor,* Paris, apud Dionysium Duvallium, 8vo

Edwardes, David (1532), *De indiciis et praecognitionibus opus,* London, ex[cudebat] Rob[ertus] Redmanns, 8vo

Emericus, Franciscus (1552), *Summaria declaratio eorum, quae ad urinarum cognitionem maxime faciunt, ex publicis Joannis Baptistae Montani praelectionibus in Patavino schola a quodam auditore excepta ... item, an urinarum vel pulsuum observatio certiores notas salutis vel mortis medico praebeat, utilis narratio,* Vienna, excudebat Egidius Aquila, 4to

Erasmus, Desiderius, *see* Galen 1989

Erastus, Thomas (1572), *Disputationum de medicina nova Philippi Paracelsi pars prima [...pars altera]*, Basle, apud Petrum Pernam, 4to

Erastus, Thomas and Mercenarius, Archangelus (1590), *Disputatio de putredine, in qua natura, differentiae et causa putredinis, ex Aristotelis, et ipsa rerum evidentia, omnia denique consensio inter philosophos et medicos declaratur...Archangeli Mercenarij de putredine adversus Thomam Erastum...Thomae Erasti ad Archangeli Mercenarii disputationem de putredine responsio...Ad Erasti responsionem Archangeli Mercenarii secunda de putredine disputatio*, Leipzig, [imprimebant haeredes Joannis Steinmanni, impensis haeredum Ernesti Voegelini], 4to

Erberus, Joannes, *see* Schegk (1579a)

Eusèbe, Jean (1566), *La philosophie rationale vulgairement appelée dialectique, pour les chirurgiens françois et autres amateurs de la langue françoyse*, Lyon, par Jean Saugrain

Fabricius, Ernestus Fridericus (1626), *Medicinae utriusque Galenicae et hermeticae anatome philosophica*, Hamburg, apud Michaelem Hering, fol.

Facciolatus, Jacobus (1757), *Fasti Gymnasii Patavini*, Padua, typis seminarii, apud Joannem Maufrè, 4to

Farinacci, Prospero (1606), *Tractatus de testibus*, Frankfurt, huius editionis auctor Zacharias Palthenius, fol.

Ferdinandus, Epiphanius (1611), *Theoremata medica et philosophica*, Venice, apud Thomam Ballionem, fol.

(1621), *Centum historiae seu observationes et casus medici*, Venice, apud Thomam Ballionem, fol.

Fernel, Jean (1610a), *De abditis rerum causis libro duo*, Hanau, impensis haeredum Claudii Marnii, fol.

(1610b), *Universa medicina*, Hanau, impensis haeredum Claudii Marnii, fol.

Ferrerius, Augerius, *see* Ferrier, Auger

Ferrier, Auger (1549a), *Liber de diebus decretoriis secundum Pythagoricam doctrinam et Astronomicam observationem*, Lyon, apud Joannem Tornaesium, 16mo

(1549b), *Liber de somniis. Hippocratis de insomniis liber. Galeni liber de insomniis. Synesii liber de insomniis*, Lyon, apud Joannem Tornaesium, 16mo

(1574), *Medendi methodus duobus libris comprehensa. Eiusdem castigationes practicae medicinae*, Lyon, ex officina Ludovici Cloquemin et Stephani Michaelis, 8vo

(1592), *Medendi methodus duobus libris comprehensa. Eiusdem castigationes practicae medicinae*, Lyon, apud Franciscum Fabrium, 8vo

Ficino, Marsiglio (1576), *Opera*, 2 vols., Basle, ex officina Henricpetrina, fol.

Fludd, Robert, (1631), *Doctor Fludd's answer unto M. Foster, or the Squeesing of Parson Foster's sponge, ordained by him wiping away of the weapon-salve*, London, for N. Butler, 4to

Foesius, Anutius (1588), *Oeconomia Hippocratis alphabetico serie distincta*, Frankfurt, apud Andreae Wecheli haeredes Claudium Marnium et Joannem Aubry, fol.

Fonseca, Pedro de (1599), *Commentarii in libros Metaphysicorum Aristotelis*, 2 vols., Frankfurt, typis Joannis Saurij, impensis Joannis Theobaldi Schonwetteri et Lazari Zetzneri, 4to

Fonseca, Rodericus, *see* Jacchinus 1615

Fontanus, Jacobus (1611), *Phisiognomia Aristotelis ordine compositorio edita ad facilitatem doctrinae . . . commentariis illustrata brevissimis et propter methodum praespicuam facillimis*, Paris, apud Joannem Paquet, 8vo

Forerus, Laurentius (1624), *Viridarum philosophicum hoc est disputationes aliquot de selectis . . . materiis partim in Ingolstadiense partim in Dilingana Universitate ad publicum certamen propositae*, Dillingen, apud Udalricum Rem, 8vo

Forestus, Petrus (1589), *De incerto, fallaci urinarum iudicio, quo uromantes, ad perniciem multorum aegrotantium, utuntur*, Leiden, ex officina Plantiniana, apud Franciscum Raphelengium, 8vo

Foster, William (1631), *Hoplocrisma-spongus, or a sponge to wipe away the weapon-salve*, London, T. Cotes for J. Grove, 4to

Foxius Morzillus, Sebastianus (1556), *De demonstratione, eiusque necessitate et vi . . .*, Basle, per Joannem Oporinum, 8vo

Fracastoro, Girolamo (1574), *Opera omnia*, 2nd edn, Venice, apud Iuntas, 4to

Frölich, Joannes Henrichus (1612), *ΣΗΜΕΙΩΤΙΚΗ ΦΟΙΒΕΙΑ paradoxis et heterodoxis D. Felicis Plateris adornata . . .*, resp. Germanus Obermeyerus, Basle, typis Johan Jacobi Genathii, 4to

Fuchs, Leonhart (1530), *Errata recentiorum medicorum lx numero adiectis eorundem confutationibus*, Hagenau, in aedibus Johannis Secerii, 4to

(1531), *Compendiaria ac succincta admodum in medendi artem εἰσαγωγὴ seu introductio*, Hagenau, per Johannem Secerium, 8vo

(1537a), *Tabulae librorum Galeni de differentiis morborum eorundem confutationibus*, Basle, fol.

(1537b), *Universae medicinae compendium, primum quidem a . . . Leonardo Fuchsio conscriptum, ac nunc demum per quendam artis studiosum in hasce tabellas collectum, et ab ipso autore postremo diligentissime recognitum*, Basle, fol.

(1546), *Paradoxorum medicinae libri tres*, Paris, apud Carolam [sic] Guillard, 8vo

(1604), *Opera didactica*, Frankfurt, prodeunt e Collegio Paltheniano, fol.

Fuchs, Samuel (1615), *Metoposcopia et opthalmoscopia*, Strasbourg, excudebat Theodosius Glaserus, sumptibus Pauli Ledertz, 8vo

Fulco, Gulielmus (1560), *Antiprognosticon contra inutiles astrologorum praedictiones Nostradami, Cuninghami, Lovi, Hilli, Vagliani et reliquorum omnium*, [London, ex officina Henrici Suttoni, impensis Humfredi Toij], 8vo

Fulke, William, *see* Fulco, Gulielmus

Furlanus, Daniel (1574), *In libros Aristotelis de partibus animalium commentarius primus*, Venice, apud Joan[nem] Baptistam Somaschum, 8vo

Galen (1531), *Opera iam recens versa* [including *De libris propriis* and *De ordine librorum suorum*, trans. Joannes Fichardus], Basle, ex aedibus Andreae Cratandri, fol.

(1533), *De paratu facilibus libellus*, trans. Hubertus Barlandus, Antwerp, ex officina Joanni Graphei, 8vo

(1540), *De praecognitione libellus*, trans. and comm. Leonardus Jacchinus, Lyon, apud Sebastianum Gryphium, 4to

(1550), *De morborum et symptomatum differentiis et causis libri sex*, ed. Guilielmus Copus, Lyon, apud Gulielmum Rouillium, 16mo

(1551), *see* Lacuna 1551

(1556a), *Opera [latina]*, 3rd edn, Venice, apud Iuntas, fol.

(1556b), *see* Brasavola 1556

(1821–33), *Opera omnia*, ed. C. G. Kühn, Leipzig

(1989), *De optimo docendi genere*, trans. Desiderius Erasmus, in *The collected works of Erasmus: literary and educational writings*, ed. Elaine Fantham and Erika Rummel, vol. 7, Toronto, Buffalo, London, pp. 240–4

(1991), *On the therapeutic method, books I and II*, ed. R. J. Hankinson, Oxford

Galilei, Galileo (1998), *Dialogi sopra i due massimi sistemi del mondo tolomeico e copernicano*, ed. Ottavio Besomi and Mario Helbing, Padua

Gallus, Paschalis (1590), *Bibliotheca medica, sive catalogus illorum, qui ex professo Artem Medicam in hunc usque annum scriptis illustrarunt*, Basle, per Conradum Waldkirch, 8vo

Gammaro, Pietro Andrea (1584), *De extensionibus*, in *Tractatus iuris universi*, Venice, 18.247–60, fol.

Gauricus, Pomponius, *see* Indagine 1603

Gavassetius, Michael (1586), *Libri duo: alter de rebus praeter naturam, alter de indicationibus curativis, seu de methodo medendi*, Venice, apud Paulum Meietum Bibliopolam Patavinum, 4to

Gemma, Cornelius (1575), *De naturae divinis characterismis: seu raris et admirandis spectaculis, causis, indiciis, proprietatibus rerum in partibus singulis universis libri ii*, Antwerp, ex officina Christophori Plantini, 8vo

Gentile da Foligno (n.d.), *De proporcionibus medicarum*, n.p., 4to

Gentile da Foligno, *see* Torrigiano 1557

Georgi, Theophilus (1742–58), *Allgemeines europäisches Bücher-Lexikon*, Leipzig, Georgi, fol.

Gessner, Conrad (1577), *Epistolae medicinales*, ed. Caspar Wolf, Zürich, excudebat Christoph[orus] Frosch[overus], 8vo

Giachini, Lionardo, *see* Jacchinus, Leonardus

Goclenius, Rodolphus (1599), *Analyses in exercitationes aliquot Julii Caesaris Scaligeri, de subtilitate*, ed. Johannes Schroderus, Marburg, excudebat Paulus Egenolphus, 1599, 8vo

(1609), *Conciliator philosophicus*, Kassel, ex officina typographica Mauritiana, opera Wilhelmi Wesselii, 4to

(1613), *Lexicon philosophicum*, Frankfurt, typis viduae Matthiae Beckeri impensis Petri Musculi et Ruperti Pistorij, 4to

(1625), *Mirabilium naturae liber, concordias et repugnantias rerum in plantis, animalibus, animaliumque morbis et partibus, manifestans*, Frankfurt, typis Egenolphi Emmelii, impensis Joannis Caroli Unckelii, 8vo

Gordon, Bernard de (1574), *Opus, lilium medicinae inscriptum, de morborum prope omnium curatione, septem particulis distributum*, Lyon, apud Guliel[mum] Rovillium, 8vo

Gorris, Jean de (1601), *Definitionum medicarum libri xxiiii literis graecis distincti*, Frankfurt, typis Wechelianis, apud Claudium Marunium et haeredes Joannis Aubrii, fol

Gratarolo, Guglielmo (1554), *Opuscula: de memoria reparanda, augenda, conservandaque, ac de reminiscentia: tutiora omnimodo remedia, praeceptiones optimae. De praedictione morum naturarumque hominum, cum ex inspectione partium corporis, tum aliis modis. De temporum omnimoda mutatione, perpetua et certissima signa et prognostica*, Basle, apud Nicolaum Episcopium iuniorem, 8vo

(1603) *see* Indagine 1603

Grawerus, Albertus (1619), *Libellus de unica veritate*, Weimar, typis Johannis Weidneri, 8vo

Grosse, Henning (1600), *Elenchus seu index generalis, in quo continentur libri omnes, qui ... post annum 1593 usque ad annum 1600 in sancto Romano imperio et vicinis regionibus novi auctive prodierunt*, Leipzig, [Henning Grosse], 4to

Gryllus, Laurentius (1566), *De sapore dulci et amaro libri duo ... accessit in fine oratio de peregrinatione studij medicinalis ergo suscepta*, first part ed. Adam Laudanus, Prague, apud Georgium Melantrichium ab Aventino, 4to

Guinther von Andernach, Joannes (1571), *De medicina veteri et nova tum cognoscenda, tum faciunda commentarii duo*, Basle, ex officina Henricpetrina, fol.

Hafenrefferus, Samuel (1640), *Monochordon symbolico-biomanticum abstrusissimam pulsuum doctrinam, ex harmoniis musicis dilucide, figurisque oculariter demonstrans*, Ulm, typis et impensis Balthasari Kühnen, 8vo

Hagecius ab Hagek, Thaddaeus (1562), *Aphorismorum metoposcopicorum libellus unus*, Prague, excudebat Georgius Melantrichius ab Aventino, 4to

(1564), *Astrologica opuscula antiqua: Fragmentum astrologicum incerto autore ... Liber Regum de significationibus planetarum ... liber Hermetis centum aphorismorum*, Prague, excudebat Georgius Melantrichius ab Aventino, 4to

(1596), *Actio medica adversus Philippum Fancellum Belgum, incolam Budvincensem, Medicastrum et Pseudoparacelsistam*, Amberg, ex officina Michäelis Forsteri, 8vo

Haly, *see* Torrigiano 1557

Harvey, William (1766), *Opera omnia a Collegio Medicorum Londinensi edita*, London, 4to, 2 vols.

(1653), *Anatomical exercitations, concerning the generation of living creatures ...*, London, for James Young and Octavian Pulleyn, 8vo

Hasfurtus Virdungus, Johannes (1533), *Nova medicinae methodus curandi morbos ex mathematica scientia deprompta*, Hagenau, [per Valentinum Korbian], 4to

Hasler, Joannes (1578), *De logistica medica, hoc est et morborum et compositorum medicaminum qualitatum gradus, purgantiumque doses atque proprietates investigandi ratione apodictica problematis novem absoluta, liber unus*, Augsburg, imprimebat Valentinus Schönigk, 4to

Herculanus, Franciscus (1584), *De negativa probanda*, in *Tractatus iuris universi*, Venice, 4.12–28, fol.

Heurnius, Joannes (1597), *Hippocratis Prolegomena et Prognosticorum libri tres cum paraphrastica versione et brevibus commentariis*, Leiden, ex officina Plantiniana, apud Franciscum Raphelengium, 4to

(1637), *Hippocratis Aphorismi Graece et Latine . . . cum historiis, observationibus, cautionibus, et remediis selectis*, Leiden, apud Joannem Maire, 12mo

Heyll, Christophorus (1534), *Artificialis medicatio, constans paraphrasi in Galeni librum de Artis Medicae constitutione . . . Methodi cognoscendorum tam particularium quam universalium morborum Betrutii . . . De idoneo auxiliorum usu Joannis de Sancto Amando*, Mainz, 4to

Hippocrates (1597), (1637), *see* Heurnius 1597, 1637
(1839–61), *Œuvres complètes*, trans. Emile Littré, Paris

Hollerius, Jacobus (1582), *In Aphorismos Hippocratis commentarii septem*, ed. Jean Liébaut, Paris, apud Jacobum du Puys, 8vo

Hornung, Joannes (1626), *Cista medica, qua in epistolae clarissimorum Germaniae medicorum, familiares, et in re medica, tam quoad hermetica et chymica . . . potissimum ex posthuma clarissimi quondam philosophiae et medicinae doctoris d[omini] Signismundi Schnitzeri Ulmensis bibliotheca*, ed. Joannes Hornung, Nuremberg, sumptibus Simonis Halbmayori, 4to

Hooke, Robert (1665), *Micrographia*, London, for J. Martyn and J. Allestry, fol

Horst, Gregor (1606), Σκέψις *physica medica de casu quodam admirando et singulari, ex quo subsequentia problemata deducuntur. I. An corpus humanum post mortem aliquot septimanis colore et habitu floridum, incorruptum, absque putridine incipiente, naturaliter, nullo artificio accidente, durare possit? II. An fluxus sanguinis cadaveris humani occisi tam in principio caedis, quam post aliquot septimanos praesentiam interfectoris indicat?* Wittenberg, typis Meisnerianis impensis Clementi Bergeri, 8vo

(1609), *Disputationum medicarum viginti: accesserunt Jacobi Horstii disputationes theoreticae et practicae*, Wittenberg, excudebat Joannes Schmidt, sumptibus Clementis Bergeri, 8vo

(1612), *De natura humana libri duo, quorum prior de corporis structura, posterior de anima tractat*, Frankfurt, typis Erasmi Kemferi, sumptibus Clementis Bergeri bibliopolae Witebergensis, 4vo

(1621), *Conciliator enucleatus seu differentiarum philosophiarum et medicarum Petri Apponensis compendium*, Giessen, impensis Casparis Chemlini, 8vo

(1629), *De morbis, eorumque causis ac symptomatibus liber, cum declaratione quaestionum controversarum*, Marburg, typis ac sumptibus Casparis Chemlini, 8vo

Horst, Jakob (1562), *see* Jokissus 1562
(1574), *Eine Vorwarnung der Krancken vor ihrem selbs eigenen Schaden und Vorseumnuss*, Görlitz, bey Ambrosio Fritsch, 4to

(1585), *Precationes medicorum piae ad varios usus tum studiorum tum etiam operum artis*, Helmstedt, excudebat Jacobus Lucius, 12mo

(1609), *see* Horst, Gregor 1609

Hotman, François (1569), *Commentarius de verbis iuris*, Lyon, apud Antonium Gryphium, fol.

Houiller, Jacques, *see* Hollerius, Jacobus

Hucher, Jean (1602), *De prognosi medica libri duo*, Lyon, apud Antonium de Harsy, 8vo

Huggelius, Joannes Jacobus (1560), *De semeiotice medicinae parte tractatus. Ex probatis collectus authoribus et in tabulae formam redactus*, Basle, per Nicolaum Brylingerum, fol.

Indagine, Joannes ab (1603), *Introductiones apotelematicae elegantes in physiologiam, astrologiam naturalem, complexiones hominum, naturas plantarum, cum periaxiomatibus de faciebus signorum et canonibus de aegritudinibus hominum: omnia ob similem materiam accessit Gulielmi Grataroli Bergomatis opuscula de memoria reparanda, augenda, conservanda; de praedictione morum naturarumque hominum; de mutatione temporum, eiusque signis perpetuis. Et Pomponii Gaurici Neapolitani tractatus de simmetriis, lineamentis et physiognomia, eiusque speciebus*, Oberursel, apud Cornelium Sutorium, impensis Lazari Zetzneri, 8vo

Infinita nature secreta (1515), *Infinita nature secreta, quibuslibet hominibus contingentias previdenda, cavenda ac prosequenda declarant in hoc libro contenta. Physionomia summi Aristotelis. Physionomia Michaelis Scoti. Physionomia Coclitis. Chyromantia eiusdem. Cum approbatione Achilini [questio de subiecto physionomie et chiromantie]*, Pavia, per B. de Garaldis, fol.

Ingolstetterus, Johannes (1596), *De aureo dente Silesii pueri, responsio ad iudicium M. Rulandi*, Leipzig, [imprimebat Michäel Lantzenberger], 8vo

    (1597), *De natura occultorum et prodigiosorum dissertatio . . . ad D. Jacobum Horstium . . . qua respondetur ipsius libello de aureo, qui putabatur, dente*, Leipzig, excudebat Abraham Lamberg, 8vo

Jacchinus, Leonardus (1534), *see Novae academiae Florentinae opuscula* 1534

    (1563), *Opuscula*, Basle, per Petrum Pernam, 4to

    (1615), *Methodus curandarum febrium*, ed. Rodericus Fonseca, Pisa, apud Joannem Fontanum, 4to

James, Thomas (1605), *Catalogus librorum Bibliothecae publicae quam vir ornatissimus Thomas Bodleius Eques Auratus in Academiae Oxoniensi nuper instituit*, Oxford, apud Josephum Barnesium, 4to

Jessenius a Jessen, Johannes, [praeses] (1599), *De sympathiae et antipathiae rerum naturalium causis disquisitio singularis quam in publico pro virili ad Cal. Iunii defendere conabitur Daniel Sennert*, praeses Johannes Jessenius a Jessen, Wittenberg, typis Meissnerianis, 4to

    (1601), *see* Campilongo 1601

    (1610), *see* Saxonia 1610

    (1628), *see* Liddel 1628

Joannitius, *see Articella* 1515, 1529, 1557; Avicenna 1608; Torrigiano 1557

Jokissus, Jacobus, [praeses] (1562), *Themata disputationis de latitudine sanitatis* συστάσει *et* διαστάσει *graduum eius cum adiecta tabula* ἐν τῆς τέχνης ἰατρικῆς *Galeni*, resp. Jakob Horst, Frankfurt an der Oder, Johann Eichorn, 4to

Joubert, Laurent (1579), *Opera*, 2 vols., Lyon, apud Stephanum Michaelum, fol.

Justus, Joannes (1618), *De indicatione*, in *Decas* 1618–31

Keckermann, Bartholomaeus (1608), *Praecognita philosophica*, Hanau, apud Gulielmum Antonium, 8vo

    (1614), *Opera*, Geneva, Jacques Aubert, fol.

Kepler, Johannes (1941), *Gesammelte Werke*, vol. 4, Munich

Kleinfeld, Nicolaus (1598), *Pathologia secundum genus hoc est de morbis eorumque causis et differentiis [et] de symptomatis eorumque causis et differentiis*, Leiden, ex officina Plantiniana, apud Christophorum Raphelengium, 16mo

Kornmannus, Henricus (1610), *De miraculis mortuorum*, [Augsburg] typis Joannis Wolfii sumptibus Jacobi Porssi, 8vo

(1614), *De miraculis vivorum, seu de varia natura, variis singularitatibus, proprietatibus, affectionibus, mirandisque virtutibus, facultatibus et signis hominum vivorum*, Frankfurt, typis viduae Matthiae Beckeri impensis Jacobi Fischeri, 8vo

Lacuna, Andreas (1551), *Epitome operum Galeni*, Basle, apud Michaelem Isingrinium, fol.

L'Alemant, Adrien (1549), *Ars parva*, Paris, apud Thomam Richardum, 8vo

(1557), *Hippocratis ... de aere aquis et locis liber ... commentariis quatuor illustratus*, Paris, apud Aegidium Gorbinum, 8vo

Landi, Bassiano (1543), *Iatrologia. Dialogi duo, in quibus de universae artis medicae, praecipue vero morborum omnium et cognoscendorum et curandorum absolutissima methodo per quam eleganter ac docte disseritur*, Basle, ex officina Johannis Oporini, 4to

Langius, Joannes (1589), *Epistolae medicinales*, Frankfurt, apud Andreae Wecheli haeredes, Claudium Marnium et Joannem Aubrium, 8vo

Laurembergius, Petrus (1621), *Laurus delphica, seu consilium, quo describitur methodus perfacilis ad medicinam. Cui adiecta universae medicinae methodus Hieronymi Thriveri*, Leiden, apud Joannem Maire, 8vo

Laurentius, Andreas, *see* du Laurens, André

Le Coq, Pascal, *see* Gallus, Paschalis

Le Pois, Nicolas (1585), *De cognoscendis et curandis praecipue internis humani corporis morbis libri tres*, Frankfurt, apud Andreae Wecheli haeredes, 8vo

Le Thielleux, François (1581), *Methodus dignoscendorum morborum, primum quidem tradita ab Argenterio, deinceps autem exemplis multis ex veteribus medicis et recentioribus desumptis adaucta*, Nantes, ex officina Joannis Gandin, 4to

Lemnius, Levinus (1582), *De habitu et constitutione corporis ... libri ii*, Erfurt, Esaias Mechlerus excudebat, 8vo

Lemosius, Ludovicus (1598), *De optimo praedicandi ratione libri sex. Item iudicii operum magni Hippocratis liber unus*, Venice, apud Robertum Meietum, 8vo

Leoniceno, Niccolò (1532), *Opuscula*, Basle, [apud Antonium Cratandrum et Joannem Bebelium], fol.

(1557), *see* Torrigiano 1557

Libau, Andreas, *see* Libavius, Andreas

Libavius, Andreas (1594), *Tractatus duo physici: prior de impostoria vulnerum per unguentum armarum sanatione Paracelsicis usitata commendataque; posterior de cruentatione cadaverum in iusta caede factorum praesente, qui occidisse creditur*, Frankfurt, excudebat Joannes Saurus, impensis Petri Kopffii, 8vo

(1599a), *Epistolicarum chymicarum liber tertius*, Frankfurt, in officina typographica Joannis Lechleri, impensis Petri Kopffii, 8vo

(1599b), *Singularium pars secunda*, Frankfurt, typis Joannis Sauri, impensis Petri Kopffii, 8vo

Liceti, Fortunio (1612), *De his qui diu vivunt sine alimento libri quatuor*, Padua, apud Petrum Bertellum, fol.

(1634), *De monstrorum caussis, natura, et differentiis libri duo*, Padua, apud Paulum Frambottum, 4to

Liddel, Duncan (1598a), *Disputatio de signis in genere, deinde de signis insalubribus diagnosticis*, Resp. Georgius Cocius, Helmstedt, excudebant haeredes Jacobi Lucij, 4to

(1598b), *De praesagiis in aegris disputatio prior*, resp. Elias Bonvinius, Helmstedt, ex officina typographica haeredum Jacobi Lucij, 4to

(1598c), *Disputationum pathologicarum quarta de symptomatibus et symptomatum differentiis*, resp. Henricus Wavenius, Helmstedt, excudebant haeredes Jacobi Lucii, 4to

(1604), *Disputatio partis prioris de praesagiis in aegris*, resp. Matthias Waltherius, Helmstedt, ex typographia Iacobi Lucij, 4to

(1624), *Operum omnium iatrogalenicorum . . . tomus unicus*, ed. Ludovicus Serranus, Lyon, Antonius Chard, 4to

(1628), *Ars medica, succincte et perspicue explicata. Accessit eiusdem tractatus de dente aureo pueri Silesii contra Horstium: ex museo Joachimi Morsii nunc primum prolatus. Adiicitur Johannis Jessenii a Jessen historica relatio de rustico Bohemo cultri-vorace*, Hamburg, ex bibliopolio Frobeniano, 8vo

Lipenius, Martin (1679), *Bibliotheca realis medica*, Frankfurt, cura et sumptibus Johannis Friderici, fol.

Lodovicus, Antonius (1540), *De occultis proprietatibus*, Lisbon, [Lodovicus Rotorigius], fol.

Lommius, Jodocus (1558), *Commentarii de sanitate tuenda in primum librum de re medica Aurel. Cornelii Celsi*, Louvain, prostant apud Antonium Maria Bergague, 8vo

Luca, Constantinus (1607), *Subtilissima in Hippocratis Aphorismos per eum in ordinem redactos expositio*, Pavia, apud Andream Vianum, 4to

Lucius, Cynacus (1597), *De medicina philosophica*, Ingolstadt, ex officina typographica Ederiana, 4to

Magirus, Joannes (1603), *Anthropologia hoc est commentarius eruditissimus in aureum Philippi Melanchthonis libellum de anima: completus et locupletatus opera Georgii Caufungeri*, Frankfurt, in officina Lichensi, excusus per Wolfgang Richterum, 8vo

Mainardi, Giovanni, *see* Manardo, Giovanni

Maioli, Lorenzo, *see* Maiolus, Laurentius

Maiolus, Laurentius (1497), *De gradibus medicinarum*, Venice, [Aldus Manutius], 4to

Maittaire, Michael (1722), *Annales typographici ab anno* MD *ad annum* MDXXXVI *continuati* (vol. 2, part 2), The Hague, apud fratres Vaillant et Nicolaeum Prevost, 4to

Maliński, Caspar, *see* Mallinus, Casparus

Mallinus, Casparus (1575), *Iatrotheologiconomicomachia. Carmen, quo medicinae excellentia, refutatis quibusdam obiectionius, ostenditur*, Strasbourg, apud Bernhardum Jobinum, 8vo

Manardo, Giovanni (1536), *In primum Artis parvae Galeni librum commentaria*, Basle, apud Jo[annem] Bebelium, 4to

Manlius, Joannes (1563), *Locorum communium collectanea*, Basle, per Joannem Oporinum, 8vo

Martinengius, Celsus (1584), *De praevidendis morborum eventibus libri tres*, Venice, apud Joan[nem] Bapt[istam] Somaschum, 4to

Martini, Cornelius (1593), *Programma cum responsione studiosorum Rameae philosophiae*, Helmstedt, excudebat Iacobus Lucius, 4to

Massarius, Dominicus (1584), *De ponderibus et mensuris medicinalibus*, ed. Conrad Gesner and Caspar Wolf, Zürich, apud Christophorum Froschoverum, 8vo

Matthaeus, Joannes (1603), *Quaestiones medicae et iucundae et lectu dignae*, Frankfurt, ex Officina Zachario-Paltheniana, 8vo

Meietus, Paulus (ed.) (1584), *Opuscula illustrium medicorum de dosibus, seu de iusta quantitate et proportione medicamentorum*, [Heidelberg], apud Joan[nem] Mareschallum, 8vo

Melanchthon, Philip (1547), *Erotemata dialectices*, Wittenberg, excusa per Johannem Luft, 8vo

(1581), *Initia doctrinae physicae*, Wittenberg, excudebant haeredes Johannis Cratonis, 8vo

(1834–60), *Opera quae supersunt omnia*, ed. C. B. Bretschneider and H. E. Bindseil, 28 vols., Halle, then Braunschweig

(1999), *Orations on philosophy and education*, ed. Sachiko Kusukawa, Cambridge

Mercenarius, Archangelus, *see* Erastus 1590

Mercuriale, Girolamo (1585), *Variarum lectionum in medicinae scriptoribus et aliis libri*, Paris, apud Nicolaum Nivellum, 8vo

Mizauld, Antoine (1554), *Memorabilium aliquot naturae arcanorum sylvula, rerum variarum sympathias et antipathias, seu naturales concordias et discordias, libellis duobus complectens*, Paris, apud Iacobum Kerver, 8vo

Mizauld, Antoine, ed. (1572), *Dioclis Carystij medici ab Hippocrate fama et aetate secundi, aurea ad Antigonum regem epistola, de morborum praesagiis et eorundem extemporaneis remediis*, Paris, apud Federicum Morellum, 8vo

Mocenius, Philippus (1588), *Tractationum philosophicarum tomus unus, in quo continentur I. Philippi Mocenici universalium institutionum ad hominum perfectionem contemplationes II. Andreae Caesalpini quaestionum peripateticarum libri v III. Bernardini Telesii de rerum natura iuxta propria principia libri xi*, [Geneva], excudebat Eustathius Vignon, fol.

Moldenarius, Christianus (1616), *Exercitationes physiognomonicae quatuor libris comprehensae*, [Wittenberg], sumptibus Zachariae Schureri Biblio[polae], 8vo

Molière, Jean-Baptiste Poquelin de (1962), *Œuvres complètes*, 2 vols., ed. R. Jouanny, Paris

Mondeville, Henri de (1892), *Die Chirurgie*, ed. Julius Pagel, Berlin

Montaigne, Michel de (1965), *Les Essais*, ed. Pierre Villey and V.-L. Saulnier, Paris

Montanus, Joannes Baptista, *see* Monte, Giambattista da

Monte, Giambattista da (1552), *see* Emericus 1552

    (1554), *In nonum librum Rhasis ad Mansorem Regem Arabum expositio*, Venice, apud Baltasarem Constantinum, 8vo

    (1556), *In artem parvam Galeni explanationes*, ed. Valentinus Lublinus, Lyon, apud Antonium Vincentum, 12mo

    (1583), *Consultationes medicae*, ed. Joannes Crato, [Basle], fol.

    (1587), *Medicina universa, ex lectionibus eius, caeterisque opusculis, tum impressis, tum scriptis collecta*, ed. Martinus Weindrichius, Frankfurt, apud Andreae Wecheli haeredes Claudium Marnium et Joannem Aubry, fol.

Montecatini, Antonio (1576), *In eam partem in libris Aristotelis de anima, quae est de mente humana, lectura*, Ferrara, ex typis haeredum Francisci Rubei, fol.

Montuus, Sebastianus (1537), *Dialexeon medicinalium libri duo*, Lyon, apud Michaelem Parmanterium, 4to

Morescottus, Alfonsus (1597), *Compendium totius medicinae: in quo de complexorum arcanis indiciis, morborum praecipuorum causis, prognosticis, et signis deque fabrica receptorum breviter tractatur*, Herborn, typis Christophori Corvini, 12mo

Moufet, Thomas (1588), *Nosomantica hippocratea, sive Hippocratis prognostica cuncta ex omnibus ipsius scriptis methodice digesta*, Frankfurt, apud Andreae Wecheli haeredes Claudium Marnium et Joannem Aubrium, 8vo

Müncerus, Paulus (1616), *XL contradictiones, quibus ratio et curatio morborum occultorum* παχυλῶς *delineata*, in *Decas* 1618–31

Nicholas of Cusa (1983), *Opera omnia*, vol. 5: *Idiota de mente*, ed. Renate Steiger, Hamburg

Nifo, Agostino (1540), *De verissimis temporum signis commentariolus*, Venice, apud Hieronymum Scotum, 8vo

Nollius, Henricus (1617), *Theoria philosophicae hermeticae . . . explicata*, Hanau, apud Petrum Antonium, 8vo

Novae academiae Florentinae opuscula (1534), *Novae academiae Florentinae opuscula adversus Avicennam et medicos neotericos qui Galeni disciplina neglecta barbaros colunt*, Lyon, excudebat Sebastianus Gryphius, 8vo [one of the authors is Leonardus Jacchinus]

Obicius, Hippolytus (1605), *De nobilitate medici contra illius obtrectatores. Dialogus*, Venice, apud Robertum Meiettum, 4to

Oddi, Marco degli (1589), *De morbi natura, et essentia tractatio dilucidissima*, Padua, apud Paulum Meiettum, 4to

Oddi, Oddo degli (1564), *In primum Aphorismorum Hippocratis sectionem elaboratissima et lucidissima expositio*, ed. Marco Oddi degli Oddi, 8vo

Paracelsus (1567), *Medici libelli: physionomia morborum . . .*, Cologne, bey Arnoldi Byrckmans Erben, 4to

    (1996), *Sämtliche Werke*, vol. 8, ed. Karl Sudhoff and Wilhelm Mattheissen, Hildesheim, Zürich, New York

Parisanus, Æmilius (1621), *Nobilium exercitationum libri duodecim de subtilitate*, Venice, apud Evangelistam Deuchinum, fol.

(1635), *De microcosmica subtilitate pars altera*, Venice, apud Marcum Antonium Brogiollum, fol.

Pascal, Blaise (1963), *Œuvres complètes*, ed. Louis Lafuma, Paris

Paulinus, Fabius, *see* Avicenna 1608

Pereira, Gometia (1558), *Novae veraeque medicinae, experimentis et evidentibus rationibus comprobatae prima pars*, [Medina del Campo], excudebat Franciscus a Canto, fol.

Peucer, Caspar (1553), *Commentarius de praecipuis divinationum generibus*, Wittenberg, 8vo

(1562), *Oratio de dignitate artis medicae*, Wittenberg, excudebat Laurentius Schrenck, 8vo

(1593), *Commentarius de praecipuis divinationum generibus, in quo a prophetijs divina autoritate traditis, et Physicis praedictionibus, separantur Diabolicae fraudes et superstitiosae observationes, et explicantur fontes ac causae*, Frankfurt, apud Andreae Wecheli haeredes Claudium Marnium et Joannem Aubrium, 8vo

Piccartus, Michael (1595), *Oratio de optima ratione interpretandi*, Nuremberg, typis Christophori Lochneri, 4to

Piccolomini, Alessandro (1600), *De rerum definitionibus*, Frankfurt, impensis Nicolai Bassaei, 4to

Pictorius, Georgius (1558), *Rei medicae totius compendiosa traditio*, Basle per Henricum Petri, 8vo

Pietro d'Abano (1548), *Conciliator controversiarum, quae inter philosophos et medicos versantur*, Venice, apud Iuntas, fol.

Pietro d'Abano, *see* Horst 1621

Piso, Nicolaus *see* Le Pois, Nicolas

Platter, Felix (1625), *Quaestiones medicae paradoxae et endoxae*, Basle, impensis Ludov[ici] Regis typis Johannis Schweteri, 4to

(1961), *Beloved son Felix: the journal of Felix Platter, a medical student in Montpellier in the sixteenth century*, trans. and introd. Seán Jennett, London

Platter, Thomas (1963), *Journal of a younger brother: the life of Thomas Platter as a medical student in Montpellier at the close of the sixteenth century*, trans. and introd. Seán Jennett, London

Polcastris, Sigismundus de (n.d.), *Questio de actuatione medicinalium . . . de appropinquatione ad equalitatem ponderalem*, n.p., 4to

Polemo (1552), *. . . Polemon Atheniensis insignis philosophi naturae signorum interpretatio*, trans. Nicolas Petreius, Venice, [ex officina Gryphii, sumptibus vero Francisci Camotii], 4to

Pomponazzi, Pietro (1567), *Opera*, ed. Guilhelmus Gratarolus, Basle, ex officina Henricpetrina, 8vo

Porta, Giambattista della (1588), *Magiae naturalis libri xx*, Naples, apud Horatium Salvianum, fol

(1593), *Physiognomia*, Hanau, apud Gulielmum Antonium, impensis Petri Fischeri, 8vo

Portius, Simon, *see* Porzio, Simone

Porzio, Simone (1598), *De rerum naturalium principiis libri duo*, Marburg, typis Pauli Egenolphi typogr[aphi] acad[emiae], 8vo

Quaestionum series (1752), *Quaestionum medicarum quae circa medicinae theoriam et praxim, ante duo saecula, in Scholis Facultatis Medicinae Parisiensis agitatae sunt et discussae, series chronologica, cum doctorum praesidum et baccalaureorum propugnantium nominibus*, Paris, apud Joannem-Thomam Hérissant, 4to

Quercetanus, Josephus, *see* du Chesne, Joseph

Rabelais, François (1973), *Œuvres complètes*, ed. Guy Demerson, Paris

Ramus, Petrus (1569), *Scholae in tres liberales artes*, Basle, per Eusebium Episcopium et Nicolai fratris haeredes, fol.

Rebuffi, Pierre (1586), *In titulum de verborum significatione commentarius*, Lyon, apud Gulielmum Rouillium, fol.

Regimen Salernitanum (1545), *De conservanda bona valetudine opusculum scholae Salernitanae, ad regem Angliae versibus conscriptum*, ed. Arnoldus Novicomensis, Joannes Curio and Jacobus Crellius, Frankfurt, apud Christianum Egenolphum, 8vo

Reinholdus, Paulus, *see* Cocus 1601

Reusnerus, Hieronymus, *see* Willichius 1582

Reynolds, John (1745), *A discourse of prodigious abstinence* (1669), reprinted in *The Harleian miscellany*, London, iv.44ff.

Rhenanus, Johannes (1614), *Urocriterium chymiatricum, sive ratio chymiatrica exacte diiudicandi urinas ex tribus principiis activis et uno passivo, hactenus neglectis aphoristice ostensa*, Frankfurt, typis Wolfgangi Richteri impensis Antonii Hummii, 8vo

Riccoboni, Antonio (1598), *De gymnasio Patavino commentariorum libri sex*, Padua, apud Franciscum Bolzetam, 4to

Riolan, Jean, the Elder (1610), *Opera omnia*, ed. Jean Riolan the Younger, Paris, ex officina Plantiniana, apud H. Périer, fol.

Roeslin, Helisaeus, *see* Schegk 1579b

Rogerius, Constantinus (1584), *Singularis tractatus de iuris interpretatione*, in *Tractatus iuris universi*, Venice, 1.386–94, fol.

Rondelet, Guillaume (1554–5), *Liber de piscibus marinis*, 2 vols., Lyon, apud Matthiam Bonhomme, fol.

  (1565), *Dispensorium sive pharmacopolarum officina*, Cologne, apud Joannem Byrkmannum, 12mo

  (1586), *Methodus curandorum omnium morborum corporis humani in tres libros distincta . . . eiusdem dignoscendis morbis liber*, Lyon, apud Gulielmum Rouillium, 8vo

Rorarius, Nicolaus (1573), *Contradictiones, dubia et paradoxa, in libros Hippocratis, Celsi, Galeni, Aetii, Aeginetae, Avicennae. Cum eorundem conciliationibus*, Venice, apud Franciscum Gasparem Bondonum et fratres, 8vo

Rosenbachius, Zacharias (1620), *De indicationibus*, in *Decas IV disputationum medicarum . . . de novo recusarum per Johannem Jacobum Genathium Acad[emiae] Basil[iensis] Typographum*, Basle, 4to

Rudius, Eustachius (1592–5), *De humani corporis affectibus dignoscendis, praedicendis, curandis et conservandis libri quinque*, Venice, apud Robertum Meiettum, fol.

Ruland, Martin, the Younger (1597a), *Nova, et in omni natura omnino inaudita historia, de aureo dente* . . . *deque eodem iudicium*, Frankfurt, excudebat Joannes Saurius impensis Petri Kopffi, 4to

(1597b), *Demonstratio iuditii de dente aureo pueri Silesii: adversus responsionem M. Johannis Ingolstetteri*, Frankfurt, apud Joannem Saurum, impensis Cornelii Sutori, 8vo

Sancto Amando, Joannes de, *see* Heyll 1534

Sanctorius, Sanctorius (1630), *Methodi vitandorum errorum omnium, qui in arte medica contingunt libri quindecim*, Geneva, apud Petrum Aubertum, 4to

(1642), *Ars de statica medicina et de responsione ad Staticomasticem aphorismorum sectionibus octo comprehensa*, Leiden, apud Davidem Lopes de Haro, 12mo

Santorre, Santori, *see* Sanctorius, Sanctorius

Santorus, Joannes Donatus (1597), *Epistolarum medicinalium lib[ri] vii*, Naples, ex typographia Stelliolae, sumptibus Scipionis Ricij, 4to

Sassone, Ercole, *see* Saxonia, Hercules

Sattler, Wolffgangus (1609), *Theses de iure et privilegiis medicorum*, Basle, a Joan[ne] Jacobo Genathio, 1609, 4to

Saubertus, Joannes, *see* Waldungus 1611

Saxonia, Hercules (1600), *Tractatus triplex, de fe[b]rium putridarum signis et symptomatibus, de pulsibus et de urinis*, ed. Petrus Uffenbachius, Frankfurt, impensis Johannis Theobaldi Schönwetteri, 1600, 8vo

(1603), *Pantheum medicinae selectum*, ed. Petrus Uffenbachius, Frankfurt, prostat in nobilis Francofurti Paltheniana, fol.

(1604), *De pulsibus*, ed. Petrus Uffenbachus, Frankfurt, prostat in nobilis Francofurti Paltheniana, fol.

(1610), *Prognoseon practicarum*, ed. Leander Vialatus, introd. Johannes Jessenius a Jessen, Frankfurt, apud Zachariam Palthenium, fol.

Scaliger, Julius Caesar (1592), *Exotericarum exercitationum liber xv, de subtilitate*, Frankfurt, apud Andreae Wecheli haeredes, Claudium Marnium et Joannem Aubrium, 8vo

Scheckius, Jacobus, *see* Schegk, Jakob

Schegk, Jakob (1540), *De causa continente*, Tübingen, apud Ulricum Morhardum, 8vo

(1564), *De demonstratione libri XV: novum opus Galeni eiusdem argumenti iacturam resarciens*, Basle, excudebant Joannes Oporinus et Eusebius Episcopius, fol.

[praeses] (1579a), *Disputatio de medendi indicationibus*, resp. Joannes Erberus, [Tübingen], 4to

[praeses] (1579b), *Disputatio instituta de his, quae pertinent ad definitionem medicinae propositam a Galeno in libello, cuius inscriptio est* τέχνη ἰατρική, resp. Helisaeus Roeslin, [Tübingen], 4to

Schenck von Grafenberg, Johannes (1609a), *Observationum medicarum rararum, novarum, admirabilium, et monstrosarum volumen, tomis septem*, Frankfurt, typis Nicolai Hoffmanni, impensis Jonae Rhodii, fol.

Schenck, Johannes Georgius (1609b), *Biblia iatrica, sive bibliotheca medica*, Frankfurt, typis Joannis Spiessij sumptibus Antonii Hummij, 8vo

Scholze, Lorenz (1589), *Aphorismi medicales cum theoretici tum practici*, Wroclaw, per haeredes Johannis Scharffenbergii, 8vo

    (1598a), *Consilia medicinalia conscriptorum a praestantiss[imis] atque exercitatiss[imis] nostrorum temproum medicis*, Frankfurt, apud Andreae Wecheli haeredes Claudium Marnium et Joannem Aubrium, fol.

    (1598b), *Epistolae philosophicae medicinales ac chymicae*, Frankfurt, apud Andreae Wecheli haeredes Claudium Marnium et Joannem Aubry, fol.

Scot, Michael (1508), *Liber phisionome*, Cologne, impressum per Cornelium de Lynch, 4to

Scribonius, Gulielmus Adolphus (1583), *Rerum naturalium doctrina methodica*, London, excudebat Henricus Mideltonus impensis G. Bishop, 8vo

    (1584), *Idea medicinae secundum logicas leges informandae et describendae*, Lemgo, apud Conradum Grothenum, 8vo

Seidelius, Bruno (1593), *Liber morborum incurabilium causas, mira brevitate summa lectionis iucunditate erudite explicans*, Frankfurt, apud Joannem Wechelum, 8vo

Sennert, Daniel (1599), *see* Jessenius a Jessen 1599

    (1650), *Opera*, 3 vols., ed. Charles Spon, Lyon, sumptibus Joannis Antonii Huguetan et Marci Antonii Ravaud, fol.

    (1676), *Opera omnia*, Lyon (cited by Eckart 1992)

Severinus, Petrus (1571), *Idea medicinae philosophicae, fundamenta continens totius doctrinae Paracelsicae, Hippocraticae et Galenicae*, Basle, ex officina Sixti Henricpetri, 4to

Silvaticus, Joannes Baptista (1601), *Controversiae medicae numero centum*, Frankfurt, apud Claudium Marnem et Joannis Aubrij haeredes, fol.

Simoneta, Petrus Paulus (1598), *Compendium totius medicinae*, Frankfurt, apud Andreae Wecheli haeredes Claudium Marnium et Joannem Aubry, 8vo

Simplicius (1882), *In Aristotelis Physicorum libros quattuor priores commentaria*, ed H. Diels, Berlin

Skalich de Lika, Paul (1556), *Occulta occultorum occulta*, [Vienna], excudebat Michael Zimmermann, 4to

Smetius a Leda, Henricus (1611), *Miscellanea*, Frankfurt, impensis Jonae Rhodii, 8vo

Spachius, Israel (1591), *Nomenclator scriptorum medicorum, hoc est, elenchus qui artem medicam suis scriptis illustrarunt, secundum locos communes ipsius medicinae conscriptus*, Frankfurt, ex officina typographica Martini Lechleri, impensis Nicolai Bassaei, 8vo

Sprat, Thomas (1667), *A history of the Royal Society*, London, T. R. for J. Martyn and J. Allestry, 4to

Struthius, Josephus (1602), *Ars sphygmica seu pulsuum doctrina super MCC annos perdita ... accessit Hieronymi Capivaccii De pulsibus elegans tractatus et Caspari Bauhini Introductio pulsuum synopsin continens*, Basle, impensis Ludovici Königs, 8vo

Stupanus, Johannes Nicolaus (1614), *Medicina theorica ex Hippocrate et Galeno Physiologicis, Pathologicis et Semeioticis, post diexodicam enarrationem summatim pro disputationibus ordinariis in theses contractas nunc demum aucta et correcta coniunctim edita*, Basle, typis Johannis Schroeteri, 8vo

Suterus, Jacobus (1584), *De rebus naturalibus dialogus*, Freiburg, typis Abrahami Gemperii, 8vo

Swineshead, Richard (1520), *Calculator*, ed. Victor Trincavellus, Venice, [Octavianus Scotus], fol.

Sydenham, Thomas (1848–50), *Works*, 2 vols., London

Sylvius, Jacobus (1539a), *Methodus sex librorum Galeni in differentiis et causis morborum et symptomatum in tabellas sex ordine suo coniecta paulo fusius, ne brevitas obscura lectorem remoretur et fallat. De signis omnibus medicis, hoc est, salubribus, insalubribus, et neutris, commentarius omnino necessarius medico futuro*, Paris, ex officina Christiani Wecheli, fol.

(1539b), *Ordo et ordinis ratio in legendis Hippocratis et Galeni libris*, Paris, ex officina Christiani Wecheli, fol.

(1554), *Methodus sex librorum Galeni in differentiis et causis morborum et symptomatum, in tabellas sex ordine suo coniecta paulo fusius, ne brevitas obscura lectorem remoretur et fallat. De signis omnibus medicis, hic est salubribus, insalubribus, et neutris, commentarius omnino necessarius medico futuro*, Venice, ex officina Erasmiana Vincentij Valgrisij, 8vo

Taisnierus, Joannes (1583), *Opus mathematicum octo libros complectens, sex priores libri absolutissimae cheiromantiae theoricam, praxim, doctrinam, artem et experientiam rarissimam continent, septimus physiognomiae dispositionem . . . octavus periaxiomata de faciebus signorum et quid sol in unaquaque domo existens natis polliceatur*, Cologne, apud Theodorum Baumium, fol.

Talpa, Petrus (1595), *Empiricus, sive indoctus medicus, dialogus*, Franeker, excudebat Aegidius Radaeus, 8vo

Taurellus, Nicolaus (1581), *Medicae praedictionis methodus*, Frankfurt, sumptibus Bernhardi Jobini per Johan[nem] Feyerabend, 4to

Telesio, Bernardino (1588), *Tractationum philosophicarum tomus unus, in quo continentur I. Philippi Mocenici universalium institutionum ad hominum perfectionem contemplationes II. Andreae Caesalpini quaestionum peripateticarum libri v III. Bernardini Telesii de rerum natura iuxta propria principia libri xi*, [Geneva], excudebat Eustathius Vignon, fol.

Thriverus, Hieremias (1592), *Universae medicinae brevissima absolutissimaque methodus*, Leiden, ex officina Plantiniana, apud Franciscum Raphelengium, 8vo

(1621), *see* Laurembergius 1621

Toletus, Franciscus (1615), *Commentaria una cum quaestionibus in octo libros Aristotelis de physica auscultatione*, Cologne, in officina Birckmannica, sumptibus Hermanni Mylii, 4to

Torrigiano, Pietro (1557), *Plusquam commentum in parvam Galeni artem Turisani*, ed. Julianus Martianus Rota, . . . *Hali qui eandem artem primum exposuit . . . Joannitii ad eandem introductio . . . Gentilis, qui primum eiusdem artis librum partim explicando, partim dubitando declaravit . . . Nicolai Leoniceni quaestio de tribus doctrinis, in capita divisa*, Venice, apud Iuntas, fol.

Tschoriderus, Ieremias (1609), *Exercitationes academicae duodecim*, Frankfurt an der Oder, typis Johannis Eichorn, 4to

Turquet de Mayerne, Théodore (1603), *Apologia in qua videre est immolatis Hippocratis et Galeni legibus, remedia chymice praeparata, tuto usurpari possi*, La Rochelle, [héritier de Jérôme Haultin], 8vo

Ulmus, Marcus Antonius (1603), *Hippocrates medicus*, Bologna, apud Jo[annem] Baptistam Bellagambam, 4to

Valerius, Cornelius (n.d.), *Anacephaleosis seu enumeratio capitum omnium totius artis dialecticae summam complectens digesta*, Antwerp, reproduced in Leon Voet, *The Plantin Press (1555–89)*, Amsterdam, 1982, v (illus. 50)

(1573), *Tabula totius dialectices*, Antwerp, ex officina Christophori Plantini, 8vo

Valleriola, Franciscus (1540), *Commentarii in sex Galeni libros de morbis*, Lyon, apud Sebastianum Gryphium, 8vo

(1554), *Enarrationum medicinalium libri sex*, Lyon, apud Sebastianum Gryphium, fol.

(1562), *Loci medicinae communes*, Lyon, apud haeredes Sebastiani Gryphii, fol.

(1573), *Observationum medicinalium libri sex*, Lyon, apud Antonium Gryphium, fol.

(1577), *Commentarii in librum Galeni De constitutione artis medicae*, Lyon, apud Carolum Pesnot, 8vo

Vallesius, Franciscus (1606), *Controversiarum medicarum et philosophicarum libri x*, Hanau, apud Claudium Marnem et haeredes Joanni Aubrij, fol.

Van Heurne, Jan, *see* Heurnius, Joannes

Varanda, Jean de (1620), *Physiologia et pathologia, quibus accesserunt eiusdem tractatus prognosticus; item tractatus de indicationibus curativis*, Montpellier, in officina Francisci Chouët, 8vo

Variolus, Constantinus (1591), *Anatomiae sive de resolutione corporis humani...libri iiii*, ed. Joannes Baptista Cortesius, Frankfurt, apud Joannem Wechelum et Petrum Fischerum consortes, 8vo

Vega, Christophorus a (1571), *Opera*, Lyon, apud Gulielmum Rouillium, fol.

Velcurio, Joannes (1553), *Commentarii in universam Physicam Aristotelis*, Tübingen, apud haeredes Ulrici Morhardi, 8vo

Velsius, Justus (1543), *Utrum in medico variarum artium et scientiarum cognitio requiratur*, Basle, ex officina Joannis Oporini, 4to

Verderius, Petrus (1600), *De morborum ac symptomatum causis occultis ac manifestis disputatio*, Venice, apud Robertum Meiettum 4to

Vettori, Benedetto, *see* Victorius, Benedictus

Vicomercatus, Franciscus (1596), *De principiis rerum naturalium libri tres*, Venice, apud Franciscum Bolzetam, 4to

Victorius, Benedictus (Faventinus) (1506), *Commentarii in tractatum proportionum Alberti de Saxonia*, Bologna, per Benedictum Hectoris, fol.

(1516), *Opus theorice latitudinum medicine ad libros tegni Galeni*, Bologna, in aedibus Benedicti Hectoris, fol.

366 Bibliography

(1551), *In Hippocratis Prognostica commentarii. Hic accessit theoricae latitudinum medicinae liber, ad Galeni scopum de arte medicinali*, Florence, apud Laurentium Torrentinum, fol.

(1598), *Medicationes empeiricae libri tres*, Frankfurt, typis Johannis Collizij sumptibus Johannis Theobaldi Schonvetteri, 8vo

(1628), *De curandis morbis ad tyrones practica magna*, ed. Petrus Uffenbachius, Frankfurt, impensis Johannis Theobaldi Schönwetteri, typis Erasmi Kempfferi, 8vo

Vigenère, Blaise de (1586), *Traicté des chiffres ou secretes manieres d'escrire*, Paris, chez Abel l'Angelier, 4to

Vimercato, Francisco, *see* Vicomercatus Franciscus

Viottus, Bartholomaeus (1560), *De demonstratione libri quinque*, Paris, apud Andream Wechelum, 8vo

Vives, Juan Luis (1555), *Opera*, 2 vols., Basle, per Nicolaum Episcopium iuniorem; apud Jacobum Parcum impensis Nicolai Episcopij iunioris, fol.

Waldungus, Wolfgangus [praeses] (1611), *Publica de monstris disputatio*, resp. Joannes Saubertus, Altdorf, apud Conradum Agricolam. 4to

Weckerus, Joannes Jacobus (1576), *Medicinae utriusque syntaxes*, Basle, ex officina Eusebii Episcopii, et Nicolai fr[atris] haeredum, fol.

(1604), *De secretis libri xvii*, Basle, typis Conradi Waldkirchii sumptibus Episcopianorum, 8vo

Weinrichius, Martinus (1595), *De ortu monstrorum commentarius, in qua essentia, differentiae, causae et affectiones mirabilium animalium explicantur*, Leipzig, sumptibus Henrici Osthusii, 8vo

Wierus, Joannes (1567), *Medicarum observationum rararum liber i*, Basle, in officina Oporiniana, 4to

Wildenbergius, Hieronymus (1585), *Totius philosophiae humanae in tres partes, nempe in rationalem, naturalem et moralem digesta*, Basle, ex officina Oporiniana, 8vo

Willichius, Jodocus (1538), *Physiognomica Aristotelis . . . additum est eiusdem interpretis oratio in laudem physiognomiae*, Wittenberg, excudebat Nicolaus Schirlentz, 8vo

(1582), *Urinarum probationes*, ed. Hieronymus Reusnerus, Basle, per Sebastianum Henricpetri, 8vo

Wittesteyn, Carolus (1588), *Vera totius medicinae forma*, Antwerp, ex officina Christophori Plantini, 8vo

Wolf, Joannes (1620), *Exercitationes semeioticae in Cl. Galeni de locis affectis libros vi*, Helmaestadi, typis haeredum Jacobi Lucii, 4to

Zabarella, Jacopo (1586–7), *Opera logica*, ed. Giulio Pace, [Heidelberg], apud Joannem Mareschallum [excudebat Joannes Wechelus], fol.

(1590), *De rebus naturalibus libri xxx*, Venice, apud Paulum Meietum, fol.

(1597), *Opera logica*, preface by Joannes Hawenreuter, Cologne, impensis Lazari Zetzneri, 4to

Zacchia, Paulo (1630), *Quaestiones medico-legales*, Leipzig, sumptibus Eliae Rehefeldii ex officina Friderici Lanckirsch [excudebat Gregorius Ritzsch], 8vo

Zaluzanius a Zaluzaniis, Adam (1606), *Animadversionum medicarum in Galenum et Avicennam libri vii, quibus singulae medicinae partes, ad totius artis logicae normam rediguntur*, Frankfurt, e Collegio Paltheniano, 8vo

Zeisoldus, Johannes, [praeses] (1638), *Teratoskopia seu contemplatio prodigiorum*, resp. Joachimus Sidelius, Jena, literis Ernesti Steinmanni, 4to

Zwinger, Jakob (1606), *Principiorum chymicorum examen ad generalem Hippocratis, Galeni caeterorumque Graecorum et Arabum consensum institutum*, Basle, apud Sebastianum Henricpetri, 8vo

Zwinger, Theodor (1561), *In artem medicinalem Galeni tabulae et commentarii*, Basle, per Joannem Oporinum, fol.

SECONDARY SOURCES

Agrimi, Jole and Crisciani, Chiara (1988), *Edocere medicos. Medicina scolastica nei secoli XIII–XV*, Naples

(1990), 'Per una ricerca su *experimentum-experimenta*: riflessione epistemologia e tradizione medica', in *Presenza del lessico greco e latino nelle lingue contemporanee*, ed. Pietro Janni and Innocenzo Mazzini, Macerata, pp. 9–49

(1994), *Les 'consilia' médicaux*, Turnhout

Amundsen, Darrel W. (1996), *Medicine, society and faith in the ancient and medieval worlds*, Baltimore and London

Arber, Agnes (1986), *Herbals: their origin and evolution; a chapter in the history of botany, 1470–1670*, ed. William T. Stearn, Cambridge

Armstrong, Elizabeth (1990), *Before copyright: the French book-privilege system 1498–1526*, Cambridge

Arrizabalaga, Jon (1998), *The Articella in the early press 1476–1534*, Cambridge

Arrizabalaga, Jon, Henderson, John, and French, R. K. (1997), *The great pox: the French disease in Renaissance Europe*, New Haven and London

Ashworth, E. J. (1988), 'Changes in logic textbooks from 1500 to 1650: the new Aristotelianism', in *Aristotle und Renaissance: In memoriam Charles B. Schmitt*, ed. Eckhard Kessler, Charles H. Lohr and Walter Sparn, Wiesbaden, pp. 75–89

(1990a), 'Domingo de Soto (1494–1560) and the doctrine of signs', in *De ortu grammaticae: studies in medieval grammar and linguistic theory in memory of Jan Pinborg*, ed. G. L. Bursill-Hall, Sten Ebbesen and K. Koerner, Amsterdam, pp. 35–48

Ashworth, Jnr, W. B. (1989), 'Light of reason, light of nature: Catholic and Protestant metaphors of scientific knowledge', *Science in Context*, 3, 89–107

(1990b), 'Natural history and the emblematic world view', in *Reappraisals of the scientific revolution*, ed. David C. Lindberg and Robert S. Westman, Cambridge, pp. 303–32

Baader, Gerhard, (1985), 'Jacques Dubois as a practitioner', in *The medical Renaissance of the sixteenth century*, ed. Andrew Wear, R. K. French and Iain M. Lonie, Cambridge, pp. 146–54

Bachelard, Gaston (1933), *Le Matérialisme rationnel*, 3rd edn, Paris

Backus, Irene (1989), 'The teaching of logic in two Protestant academies at the end of the sixteenth century: the reception of Zabarella in Strasbourg and Geneva', *Archiv für Reformationsgeschichte*, 80, 240–51

Baldi, Marialuisa and Canziano, Guido, eds. (1999), *Girolamo Cardano. Le opere, le fonti, la vita*, Milan

Baldini, Ugo (1997), 'Reflections on a changing field', in *Marcello Malpighi: anatomist and physician*, ed. Domenico Bertolini Meli, Florence, pp. 193–246

Barker, Peter (1997), 'Kepler's epistemology', in *Method and order in Renaissance philosophy of nature*, ed. Daniel A. Di Liscia, Eckhard Kessler and Charlotte Methuen, Aldershot, pp. 355–68

Barnes, Jonathan (1991), 'Galen on logic and therapy', in *Galen's method of healing*, ed. Fridolf Kudlien and Richard J. Durling, Leiden, New York, Copenhagen and Cologne, pp. 50–102

Barona, Josep Lluís (1993), *Sobre medicina y filosofía natural en el Renacimento*, Godella
  (1994), *Ciencia e historia: debates y tendencias en la historiografía de la ciencia*, Godella

Barondess, J. A. (1986), 'Diagnosis', in *The Oxford Companion to Medicine*, ed. John Walton and Paul B. Beeston, Oxford, pp. 308–11

Barton, Tamsyn (1994), *Power and knowledge: astrology, physiognomics and medicine under the Roman Empire*, Ann Arbor

Bates, Don (1998), 'Closing the circle: how Harvey and his contemporaries played the game of truth', *History of Science*, 36, 213–32; 36, 245–67

Bates, Don, ed. (1995), *Knowledge and the scholarly medical traditions*, Cambridge

Baudrier, Henri Louis (1895–1921), *Bibliographie lyonnaise*, 12 vols., Lyon

Beck, Eric R., Francis, John L., and Souhami, Robert L. (1974), *Tutorials in differential diagnosis*, London

Béhar, Pierre (1996), *Les Langues occultes de la Renaissance: essai sur la crise intellectuelle de l'Europe au XVIe siècle*, Paris

Bennett, Jim (1998), 'Operative knowledge', *Configurations*, 6, 195–222

Bergdolt, Klaus (1992), *Arzt, Krankheit und Therapie bei Petrarca*, Weinheim

Bertolaso, B. (1959–60), 'Ricerche d'archivio su alcuni aspetti dell'insegnamento medico presso l'Università di Padova nel cinque- e seicento', *Acta medicae historiae patavina*, 6, 17–38

Bertolis, G. de (1956–7), 'Alessandro Benedetti: il primo teatro anatomico padovano', *Acta medicae historiae patavina*, 3, 1–14

Bianchi, Massimo Luigi (1987), *Signatura rerum: segni, magia e cognoscenza da Paracelso a Leibniz*, Rome

Biraben, Jean-Noël (1975–6), *Les Hommes et la peste en France et dans les pays européens et méditerranéens*, 2 vols., Paris and The Hague

Blackwell, Constance and Kusukawa, Sachiko, eds. (1999), *Philosophy in the sixteenth and seventeenth centuries: conversations with Aristotle*, Aldershot

Blair, Ann (1997), *The theater of nature: Jean Bodin and Renaissance science*, Princeton
  (1999), 'The problemata as a natural philosophical genre', in *Natural particulars: nature and the disciplines in Renaissance Europe*, ed. Anthony Grafton and Nancy Siraisi, Cambridge, Mass. and London, pp. 171–204

(2000), 'Mosaic physics and the search for a pious natural philosophy in the late Renaissance', *Isis*, 91, 32–58

Blum, Paul Richard (1992), 'Qualitates occultae: zur philosophischen Vorgeschichte eines Schlüsselbegriffs zwischen Okkultismus und Wissenschaft', in *Die okkulten Wissenschaften in der Renaissance*, ed. August Buck, Wiesbaden, pp. 45–64

Blum, Paul Richard, ed. (1999), *Sapientiam amemus: Humanismus und Aristotelismus in der Renaissance: Festschrift für Eckhard Kessler*, Munich

Blumenberg, Hans (1989), *Die Lesbarkeit der Welt*, Frankfurt

Bogner, Ralf-Georg (1994), 'Paracelsus auf dem Index', in *Analecta Paracelsica*, ed. Joachim Telle, Stuttgart, pp. 489–530

Boh, Ivan (1982), 'Consequences', in *The Cambridge history of later medieval philosophy*, ed. Norman Kretzmann, Anthony Kenny and Jan Pinborg, Cambridge, pp. 300–15

Bono, James J. (1995), *The Word of God and the languages of man: interpreting nature in early modern science and culture*, vol. 1, Madison

Bonuzzi, Luciano (1975–6), 'Galilei e la medicina padovana', *Acta medicae historiae patavina*, 22, 33–6

Boriaud, Jean-Yves (1999), 'La Place du *Traité des songes* dans la tradition oniro-critique. Le problème de l'image onirocritique', in *Girolamo Cardano. Le opere, le fonti, la vita*, ed. Marialuisa Baldi and Guido Canziano, Milan, pp. 215–26

Bos, Gerrit and Burnett, Charles (1998), *Scientific weather forecasting in the Middle Ages: the writings of Al Kindi*, London and New York

Bosatra, Andrea (1955–6), 'British doctors at Padua University', *Acta medicae historiae patavina*, 2, 1–14

Brigi, B. and Andrich, A. (1892), *Rotulus et matricula dd iuristarum et artistarum Gymnasii Patavini anno 1592–3*, Padua

Brockliss, Laurence (1993), 'Seeing and believing: contrasting attitudes towards observational autonomy among French Galenists in the first half of the seventeenth century', in *Medicine and the five senses*, ed. Roy Porter and W. F. Bynum, Cambridge, pp. 63–84

Brockliss, Laurence and Jones, Colin (1997), *The medical world of early modern France*, Oxford

Bruyère, Nelly (1984), *Méthode et dialectique dans l'œuvre de La Ramée*, Paris

Buck, August, ed. (1992), *Die okkulten Wissenschaften in den Renaissance*, Wiesbaden

Burnett, Charles (1999), 'Al-Kindi in the Renaissance', in *Sapientiam amemus: Humanismus und Aristotelismus in der Renaissance: Festschrift für Eckhard Kessler*, ed. Paul Richard Blum, Munich, pp. 13–30

Burnett, Charles and Mendelsohn, Andrew (1997), 'Aristotle and Averroes on method in the Middle Ages and the Renaissance: the "Oxford gloss" to the *Physics* and Pietro d'Afeltro's *Expositio proemii Averroys*', in *Method and order in Renaissance philosophy of nature*, ed. Daniel A. Di Liscia, Eckhard Kessler and Charlotte Methuen, Aldershot, pp. 53–111

Burnyeat, M. F. (1982), 'The origins of non-deductive inference', in *Science and speculation: studies in Hellenistic theory and practice*, ed. Jonathan Barnes,

Jacques Brunschvig, M. F. Burnyeat and Malcolm Schofield, Cambridge, pp. 193–238

(1994), 'Enthymeme: Aristotle on the logic of persuasion', in *Aristotle's Rhetoric: philosophical essays*, ed. David J. Furley and Alexander Nehamas, Princeton, pp. 3–53

(unpublished), 'Other minds, other faces: philosophy and physiognomonics in the ancient world'

Bylebyl, Jerome J. (1971), 'Galen on the non-natural causes of variation in the pulse', *Bulletin of the History of Medicine*, 45, 482–5

(1979), 'The School of Padua: humanistic medicine in the sixteenth century', in *Health, medicine and mortality in the sixteenth century*, ed. Charles Webster, Cambridge, 1979, pp. 335–70

(1985a), 'Disputation and description in the Renaissance pulse controversy', in *The medical Renaissance of the sixteenth century*, ed. A. Wear, R. K. French and Iain M. Lonie, Cambridge, pp. 223–45

(1985b), 'Medicine, philosophy, and humanism in Renaissance Italy', in *Science and the arts in the Renaissance*, ed. J. W. Shirley and F. D. Hoeniger, Washington D.C. and London, pp. 27–49.

(1990), 'The medical meaning of "physician"', *Osiris*, 2nd series, 6, 15–41

(1991), 'Teaching *Methodus Medendi* in the Renaissance', in *Galen's method of healing*, ed. F. Kudlien and Richard J. Durling, Leiden, pp. 157–89

Bynum, W. F. and Porter, Roy (1993), *Companion encyclopaedia of the history of medicine*, London and New York

Cadden, Joan (1986), 'Medieval scientific and medical views of sexuality: questions of propriety', *Medievalia et humanistica*, n.s., 14, 157–71

(1998), 'Just like a woman: authority and comparison in the anatomy of an argument', paper circulated at the conference of the Max-Planck-Institut für Wissenschaftsgeschichte on Demonstration, Test, Proof

Canziani, Guido (1988), 'Causalité et analogie dans la théorie physiognomique', *Revue des Sciences Philosophiques et Théologiques*, 72, 209–25

Carlino, Andrea (1994a), 'Corpi di carta. Fogli volanti e diffusione delle conoscenze anatomiche nell'Europa moderna', *Physis*, 31, 731–69

(1994b), *La fabbrica del corpo: Libri e dissezione ne Rinascimento*, Turin

(1995), '"Knowe Thyself". Graphic communication and anatomical knowledge in early modern Europe', *Res*, 27, 52–69

(1999a), *Books of the body: anatomical ritual and Renaissance learning*, Chicago

(1999b), *Paper bodies: a catalogue of anatomical fugitive sheets 1538–1687*, London

Caroti, Stefano (1983), *L'astrologia in Italia*, Rome

Carruthers, Mary (1997), *The book of memory*, Cambridge

Cassirer, Ernst (1963), *The individual and the cosmos in Renaissance philosophy*, trans. Mario Domandi, New York and Evanston

Céard, Jean (1994), 'Inventions et inventeurs selon Polydore Vergile', in *Inventions et découvertes au temps de la Renaissance*, ed. M. T. Jones-Davies, Paris, pp. 109–22

(1996), *La Nature et les prodiges: l'insolite au XVIe siècle*, Geneva

Ceseracciu, Elda Veronese (1978), 'Spagnoli e portughesi all'Università di Padova nel ventenno 1490–1510', *Quaderni per la storia dell'università di Padova*, 11, 39–86

Chapman, Alan (1979), 'Astrological medicine', in *Health, medicine and mortality in the sixteenth century*, ed. Charles Webster, Cambridge, pp. 275–300

Chaunu, Pierre and Gascon, Richard (1977), *Histoire économique st sociale de la France*, vol. 1, part 1, Paris

Christie, J. R. R. (1998), 'The Paracelsian body', in *Paracelsus: the man and his reputation, his ideas and their transformation*, ed. Ole Peter Grell, Leiden, Boston, Cologne, pp. 270–91

Clark, Michael and Crawford, Catherine (1994), *Legal Medicine in History*, Cambridge

Clark, Stuart (1983), 'French historians and early modern culture', *Past and Present*, 100, 62–99

   (1997), *Thinking with demons: the idea of witchcraft in early modern Europe*, Oxford

Clulee, Nicholas H. (1971), 'John Dee's mathematics and the grading of compound qualities', *Ambix*, 18, 178–211

   (1984), 'At the crossroads of magic and science: John Dee's Archemastrie', in *Scientific and Occult Mentalities in the Renaissance*, ed. Brian Vickers, Cambridge, pp. 57–72

Cochrane, Eric (1976), 'Science and humanism in the Italian Renaissance', *Historical Review*, 81, 1039–57

Cohen, L. Jonathan (1980), 'Some historical remarks on the Baconian conception of probability', *Journal of the History of Ideas*, 41, 219–31

Conan Doyle, Arthur (1950), *The memoirs of Sherlock Holmes*, Harmondsworth

Conrad, Laurence I., Neve, Michael, Nutton, Vivian, Porter, Roy, and Wear, Andrew (1995), *The Western medical tradition 800 BC to AD 1800*, Cambridge

Cooper, Richard (1987), 'Bibliographie sommaire d'ouvrages sur le songe publiés en France et en Italie jusqu'en 1600', in *Le songe à la Renaissance: colloque international de Cannes 29–31 mai 1987*, Saint-Etienne, pp. 255–71

Copenhaver, Brian P. (1978), *Symphorien Champier and the reception of the occultist tradition in Renaissance France*, The Hague, Paris, New York

   (1988), 'Astrology and magic', in *The Cambridge history of Renaissance philosophy*, ed. Charles B.Schmitt and Quentin Skinner, pp. 264–300

   (1992), 'Did science have a Renaissance?', *Isis*, 83, 387–407

Copenhaver, Brian P. and Schmitt, Charles B. (1992), *Renaissance philosophy*, Oxford

Cranefield, Paul (1970), 'On the origin of the phrase "Nihil est in intellectu quod non prius fuerit in sensu"', *Journal of the History of Medicine*, 25, 77–80

Cranz, F. Edward (1976), 'Editions of the Latin Aristotle accompanied by the commentaries of Averroes', in *Philosophy and humanism*, ed. E. P. Mahoney, Leiden, pp. 117–28

Cranz, F. Edward and Schmitt, Charles B. (1984), *A bibliography of Aristotle editions 1501–1600*, Baden-Baden

Crawford, C. (1994), 'Legalizing medicine: early modern legal systems and the growth of medico-legal knowledge', in *Legal medicine in history*, ed. C. Crawford and M. Clark, Cambridge, pp. 89–116

Crisciani, Chiara (1990), 'History, novelty, and progress in scholastic medicine', *Osiris*, 2nd series, 6, 118–39

    (1996a), 'Alchemy and medicine in the Middle Ages: recent studies and projects of research', *Bulletin de Philosophie Médiévale*, 38, 9–21

    (1996b), 'L'individuale nella medicina tra medioevo e umanesimo: i "consilia"', in *Umanesimo e medicina: il problema dell'"individuale"*, ed. Roberto Cardini and Mariangela Regoliosi, Rome, pp. 1–32

    (1998), 'Esperienza, comunicazione e scrittura in alchimia (secolo XIII–XIV)', in *Le forme della comunicazione scientifica*, ed. Massimo Galuzzi, Gianni Michele and Maria Teresa Monti, Milan, pp. 85–110

Crombie, A. C. (1994), *Styles of scientific thinking in the European tradition*, London

Culler, Jonathan (1975), *Structuralist poetics*, London and Henley

Cunningham, Andrew (1985), 'Fabricius and the "Aristotle project" in anatomical teaching and research at Padua', in *The medical Renaissance of the sixteenth century*, ed. A. Wear, R. K. French and Iain M. Lonie, Cambridge, pp. 195–222

    (1992), 'Transforming plague: the laboratory and the identity of infectious disease', in *The laboratory revolution in medicine*, ed. Andrew Cunningham and Perry Williams, Cambridge, pp. 209–44

    (1997), *The anatomical Renaissance*, Aldershot

Cunningham, Andrew, and Williams, Perry, eds. (1992), *The laboratory revolution in medicine*, Cambridge

Dale, Henry Hallett (1962), *A catalogue of printed books in the Wellcome Historical Medical Library 1: Books printed before 1641*, London

Daston, Lorraine (1988), *Classical probability in the Enlightenment*, Princeton

    (1997), *Recherches en l'épistémologie historique des sciences: empirisme et objectivité*, Max-Planck-Institut für Wissenschaftsgeschichte, Berlin, preprint 64

    (2000), 'Can scientific objectivity have a history?', *Alexander von Humboldt Stiftung Mitteilungen*, 75, 31–40

Daston, Lorraine and Park, Katharine (1998), *Wonders and the order of nature, 1150–1750*, New York

Davis, Natalie Zemon (1975), *Society and culture in early modern France*, London

De Renzi, Silvia (forthcoming), 'Nature brought to trial: judges, physicians and the Tribunal of the Sacra Rota in seventeenth-century Rome'

Dear, Peter (1987), 'Jesuit mathematical science and the reconstitution of experience in the early seventeenth century', *Studies in the History and Philosophy of Science*, 18, 131–75

    (1990), 'Miracles, experiments and the ordinary course of nature', *Isis*, 81, 663–83

    (1995), *Discipline and experience: the mathematical way in the Scientific Revolution*, Chicago and London

Debus, Allen G. (1977), *The chemical philosophy*, New York

(1991), *The French Paracelsians. The chemical challenge to medical and scientific tradition in early modern France*, Cambridge, New York, Port Chester, Melbourne and Sydney

Debus, Arnelle (1999), 'The classical origins of medical ethics', *European Review* 7.4, 479–85

Demonet, Marie-Luce (1992), *Les Voix du signe: nature et origine du langage à la Renaissance: 1480–1580*, Paris and Geneva

(1994), '*Si les signes vous fâchent*. . .: inférence naturelle et science des signes à la Renaissance', *Renaissance, Humanisme, Réforme*, 38, 7–44

(1995), 'Les Marques insensibles ou les nuages de la certitude', *Littératures Classiques*, 25, 97–134

(2001), 'Les Signes probables (*eikota*) au temps de Montaigne', *Bibliothèque d'Humanisme et Renaissance*, 64, 7–29

(forthcoming), 'Du signe au symptôme: la séméiotique d'Ambroise Paré', in *Actes du colloque Ambroise Paré*, ed. Evelyne Berriot-Salvatore

Derrida, Jacques (1967), *De la grammatologie*, Paris

Des Chene, Dennis (1996), *Physiologia: natural philosophy in late Aristotelian and Cartesian thought*, Ithaca and London

Dewhurst, Kenneth (1966), *Dr Thomas Sydenham (1624–89): his life and original writings*, London

Di Liscia, Daniel A., Kessler, Eckhard and Methuen, Charlotte, eds. (1997), *Method and order in Renaissance philosophy of nature*, Aldershot

Dilg, Peter (1991), 'Johann Agricola Ammonius' Kommentar zu Galens *Methodus medendi*', in *Galen's method of healing*, ed. Fridolf Kudlien and Richard J. Durling, Leiden, New York, Copenhagen and Cologne, pp. 190–8

Dulieu, Louis (1979), *La Médecine à Montpellier. II. La Renaissance*, Avignon

Durling, Richard J. (1961), 'A chronological census of Renaissance editions and translations of Galen', *Journal of the Warburg and Courtauld Institutes*, 24, 230–305

(1990), 'Girolamo Mercuriale's *De modo studendi*', *Osiris*, 2nd series, 6, 181–95

Eamon, William (1993), '"With the rules of life and an enema": Leonardo Fioravanti's medical primitivism', in *Renaissance and revolution: humanists, scholars, craftsmen and natural philosophers in early modern Europe*, ed. J. V. Field and Frank A. J. L. James, Cambridge, pp. 29–44

(1994), *Science and the secrets of nature. Books of secrets in early modern culture*, Princeton

Eckart, Wolfgang U. (1992), 'Antiparacelsismus, okkulte Qualitäten und medizinisch-wissenschaftliches Erkennen im Werk Daniel Sennerts', in *Die okkulten Wissenschaften in der Renaissance*, ed. August Buck, Wiesbaden, pp. 139–58

(1998), 'Philipp Melanchthon und die Medizin', in *Melanchthon und die Naturwissenschaften*, ed. Günter Frank und Stefan Rhein, Sigmaringen, 1998, pp. 183–202

Edgerton, Jnr, Samuel Y., (1980), 'The Renaissance artist as quantifier', in *The perception of pictures*, ed. Margaret A. Hagen, New York, I.179–212

(1985), 'The Renaissance development of scientific illustration', in *Science and arts in the Renaissance*, ed. J. W. Shirley and F. D. Hoeniger, Washington D.C. and London, pp. 168–97

Edwards, W. F. (1976), 'Leoniceno and humanist discussion of method', in *Philosophy and humanism*, ed. E. P. Mahoney, Leiden, 1976, pp. 283–305

Efron, John M. (1998), 'Interminably maligned: the conventional lies about Jewish doctors', in *Jewish history and Jewish memory*, ed. Elisheva Carlebach, John M. Efron and David N. Myers, Hanover, N. H. and London, pp. 296–310

Eisenhardt, Ulrich (1970), *Die kaiserliche Aufsicht über Buchdruck, Buchhandel und Presse im Heiligen Römischen Reich Deutscher Nation (1496–1806)*, Karlsruhe

Eisenstein, Elizabeth (1979), *The printing press as an agent of change*, Cambridge

Engel, Pascal (1990), 'Interpretation without hermeneutics: a plea against ecumenism', *Topoi*, 10, 137–46.

Evans, M. (1980), 'The geometry of the mind', *Architectural Association Quarterly*, 12.4, 32–55

Evans. R. J. W. (1975), *The Wechel presses: humanism and Calvinism in central Europe 1572–1627*, *Past and Present*, supplement no. 2, Oxford

(1981), 'German Universities after the Thirty Years War', *History of Universities*, 1, 169–90

Fabian, Bernhard, ed. (1972–8), *Die Messkataloge des sechzehnten Jahrhunderts 1564–92*, Hildesheim and New York

Ferrari, Giovanna, (1976), 'Public anatomy lessons and the carnival', *Past and Present*, 73, 50–106

Fichtner, Gerhard (1972–3), 'Padova e Tübingen: la formazione medica nei secoli XVI e XVII', *Acta medicae historiae patavina*, 19, 43–62

Field, J. V. and James, Frank A. J. L. (1993), *Renaissance and revolution: humanists, scholars, craftsmen and natural philosophers in early modern Europe*, Cambridge

Findlen, Paula (1990), 'Jokes of nature and jokes of knowledge: the playfulness of scientific discourse in Early Modern Europe', *Renaissance Quarterly*, 43, 292–331

(1994), *Possessing nature: museums, collecting and scientific culture in Early Modern Italy*, Berkeley

(1996), 'Courting nature', in *Cultures of natural history*, ed. N. Jardine, J. A. Secord and E. C. Spary, Cambridge, pp. 57–74

(1999), 'The formation of a scientific community: natural history in sixteenth-century Italy', in *Natural particulars*, ed. Anthony Grafton and Nancy Siraisi, pp. 369–400

Fleck, Ludwik (1979), *Genesis and development of a scientific fact*, trans. Thaddeus J. Trenn, introd. Thomas S. Kuhn, Chicago and London

Flood, John L. (forthcoming), *The English sweating sickness of 1529 on the continent*

Flood, John L. and Kelly, W. A., eds. (1995), *The German book, 1450–1750: studies presented to David L. Paisey*, London

Flood, John L. and Shaw, David J. (1997), *Johannes Sinapius (1505–1560): hellenist and physician in Germany and Italy*, Geneva

Fondscatalogus (1988–9), *Plantins Fondscatalogus uit 1567*, ed. Chris Coppens, *De gulden Passer*, 66–7, 277–99

Foucault, Michel (1966), *Les Mots et les choses*, Paris

Franklin, James (2000), 'Diagrammatic reasoning and modelling in the imagination: the secret weapons of the Scientific Revolution', in *1543 and All That: image and word, change and continuity in the proto-scientific revolution*, ed. Guy Freeland and Anthony Corones, London, Dordrecht, Boston, pp. 53–115

Freedman, Joseph S. (1988), *European academic philosophy in the late sixteenth and early seventeenth centuries: the life, significance, and philosophy of Clemens Timpler (1563/4–1624)*, Hildesheim, Zürich and New York

Freeland, Guy and Corones, Anthony (2000), *1543 and All That: image and word, change and continuity in the proto-scientific revolution*, London, Dordrecht, Boston

French, R. K. (1979), 'A note on the anatomical accessus of the Middle Ages', *Medical History*, 23, 461–8

(1985a), 'Berengario da Carpi and the use of commentary in anatomical teaching', in *The medical Renaissance of the sixteenth century*, ed. A. Wear, R. K. French and Iain M. Lonie, Cambridge, pp. 42–74

(1985b), 'Gentile da Foligno and the via medicorum', in *The light of nature: essays in the history and philosophy of science presented to A. C. Crombie*, ed. J. D. North and J. J. Roche, Dordrecht, pp. 21–34

(1993), 'The medical ethics of Gabriele de Zerbi', in *Doctors and ethics: the earlier historical setting of professional ethics*, ed. Andrew Wear, Johanna Geyer-Kordesch and R. K. French, Amsterdam, pp. 72–97

(1994), *William Harvey's natural philosophy*, Cambridge

French, R. K., and Arrizabalaga, Jon (1998), 'Coping with the French disease: university practitioners' strategies and tactics in the transition from the fifteenth to the sixteenth century', in *Medicine from the Black Death to the French disease*, ed. R. K. French, Jon Arrizabalaga, Andrew Cunningham and Luis García Ballester. Aldershot, pp. 248–87

French, R. K., Arrizabalaga, John, Cunningham Andrew and GarcíaBallester, Luis, eds. (1998), *Medicine from the Black Death to the French disease*, Aldershot

Friedensburg, Walter (1926), *Urkundenbuch der Universität Wittenberg I: 1502–1611*, Magdeburg

Fuggles, John (1975), 'A history of the library of St John's College, Oxford', unpublished Oxford B.Litt. thesis

Gabbey, Alan (1993), 'Between *ars* and *philosophia naturalis*: reflections on the historiography of early modern mechanics', in *Renaissance and revolution: humanists, scholars, craftsmen and natural philosophers in early modern Europe*, ed. J. V. Field and Frank A. J. L. James, Cambridge, pp. 133–45

Gadamer, Hans Robert (1962), *Wahrheit und Methode*, Tübingen

(1979), *Truth and method*, trans. W. Glen-Doepel, London

Gambacorta, G., and Giordano, A. (1983), *Regimen sanitatis salernitanum: bibliographia*, Milan

García Ballester, Luis (1981), 'Galen as a medical practitioner: problems in diagnosis', in *Galen: problems and prospects*, ed. Vivian Nutton, London, pp. 13–46

(1988), 'Soul and body, disease of the soul and disease of the body in Galen's medical thought', in *Le opere psicologiche di Galeno*, ed. Paola Manuli and Mario Vegetti, Pavia, pp. 117–52

(1993a), 'The Inquisition and minority medical practitioners in Counter-Reformation Spain: Judaizing and Morisco practitioners 1560–1610', in *Medicine and the Reformation*, ed. Ole Peter Grell and Andrew Cunningham, London and New York, pp. 156–91

(1993b), 'Medical ethics in transition in the Latin Medicine of the thirteenth and fourteenth centuries: new perspectives on the physician–patient relationship and the doctor's fee', in *Doctors and ethics: the earlier historical setting of professional ethics*, ed. Andrew Wear, Johanna Geyer-Kordesch and R. K. French, Amsterdam, pp. 38–71

(1993c), 'On the origins of the "Six non-natural things" in Galen', in *Galen und das hellenistische Erbe*, ed. Jutta Kollesch and Diethard Nickel, Stuttgart, pp. 105–15

(1995), 'Artifex factivus sanitatis: health and medical care in medieval Latin Galenism', in *Knowledge and the scholarly medical traditions*, ed. Don Bates, Cambridge, pp. 127–50

Garin, Eugenio (1983), *Astrology in the Renaissance: the zodiac of life*, trans. Carolyn Jackson and June Allen, revised by Eugenio Garin and Clare Robertson, London, Boston, Melbourne and Henley

Garin, Eugenio, ed. (1947), *La disputa delle arti*, Florence

Geertz, Clifford (1973), *The interpretation of cultures*, New York

Gehl, Paul F. (1997), 'Credit sales strategies in the late cinquecento book trade', in *Libri, tipografi, biblioteche; ricerche storiche dedicate a Luigi Balsamo*, Florence, pp. 193–206

Gentilcore, David (1993), 'The church, the Devil, and the healing activities of living saints in the Kingdom of Naples after the Council of Trent', in *Medicine and the Reformation*, ed. Ole Peter Grell and Andrew Cunningham, London and New York, pp. 134–55

(1995), 'Contesting illness in early modern Naples: miracolati, physicians and the Congregation of Rites', *Past and Present*, 148, 117–48

Gilbert, Neil W. (1960), *Renaissance concepts of method*, New York

Gillespie, C. C., ed. (1970–80), *The dictionary of scientific biography*, 16 vols., New York

Glucker, John (1995), '*Probabile, veri simile* and related terms', in *Cicero the philosopher*, ed. J. G. F. Powell, Oxford, pp. 115–44

Goldammer, Kurt (1991), *Der göttliche Magier und die Magierien Natur. Religion, Naturmagie und die Anfänge der Naturwissenschaft vom Spätmittelalter bis zur Renaissance*, Stuttgart

Göpfert, Herbert G., Vodosek, Peter, Weyrauch, Erdmann and Wittmann, Reinhard, eds. (1985), *Beiträge zur Geschichte des Buchwesens im konfessionellen Zeitalter*, Wiesbaden

Goyet, Francis (1996), *Le Sublime du "lieu commun": l'invention rhétorique dans l'Antiquité et à la Renaissance*, Paris

Grafton, Anthony (1998), 'Girolamo Cardano and the tradition of classical astrology', *Proceedings of the American Philosophical Society*, 142, 323–54

(1999), *Cardano's cosmos: the worlds and works of a Renaissance astrologer*, Cambridge, Mass. and London

Grafton, Anthony, and Siraisi, Nancy G. (forthcoming), 'Between the election and my hopes: Girolamo Cardano and medical astrology', *Archimedes*

Grafton, Anthony, and Siraisi, Nancy, eds. (1999), *Natural particulars: nature and the disciplines in Renaissance Europe*, Cambridge, Mass. and London

Grant, Edward (1978), 'Aristotelianism and the longevity of the medieval world view', *History of Science*, 16, 93–106

(1996), *The foundations of modern science in the Middle Ages*, Cambridge

Gregory, Tullio (1988), 'Forme di conoscenza e ideali di sapere nella cultura medievale', *Giornale critico della filosofia italiana*, 67, 1–62

Grell, Ole Peter (1993), 'Caspar Bartholin and the education of a pious physician', in *Medicine and the Reformation*, ed. Ole Peter Grell and Andrew Cunningham, London and New York, pp. 78–100

Grell, Ole Peter, ed. (1998), *Paracelsus: the man and his reputation, his ideas and their transformation*, Leiden, Boston, Cologne

Grell, Ole Peter and Cunningham, Andrew, eds. (1993), *Medicine and the Reformation*, London and New York

Gremer, Mirko D., and Fantini, Bernadino (1995), *Histoire de la pensée médicale en occident: l'antiquité et moyen âge*, Sens

Grendler, Paul F. (1977), *The Roman Inquisition and the Venetian press 1540–1605*, Princeton

Guerlac, Henri de (1978), 'Amicus Plato and other friends', *Journal of the History of Ideas*, 39, 627–33

Gunther, R. T. (1921), 'The row of books of Nicholas Gibbard of Oxford', *Annales of Medical History*, 3, 324–6

Hacking, Ian (1975), *The emergence of probability*, Cambridge

(1990), *The taming of chance*, Cambridge

(1999), *Mad travelers*, Charlottesville and London

Hale, J. R. and Highfield, J. R. L. (1965), *Europe in the late Middle Ages*, London

Hallyn, Fernand (1995), 'Une "feintise"', in *Les Olympiques de Descartes*, ed. Fernand Hallyn, Geneva, pp. 91–111

Hankinson, Robert James (1994), 'Galen on the use and abuse of language', in *Language*, ed. Stephen Everson, Cambridge, pp. 166–87

(1995), 'The growth of medical empiricism', in *Knowledge and the scholarly medical traditions*, ed. Don Bates, Cambridge, pp. 60–83

Hannaway, Owen (1975), *The chemists and the word: the didactic origins of chemistry*, Baltimore and London

Hase, Martin von (1968), *Bibliographie der Erfurter Drucke von 1501–1550*, Nieuwkoop

Heath, Terrence (1971), 'Logical grammar, grammatical logic, and humanism in three German universities', *Studies in the Renaissance*, 18, 9–64

Hecht, Louis-Emile (1864–86), 'Le Diagnostic ou la diagnose', in *Dictionnaire encyclopédique des sciences médicales*, ed. A. Dechambre, 100 vols., Paris, 2.28, pp. 685–93

Helbing, Mario Otto (1989), *La filosofia di Francesco Buonamici*, Pisa

Helm, Jürgen (1998), 'Die "spiritus" in der medizinalhistorischen Tradition und in Melanchthons "Liber de anima"', in *Melanchthon und die Naturwissenschaften*, ed. Günter Frank and Stefan Rhein, Sigmaringen, pp. 219–38

Henry, John (1997), *The Scientific Revolution and the origins of modern science*, Basingstoke

Henry, John and Hutton, Sarah, eds. (1990), *New perspectives on Renaissance thought: essays in the history of science, education and philosophy in memory of Charles B. Schmitt*, London

Herberger, Maximilian (1981), *Dogmatik: zur Geschichte von Begriff und Methode in Medizin und Jurisprudenz*, Frankfurt

Hieronymus, Frank (1995), 'Physicians and publishers: the translations of medical works in sixteenth-century Basle', in *The German book 1450–1750*, ed. John L. Flood and William A. Kelly, London, pp. 95–110

    (1997), *1488 Petri: Schwabe 1988: eine traditionsreiche Basler Offizin im Spiegel ihrer frühen Drucke*, Basle

Hirsch, Rudolf (1967), *Printing, selling and reading 1450–1550*, Wiesbaden

Höltgen, Karl Josef (1965), 'Synoptische Tabellen in der medizinischen Literatur und die Logik Agricolas und Ramus', *Sudhoffs Archiv*, 49, 371–90.

Horden, Peregrine (ed.) (2000), *Music as medicine: the history of music therapy since antiquity*, Aldershot, Brookfield, Singapore and Sydney

Hudson, Robert P. (1983), *Disease and its control: the shaping of modern thought*, London and Westport

Husner, Fritz (1942), *Verzeichnis der Baseler Medizinischen Universitätsschriften von 1575–1829*, Basle

Hutchinson, Keith (1982), 'What happened to occult qualities in the Scientific Revolution?', *Isis*, 73, 233–53

Iliffe, Rob (1998), 'Rational artistry: Crombie's Magnum Opus', *History of Science*, 36, 329–57

Ingegno, Alfonso (1988), 'The new philosophy of nature', in *The Cambridge history of Renaissance philosophy*, ed. Charles B. Schmitt and Quentin Skinner, pp. 236–63

Iskandar, A. Z. (1976), 'An attempted reconstruction of the late Alexandrian medical curriculum', *Medical History*, 20, 235–58

Jacquart, Danielle (1998), *La Médecine médiévale dans le cadre parisien, XIVe–XVe siècle*, Paris

Jardine, Lisa (1974), *Francis Bacon: discovery and the art of discourse*, Cambridge

Jardine, Nicholas (1988), 'Epistemology of the sciences', in *The Cambridge history of Renaissance philosophy*, ed. Charles B. Schmitt and Quentin Skinner, Cambridge, pp. 685–711

    (1997), 'Keeping order in the School of Padua: Jacopo Zabarella and Francesco Piccolomini on the offices of philosophy', in *Method and order in Renaissance philosophy of nature*, ed. Daniel A. Di Liscia, Eckhard Kessler and Charlotte Methuen, Aldershot, pp. 183–210

Jardine, Nicholas and Frasca-Spada, Marina (1997), 'Splendours and miseries of the science wars', *Studies in the History and Philosophy of Science*, 28, 219–35

Jardine, Nicholas and Segonds, Alain (1999), 'Kepler as reader and translator of Aristotle', in *Philosophy in the sixteenth and seventeenth centuries: conversations with Aristotle*, ed. Constance Blackwell and Sachiko Kusukawa, Aldershot, pp. 206–33

Jensen, Kristian (1990), *Rhetorical philosophy and philosophical grammar: Julius Caesar Scaliger's theory of language*, Munich

(2000), 'Description, division, definition – Caesalpinus and the study of plants as an independent discipline', in *Renaissance readings of the corpus Aristotelicum*, ed. Marianne Pade, Copenhagen, pp. 185–206

Jones, J. W. (1940), *Historical introduction to the theory of law*, Oxford

Jones, Peter Murray (2000), 'Medical libraries and medical Latin', in *Medical Latin from the late middle ages to the eighteenth century*, ed. Wouter Bracke and Herwig Deumens, Brussels, pp. 115–36

Joutsivuo, Timo (1999), *Scholastic tradition and humanist innovation: the concept of neutrum in Renaissance medicine*, Helsinki

Kantola, Ilkka (1994), *Probability and moral uncertainty in late medieval and early modern times*, Helsinki

Kapp, Friedrich (1886), *Geschichte des deutschen Buchhandels*, Leipzig

Keil, Gundolf (1992), '*Virtus occulta*: der Begriff des "empiricum" bei Nikolaus von Polen', in *Die okkulten Wissenschaften in der Renaissance*, ed. August Buck, Wiesbaden, pp. 159–96

(2000), 'Zwei altdeutsche Übersetzungen der *Diaetae particulares* von Isaak Judäs', in *Medical Latin from the late Middle Ages to the eighteenth century*, ed. Wouter Bracke and Herwig Deumens, Brussels, pp. 197–222

Kelley, Donald R., ed. (1997), *History and the disciplines: the reclassification of knowledge in early modern Europe*, Rochester

Kemp, Martin (2000), 'Vision and visualisation in the illustration of anatomy and astronomy from Leonardo to Galileo', in *1543 and All That: image and word, change and continuity in the proto-scientific revolution*, ed. Guy Freeland and Anthony Corones, London, Dordrecht, Boston, pp. 17–51

Kennedy, George A. (1980), *Classical rhetoric and its Christian and secular tradition from ancient to modern times*, London

Kenny, Neil (1998), *Curiosity in early modern Europe: word histories*, Wiesbaden

Kessler Eckhard (1988), 'Physik oder Metaphysik: zum Begriff einer Wissenschaft von der Natur in der Methodendiskussion der "Schule von Padua" im beginnenden 16. Jahrhundert', in *Aristotelismus und Renaissance: in memoriam Charles B. Schmitt*, ed. Eckhard Kessler, Charles Lohr and Walther Sparn, Wiesbaden, pp. 223–44

(1994b), 'Naturverständnisse im 15. und 16. Jahrhundert', in *Naturauffassungen in Philosophie, Wissenschaft, Technik*, ed. Lothar Schäfer and Elisabeth Ströker, Munich, pp. 13–57

(1995), 'Clavius entre Proclus et Descartes', in *Les Jésuites à la Renaissance*, ed. Luce Giard, Paris, pp. 285–308

(1999), 'Introducing Aristotle to the sixteenth century: the Lefevre enterprise', in *Philosophy in the sixteenth and seventeenth centuries*, ed. Constance Blackwell and Sachiko Kusukawa, Aldershot, pp. 1–21

(forthcoming), 'Die verborgene Gegenwart und Funktion des Nominalismus in der Renaissance-Philosophie: das Problem der Universalien', in *Res et verba in the Renaissance*, ed. Eckhard Kessler and Ian Maclean, Wiesbaden

Kessler, Eckhard, ed. (1994a), *Girolamo Cardano: Philosoph, Naturforscher, Arzt*, Wiesbaden

Kessler, Eckhard, Lohr, Charles and Sparn, Walther, eds. (1988), *Aristotelismus und Renaissance: in memoriam Charles B. Schmitt*, Wiesbaden

Keynes, Geoffrey, ed. (1968), *The apology and treatise of Ambroise Paré*, London

King, Lester S. (1982), *Medical thinking: a historical preface*, Princeton

Kneale, William and Martha (1962), *The development of logic*, Oxford

Koch, Theodor (1998), 'Melanchthon und die Vesal-Rezeption in Wittenberg', in *Melanchthon und die Naturwissenschaften*, ed. Günter Frank and Stefan Rhein, Sigmaringen, pp. 203–18

Kolb, Robert (1976), *Caspar Peucer's library*, St Louis

Koyré, Alexandre (1958), *From a closed world to an infinite universe*, Baltimore

Kretzmann, Norman, Kenny, Anthony, and Pinborg, Jan, eds. (1982), *The Cambridge history of later medieval philosophy*, Cambridge

Kristeller, Paul O. (1961), *Renaissance thought: the classic, scholastic and humanist strains*, New York, Hagerstown, San Francisco, London

    (1978), 'Philosophy and medicine in medieval and Renaissance Italy', in *Organism, medicine, and metaphysics*, ed. S. F. Spicker, Dordrecht, pp. 29–36

    (1988), 'Humanism', in *The Cambridge history of Renaissance philosophy*, ed. Charles B. Schmitt and Quentin Skinner, Cambridge, pp. 113–38

Kudlien, Fridolf (1991), '"Endeixis" as a scientific term: Galen's usage of the word in medicine and logic', in *Galen's method of healing*, ed. Fridolf Kudlien and Richard J. Durling, Leiden, New York, Copenhagen and Cologne, pp. 103–11

Kudlien, Fridolf and Durling, Richard J., eds. (1991), *Galen's method of healing*, Leiden

Kühlmann, Wilhelm (1992), 'Oswald Crollius und seine Signaturenlehre: zum Profil hermetischer Naturphilosophie in der Ära Rudolphs II', in *Die okkulten Wissenschaften in den Renaissance*, ed. August Buck, Wiesbaden, pp. 103–24

Kuhn, Heinrich C. (1997), 'Non-regressive methods (and the emergence of modern science)', in *Method and order in Renaissance philosophy of nature*, ed. Daniel A. Di Liscia, Eckhard Kessler and Charlotte Methuen, Aldershot, pp. 319–36

Kuhn, Michael (1996), *De nomine et vocabulo: der Begriff der medizinischen Fachsprache und die Krankheitsnamen bei Paracelsus, 1493–1541*, Heidelberg

Kuhn, Thomas S. (1970), *The structure of scientific revolutions*, 2nd edn, Chicago and London

Kusukawa, Sachiko (1993), *'Aspectio divinorum operum*: Melanchthon and astrology for Lutheran medics', in *Medicine and the Reformation*, ed. Ole Peter Grell and Andrew Cunningham, London and New York, pp. 33–56

  (1995a), *The transformation of natural philosophy: the case of Philip Melanchthon*, Cambridge

  (1995b), *A Wittenberg University Library catalogue of 1536*, Cambridge

  (1997), 'Leonhart Fuchs on the importance of pictures', *Journal of the History of Ideas*, 58, 403–27

  (1998), 'Between the *De anima* and dialectics: a prolegomenon to Philippo-Ramism', in *Sapientiam Amemus: Festschrift für Eckhard Kessler*, ed. Paul Richard Blum, Munich, pp. 127–39

  (1999), 'Lutheran uses of Aristotle: a comparison between Jacob Schegk and Philip Melanchthon', in *Philosophy in the sixteenth and seventeenth centuries: conversations with Aristotle*, ed. Constance Blackwell and Sachiko Kusukawa, Aldershot, pp. 169–88

  (forthcoming a), 'Varieties of illustration in sixteenth-century *materia medica*'

  (forthcoming b), 'Melanchthon's influence in England', in *Melanchthon in Südwest Europa*, ed. Günther Frank, Sigmaringen

Lawrence, Christopher and Shapin, Steven, eds. (1998), *Science incarnate: historical embodiments of natural knowledge*, Chicago and London

Le Brun, Jacques (1994), 'Jérôme Cardan et l'interprétation des songes', in *Girolamo Cardano: Philosoph, Naturforscher, Arzt*, ed. Eckhard Kessler, Wiesbaden, pp. 185–205

Le Roy Ladurie, Emmanuel and Morineau, Michel (1977), *Histoire économique et sociale de la France*, vol. 1, part 2, Paris

Lee, H. D. P. (1935), 'Geometrical method and Aristotle's account of first principles', *Classical Quarterly*, 29, 113–24

Leedham-Green, E. S. (1986), *Books in Cambridge inventories: book lists from Vice-Chancellor's court probate inventories of the Tudor and Stuart periods*, 2 vols., Cambridge

Lehoux, Françoise (1976), *Le Cadre de vie des médecins parisiens aux XVIe et XVIIe siècles*, Paris

Leijenhorst, Cees (forthcoming), '"Insignificant speech": Thomas Hobbes and late Aristotelianism on words, concepts and things', in *Res et verba in the Renaissance*, ed. Eckhard Kessler and Ian Maclean, Wiesbaden

Lennox, J. G. (1985), 'Theophrastus and the limits of teleology', in *Theophrastus of Eresus*, ed. William Fortenbaugh *et al.*, New Brunswick, pp. 143–64

Lenoble, R. (1968), *Esquisse d'une histoire de l'idée de Nature*, Paris

Lévi-Strauss, Claude (1962), *La Pensée sauvage*, Paris

Lightfoot, Jane (1999), *Parthenios of Nicaea*, Oxford

Linden, David E. J. (1999), 'Gabriele Zerbi's *De cautelis medicorum* and the tradition of medical prudence', *Bulletin of the History of Medicine*, 73, 19–37

Lines, David (forthcoming), 'The institutional context of the teaching of natural philosophy and medicine in Italian universities of the Renaissance, with special reference to Padua'

Lloyd, Geoffrey E. R. (1979), *Magic, reason and science*, Cambridge

(1988), 'Scholarship, authority and argument in Galen's "Quod animi mores"', in *Le opere psicologiche di Galeno*, ed. Paola Manuli and Mario Vegetti, Pavia, pp. 11–42

Lohr, Charles (1988), 'Metaphysics', in *The Cambridge history of Renaissance philosophy*, ed. Charles B. Schmitt and Quentin Skinner, Cambridge, pp. 537–638

Lonie, Iain M. (1981), 'Fever pathology in the sixteenth century: tradition and innovation', in *Theories of fever from antiquity to the Enlightenment*, ed. W. F. Bynum and V. Nutton, *Medical History*, Supplement no. 1, London, 19–44

(1985), 'The "Paris Hippocratics": teaching and research in Paris in the second half of the sixteenth century', in *The medical Renaissance of the sixteenth century*, ed. Andrew Wear, R. K. French and Iain M. Lonie, Cambridge, pp. 155–72

Lovejoy, Arthur O. (1936), *The great chain of being*, Cambridge, Mass.

Luyendijk-Elshout, A. M. (1991), 'Der Einfluss der italienischen Universitäten auf die medizinische Fakultät Leiden (1575–1620)', in *Die Renaissance im Blick der Nationen Europas*, ed. Georg Kauffmann, Wiesbaden, pp. 339–54

Lynch, John (1964–9), *Spain under the Hapsburgs*, Oxford, 2 vols.

Macdonald, Michael (1981), *Mystical bedlam: madness, anxiety and healing in seventeenth-century England*, Cambridge

McGinn, Colin (2000), 'Sign language', *The New York Review of Books*, 48.10, 62–5

Mack, Peter (1990), *Renaissance argument: Valla and Agricola in the traditions of rhetoric and dialectic*, Leiden, New York and Cologne

Mackinney, L. (1938), 'Medieval medical dictionaries and glossaries', in *Medieval and historiographical essays in honor of James Westfall*, ed. J. L. Cate and E. N. Anderson, Chicago, pp. 240–58

Maclean, Ian (1980), *The Renaissance notion of woman: a study in the fortunes of scholasticism and medical science in European intellectual life*, Cambridge

(1984), 'The interpretation of natural signs: Cardano's *De subtilitate* versus Scaliger's *Exercitationes*', in *Occult and scientific mentalities in the Renaissance*, ed. Brian Vickers, Cambridge, pp. 231–52

(1988), 'André Wechel at Frankfurt: 1572–1581', *Gutenberg Jahrbuch*, 63, 146–76

(1990), 'Philosophical books in European markets, 1570–1630: the case of Ramus', in *New perspectives on Renaissance thought: essays in the history of science, education and philosophy in memory of Charles B. Schmitt*, ed. John Henry and Sarah Hutton, London, pp. 253–63

(1991), 'The market for scholarly books and conceptions of genre in Northern Europe 1570–1630', in *Die Renaissance im Licht der Nationen Europas*, ed. Georg Kauffmann, Wiesbaden, pp. 16–31

(1992), *Interpretation and meaning in the Renaissance: the case of law*, Cambridge

(1994), 'Cardano and his publishers, 1534–1663', in *Girolamo Cardano: Philosoph, Naturforscher, Arzt*, ed. Eckhard Kessler, Wiesbaden, pp. 305–33

(1996), *Montaigne philosophe*, Paris

(1998a), 'Foucault's Renaissance episteme reassessed: an Aristotelian counterblast', *Journal of the History of Ideas*, 59, 149–66

(1998b), 'Naturalisme et croyance personnelle dans le discours médical à la fin de la Renaissance', *Journal of the Institute of Romance Studies*, 6, 177–92

(1998c), 'The process of intellectual change: a post-Foucauldian hypothesis', *Arcadia*, 33, 168–81

(1999a), 'Interpreting the *De Libris Propriis*', in *Girolamo Cardano. le opere, le fonti, la vita*, ed. Marialuisa Baldi and Guido Canziani, Milan, pp. 13–33

(1999b), 'Language in the mind: reflexive thinking in the late Renaissance', in *Philosophy in the Sixteenth and Seventeenth Centuries: Conversations with Aristotle*, ed. Constance Blackwell and Sachiko Kusukawa, Aldershot, pp. 296–321

(1990c), 'Legal fictions and fictional entities in Renaissance jurisprudence', *The Journal of Legal History*, 20, 1–24

(2000a), 'The diffusion of learned medicine in the sixteenth century through the printed book', in *Medical Latin from the late Middle Ages to the eighteenth century*, ed. Wouter Bracke and Herwig Deumens, Brussels, pp. 93–114

(2000b), 'Evidence, logic, the rule and the exception in Renaissance law and medicine', *Early Science and Medicine*, 5, 227–57

(2001), 'Logical division and visual dichotomies: Ramus in the context of Renaissance legal and medical writing', in *The influence of Petrus Ramus, 1570–1630*, ed. Mordecai Feingold, Joseph Freedman and Wolfgang Rother, Basle, pp. 229–49

(forthcoming a), 'Mediations of Zabarella in Northern Germany, 1586–1623', in *The presence of Paduan philosophy in Northern Europe*, ed. Gregorio Piaia

(forthcoming b), 'Melanchthon at the book fairs', in *Melanchthon in Südwest Europa*, ed. Günther Frank, Sigmaringen

(forthcoming c), 'Textauslegung und Hermeneutik in den juristischen und medizinischen Fächern der späten Renaissance: auctoritas, ratio, experientia', in *Theorie der Interpretation*, ed. Jan Schröder, Tübingen

(forthcoming d), 'Aristotle's infinities in the Renaissance', in *Aristotle, literature, Renaissance*, ed. Ullrich Langer, Geneva

McVaugh, Michael R. (1969), 'Quantified medical theory and practice at fourteenth-century Montpellier', *Bulletin of the History of Medicine*, 43, 397–413

(1990), 'The nature and limits of medical certitude at early fourteenth-century Montpellier', *Osiris*, 2nd series, 6, 62–84

(1997), 'Bedside manners in the Middle Ages', *Bulletin of the History of Medicine*, 71, 201–23

Madden, E. H. (1957), 'Aristotle's treatment of probability and signs', *Philosophy of Science*, 24, 167–72

Maddison, Francis, Pelling, Margaret and Webster, Charles, eds. (1977), *Essays on the life and work of Thomas Linacre, c. 1460–1524*, Oxford

Madonia, Claudio (1988), 'Simone Simoni', in *Bibliotheca dissidentium: répertoire des non-conformistes religieux des seizième et dix-septième siècles*, ed. André Ségenny,

Irena Backus and Jean Rott, vol. 9, Baden-Baden and Bouxwiller, pp. 25–110

Mahoney, M. S. (1985), 'Diagrams and dynamics: mathematical perspectives on Edgerton's thesis', in *Science and the arts in the Renaissance*, ed. J. W. Shirley and F. D. Hoeniger, Washington D.C. and London, pp. 198–220

Mancosu, Paolo (1996), *Philosophy of mathematics and mathematical practice in the seventeenth century*, New York and Oxford

Manetti, Giovanni (1987), *Le teorie del segno nell'antichità classica*, Milan

Mani, Nikolaus (1956), 'Die griechische *editio princeps* des Galenos (1525), ihre Entstehung und ihre Wirkung', *Gesnerus*, 13, 29–52

Mardersteig, G. (1967), *The remarkable story of a book made in Padua in 1477: Gentile da Foligno's commentary on Avicenna printed by Petrus Maufer*, London

Margolin, Jean-Claude (1994), 'Inventer et découvrir à la Renaissance', in *Inventions et découvertes au temps de la Renaissance*, ed. M. T. Jones-Davies, Paris, pp. 123–45

Martellozzo, Forin and Veronese, Elda (1969), *Acta graduum academicorum ab anno 1501 ad annum 1550*, 3 vols., Padua

(1971), 'Studenti e dottori tedeschi a Padova nei secoli XV e XVI', *Quaderni per la storia dell'università di Padova*, 4, 49–102

Martín Ferreira, Ana Isabel (1995), *El humanismo médico en la Universidad de Alcalá (siglo XVI)*, Alcalá

Matsen, H. S. (1968), 'Alessandro Achillini (1468–1512) as professor of philosophy in the "studio" of Padua (1506–8)', *Quaderni per la storia dell'università di Padova*, 1, 91–110

Meier-Oeser, Stephan (1997), *Die Spur des Zeichens: das Zeichen und seine Funktion in der Philosophie des Mittelalters und der frühen Neuzeit*, Berlin and New York

Meinel, Christoph (1992), 'Okkulte und exakte Wissenschaften', in *Die okkulten Wissenschaften in der Renaissance*, ed. August Buck, Wiesbaden, pp. 21–44

Mignucci, M. (1981), 'Hōs epi to polu et nécessaire dans la conception aristotélicienne de la science', in *Aristotle on Science: Posterior analytics*, ed. E. Perti, Padua, pp. 173–203

Mikkeli, Heikki (1992), *An Aristotelian response to Renaissance humanism: Jacopo Zabarella on the nature of the arts and the sciences*, Helsinki

(1998), 'The status of the mechanical arts in the Aristotelian classifications of knowledge in the early sixteenth century', in *Sapientiam Amemus: Festschrift für Eckhard Kessler*, ed. Paul R. Blum, Munich, pp. 109–26

(1999), *Hygiene in the early modern medical tradition*, Helsinki

(forthcoming), 'Paduan Aristotelians on the question of subalternation between philosophy of nature and medicine', in *The dynamics of natural philosophy in the Aristotelian tradition*, ed. Hans Thijssen, Cees Leijenhorst and Christoph Lüthy

Momigliano, Arnaldo (1985), *Tra storia e storicismo*, Pisa

Montefusco, Lucia Calboli (1998), 'Omnis autem argumentatio... aut probabilis aut necessaria esse debebit (Cic. Inv. 1.44)', *Rhetorica*, 16, 1–24

Montfort, Marie-Laure (2000), 'La Notion de vulgate hippocratique' in *Medical Latin from the late Middle Ages to the eighteenth century*, ed. Wouter Bracke and Herwig Deumens, Brussels, pp. 53–66

Monti, Maria Theresa (2000), 'Epigenesis of the monstrous form and preformistic "genetics"', *Early Science and Medicine*, 5, 3–32

Moran, Bruce (1998), 'Medicine, alchemy, and the control of language: Andreas Libavius versus the neoparacelsians', in *Paracelsus: the man and his reputation, his ideas and their transformation*, ed. Ole Peter Grell, Leiden, Boston, Cologne, pp. 135–49

Moraux, Paul (1981), 'Galien comme philosophe: la philosophie de la nature', in *Galen: problems and prospects*, ed. Vivian Nutton, London, pp. 86–116

Morrison, Donald (1997), 'Philoponus and Simplicius on tekmeriodic proof', in *Method and order in Renaissance philosophy of nature*, ed. Daniel A. Di Liscia, Eckhard Kessler and Charlotte Methuen, Aldershot, pp. 1–22

Moss, Ann (1996), *Printed commonplace-books and the structuring of Renaissance thought*, Oxford

Mugnai Carrara, Daniela (1999), 'Epistemological problems in Giovanni Mainardi's commentary on Galen's *Ars parva*', in *Natural particulars: nature and the disciplines in Renaissance Europe*, ed. Anthony Grafton and Nancy Siraisi, Cambridge, Mass. and London, pp. 251–74

Müller-Jahnke, Wolf-Dieter (1992), 'Kaspar Peucers Stellung auf Magie', in *Die okkulten Wissenschaften in der Renaissance*, ed. August Buck, Wiesbaden, pp. 91–102

  (1994), 'Georg am Wald (1554–1616), Arzt und Unternehmer', in *Analecta paracelsica*, ed. Joachim Telle, Stuttgart, pp. 213–304

Murdoch, John E. (1984), *Album of science: antiquity and the Middle Ages*, New York

Murphy, James J. (1974), *Rhetoric in the Middle Ages*, Berkeley and London

Nance, Brian K. (1993), 'Determining the patient's temperament: an excursion into seventeenth-century medical semeiology', *Bulletin of the History of Medicine*, 67, 417–38

Nardi, Bruno (1958), *Saggi sull'Aristotelismo padovano dal secolo XIV al XVI*, Florence

Nauck, E. Th. (1954), 'Die Zahl der Medizinstudenten deutscher Hochschulen vom 14. bis 18. Jahrhundert', *Sudhoffs Archiv*, 38, 175–86

Needham, Rodney (1975), 'Polythetic classification: convergence and consequences', *Man*, n.s., 10, 349–69

Newman, William R. (1996), 'The alchemical sources of Robert Boyle's corpuscular philosophy', *Annals of Science*, 53, 567–85

  (1997), 'Art, nature and experiment among some Aristotelian alchemists', in *Texts and contexts in ancient and medieval science; studies on the occasion of John E. Murdoch's seventieth birthday*, ed. Edith Sylla and Michael McVaugh, pp. 305–17

  (1998), 'Alchemical and Baconian views of the art–nature division', in *Reading the Book of Nature: the other side of the scientific revolution*, ed. Allen. G. Debus and Michael T. Walton, Kirksville, pp. 81–90

Niebyl, Peter H. (1971), 'The non-naturals', *Bulletin of the History of Medicine*, 45, 489–92

Niewöhner, Friedrich, and Pluta, Olaf, eds. (1999), *Atheismus im Mittelalter und in der Renaissance*, Wiesbaden

Nischan, Bodo (1994), *Prince, people and confession: the second Reformation in Brandenburg*, Philadelphia

Noreña, Carlos G. (1970), *Juan Luis Vives*, The Hague

Nörr, Dieter (1972), *Divisio und Partitio: Bemerkungen zur römischen Rechtsquellenlehre und zur antiken Wissenschaftstheorie*, Berlin

Nutton, Vivian (1979), 'John Caius and the Linacre tradition', *Medical History*, 23, 373–91

(1983), 'The seeds of disease: an explanation of contagion and infection from the Greeks to the Renaissance', *Medical History*, 27, 1–34

(1985a), 'Humanist surgery', in *The medical Renaissance of the sixteenth century*, ed. Andrew Wear, R. K. French and Iain M. Lonie, Cambridge, pp. 75–99

(1985b), 'Murder and miracles: lay attitudes to medicine in classical antiquity', in *Patients and practitioners*, ed. Roy Porter, Cambridge, pp. 23–53

(1987), *John Caius and the manuscripts of Galen*, Cambridge

(1988), '*De Placitis Hippocratis et Platonis* in the Renaissance', in *Le opere psicologiche di Galeno*, ed. Paola Manuli and Mario Vegetti, Pavia, pp. 281–309

(1989), 'Hippocrates in the Renaissance', *Sudhoffs Archiv*, Beiheft 27, 420–39

(1990a), 'Medicine, diplomacy and finance: the prefaces to a Hippocratic commentary of 1541', in *New perspectives on Renaissance thought: essays in the history of science, education and philosophy in memory of Charles B. Schmitt*, ed. John Henry and Sarah Hutton, London, pp. 230–43

(1990b), 'The reception of Fracastoro's theory of contagion: the seed that fell among thorns?', *Osiris*, 2nd series, 6, 196–234

(1990c), 'Anatomy of the soul', in *The human embryo: Aristotle and the Arabic and European traditions*, ed. G. R. Dunstan, Exeter, pp. 136–57

(1993a), 'Galen at the bedside: the methods of a medical detective', in *Medicine and the five senses*, ed. Roy Porter and W. F. Bynum, Cambridge, pp. 7–16

(1993b), 'Greek science in the sixteenth-century Renaissance', in *Renaissance and revolution: humanists, scholars, craftsmen and natural philosophers in early modern Europe*, ed. J. V. Field and Frank A. J. L. James, Cambridge, pp. 15–28

(1993c), 'Medicine and printing in the sixteenth century' (Bishop Memorial lecture)

(1993d), 'Wittenberg anatomy', in *Medicine and the Reformation*, ed. Ole Peter Grell and Andrew Cunningham, London and New York, pp. 11–32

(1995), 'The changing language of medicine 1450–1550', in *Vocabulary of teaching and research between the Middle Ages and Renaissance*, ed. Olga Weijers, Turnhout, pp. 184–98

(1996), 'Idle old trots, coblers and costardmongers: Pieter van Foreest on quackery', in *Petrus Forestus Medicus*, ed. Henrietta A. Bosman-Jelgersma, Amsterdam, pp. 243–56

(1997a), 'Hellenism postponed: some aspects of Renaissance medicine 1490–1530', *Sudhoffs Archiv*, 81, 158–170

(1997b), 'The rise of medical humanism: Ferrara 1464–1555', *Renaissance Studies*, 11, 2–19

Nutton, Vivian, ed. (1981), *Galen: problems and prospects*, London

Olivieri, Luigi (1983a), *Aristotelismo veneto e scienza moderna*, Atti del 250 anno accademico del centro per la storia della tradizione aristotelica nel Veneto, 2 vols., Padua

(1983b), *Certezza e gerarchia del sapere*, Padua

O'Malley, Charles D. (1964), *Andreas Vesalius of Brussels, 1514–1564*, Berkeley and Los Angeles

(1970), 'Medical education during the Renaissance', in *The history of medical education*, ed. C. D. O'Malley, UCLA Forum in Medical Sciences, xii, Berkeley, Los Angeles and London, pp. 89–102

O'Neill, Ynez Violé (1975), 'Giovanni Michele Savonarola: an atypical Renaissance practitioner', *Clio medica*, 10, 77–93

Ong, Walter J. (1974), *Ramus: method and the decay of dialogue*, New York

Ongaro, Giuseppe (1994), 'L'insegnamento clinico di Giovan Battista da Monte (1489–1551): una revisione critica', *Physis*, 31, 3547–69

Osler, Sir William (1923), *Incunabula medica: a study of the earliest printed medical books, 1467–1480*, Oxford

Ott, Hugo and Fletcher, John M., eds. (1964), *The medieval statutes of the Faculty of Arts of the University of Freiburg im Breisgau*, Notre Dame

Otto, Stephan (1992), *Das Wissen des Ähnlichen: Michel Foucault und die Renaissance*, Frankfurt, Berne, New York and Paris

Ottosson, Per-Gunnar (1984), *Scholastic medicine and philosophy: a study of commentaries on Galen's Tegni (ca. 1300–1450)*, Naples

Pagel, Walter (1935), 'Religious motives in the medical biology of the xviith century', *Bulletin of the History of Medicine*, 3, 97–128, 213–31, 265–312

(1958), *Paracelsus: an introduction to philosophical medicine of the era of the Renaissance*, Basle and New York

(1967), *William Harvey's biological ideas*, Basle and New York

(1985), *Religion and neoplatonism in Renaissance medicine*, ed. Marianne Winder, London

(1986), *From Paracelsus to Van Helmont: studies in Renaissance medicine and science*, ed. Marianne Winder, London

Pallmann, Heinrich (1881), *Sigismund Feyerabend: sein Leben und seine geschäftlichen Verbindungen nach archivalistischen Quellen*, Frankfurt

Palmer, Richard (1981), 'Physicians and the state in post-mediaeval Italy', in *The town and state physician in Europe from the Middle Ages to the Enlightenment*, ed. A. W. Russell, Wolfenbüttel, pp. 47–60

(1983), *The Studio of Venice and its graduates in the sixteenth century*, Padua

(1985), 'Pharmacy in the republic of Venice in the sixteenth century', in *The medical Renaissance of the sixteenth century*, Andrew Wear, R. K. French and Iain M. Lonie, Cambridge, pp. 100–17

(1993), 'Physicans and the Inquisition in sixteenth-century Venice', in *Medicine and the Reformation*, ed. Ole Peter Grell and Andrew Cunningham, London and New York, pp. 118–33

Panizza, Letizia (1999), 'Learning the syllogisms: Byzantine visual aids in Renaissance Italy – Ermolao Barbaro', in *Philosophy in the sixteenth and seventeenth centuries: conversations with Aristotle*, ed. Constance Blackwell and Sachiko Kusukawa, Aldershot, pp. 22–47

Panofsky, Erwin (1924–5), *Die Perspective als 'symbolische Form'*, Berlin

Pantin, Isabelle (forthcoming), 'Melanchthon's *Initia doctrinae physicae* and France', in *Melanchthon in Südwest Europa*, ed. Günther Frank, Sigmaringen

Papy, Jean (1999), 'The attitude towards Aristotelian biological thought in the Louvain medical treatises during the sixteenth and early seventeenth century: the case of embryology', in *Aristotle's animals in the Middle Ages and Renaissance*, ed. Carlos Steel, Guy Guldentops and Pieter Beullens, Louvain, pp. 317–37

Park, Katharine (1985), *Doctors and medicine in early Renaissance Florence*, Princeton

(1995), 'The life of the corpse: division and dissection in late medieval Europe', *Journal of the History of Medicine*, 50, 11–32

Peirce, C. S. (1931–58), 'Icon, index, symbol', in *Collected papers*, ed. Charles Hartshore and Paul Weiss (vols. 7 & 8 ed. Arthur W. Burks), Cambridge, Mass., 8 vols., vol. 2, pp. 156–73

Pelling, Margaret (1995), 'Knowledge common and acquired: the education of unlicensed medical practitioners in early modern London', in *The history of medical education in Britain*, ed. Vivian Nutton and Roy Porter, London, *Clio medica*, 30, 250–79

Perfetti, Stefano (1999a), '*Docebo vos dubitare*. Il commento inedito di Pietro Pomponazzi al *De partibus animalium* (Bologna 1521–1524)', *Documenti e studi sulla tradizione filosofica medievale*, 10, 439–66

(1999b), 'Three different ways of interpreting Aristotle's *De partibus animalium*: Pietro Pomponazzi, Niccolò Leonico Tomeo and Agostino Nifo', in *Aristotle's animals in the Middle Ages and Renaissance*, ed. Carlos Stell, Guy Guldentops and Pieter Beullens, Louvain, pp. 299–316

Pesenti, Tiziana (1984), *Professori e promotori di medicina nello studio di Padova dal 1405 al 1509: repertorio bibliografico*, Padua

(2000), 'How did early printers choose medical commentaries for the press?', in *Medical Latin from the late Middle Ages to the eighteenth century*, ed. Wouter Bracke and Herwig Deumens, Brussels, pp. 67–92

Pettas, William (1997), 'The Giunti and the book trade in Lyon', in *Libri, tipografi, biblioteche; ricerche storiche dedicate a Luigi Balsamo*, Florence, pp. 169–92

Piaia, G (1973), 'Aristotelismo, "heresia" e giurisdizionalismo nella polemica del p. Antonio Possevino contro lo Studio di Padova', *Quaderni per la storia dell'università di Padova*, 6, 125–48

Pic, Pierre (1911), *Guy Patin*, Paris

Pickering, A. (1995), 'Beyond constraint: the temporality of practice and the historicity of knowledge', in *Scientific practice*, ed. Jed Z. Buchwald, Chicago and London, pp. 42–55

Pittion, Jean-Paul (1987), 'Scepticism and medicine in the Renaissance', in *Scepticism from the Renaissance to the Enlightenment*, ed. Richard H. Popkin and Charles B. Schmitt, Wiesbaden, pp. 103–32

Pluta, Olaf (1991), 'Ewigkeit der Welt, Sterblichkeit der Seele, Diesseitigkeit des Glücks: Elemente einer materialistischen Philosophie bei Johannes Buridan', in *Historia philosophiae medii aevi*, ed. Burkhard Mojsisch and Olaf Pluta, Amsterdam, pp. 847–72

Pollard G. and A. Ehrmann A. (1965), *The distribution of books by catalogue from the invention of printing to AD 1800, based on material in the Broxbourne Library*, Cambridge, 1965

Popper, K. R. (1970), 'Normal science and its dangers', in *Criticism and the growth of knowledge*, ed. Imre Lakatos and Alan Musgrave, Cambridge, pp. 51–8

Porter, Martin (1997), 'English treatises on physiognomy', Oxford D. Phil. thesis

Pozzo, Ricardo (forthcoming), 'Petrus Ramus' metaphysics and its criticism by the Aristotelians at Helmstedt', in *The influence of Petrus Ramus, 1570–1630*, ed. M Feingold, J. Freedman and W. Rother, Basle

Premuda, Loris (1961–2), 'Prospero Alpini: il rilancio delle antiche dottrine fisiche in medicina nella Padova di Galileo Galilei', *Acta medicae historiae patavina*, 8, 9–63

(1963), 'Die Natio Germanica an der Universität Padua', *Sudhoffs Archiv*, 47, 97–105

(1987–8), 'L'Universalité de la pensée de l'école médicale de Padoue entre le seizième et le dix-huitième siècle', *Acta medicae historiae patavina*, 36, 199–24

Prestwich, Menna, ed. (1985), *International Calvinism*, Oxford

Priest, Graham (1995), *Beyond the limits of thought*, Cambridge

Pumfrey, Steve (1998), 'The spagyric art: on the impossible work of separating pure from impure Paracelsianism: a historiographical analysis', in *Paracelsus: the man and his reputation, his ideas and their transformation*, ed. Ole Peter Grell, Leiden, Boston, Cologne, pp. 21–51

Putnam, George Haven (1906–7), *The censorship of the Church of Rome and its influence upon the production and distribution of literature*, 2 vols., New York

Randall, J. H. (1961), *The School of Padua and the emergence of modern science*, Padua

(1976), 'Paduan Aristotelianism reconsidered', in *Philosophy and humanism*, ed. E. P. Mahoney, Leiden, 1976, pp. 275–82

Redondi, Pietro (1987), 'Science: the renaissance of a history. Proceedings of the International Conference Alexandre Koyré, Paris, Collège de France, 10–14 June 1986', *History and technology*, 4, special issue, ed. Pietro Redondi

Reeds, Karen M. (1991), *Botany in medieval and Renaissance universities*, New York and London

Rener, Frederick M. (1989), *Interpretatio: language and translation from Cicero to Tyler*, Amsterdam and Atlanta

Rhodes, Dennis E. (1987), 'Some neglected aspects of the career of Giovanni Battista Ciotti', *The Library*, 6th series, 9, 225–39

Rice, Jnr, Eugene F. (1976), 'The *De magia naturali* of Jacques Lefèvre d'Etaples', in *Philosophy and humanism*, ed. E. P. Mahoney, Leiden, 1976, pp. 20–9

Richardson Linda Deer (1985), 'The generation of disease: occult causes and diseases of the total substance', in *The medical Renaissance of the sixteenth century*, ed. Andrew Wear, R. K. French and Iain M. Lonie, Cambridge, pp. 175–94

Ridder-Symoens, H. D. (1996), *The history of the university in Europe*, Cambridge

Risse, Wilhelm (1964), *Die Logik der Neuzeit, 1: 1500–1640*, Stuttgart

Roger, Jacques (1960), *Jean Fernel et les problèmes de la médecine de la Renaissance*, Paris

(1997), *The life sciences in eighteenth-century French thought*, trans. Robert Ellrich, ed. Keith R. Benson, Stanford

Rojo Vega, A. (1997), 'Les Livres des Espagnols à l'époque moderne', *Bulletin Historique*, 99, 193–210

Rosenberg, C. E. (forthcoming), 'The tyranny of diagnosis', in *Health in America: the past one hundred years*, ed. Judith Sealander, Berkeley and Los Angeles

Rossetti, Lucia (1969), 'Le bibliotheche delle "natione" nello studio di Padova', *Quaderni per la storia dell'università di Padova*, 2, 53–70

(1986), *Matricula nationis Germanicae artistarum in Gymnasio Patavino (1553–1721)*, Padua

Rossi, Paolo (1960), *Clavis universalis; arti mnemoniche e logica combinatoria da Lullo a Leibniz*, Milan

(1970), *Philosophy, technology and the arts in the early modern era*, New York

Roth, Rudolph (1973), *Urkunden zur Geschichte der Universität Tübingen 1476–1550*, Aalen

Rupp, Jan C. C. (1990), 'Matters of life and death: the social and cultural conditions of the rise of anatomical theatres', *History of Science*, 28, 263–87

Russell, A. W., ed. (1981), *The town and state physician in Europe from the Middle Ages to the Enlightenment*, Wiesbaden

Rütten, Thomas (1996), 'Receptions of the Hippocratic oath in the Renaissance. The prohibition of abortion as a case study in reception', in *Journal of the History of Medicine and Allied Sciences*, 51, 456–83

(1999), 'Ärztliche Ethik in der Renaissancemedizin: Mechanismen der Neukontextuierung des hippokratischen Eides in der späthumanistischen Kommentarliteratur zwischen 1540 und 1640', in *Aspetti della terapia nel Corpus Hippocraticum*, ed. Ivan Garofalo, Alessandro Lami, Daniela Manetti and Amneris Roselli, Florence, pp. 517–42

Sackett, David L., Richardson, W. Scott, Rosenberg, William, and Haynes, R. Brian (1997), *Evidence-based medicine: how to practice and teach EBM*, New York, Edinburgh, London, Madrid, Melbourne, San Francisco, Tokyo

Sarton, George (1953), *Introduction to the history of science*, Baltimore

Saunders, J. B. de C. M., and O'Malley, Charles D. (1950), *The illustrations from the works of Andreas Vesalius of Brussels*, Cleveland

Sayle, C. (1921), 'The library of Thomas Lorkyn', *Annals of Medical History*, 3, 310–23

Schaffer, Simon (1996), 'Piety, physic and prodigious abstinence', in *Religio medici: medicine and religion in seventeenth-century England*, ed. Ole Peter Grell and Andrew Cunningham, Aldershot, pp, 171–203

Schleiner, Winfried (1995), *Medical ethics in the Renaissance*, Washington D.C.

Schmidt, Imke (1996), *Die Bücher aus der Frankfurter Offizin Gülfferich-Han Weigand Han Erben*, Wiesbaden

Schmidt-Biggemann, Wilhelm (1983), *Topica universalis: eine Modellgeschichte humanistischer und barocker Wissenschaft*, Hamburg

Schmitt, Charles B. (1967), 'Giulio Castellani (1528–1586): a sixteenth-century opponent of scepticism', *Journal of the History of Philosophy*, 5, 15–39

    (1969), 'Experience and experiment: a comparison of Zabarella's view with Galileo's in *De motu*', *Studies in the Renaissance*, 16, 80–138

    (1972), 'The faculty of arts at Pisa at the time of Galileo', *Physis*, 14, 243–72

    (1974), 'The university of Pisa in the Renaissance', *History of Education*, 3, 3–17

    (1976a), 'Girolamo Borro's *Multae sunt nostrarum ignorationum causae* (Ms Vat. Ross. 1009)', in *Philosophy and humanism*, ed. E. P. Mahoney, Leiden, pp. 462–76

    (1976b), 'L'Introduction de la philosophie platonicienne dans l'enseignement des universités à la Renaissance', *Platon et Aristote à la Renaissance: XVIe Colloque international de Tours*, Paris, pp. 93–106

    (1977), 'The correspondence of Jacques Daléchamps (1513–1588)', *Viator*, 8, 399–434

    (1978), 'Filippo Fabri's *Philosophia naturalis Io. Duns Scoti* and its relation to Paduan Aristotelianism', in *Regnum hominis et regnum Dei*, ed. C. Bérubé, Rome, vol. 2, pp. 305–12

    (1979), 'Renaissance Averroism studied through the Venetian editions of Aristotle-Averroes (with particular reference to the Giunta edition of 1550–2)', in *L'Averroismo in Italia*, Atti dei Convegni Lincei 40, Rome, pp. 121–41

    (1981), *Studies in Renaissance Philosophy and Science*. London

    (1983a), *Aristotle in the Renaissance*, Harvard

    (1983b), 'Aristotelianism in the Veneto and the origins of modern science: some considerations of continuity', in *Aristotelismo veneto e scienza moderna, Atti del 250 anno accademico del centro per la storia della tradizione aristotelica nel Veneto*, ed. Luigi Olivieri, 2 vols., Padua, vol. 2, pp. 104–25

    (1983c), 'Recent trends in the study of medieval and Renaissance science', in *Information sources in the History of Medicine*, ed. Pietro Corsi and Paul Weindling, London, Boston, Durban, Singapore, Sydney, Toronto, Wellington, pp. 221–42

    (1984a), *The Aristotelian tradition and Renaissance universities*, London

    (1984b), 'William Harvey and Renaissance Aristotelianism: a consideration of the Praefatio to *De generatione animalium*, 1651', in *Humanismus und Medizin*, ed. Rudolf Schmitz and Gundolf Keil, Weinheim, pp. 117–38

(1985), 'Aristotle among the physicians', in *The medical Renaissance of the sixteenth century*, ed. Andrew Wear, R. K. French and Iain M. Lonie, Cambridge, pp. 1–15 and notes

(1987), 'Philoponus's commentary on Aristotle's *Physics* in the sixteenth century', in *Philoponus and the rejection of Aristotelian science*, ed. Richard Sorabji, London, pp. 210–30

(1988a), 'The rise of the philosophical textbook', in *The Cambridge history of Renaissance philosophy*, ed. Charles B. Schmitt and Quentin Skinner, Cambridge, pp. 792–804

(1988b), 'Towards a history of Renaissance philosophy', *Aristotelismus und Renaissance: in memoriam Charles B. Schmitt*, ed. Eckhard Kessler, Charles Lohr and Walter Sparn, Wiesbaden, pp. 9–16

Schmitt, Charles B. and Skinner, Quentin, eds. (1988), *The Cambridge history of Renaissance philosophy*, Cambridge

Schneider-Hiltbrunner, Verena (1976), *Wilhelm Fabry von Hilden 1560–1634: Verzeichnis der Werke und des Briefwechsels*, Berne, Stuttgart and Vienna

Schottenloher, K. (1933), 'Die Druckprivilegien des 16 Jahrhunderts', *Gutenberg Jahrbuch*, 94–110

Schüling, H., ed. (1967), *Bibliographie der psychologischen Literatur des 16. Jahrhunderts*, Hildesheim

Schwetschke, Gustav (1850–77), *Codex nundinarius Germaniae literatae bisecularis*, Halle

Sdzui, Reimund (1997), *Historische Studien zur Interpretationsmethodologie der frühen Neuzeit*, Würzburg

Sedley, David (1982), 'On signs', in *Science and speculation: studies in Hellenistic theory and practice*, ed. Jonathan Barnes, Jacques Brunschwig, Myles Burnyeat and Malcolm Schofield, Cambridge, pp. 239–72

Shapin, Steven (1994), *A social history of truth: civility and science in seventeenth-century England*, Chicago and London

Shapiro, Barbara (1999), *A culture of fact: England 1550–1720*, Ithaca and London

Sherman, William H. (1995), *John Dee: the politics of reading and writing in the English Renaissance*, Amherst

Simon, Josef (1989), *Philosophie des Zeichens*, Berlin and New York

Singh Gill, Harjeet and Manetti, Giovanni (1999–2000), *Signs and signification*, New Delhi

Siraisi, Nancy G. (1981), *Taddeo Alderotti and his pupils: two generations of Italian medical learning*, Princeton

(1987a), *Avicenna in Renaissance Italy: the Canon and the medical teaching in Italian universities after 1500*, Princeton

(1987b), 'The physician's task: medical reputations in humanist collective biographies', in *The traditional arts of living: Smith College Studies in History*, 50, pp. 105–33

(1990a), 'Giovanni Argenterio and sixteenth-century medical innovation, between princely patronage and academic controversy', *Osiris*, 2nd series, 6, 161–80

(1990b), 'Medicine, physiology and anatomy in early sixteenth-century critiques of the arts and the sciences', in *New perspectives on Renaissance thought: essays in the history of science, education and philosophy in memory of Charles B. Schmitt*, ed. John Henry and Sarah Hutton, London, pp. 214–29

(1990c), *Medieval and early Renaissance medicine*, Chicago

(1991), 'Girolamo Cardano and the art of medical narrative', *Journal of the History of Ideas*, 52, 581–602

(1994a), 'Cardano, Hippocrates and Criticism of Galen', in *Girolamo Cardano: Philosoph, Naturforscher, Arzt*, ed. Eckhard Kessler, Wiesbaden, pp. 131–55

(1994b), 'Vesalius and Human diversity in *De humani corporis fabrica*', *Journal of the Warburg and Courtauld Institutes*, 57, 60–88

(1997), *The clock and the mirror: Girolamo Cardano and Renaissance medicine*, Princeton

(1998), 'La communicazione del sapere anatomico ai confini tra diritto e agiografia: due casi del secolo XVI', in *Le forme della comunicazione scientifica*, ed. Massimo Galuzzo, Gianni Michele and Maria Teresa Monti, Milan, pp. 419–38

(1999), 'Cardano and the history of medicine', in *Girolamo Cardano. Le opere, le fonti, la vita*, ed. Marialuisa Baldi and Guido Canziani, Milan, pp. 342–62

(2000), 'Anatomizing the past: physicians and history in Renaissance culture', *Renaissance Quarterly*, 53, 1–30

(forthcoming), 'Disease and symptom as problematic concepts in Renaissance medicine', *Res et verba in the Renaissance*, ed. Eckhard Kessler and Ian Maclean, Wiesbaden

Skinner, Quentin (1996), *Reason and rhetoric in the philosophy of Hobbes*, Cambridge

Slack, Paul (1979), 'The use of vernacular medical literature in Tudor England', in *Health, medicine and mortality in the sixteenth century*, ed. Charles Webster, Cambridge, pp. 237–73

Smith, Wesley D. (1979), *The Hippocratic tradition*, Ithaca

Specht, Rainer (1998), 'Autoritätsargument und Erfahrungsargument im 17. Jahrhundert', in *Entwicklung der Methodenlehre in Rechtswissenschaft und Philosophie vom 16. bis zum 18. Jahrhundert*, ed. Jan Schröder, Stuttgart, pp. 47–64

Starobinski, Jean (1982), *Montaigne en mouvement*, Paris

Stone, Howard (1953), 'The French language in Renaissance medicine', *Bibliothèque d'Humanisme et Renaissance*, 15, 315–46

Straus, Jnr, William L. and Temkin, Owsei (1943), 'Vesalius and the problem of variability', *Bulletin of the History of Medicine*, 14, 609–33

Stübler, E. (1926), *Geschichte der medizinischen Fakultät der Universität Heidelberg*, Heidelberg

Stump, Eleonore (1982), 'Topics: their development and absorption into consequences', in *The Cambridge history of later medieval philosophy*, ed. Norman Kretzmann, Anthony Kenny and Jan Pinborg, Cambridge, pp. 273–99

Sudhoff, Karl (1894), *Bibliographia Paracelsica*, Berlin

Taub, Liba (1997), 'The rehabilitation of wretched subjects', *Early Science and Medicine*, 2, 74–87

Temkin, Oswei (1973), *Galenism: rise and decline of a medical philosophy*, Ithaca and London

(1977), *The double face of Janus*, Baltimore

Thorndike, Lynn (1923–58), *A history of magic and experimental science*, 8 vols., New York

Towaide, Alan (2000), '*Loquantur ipsi ut velint . . . modo quis serpens sit tirus . . . non ignorent*: Leoniceno's contribution to Renaissance epistemological approach to scientific lexicography', in *Medical Latin from the late Middle Ages to the eighteenth century*, ed. Wouter Bracke and Herwig Deumens, Brussels, pp. 151–74

Trinkaus, C. (1985), 'The astrological cosmos and rhetorical culture of Giovanni Gioviano Pontano', *Renaissance Quarterly*, 38, 446–72

Truman, Ronald (1994), 'Analogy and argument in Jerónimo Merola's *República original*', in *The discerning eye: studies presented to Robert Pring-Mill on his seventieth birthday*, ed. Nigel Griffin *et al.*, Llangrannog, pp. 47–56

Tuilier, André (1998), 'Ramus, lecteur royal, et l'enseignement universitaire à Paris au milieu du XVI siècle', in *Les Origines du Collège de France*, ed. Marc Fumaroli, pp. 375–90

Vasoli, Cesare (1968), *La dialettica e la retorica dell'Umanesimo, 'invenzione', 'metodo' nella cultura del XV e del XVI secolo*, Milan

Veyne, Paul (1978), *Comment on écrit l'histoire*, Paris

Vickers, Brian (1968), *Francis Bacon and Renaissance prose*, Cambridge

(1979), 'Frances Yates and the writing of history', *Journal of Modern History*, 51, 287–316

(1984a), 'Analogy versus identity: the rejection of occult symbolism, 1580–1680', in *Occult and scientific mentalities in the Renaissance*, ed. Brian Vickers, Cambridge, pp. 95–164

(1988a), *In defence of rhetoric*, Oxford

(1988b), 'On the function of analogy in the occult', in *Hermeticism and the Renaissance*, ed. Ingrid Merkel and Allen G. Debus, Washington D.C., pp. 265–91

Vickers, Brian, ed. (1984b), *Occult and scientific mentalities in the Renaissance*, Cambridge

Voet, Leon (1969–72), *The golden compasses*, 2 vols., Amsterdam

Voet, Leon and Voet-Grisolle, Jenny (1980–3), *The Plantin Press 1555–1589: a bibliography of the works printed and published by Christopher Plantin at Antwerp and Leiden*, 6 vols., Amsterdam

von Staden, Heinrich (1998), 'The rule and the exception; Celsus on a scientific conundrum', in *Maladie et maladies dams les textes latins antiques et médiévaux*, ed. Carl Deroux, Brussels, pp. 108–28

Walker, D. P. (1958), *Spiritual and demonic magic from Ficino to Campanella*, London

Wallace, William (1988), 'Traditional natural philosophy', in *The Cambridge history of Renaissance philosophy*, ed. Charles B. Schmitt and Quentin Skinner, Cambridge, pp. 201–35

Wallis, Faith (1995), 'The experience of the book: manuscripts, texts and the role of epistemology in early medieval medicine', in *Knowledge and the scholarly medical traditions*, ed. Don Bates, Cambridge, pp. 101–26

Wear, Andrew (1973), 'Contingency and logic in Renaissance anatomy and physiology', Ph.D. thesis, Imperial College, London

(1981), 'Galen in the Renaissance', in *Galen: problems and prospects*, ed. Vivian Nutton, London, pp. 229–67

(1985), 'Explorations in Renaissance writings on the practice of medicine', in *The medical Renaissance of the sixteenth century*, ed. Andrew Wear, R. K. French and Iain M. Lonie, Cambridge, pp. 118–45

(1995a), 'Epistemology and learned medicine in early modern England', in *Knowledge and the scholarly medical traditions*, ed. Don Bates, Cambridge, pp. 151–73

(1995b), 'Medicine in early modern Europe, 1500–1700', in *The Western medical tradition 800 BC to AD 1800*, ed. Laurence I. Conrad, Michael Neve, Vivian Nutton, Roy Porter and Andrew Wear, Cambridge, pp. 215–70

(1996), 'Religious beliefs and medicine in early modern England', in *The task of healing*, ed. H. Marland and M. Pelling, Rotterdam, pp.145–69

Wear, Andrew, French, R. K., and Lonie, Iain M., eds. (1985), *The medical Renaissance of the sixteenth century*, Cambridge

Weber, Max (1991), *From Max Weber: essays on sociology*, ed. Hans Heinrich Gerth and C. Wright Mills, London

Webster, Charles (1967), 'Harvey's *De generatione*: its origins and relevance to the theory of the circulation', *British Journal of the History of Science*, 3, 262–74

(1979), 'Alchemical and Paracelsian medicine', in *Health, medicine and mortality in the sixteenth century*, ed. C. Webster, Cambridge, pp. 301–34

(1982), *From Paracelsus to Newton: magic and the making of modern science*, Cambridge and New York

(1990), 'Conrad Gesner and the infidelity of Paracelsus', in *New Perspectives on Renaissance thought: essays in the history of science, education and philosophy in memory of Charles B. Schmitt*, ed. John Henry and Sarah Hutton, London, pp. 13–23

(1995), 'Paracelsus confronts the saints: miracles, healing and the secularization of magic', *Social History of Medicine*, 8, 403–21

(1998), 'Bare heads against red hats: a portrait of Paracelsus', in *From physico-theology to bio-technology*, ed. K. Bayertz and Roy Porter, Amsterdam, pp. 54–75

Webster, Charles, ed. (1979b), *Health, medicine and mortality in the sixteenth century*, Cambridge

Weidmann, H (1989), 'Aristotle on inferences from signs', *Phronesis*, 34, 342–51

Westman, R. S. (1993), 'Copernicus and the prognosticators: the Bologna period 1496–1500', *Universitas*, 5, 1–5

White, Hayden (1987), *The content of the form*, Baltimore and London

Whitteridge, Gweneth (1981), 'Introduction', to *William Harvey: Disputations touching the generation of animals*, trans. and introd. Gweneth Whitteridge, Oxford, London, Edinburgh, Boston, Melbourne, pp. i–lxv

Widmann, Reinhart, ed. (1984), *Bücherkataloge als buchgeschichtliche Quellen in der frühen Neuzeit*, Wiesbaden

Wightman, William P. D. (1962), *Science and the Renaissance*, 2 vols., Edinburgh and London

(1964), 'Quid sit methodus? Method in sixteenth-century medical teaching and discovery', *Journal of the History of Medicine and Allied Sciences*, 19, 360–76

Wippel, J. F. (1977), 'The condemnations of 1270 and 1277 at Paris', *Journal of Medieval and Renaissance Studies*, 7, 169–201

Woolfson, Jonathan (1998), *Padua and the Tudors: English students in Italy 1483–1603*, Toronto and Buffalo

Worth, Valerie (1988), *Practising translation in Renaissance France: the example of Etienne Dolet*, Oxford

Yates, Frances (1967), 'The Hermetic tradition in Renaissance science', in *Art, science and history in the Renaissance*, ed. Charles S. Singleton, Baltimore, pp. 255–74

Zambelli, Paolo (1992), 'Cornelius Agrippa, ein kritischer Magus', in *Die okkulten Wissenschaften in der Renaissance*, ed. August Buck, Wiesbaden, pp. 65–90

Zanier, Giancarlo (1983), *Medicina e filosofia tra '500 e '600*, Milan

(1985), 'La medicina paracelsiana in Italia: aspetti di un'accoglienza particolare', *Rivista di storia della filosofia*, 4, 627–53

Index of names and terms

Secondary sources appearing in footnotes have not been recorded, unless in acknowledgement of specific help given.

IDEAS IN CONTEXT

Edited by
Quentin Skinner (*General Editor*),
Lorraine Daston, Dorothy Ross and James Tully

(Form L-9)   W   M-719